D0532678

GOOD HOUSEKEEPING

FAMILY

HEALTH

ENCYLOPAEDIA

GOOD HOUSEKEEPING

FAMILY HEALTH ENCYLOPAEDIA

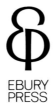

EBURY
PRESS

A QUARTO BOOK

Published by Ebury Press
an imprint of Century Hutchinson
Limited
Brookmount House
62-65 Chandos Place
Covent Garden
London WC2N 4NW

Copyright © 1989 Quarto Publishing
plc

All rights reserved. No part of this
publication may be reproduced, stored
in a retrieval system, or transmitted in
any form or by any means, electronic,
mechanical, photocopying, recording
or otherwise, without the prior
permission of the publisher and
copyright holder. The expression
GOOD HOUSEKEEPING as used in
the title of this book is the trade mark
of The National Magazine Company
Limited and The Hearst Corporation,
registered in the United Kingdom and
the USA and other principal countries
in the world and is the absolute
property of The National Magazine
Company and The Hearst Corporation.
The use of this trade mark other than
with the express permission of The
National Magazine Company Limited
or The Hearst Corporation is strictly
prohibited.

British Library Cataloguing in
Publication Data

Good Housekeeping family health
encyclopedia. – Rev.
ed
1. Man. Health
613
ISBN 0 85223 764 2

This book was designed and produced
by Quarto Publishing plc, The Old
Brewery, 6 Blundell Street, London
N7 9BH with the editorial and
conceptual assistance of The Paul
Press, whose help is gratefully
acknowledged.

Quarto wish to acknowledge the
assistance of the following: Dr.
Anthony Campbell, *revisions editor*,
Sheila Bingham SRD, *nutritionist*, Dr.
Ingvar Bjarrnason MD, Linda Coffey,
medical writer, Jill Frankham, *medical
writer*, Judy Graham, *medical writer*,
Dr. Anthony Grewel MB BS, Dr.
Patricia Grewel MB BS MRCP, Dr.
Mark Harries MD BS MRCP MRCS,
Dr. Finbarr Martin MB BS MSc
MRCP, Dr. Nicola McClure MS BS,
Fiona Roderick SRN NDN, Fiona
Ross BSc SRN NDN, Peter Saugman,
medical writer, Rose Shapiro, *medical
writer*, Michael Simmons, *ophthalmic
optician*, Jeremy Walker, *social worker*,
Dr. Jennifer Wilson-Barnett PhD, Dr.
Theresa Wilkinson MB BS, Dr. Luke
Zander MB BS MRCGP DRCOG
DCH. They would like to thank Julia
Bard, Sharron Brown, Jemima Kallas,
Jeanie Simmons, Jean Train and Janet
Wilson for their assistance and
especially Yvonne McFarlane and Jean
Shapiro for their invaluable help.

Project Director: Nigel Perryman
(The Paul Press)
Editorial: Don Clarke, Nancy Duin,
Pip Morgan, Helen Varley
Art Editor: Moira Clinch
Designer: Joanna Swindell
Illustrators: Lindsay Blow, Paul
Cooper, Chris Forsey, Arka Graphics,
Hussien Hussien, Edwina Keene, Aziz
Khan, Ted Kinsey, Sally Launder,
David Lawrence, David Mallott,
Simon Roulstone, Charlotte Styles,
Roger Twinn, David Worth
Photography: John Watney
Photographic Library, London
Scientific Fotos
Art Director: Robert Morley
Editorial Director: Jeremy Harwood

Typeset in Great Britain by
Wordsmiths, Street, Somerset, QV
Typesetting, London, Text
Filmsetters Ltd, Talisman Litho
Studios Ltd, London
Manufactured in Hong Kong by
Regent Publishing Services Ltd
Printed in Hong Kong by Leefung
Asco Printers Ltd

Contents

Foreword

AS FAR AS the majority of laypeople are concerned, medicine is a baffling and complex subject, full of technical jargon and terms that no one lacking a medical or nursing qualification could possibly fully understand. There is no reason why this should be so, and, thus the *Good Housekeeping Family Health Encyclopaedia* has been planned, written and illustrated to blow away the cobwebs, throw open the closed doors of the confessional consulting room and strip the subject bare of technical mumbo-jumbo. Its aim is simple — to help people enjoy their health to the full, by showing them what practical steps they can take to preserve it, and, in cases of illness and disease, how to understand what can be done to help them regain their normal level of fitness.

Throughout, the aim has been to demystify — to explain in clear, down-to-earth terms everything your doctor would tell you if he or she had the time. The book takes as its basic philosophy the desire most people show, when they visit their doctors, for reassuring explanation — statistics actually demonstrate that many people enter a doctor's surgery with this in mind. Worry and stress are contributory factors to quite a few illnesses — physical as well as psychological ones — and any good doctor's aim is to tackle these problems as well as the ones posed by actual physical disease. The doctor today is as much counsellor as diagnostician. In addition, the modern surgery has social, as well as medical, back-up, in the form of ancillary staff of all kinds, who are concerned as much with general welfare as with specific medical problems.

Remember a few things. Firstly, there is a lot you can do yourself to preserve your health, as *You and Your Health* shows. Secondly, there is much you can do to ease the impact of disease, as demonstrated in *Home Nursing*. Thirdly, and most importantly, you should never be afraid to ask questions, whether a doctor is visiting you at home, or you are in the local surgery, or in hospital. Most doctors are happy to sit down and talk through a problem if you really want them to, and this should be your opportunity to ask them to explain anything you feel unsure of, or do not follow. Do not be afraid that you will show your ignorance. After all, many doctors are equally ignorant of technical subjects outside their profession.

One thing this book is not is a guide to self-diagnosis and treatment. Encouraging this could well be dangerous. If you feel ill, never, ever, think it is not worth bothering a doctor; any doctor would far rather treat a minor complaint than be faced with one that has grown into a major problem.

Finally, a word about the writers. The Medical Consultant is a busy general practitioner, who, on average, sees 500 patients a month. Other sections have been written by a team of young, up-to-date general practitioners, supported by experts in particular specialist fields. All have been advised by an Editorial Board of prominent medical authorities. We hope we have fulfilled the aims outlined here and that the *Good Housekeeping Family Health Encyclopaedia* will inform and enlighten you.

Nora McClure

How to use this book

THIS BOOK is planned and designed to help you unravel the mysteries of medicine. In clear and simple language, it explains how more than 1,000 diseases develop, how they affect the body, and what course they are likely to take — all the information that your family doctor would give you, if he or she had the time. It also describes the special tests and investigations that may be needed to make a firm diagnosis, and the possible forms of treatment in each case.It shows you the simple techniques that can be used to save life in an emergency. It tells you how to cope with sickness in the home and how to reduce the risk of disease by sensible living.

The book is divided into four sections: the Systems of the Body, the Language of Medicine, You and Your Health, and First Aid. Each is concerned with a different aspect of medicine, but no single section stands in isolation. All are connected by a simple system of cross-references, making it easy to find the information you need to fully understand the implications of any disorder.

The first section — the Systems of the Body — describes how the healthy body works. This information is vital to an understanding of how diseases affect the body's functions, and how they can be fought. Section Two — the Language of Medicine — describes how doctors make a diagnosis, explains the functions of specialists, and the organization and routine of hospitals and doctor's surgeries. This is followed by the core of the book — an A-Z of Medicine, in which medical terms and diseases are defined and explained; an A-Z of Alternative Medicine; and an A-Z of Special Tests and Laboratory Investigations. You and Your Health, the third section, explains how you can help to keep youself healthy by paying close attention to diet, exercise, hygiene and routine health checks, and by avoiding stress; it also shows how to cope with sickness in the home and care for both disabled people and old people.

The final section — First Aid — shows how, by acting promptly, you can help save life and prevent serious injury in an emergency. The book is completed by a list of useful addresses, a bibliography and a comprehensive index.

Understanding medicine

At the start, you should first read one very important section — The Doctor, The Patient and Disease. This explains the nature of disease and of diagnosis; it shows the whole range of factors other than the symptoms experienced by the patient that have to be taken into account before diagnosis and treatment can begin. Reliable self-diagnosis is almost impossible and can often be dangerous for these reasons, which is why, if you feel ill, you should always consult a doctor.

Cross references

Throughout the book, cross-references are given within the text in italic type. Within the A-Z of Medicine, a word is printed in italic type when there is an entry for that word in the A-Z. Cross-reference to other parts of the book gives, the page number of the first page of the relevant section within which the information is to be found. Outside the A-Z of diseases, A-Z entries are listed in 'Connection boxes' in each sub-section.

To get the full benefit from this book, you should use the cross-reference system. The examples here show you how this works. If, for instance, you want to know about *Bronchitis*, look up the headword in the *A-Z of Medicine* in Section Two. The entry here tells you what the disease is, how it affects you, why it happens and how it is treated. Cross-references in *italic* pick out other diseases in the A-Z which are related to *Bronchitis*. You are also referred to other sections of the book.

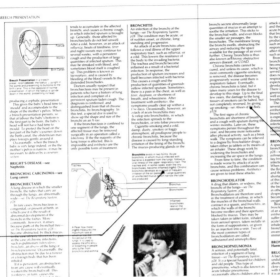

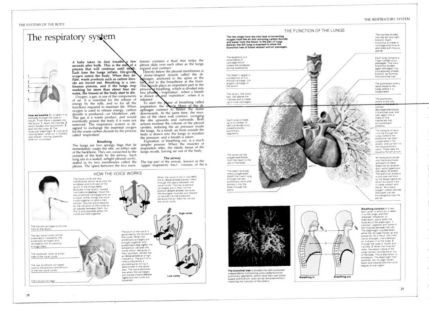

The reference forward to Section Three — *You and Your Health* — similarly takes you straight to the pages dealing with *Abuses of the Body*. Here, you are shown what steps you can take for yourself to lessen the chances of contracting bronchitis.

The reference back to **The respiratory system** in Section One — *The Systems of the Body* — takes you to the introductory pages where the normal working of the lungs and their importance to the body is explained. This information is vital to a full understanding of the problem. Here, too, you will find a connections box on the last page. This enables you to work forward from Seciton One to the *A-Z of Medicine.*

THE SYSTEMS OF THE BODY

THE HUMAN BODY is an incredibly complex piece of machinery. It is divided into a number of key systems, the proper functioning of which is essential to life. These systems, however, do not function in isolation. They are all interrelated, so that a defect in one can have repercussions on another. This section of the book not only explains how each individual system works independently; it explains the relationships between them, so you can see how the body works and how a disease in one part of it can affect the health of another.

The embryology of the body

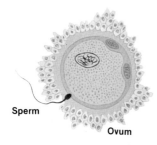

Sperm

Ovum

The basic units of life Human life starts when a male sperm and female ovum are brought together by the act of sexual intercourse. After ejaculation, sperm enter the womb and swim up the Fallopian tube where they meet the ovum which has been released from an ovary at ovulation. Both the sperm and ovum contain a set of 23 chromosomes, which hold a blueprint of the life that will be formed. At fertilization, chromosomes from the sperm pair off with chromosomes from the ovum. As soon as this has happened, the physical characteristics and the basic intelligence of the child are established.

The starting point for all human life is the moment of fertilization, when a sperm from a man meets the egg from a woman. At this time the new life consists of just one cell. Nine months later, when the baby is born, this has multiplied millions and millions of times. The new cells have assumed specialized functions and have become organized to form a complete, complex, human being.

Embryology tells the story of these extraordinary changes. It shows how many of the body's systems are linked by a common origin, and how outside influences can affect the baby's development. To understand the human body is to have unravelled a complicated tangle of relationships between the shape, structure and function of organs and tissues: the task is not easy, but, without a knowledge of the basic principles of embryology, it becomes impossible.

The starting point

Though it affects so many aspects of life, in biological terms, sex is simply a reproductive device (p54). Its object is to make possible the fertilization of an egg, or ovum, from the mother by a sperm from the father. The sperm and the egg each have one set of chromosomes, carrying genes, the basic units of heredity. On fertilization the two sets of chromosomes join to form a complete and unique blueprint for the child that has been conceived. Once this has happened the fertilized egg begins to grow by division.

The fertilized ovum, about 0.2mm (1/160in) in diameter, starts to divide on the day after fertilization. With each division, called a cleavage, the number of cells inside the egg doubles. At this time the ovum is in the Fallopian tube, and as cleavage takes place it is wafted down the tube towards the womb by a mass of cilia, or tiny hairs, that line the wall of the tube. By the fourth or fifth day, the egg reaches the womb; it has turned into a hollow ball called a blastocyst, with an outer layer of about 50 or 60 cells surrounding a central cavity filled with fluid.

A rich and plentiful supply of food and oxygen is essential for the intensive growth and development that follow. In order to obtain these basic requirements, the blastocyst must form a direct link with the mother, by implantation.

Joined to the mother

Implantation is a delicate and complicated process that takes almost a week to complete. The outer layer of the blastocyst eats away the inside wall of the womb, known as the endometrium, while the cells inside the blastocyst divide into two layers, called the ectoderm and endoderm. The endoderm spreads around the inner surface of the ball to enclose a large cavity called the yolk sac—a smaller version of the yolk of a hen's egg and, like the hen's egg, filled with nutrients. The ectoderm encloses a smaller cavity on the mother's side of the ball, forming a membrane called the amnion that will protect a developing baby.

As the outer cells of the blastocyst eat away the mother's tissues they break down blood vessels, providing the developing cells with a source of food and oxygen. (Sometimes this process causes a slight spotting of blood that can mimic menstruation, and confuse a pregnant woman about the date of her last period.) The cells then organize themselves into a mass of finger-like projections called villi, which spread into the wall of the womb and link up with the mother's blood vessels to form the placenta.

The villi are connected to the cavity surrounded by the amnion, in which the baby will develop, by a single piece of tissue called the body stalk. Eventually this piece of tissue grows into the umbilical cord. Most of the food needed for growth is supplied by the yolk sac until the umbilical cord and placenta are fully developed: after that the mother's blood carries a rich supply of nutrients to the growing baby.

The germ of life

By the end of the second week after conception, implantation is complete. The blastocyst is now called an embryo, and consists of a two-layered disc of cells. The layers, the endoderm and ectoderm, have each grown outwards from the edges of the disc to surround a cavity—the yolk sac and the amniotic cavity respectively. The embryo has an established and increasing supply of food and oxygen from the growing placenta, so everything is ready for the spurt of growth that is to take place over the next few weeks.

During the third week, a new layer of tissue develops. Cells from the ectoderm thicken in the middle of the embryo to form the 'primitive streak'; from this a new layer of cells called the mesoderm spreads out, between and around the original two layers. All the tissues and organs of the body develop from one of these three layers—the ectoderm will form the skin, hair, teeth, nails, the nervous system and sense organs; the endoderm will supply the lining of the digestive system, the liver, pancreas, gall bladder and the lungs; and the mesoderm will form muscle, bone, cartilage, connective tissue, the kidneys and the sex glands.

The structures of the body start to

THE BEGINNING OF LIFE

A woman's reproductive organs *(left)* are protected by the pelvic bones. Soon after the ovum leaves the ovary *(right and below)* it is fertilized by a sperm in the Fallopian tube. As the newly-fertilized ovum moves down the tube, it divides several times and doubles the number of cells, before implanting itself in the lining of the uterus.

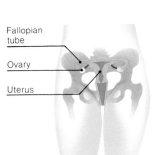

Fallopian tube

Ovary

Uterus

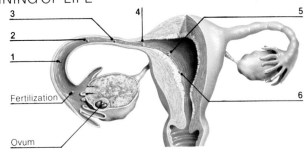

3
2
1
4
5
6

Fertilization

Ovum

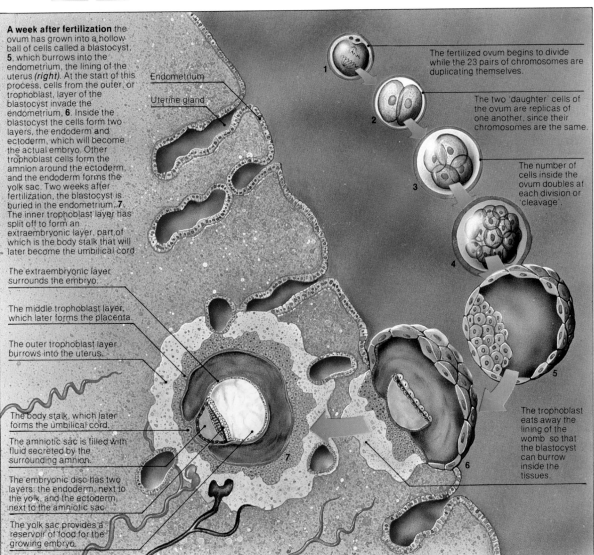

A week after fertilization the ovum has grown into a hollow ball of cells called a blastocyst, **5**, which burrows into the endometrium, the lining of the uterus *(right)*. At the start of this process, cells from the outer, or trophoblast, layer of the blastocyst invade the endometrium, **6**. Inside the blastocyst the cells form two layers, the endoderm and ectoderm, which will become the actual embryo. Other trophoblast cells form the amnion around the ectoderm, and the endoderm forms the yolk sac. Two weeks after fertilization, the blastocyst is buried in the endometrium, **7**. The inner trophoblast layer has split off to form an extraembryonic layer, part of which is the body stalk that will later become the umbilical cord.

The extraembryonic layer surrounds the embryo.

The middle trophoblast layer, which later forms the placenta.

The outer trophoblast layer burrows into the uterus.

The body stalk, which later forms the umbilical cord.

The amniotic sac is filled with fluid secreted by the surrounding amnion.

The embryonic disc has two layers: the endoderm, next to the yolk, and the ectoderm, next to the amniotic sac.

The yolk sac provides a reservoir of food for the growing embryo.

Endometrium

Uterine gland

The fertilized ovum begins to divide while the 23 pairs of chromosomes are duplicating themselves.

The two 'daughter' cells of the ovum are replicas of one another, since their chromosomes are the same.

The number of cells inside the ovum doubles at each division or 'cleavage'.

The trophoblast eats away the lining of the womb so that the blastocyst can burrow inside the tissues.

differentiate from the layers of cells while the mesoderm is growing. A slight thickening of endoderm at one end of the disc has already given the embryo an axis—the thickening represents the position of the head. But now the axis is further defined by the growth of the notochordal process, the first stage in the formation of the spine. This spreads towards the head of the embryo from the primitive streak, which itself starts to grow towards the embryo's tail. Soon the notochord has become a rod of cells that extends the length of the embryo, from a gap in the mesoderm at the head that will form the mouth (called the oral membrane), to a gap at the tail that will form the anus (called the cloacal membrane). The layer of ectoderm that lies over the notochord grows downwards towards it in a U-bend; eventually this closes at the top to form the neural tube, which will develop into the spinal canal.

While this is happening the embryo continues to grow, and at the same time ▷

folds in on itself—as if the edges of a soup plate were turned downwards while it became larger and longer, until it looked like a rolling-pin. All the time, the tissues inside the embryo are differentiating, and becoming more specialized. On the 20th day, for example, the mesoderm becomes organized into paired blocks of tissue called somites, which are positioned on each side of the neural tube. By the fourth week there are 25 pairs of somites; eventually there will be 42. These blocks of mesoderm divide the embryo into segments, and form the pattern for the segmental development of vertebrae and ribs.

At the end of the third week the embryo is about 2.5mm (1/10in) long. It has a rudimentary spinal cord and brain, the first few pairs of somites, and an opening for the mouth and anus. Its tissues have started to differentiate—the heart, for example, is just beginning to develop at the very top of the embryo. In the next few weeks all the baby's organs and structures are built. It is the most critical and sensitive period of pregnancy.

The critical weeks

By the beginning of the fourth week, the embryo is a cylinder of cells, connected to the mother by the body stalk and placenta. It is protected by the amniotic sac on one side, and nourished by the yolk sac on the other. In order to achieve a human shape, and to form an inner cavity that will eventually become the gut, the embryo must fold in on itself again twice. The process is ingenious. The sides and ends of the cylinder curl underneath the main body of the tube, growing larger all the time. As they do this they enclose a cylindrical space with the oral membrane, the future mouth, at the top, and the cloacal membrane, the future anus, at the bottom. A rudimentary digestive tract has been created. The body stalk is trapped between these folds, to form the umbilical cord. The opening to the yolk sac, which is also trapped, shrinks and eventually disappears.

As a result of these folds, the embryonic heart is moved from the top of the embryo to its correct position halfway down the body. It grows rapidly; by the 25th day it makes up almost half the bulk of the embryo. At first the heart is just a thickened tube of tissue, but over the next few weeks chambers are formed within the tube, and the organ becomes linked to a complex network of blood vessels that run through the developing baby and the placenta.

At the head of the embryo the brain grows quickly, linking up with the somites and neural tube, the primitive backbone, to establish the nervous system. Behind the head the tissues thicken to form a series of linked arches, each with a nerve and an artery. These structures are similar to the gills of a fish, though they do not

THE FOLDS OF THE EMBRYO

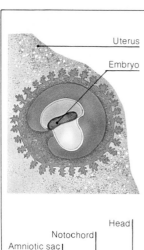

The third and fourth week of pregnancy are critical for the embryo, for it must fold in on itself several times and lay the foundations for the major systems of the body. The embryonic disc *(top left)* folds downwards from its edges and becomes longer, larger and cylindrical, like a rolling pin. Rudimentary vertebrae and ribs take shape as paired blocks of tissue either side of the axis or notochord *(below left)*. Two folds of ectodermal tissue then rise up above this notochord *(red arrows, right)*, forming a U-bend which soon closes to become the neural tube.

The ectodermal tissue at the side of the embryo folds downwards *(blue arrows, right)*, trapping the body stalk and yolk sac, and creating a primitive digestive tract. At the same time, the ends of the embryo also fold downwards. The fold at one end *(dark green arrow, right)* moves the rudimentary heart to its correct position and begins to develop into the brain and head. The fold at the tail end *(light green arrow, right)* curls down and underneath the main body, creating the cloacal membrane. This later becomes the anus.

Uterus

Embryo

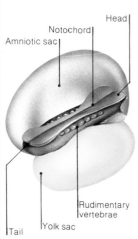

Head

Notochord

Amniotic sac

Tail

Yolk sac

Rudimentary vertebrae

A three-dimensional view of an embryo, shown in section below.

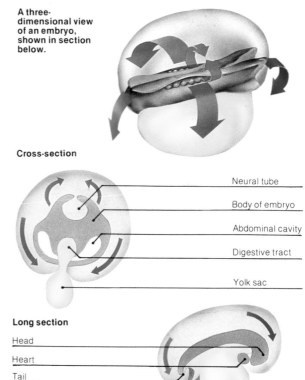

Cross-section

Neural tube

Body of embryo

Abdominal cavity

Digestive tract

Yolk sac

Long section

Head

Heart

Tail

Yolk sac

THE SYSTEMS OF THE EMBRYO

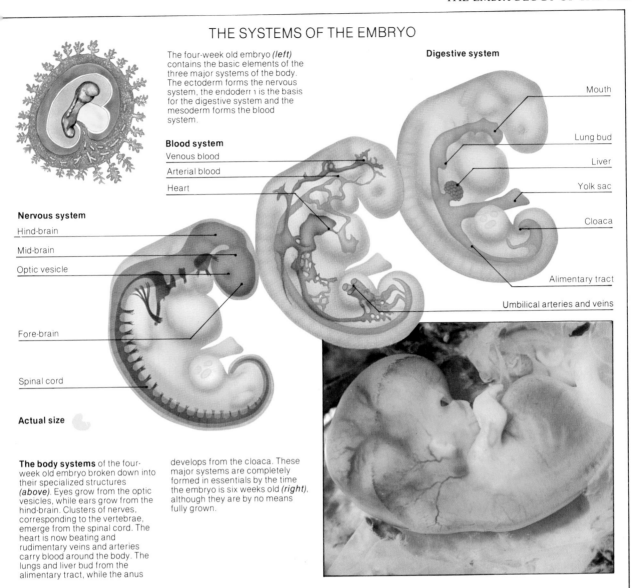

The four-week old embryo *(left)* contains the basic elements of the three major systems of the body. The ectoderm forms the nervous system, the endoderm is the basis for the digestive system and the mesoderm forms the blood system.

Digestive system

- Mouth
- Lung bud
- Liver
- Yolk sac
- Cloaca
- Alimentary tract
- Umbilical arteries and veins

Blood system

- Venous blood
- Arterial blood
- Heart

Nervous system

- Hind-brain
- Mid-brain
- Optic vesicle
- Fore-brain
- Spinal cord

Actual size

The body systems of the four-week old embryo broken down into their specialized structures *(above)*. Eyes grow from the optic vesicles, while ears grow from the hind-brain. Clusters of nerves, corresponding to the vertebrae, emerge from the spinal cord. The heart is now beating and rudimentary veins and arteries carry blood around the body. The lungs and liver bud from the alimentary tract, while the anus develops from the cloaca. These major systems are completely formed in essentials by the time the embryo is six weeks old *(right)*, although they are by no means fully grown.

have an opening to the outside of the embryo, and are merely a reminder of our common origin millions of years ago. Eventually the arches form the skeleton, muscles and blood vessels of the jaws, palate, larynx and pharynx.

During the fifth week after fertilization the sense organs begin to grow from the brain tissue, and pits can be seen at the site of the eyes and ears. At this time the limb buds develop, making the embryo recognizably human in shape, though still only just over 10mm (⅖in) long. Inside the embryo, the organ systems are growing. The lungs start to develop from an outgrowth of the gut; the kidneys form at the tail and then migrate to their adult position in the low back; the liver, pancreas and spleen become defined structures.

By the end of the sixth week all the major systems of the body are present and can be easily identified, though they are not full-grown and are not always in the same position as in an adult. The only exceptions are the sex organs, which at this time are present in a form that is common to both males and females—these organs do not start to differentiate until the 14th week. But the embryo is now a recognizable human being, though only eight weeks old, and from this time is called a foetus. It is almost 22.5mm (1in) long, and has all its internal organs, a face, a trunk and limbs.

Common origins

Over the next 30 weeks until the foetus is born there is steady growth. The organs and systems develop until the baby is able to cope with life outside the mother's womb. The baby that started life from a single fertilized egg now has countless millions of cells, each with a specific function. The original three layers of tissue — the endoderm, ectoderm and mesoderm—have turned into muscle, bone, connective tissue, blood, nerves, organs and body systems. All of these are linked in the adult as in the foetus by their origin in one of the three tissue layers. The link is of vital significance to the body in health and in disease.

Connections
Chromosome
Gene

Bone and muscle

Like any other structure, the human body needs a system of firm supports to give it shape, hold it together and protect any delicate internal parts. As the walls of a building are constructed around a framework of girders, so muscle and connective tissue surround a solid skeleton of bone and cartilage. Unlike a building, though, where the beams and girders are rigid, the body must be able to move. To allow such mobility, the bones are connected to each other by articulated joints, operated by muscles.

The prototype of the skeleton starts to develop after conception as the foetus begins its development in the womb. At this stage, the chief constituent is cartilage, but, as time passes, most of this cartilage hardens, grows and turns into bone.

The cartilage is formed by specialized cells called chondroblasts, which divide to produce a mesh, or matrix, of fibrous strands of the proteins collagen and elastin. This mesh binds together a gel of water and chemicals. At first the cartilage develops in a column which grows in

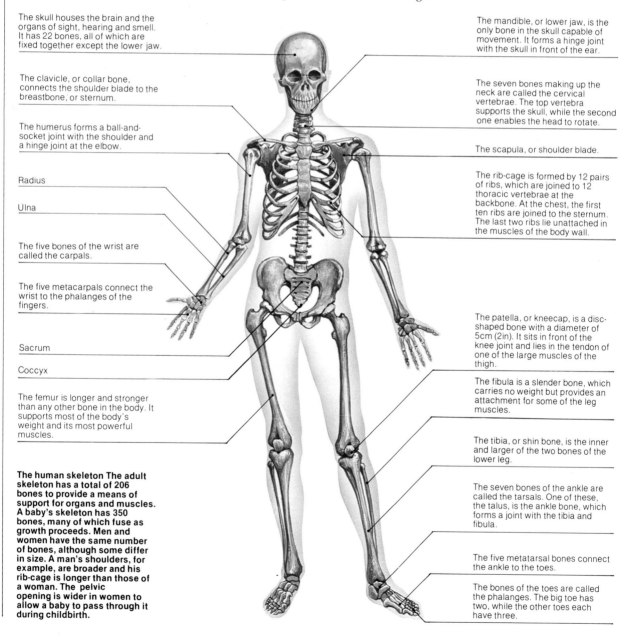

The skull houses the brain and the organs of sight, hearing and smell. It has 22 bones, all of which are fixed together except the lower jaw.

The clavicle, or collar bone, connects the shoulder blade to the breastbone, or sternum.

The humerus forms a ball-and-socket joint with the shoulder and a hinge joint at the elbow.

Radius

Ulna

The five bones of the wrist are called the carpals.

The five metacarpals connect the wrist to the phalanges of the fingers.

Sacrum

Coccyx

The femur is longer and stronger than any other bone in the body. It supports most of the body's weight and its most powerful muscles.

The human skeleton The adult skeleton has a total of 206 bones to provide a means of support for organs and muscles. A baby's skeleton has 350 bones, many of which fuse as growth proceeds. Men and women have the same number of bones, although some differ in size. A man's shoulders, for example, are broader and his rib-cage is longer than those of a woman. The pelvic opening is wider in women to allow a baby to pass through it during childbirth.

The mandible, or lower jaw, is the only bone in the skull capable of movement. It forms a hinge joint with the skull in front of the ear.

The seven bones making up the neck are called the cervical vertebrae. The top vertebra supports the skull, while the second one enables the head to rotate.

The scapula, or shoulder blade.

The rib-cage is formed by 12 pairs of ribs, which are joined to 12 thoracic vertebrae at the backbone. At the chest, the first ten ribs are joined to the sternum. The last two ribs lie unattached in the muscles of the body wall.

The patella, or kneecap, is a disc-shaped bone with a diameter of 5cm (2in). It sits in front of the knee joint and lies in the tendon of one of the large muscles of the thigh.

The fibula is a slender bone, which carries no weight but provides an attachment for some of the leg muscles.

The tibia, or shin bone, is the inner and larger of the two bones of the lower leg.

The seven bones of the ankle are called the tarsals. One of these, the talus, is the ankle bone, which forms a joint with the tibia and fibula.

The five metatarsal bones connect the ankle to the toes.

The bones of the toes are called the phalanges. The big toe has two, while the other toes each have three.

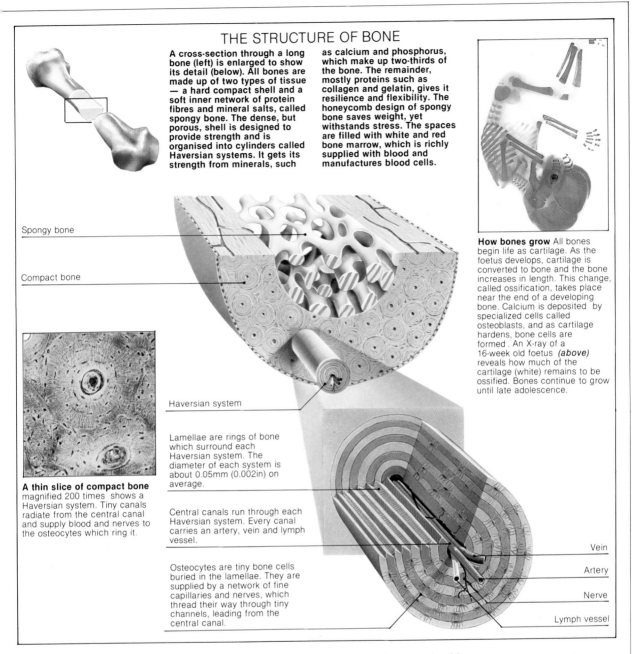

THE STRUCTURE OF BONE

A cross-section through a long bone (left) is enlarged to show its detail (below). All bones are made up of two types of tissue — a hard compact shell and a soft inner network of protein fibres and mineral salts, called spongy bone. The dense, but porous, shell is designed to provide strength and is organised into cylinders called Haversian systems. It gets its strength from minerals, such as calcium and phosphorus, which make up two-thirds of the bone. The remainder, mostly proteins such as collagen and gelatin, gives it resilience and flexibility. The honeycomb design of spongy bone saves weight, yet withstands stress. The spaces are filled with white and red bone marrow, which is richly supplied with blood and manufactures blood cells.

Spongy bone

Compact bone

How bones grow All bones begin life as cartilage. As the foetus develops, cartilage is converted to bone and the bone increases in length. This change, called ossification, takes place near the end of a developing bone. Calcium is deposited by specialized cells called osteoblasts, and as cartilage hardens, bone cells are formed. An X-ray of a 16-week old foetus *(above)* reveals how much of the cartilage (white) remains to be ossified. Bones continue to grow until late adolescence.

Haversian system

A thin slice of compact bone magnified 200 times shows a Haversian system. Tiny canals radiate from the central canal and supply blood and nerves to the osteocytes which ring it.

Lamellae are rings of bone which surround each Haversian system. The diameter of each system is about 0.05mm (0.002in) on average.

Central canals run through each Haversian system. Every canal carries an artery, vein and lymph vessel.

Osteocytes are tiny bone cells buried in the lamellae. They are supplied by a network of fine capillaries and nerves, which thread their way through tiny channels, leading from the central canal.

Vein

Artery

Nerve

Lymph vessel

length at both ends. It soon starts to increase in thickness, however, with new sheets of tissue being laid down in concentric rings, like the trunk of a tree.

Ossification—the process by which cartilage is replaced by bone—begins in the seventh week after conception. First of all the cartilage at the centre of the bone degenerates, leaving spaces called lacunae in the mesh of fibres. In the lacunae, bone-producing cells develop. These lay down the mineral calcium, obtained from the blood, on to the protein mesh, to form a strong, rigid scaffolding.

A network of blood vessels then develops and enters the matrix, supplying the bone-producing cells with food and oxygen. This honeycomb of calcium and protein in the centre of the cartilage prototype is called 'spongy bone'. Its structure combines lightness with considerable strength.

Hard, or 'compact' bone is formed in sheets outside the spongy bone. As in the case of the cartilage these sheets, too, develop in concentric rings like the trunk of a tree. In each sheet of bone the protein mesh runs in a different direction, giving it extra strength, while the rings are arranged round a canal containing blood vessels, lymph vessels and a nerve. The resulting bone is flexible, yet so strong that the thigh bone of a young adult could support a vertical load of one ton.

Growth

The ossification of cartilage to form bone is a gradual process. During life in the womb, the bone that starts to form at the centre of the cartilage spreads outwards ▷

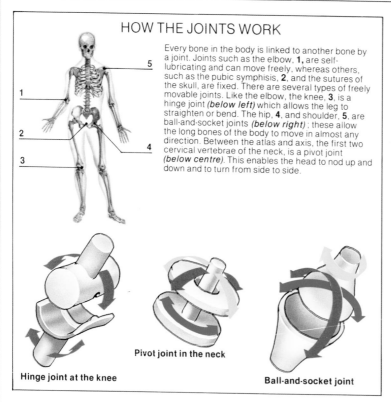

HOW THE JOINTS WORK

Every bone in the body is linked to another bone by a joint. Joints such as the elbow, **1**, are self-lubricating and can move freely, whereas others, such as the pubic symphisis, **2**, and the sutures of the skull, are fixed. There are several types of freely movable joints. Like the elbow, the knee, **3**, is a hinge joint *(below left)* which allows the leg to straighten or bend. The hip, **4**, and shoulder, **5**, are ball-and-socket joints *(below right)*; these allow the long bones of the body to move in almost any direction. Between the atlas and axis, the first two cervical vertebrae of the neck, is a pivot joint *(below centre)*. This enables the head to nod up and down and to turn from side to side.

Hinge joint at the knee

Pivot joint in the neck

Ball-and-socket joint

How the knee works The knee, the largest joint of the body, is shown *(below)* with the knee-cap, or patella, removed. The knee takes much of the body's weight, but allows the femur, **1**, and tibia, **2**, to move freely in relation to each other. The femur is linked to the fibula, **3**, and tibia by the fibular, **4**, and tibial, **5**, ligaments. These ligaments, which do not extend, provide most of the knee's strength and prevent it from dislocating to one side or the other. The medial meniscus, **6**, and the lateral meniscus, **7**, are made of cartilage. They reduce friction between the bones and act as shock absorbers during running and walking. The cruciate ligaments, **8**, linked to both tibia and femur, stop the knee from dislocating to the front or back.

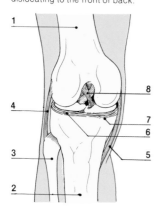

are rubbed together, there is three times less friction than if ice is rubbed on ice. But as people get older, calcium is deposited in the cartilage, making the joints stiff and the bones brittle.

Joints

The skeleton is the framework that supports the body, with the individual bones linked in such a way that they can move in relation to one another. These joints are highly sophisticated. Many of them allow a wide range of movement, are self-lubricating, contain shock absorbers and have their own protection and supports.

There are several different types of joint. In each type which allows movement, the bones concerned move in a different way and in different directions. Friction between the bones is reduced to a minimum by the hyaline cartilage that lines all the articulating parts, and also by synovial fluid—a liquid secreted by the synovial membrane. Fibrous ligaments tie the bones together in large joints and, in the case of the knee and vertebral joints, cartilage pads help to smooth movement and cushion the joint—in the knee joint these are called menisci, and in the inter-vertebral joints, discs.

Some joints are not designed to move. The pubic bones in the groin, for example, are connected by cartilage, and provide a rigid framework to protect the delicate internal organs. This joint is called the pubic symphisis. In women it expands during childbirth just enough to allow the baby's head to pass through, the bones then returning to their original positions. The bones in the skull are also connected by rigid joints called sutures. In a newborn child some of these sutures are still open, leaving gaps called fontanelles; these do not close completely for a year.

Muscles

To allow the body to move, a physical force must be exerted over the joints. This force is supplied by the muscles.

If the skin were peeled off a human body, and the packing tissue removed, a mass of fibrous bundles would be revealed. These are muscles. Each muscle has a particular function, and each is responsible for movement of a different bone in a different direction. When a muscle contracts, the bones to which it is connected at either end move through the joint that articulates them. This is movement at its most basic. In fact, even simple movements are the result of the action of whole groups of muscles—each muscle anchors a bone, and contracts or relaxes, depending on the movement, like a system of pulleys and levers.

There are several different types of muscle. Those that move the bones of the skeleton are called skeletal or voluntary muscles. They are under the conscious control of the brain, which passes instructions to them through the nervous system *(p32)*. The voluntary muscles are made up of bundles of fibres. Each long, thin fibre is ▷

until, by the time the child is born, only the ends of the bones are still made of cartilage.

The bones continue to grow throughout childhood and adolescence, this growth being controlled by the hormones of the endocrine system *(p48)*. Cartilage grows out at the end of each piece of the skeleton at the point at which it interfaces with bone—the cartilage side of this interface is known as an epiphysis—while bone slowly replaces the cartilage from its side, called the diaphysis. As this cartilage ossifies, more cartilage is formed, making the bone longer. This growth is not complete until the age of about 18 in boys and 16 in girls. Because the development is so precise, it is possible to pinpoint the age of a bone on an X-ray by the presence or absence of an epiphysis.

There are three types of cartilage in the body of an adult. The nature of each protein matrix differs slightly, depending on the function of the cartilage. Fibrocartilage—the name given to the strong cartilage of the knee joint and the discs between the vertebrae—has a high proportion of the protein collagen and not much elastin. As a result, it is very resilient, but does not have much 'give'. In contrast, elastic cartilage, found in the ear and the throat, has a high proportion of elastin and thus is extremely flexible. Hyaline cartilage is simply gristle. It lines the articulating surfaces of all the joints, connects the breastbone to the ribs, holds open the windpipe or trachea and forms the end of the nose. Hard, clear and with a bluish tinge, hyaline cartilage is one of the most friction-free materials known. If two pieces

THE MUSCLES OF THE BODY

Over 650 muscles, attached to the bones of the skeleton, coordinate all the movements of the body and help to maintain its posture against the force of gravity.

The trapezius muscle covers the shoulder blade, holding it in position. It can rotate the shoulder blade, and also draw the head back or to the side.

The deltoid muscle covers the shoulder joint. It raises and rotates the arm.

The triceps muscle joins the shoulder to the elbow and contracts to extend the forearm.

The brachioradialis muscle helps to turn the palm of the hand upwards.

Latissimus dorsi is a large muscle which connects the backbone to the humerus of the arm.

Gluteus maximus is the large muscle of the buttock. It extends and rotates the thigh around the hip joint and also raises the trunk of the body from a stooping position.

Semitendinosus is a hamstring muscle which runs from the pelvis to the tibia below the knee.

Biceps femoris is one of the three hamstring muscles of the thigh which flex the knee and rotate it outwards.

The gastrocnemius muscle has two parts which together form nearly all of the calf.

The tendo calcaneus, or Achilles tendon, is the strongest tendon in the body and connects the calf muscles to the ankle.

Orbicularis oculi lies in the orbit of the eye and surrounds it. This muscle closes the eyelid, wrinkles the forehead and squeezes tears into the eye.

The sternomastoid muscle runs down the side of the neck and stands out when it contracts. It either inclines the head towards the shoulder of the same side or rotates it towards the other side.

Pectoralis major is the large shoulder muscle which lies across the chest. It can either draw the arm forward or rotate it.

Biceps brachii runs from the shoulder to the ulna in the forearm. It bends the arm at the elbow and helps to turn the palm upwards.

The two rectus abdominis muscles run down the front of the abdomen and bend the trunk of the body forward or to the side.

Sartorius is the longest muscle in the body, extending from the pelvis to the tibia. It rotates the thigh or raises it up to the abdomen, and also helps to bend the knee.

Vastus lateralis runs down the outside of the thigh. The fourth part of the quadriceps muscle, the vastus intermedius, lies between the vastus lateralis and medialis below the rectus femoris.

Rectus femoris is a long straight muscle at the front of the thigh which helps to raise the leg from the hip. Together with the three vastus muscles, it forms the quadriceps. This powerful group of muscles straightens out the leg and locks it in position when standing.

Vastus medialis runs down the inside of the thigh.

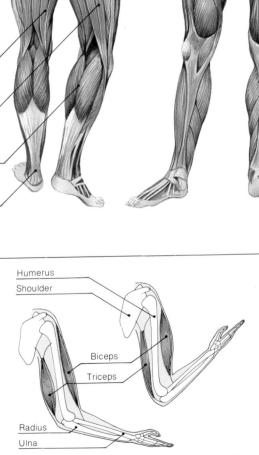

The arm bends and straightens as a result of the opposing action of two muscles over the hinge joint of the elbow. The biceps muscle is attached to the shoulder and to the radius, one of the bones in the forearm. The triceps muscle is attached to both the shoulder and the humerus at one end, and to the ulna at the other. As one muscle contracts, the other relaxes and stretches. When the biceps contracts it bulges and shortens, pulling up the forearm. When the triceps contracts it pulls in the opposite direction and so straightens the forearm.

Humerus
Shoulder
Biceps
Triceps
Radius
Ulna

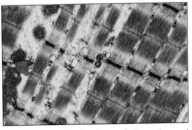

Each fibre of a skeletal muscle is made up of many smaller fibres, shown magnified 6,000 times *(above)*. Thin actin filaments, extending from each side of the solid black bands, overlap the thicker myosin filaments in the centre and create a wider band called a striation.

THE FUNCTION OF SKIN

The skin is more than just a covering for the body. The hairs, **1**, and sweat glands, **3**, help to regulate the body temperature. Stimulated by nerves, muscles, **4**, in the hair follicles, **2**, contract, making the hairs 'stand on end' and 'goose pimples' appear. The sebaceous glands, **5**, make oils which lubricate the skin; they are especially productive during puberty. The epidermis, **6**, is waterproof, protects the underlying tissues and is a barrier to harmful bacteria. Its cells are continually shed and replaced from below. The dermis, **7**, beneath it contains connective tissues, elastic fibres, blood vessels, carried in arterioles, **8**, and venules, **9**, and fat, **10**. Sensory cells, **11**, respond to touch and temperature; when the hand touches boiling water, for example, the cells alert the brain which moves the hand away via a nerve reflex.

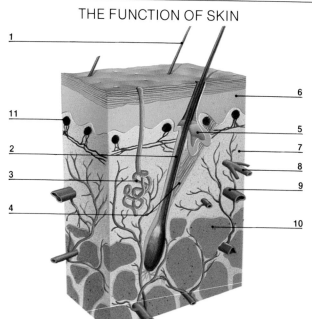

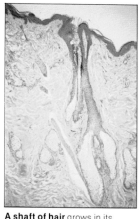

A shaft of hair grows in its follicle in a cross-section of a piece of skin, magnified 60 times *(above)*. A large sebaceous gland, full of oily sebum, extends downwards to the right of the follicle. During puberty, hormones from sex glands cause large amounts of sebum to be made.

a single cell, the fibres being arranged in different patterns depending on what the muscle is designed to do. In muscles that twist the body, such as the trapezius in the back, the bundles of fibres are arranged in spirals. In short, powerful muscles, such as the deltoid in the shoulder, the bundles make a pattern somewhat like the feathers in a bird's wing.

Smooth and striated

In voluntary muscle, the fibres are made up of two different types of short strand, or filament. One type of filament contains the protein actin, the other myosin. A single fibre examined under the microscope has alternate light and dark bands, or striations. The dark bands indicate where the two kinds of filament overlap. Because of this banded pattern, voluntary muscle is also known as striated muscle.

In order for a muscle to contract, it must receive a signal from the nervous system. A chemical called acetylcholine is released from the appropriate nerve ending in response to the signal; this chemical triggers a chemical reaction between the two proteins. The myosin filaments pull the thinner actin filaments towards them, shortening the muscle and using up energy—*see Metabolism, p44*. A by-product of this reaction is lactic acid. This acid can be broken down only by the oxygen that is carried to the muscle in the blood. In strenuous exercise the oxygen supply does not keep up with the production of lactic acid, and the acid that accumulates causes cramp and muscle fatigue. Regular exercise and fitness training increases the amount of lactic acid that can be tolerated in the muscles.

There are two other types of muscle: cardiac muscle, which contracts to make the heart beat, and involuntary, or 'smooth' muscle. Involuntary muscles contract without the conscious knowledge of the brain—they are controlled by the autonomic nervous system *(p33)*. These muscles are found throughout the body. Among their functions, they constrict and dilate the blood vessels, and the bronchi of the lungs; they contract rhythmically to move food through the digestive system; and they control the sphincters of the bladder and anus.

Involuntary muscle fibres are not striated, as the arrangement of filaments is different from that in voluntary muscles. Smooth muscle contracts in much the same way, however, but the contraction is more as a response to the muscle being stretched than to a signal from the brain. The fibres of cardiac muscle are branched, and their contraction is controlled by the pacemaker of the heart *(p27)*. These fibres have an independent rhythm, which allows contractions to spread through the heart in waves during each beat.

Covering and packing

To complete the physical framework of the body, an outer covering and an inner packing material are necessary. The outer covering is the skin which, if laid out flat, would measure 1½ square metres (17 sq ft). Skin is a tough, waterproof barrier that also acts as a sense organ, an insulator and a protective wall. The packing material is connective tissue, made up of a variety of different cells and fibres. All the nooks and crannies of the body are filled with 'loose' or 'areolar' connective tissue, which is sometimes called 'fascia'. It forms a sheath around the muscles, nerves and blood vessels, and packing round the organs and intestines.

The blood and lymph systems

The human body is made up of countless tiny cells. To co-ordinate the activities of each cell, there must be effective communication between them. The blood and lymph system provide this means of communication in the form of a vast network of channels, or vessels. The vessels branch again and again, until they are so fine that they can reach every individual cell, providing vital chemicals and carrying away waste. But as well as providing a means of transport, the blood and lymph systems are essential in the defence of the body against disease.

What blood is

The ancient Greek physician Galen believed that blood carried the spirit of life, and distributed it through the body. This is exactly what it does—the 5 litres (8½ pints) of blood carry around the body oxygen, waste products, chemical messengers, heat and the essential ingredients of the body's defence system against disease. In order to fulfil all these functions, blood is made up of a number of different components, each with its own specialized role.

Some of these components are visible to the naked eye. When the skin is cut, for instance, a red liquid oozes out. But, in fact, blood consists primarily of a straw-coloured liquid called plasma, white blood cells (leucocytes), and red blood cells (erythrocytes).

The red and white blood cells are suspended in the plasma, together with a number of chemicals and particles described later in this section. The white cells are the 'soldier' cells of the body, forming a defensive barrier against the foreign bodies that cause infection; the red blood cells transport life-giving oxygen to all the other cells of the body.

Red blood cells

In one cubic millimetre of blood, there are about five million red blood cells. This number might seem staggering, but each cell has an essential role to play. The cells are created continuously. Old cells normally wear out after about 120 days; they are broken down by the liver and spleen, and others take their place. In adults the replacement cells are manufactured in the bone marrow, and in babies are made in the spleen as well.

The stimulus for the manufacture of new cells is given by a chemical called erythropoietin. This is produced and released by the kidneys when the oxygen ▷

THE CONSTITUENTS OF BLOOD

The separated plasma contains the blood's platelets.

Though white cells make up a small part of the blood, they have a vital role in the fight against disease.

Red cells make up about 45 per cent of blood.

If it stands in a test tube, blood separates into three layers and is prevented from clotting *(left)*. The percentage of red cells by volume of the total fluid is called the haematocrit and is normally between 40—47%. An abnormal figure may be a symptom of disease; in cholera, for example, the victims have a haematocrit of 65%.

Blood has three main constituents — red cells, white cells, and platelets. Red cells, **1**, contain the oxygen carrier, haemoglobin, and are the most numerous. The five kinds of white cell all defend the body against foreign bodies and infections. The neutrophils, **2**, basophils, **3**, and eosinophils, **4**, get their names from the way they take up laboratory stains. They all contain granules — they are collectively called granulocytes — whereas the other two kinds, monocytes, **5**, and lymphocytes, **6**, do not. Like red cells platelets, **7**, they do not have a nucleus. They play a vital role in blood clotting, by clumping together to plug a hole in a blood vessel.

Blood clotting A complex chain of events is set in motion when the skin is cut. Blood starts to clot almost at once, and in about two hours the wound is sealed. Both red blood cells and platelets (*below*) are crucial to this process.

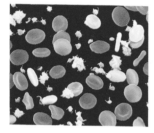

The most important role is played by the platelets (*below*). These clump together to form a plug at the site of the injury, then break down and release two substances. One, serotonin, reduces the flow of blood.

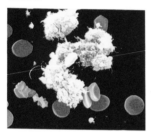

The other, thromboplastin, the first of the 'blood-clotting factors' converts prothrombin, a protein in the blood plasma, into thrombin. This changes another protein, fibrinogen, into strands of fibrin which trap red blood cells (*below*).

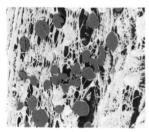

The sticky fibrin mesh attaches itself to the surrounding tissues to form a clot. At first this is soft, but it soon begins to contract and exude serum. If the clot is exposed to the air, it will harden, sealing the wound until the damage has been repaired. Ten more chemical blood clotting factors play an essential part in the process. When one or more factors are missing, as in inherited diseases such as haemophilia or Christmas disease, blood does not clot effectively, and wounds take a long time to heal.

content of the blood falls. Two other substances are needed for the manufacturing process: Vitamin B12 and iron. A deficiency of these substances, or of erythropoietin; leads to anaemia, a disease in which the number of red blood cells circulating in the body, or their ability to carry oxygen, is reduced.

Vitamin B12 is absorbed from food during digestion (*p40*). Without it, the red cells fail to mature and the result is a serious type of anaemia called pernicious anaemia. Iron is also absorbed from food. It is the essential constituent in haemoglobin, the pigment found in red blood cells that plays a vital part in the transport of oxygen around the body.

When haemoglobin links up with oxygen in the lungs—*see Respiration, p28*—or when the blood is exposed to the air as a result of a wound, its chemical structure changes. This is reflected in a change in colour—the dark-blue haemoglobin combines with the oxygen to become bright red oxyhaemoglobin. As oxygen passes out of the blood and into the cells, the reverse takes place, with the oxyhaemoglobin turning back into haemoglobin.

If the body's diet contains too little iron, not enough haemoglobin is produced. The result is another type of anaemia, known as iron-deficiency anaemia.

White blood cells

The blood contains far fewer white cells than red—between 4,000 and 10,000 in one cubic millimetre of blood. While the red cells are all of the same size and type, there are five different types of white cell, each with a specific function.

All white cells have a number of characteristics in common—unlike red cells, they can move and, in some circumstances, reproduce themselves. Above all, each type plays a vital, though different, role in the body's continual fight against disease and infection.

About 25 per cent of white cells belong to the type known as lymphocytes. Like red cells, they are manufactured in the bone marrow, but are also produced in large numbers by the various organs of the lymph system, such as the tonsils, spleen and thymus, especially when a long-standing infection is present. The cells surround foreign bodies, such as bacteria and release antibodies to deal with them. They form a vital part of the body's defences against disease in the elaborate workings of the immune system (*p52*).

Monocytes, the second type of white cell, form another line of defence. These are 'phagocytic'—they surround foreign bodies and digest them. Neutrophils, the third type, work in the same way, but die when their digestive powers have been exhausted; the pus in a pimple, for instance, contains large numbers of dead neutrophils. Eosinophils combat allergies and parasites, by acting as a natural anti-histamine; while basophils, the least numerous of the white cells, produce vital chemicals, such as heparin. These

inhibit blood-clotting inside the body, allowing the blood to flow smoothly.

The role of plasma

Plasma carries the red and white cells through the blood stream, but it also has a vitally important role of its own. In addition to blood cells it contains millions of particles, called platelets, and a wide range of chemicals that are essential to the functioning of the body.

Platelets are tiny particles, each about two and a half thousandths of a millimetre in size; there are around 250,000 in one cubic millimetre of blood. Like red cells, they are manufactured in the bone marrow. Their job is simple; they are essential if blood is to clot properly to seal off an internal or external wound.

The other substances that plasma carries are present in solution, just as sugar is dissolved in coffee or tea (the small globules of fat that may slightly cloud the blood after a heavy meal are an exception—*see Metabolism, p44*). The list of these substances is enormous. It includes: minerals; carbon dioxide (the end-product of energy production by the cells); blood-clotting chemicals in addition to the platelets; the products of digestion and metabolism, such as amino acids (*p44*) and glucose (*p44*); and chemical messengers, called hormones (*p48*).

Plasma transports one further range of substances by linking them to carrier-chemicals called the plasma proteins. Substances carried in this way are many and varied. They include: Vitamins A, K, D and B12; cholesterol; iron; some fats; histamine; antigens and antibodies; and the three hormones insulin, cortisol and thyroxine.

The transport network

A vast, intricate network of blood vessels—the cardiovascular system—carries blood throughout the body. The pivot of this network is the heart, the biological pump that forces blood through the system. Vessels taking blood away from the heart are called arteries, and those carrying blood back to the heart are called veins.

When the heart beats, newly oxygenated blood from the lungs—*see Respiration, p28*—is forced out under pressure into the great arteries of the body. This pressure is called the 'blood pressure'. During the pumping phase of the heart beat, called systole, the pressure in a young healthy adult is between 90mm and 120mm of mercury; when the heart fills with blood, in the phase called diastole, the pressure is between 60mm and 80mm. These values, which can be measured by an instrument called a sphygmomanometer, are written in the form '120/80' and '90/60'. The values tend to increase with age—as a rough guide, the systolic pressure is equivalent to the person's age plus 100—and sometimes become dangerously high in people who suffer from conditions such as atherosclerosis and arteriosclerosis.

To cope with the pressure, arteries have

BLOOD GROUPS AND HEREDITY

Blood transfusions became a safe medical procedure when blood was classified into groups at the turn of the century. Two substances, called antigen A and antigen B, are either present or absent on the surface of red blood cells. People with antigen A on their cells belong to group A; people with B belong to group B; people with neither belong to group O; and people with both belong to group AB. The plasma of each group except AB has antibodies which agglutinate, or clump together, the red cells of another group. The chart *(below)* sums up this relationship and shows the typical distribution of blood groups — the proportions change according to race and colour.

The group of any blood can be established by a simple test *(right)*. Two drops of blood are put on a glass plate: anti-A antibodies are added to one, and anti-B antibodies are added to the other. Anti-A antibodies agglutinate the cells of groups A and AB; anti-B antibodies agglutinate cells of groups B and AB. Group O cells are not agglutinated by either. On the glass plate, the red cell has clumped where the blood is speckled.

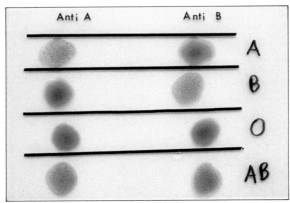

Blood Group	A	B	O	AB
% population	42%	9%	46%	3%
Antigen	A	B	None	AB
Antibody	Anti-B	Anti-A	Anti-A & Anti-B	None

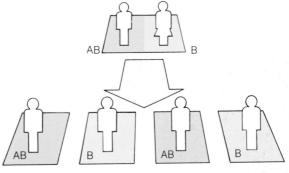

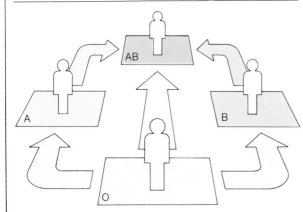

Which blood group is used for whom is shown diagrammatically *(left)*. Group O is the universal donor. Blood groups are determined by heredity. An AB man and B woman can produce only AB or B children *(above)*. Group O children can be born if either parent has O blood, or both parents carry the O gene. Another genetic factor, which applies to all blood groups, is the individual rhesus grouping. This can be positive or negative. One problem that can arise from this is rhesus incompatibility in pregnancy. If an RH negative mother gives birth to an Rh positive child — the positive gene coming from the father — the mother can develop antibodies to Rh positive blood. These can destroy the red cells of a second Rh positive baby. Modern treatment, however, means that the problem is rarely insoluble.

a thick muscular wall that helps to contain and smooth out the fluctuations of blood flow as the heart beats. Nevertheless, these pressure waves can still be felt in certain parts of the body as pulses.

The main artery of the body, the aorta, carries blood from the heart and then forms tributaries which take oxygenated blood to all parts of the body. The tributaries branch in their turn, becoming smaller and smaller. These tiny arteries, called arterioles, still have muscular walls and can expand and contract in response to nerve impulses *(p32)*. In this way blood can be directed towards or away from vital areas. In cold conditions, for example, the skin becomes pale, because the arterioles near the surface contract to reduce the loss of heat from the blood.

As the arterioles branch again and again, they change into tiny tubes called capillaries. These are only about 10 thousandths of a millimetre in diameter—just wide enough to allow the passage of a red blood cell—and have a wall that is only one cell thick, with tiny slits between each cell. When the blood reaches the capillaries, it delivers its chemical nutrients and messengers to their eventual destination, the cell.

Between arteries and veins

Blood does not come into direct contact with the cells, which are on the other side of the capillary wall. The spaces between the cells of the body are filled with a liquid known as 'tissue fluid'—a watery fluid similar to plasma. Tissue fluid is forced out of the blood, through the thin capillary wall and into the spaces between cells by the pressure inside the bloodstream.

The blood in the capillaries contains a high concentration of dissolved chemicals, such as glucose *(p44)*, which diffuse through the capillary membrane to supply the cell. At the same time, large molecules and white cells pass through the slits in the capillary wall. But the cell in its turn is producing chemicals as a by-product of the ▷

THE CIRCULATION OF THE BLOOD

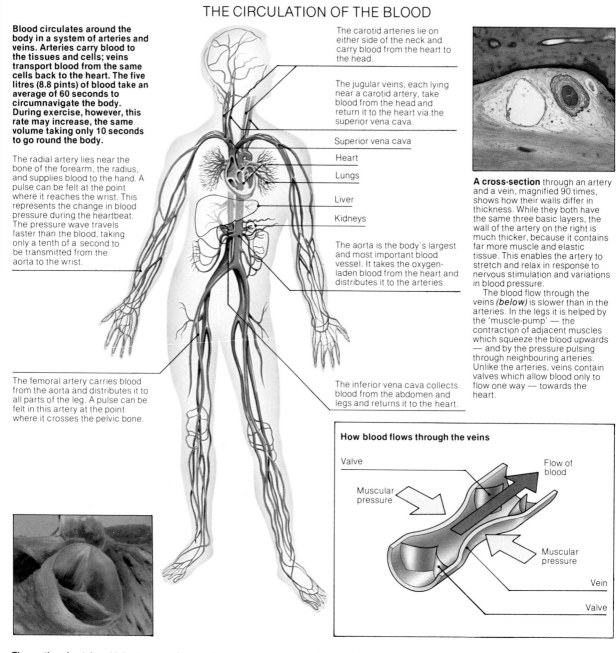

Blood circulates around the body in a system of arteries and veins. Arteries carry blood to the tissues and cells; veins transport blood from the same cells back to the heart. The five litres (8.8 pints) of blood take an average of 60 seconds to circumnavigate the body. During exercise, however, this rate may increase, the same volume taking only 10 seconds to go round the body.

The radial artery lies near the bone of the forearm, the radius, and supplies blood to the hand. A pulse can be felt at the point where it reaches the wrist. This represents the change in blood pressure during the heartbeat. The pressure wave travels faster than the blood, taking only a tenth of a second to be transmitted from the aorta to the wrist.

The femoral artery carries blood from the aorta and distributes it to all parts of the leg. A pulse can be felt in this artery at the point where it crosses the pelvic bone.

The carotid arteries lie on either side of the neck and carry blood from the heart to the head.

The jugular veins, each lying near a carotid artery, take blood from the head and return it to the heart via the superior vena cava.

Superior vena cava

Heart

Lungs

Liver

Kidneys

The aorta is the body's largest and most important blood vessel. It takes the oxygen-laden blood from the heart and distributes it to the arteries.

The inferior vena cava collects blood from the abdomen and legs and returns it to the heart.

A cross-section through an artery and a vein, magnified 90 times, shows how their walls differ in thickness. While they both have the same three basic layers, the wall of the artery on the right is much thicker, because it contains far more muscle and elastic tissue. This enables the artery to stretch and relax in response to nervous stimulation and variations in blood pressure.
The blood flow through the veins (below) is slower than in the arteries. In the legs it is helped by the 'muscle-pump' — the contraction of adjacent muscles which squeeze the blood upwards — and by the pressure pulsing through neighbouring arteries. Unlike the arteries, veins contain valves which allow blood only to flow one way — towards the heart.

How blood flows through the veins

Valve

Flow of blood

Muscular pressure

Muscular pressure

Vein

Valve

The aortic valve (above) links the aorta, the artery through which blood is pumped from the heart around the body, with the left ventricle. Such valves are more complex than the valves in the veins, since they have to function in a precise sequence to seal the heart chambers, keep the blood flowing the right way and stop it rushing back into the heart. The three flaps here are closed to prevent this.

release of energy—see Metabolism, p46. As the capillary runs its short course through the cells, the concentration of chemicals in the tissue fluid is increased by these waste-products until it is greater than that in the capillaries. The concentration of the chemicals in the tissue fluid is now stronger than in the blood, so chemicals seep back into the capillaries, to be carried back towards the heart by the veins.

At the same time, tissue fluid is forced back into the capillaries. This process depends on a biological principle called osmosis, according to which chemical units, or molecules, will move through a semi-permeable membrane from a strong solution to one that is weaker.In this manner waste products, such as carbon dioxide, are transported through the sys-

tem to be be excreted from the body.

The process of capillary exchange depends on a number of factors. If the arteries are dilated, or expanded, the increased pressure in the capillaries will force more fluid across the membrane. If the veins are obstructed so that blood cannot flow properly, the venous capillaries will not be able to reabsorb fluid. In some diseases, such as kidney failure, the concentration of plasma proteins in the blood is reduced. This, in turn, reduces the amount of fluid that seeps back into the venous capillaries. Alternatively, damage to the capillaries from a blow may allow plasma proteins to pass across the membrane too freely. The physical sign of all these problems is a condition called oedema, sometimes known as 'dropsy'. In this, ▷

THE LYMPHATIC SYSTEM

The lymphatic system consists of a network of vessels which link together the spleen, tonsils, thymus gland and a multitude of lymph nodes. The system filters the body's tissue fluid and returns it to the blood. The lymph tissues also produce lymphocytes and antibodies which are crucial to the defence of the body against infection.

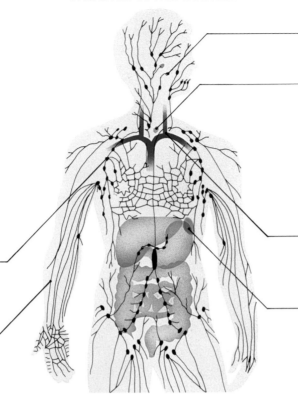

Lymphocytes from the two tonsils in the throat engulf bacteria and microorganisms.

The thymus gland is an important source of lymphocytes for children, but it shrinks after puberty.

The thoracic lymph duct leads into a large vein just above the heart. It is one of the main channels by which tissue fluid is returned to the blood.

A lymph node is a small mass of tissue which filters lymph fluid and produces lymphocytes. Important groups of nodes are found in the groin, around the lungs, in the armpit and behind the ear.

The spleen breaks down worn out red blood cells and produces lymphocytes, especially in babies.

A lymph vessel.

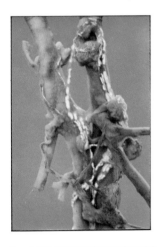

Lymph nodes vary in size from a pin-head to a pea, *(right)*. Lymph vessels feed lymph into the node where foreign particles and bacteria are removed. Germinal centres make lymphocytes which mix with the freshly filtered lymph as it percolates into the outgoing vessels. Strings of white lymph nodes are often found closely linked with blood vessels *(left)*.

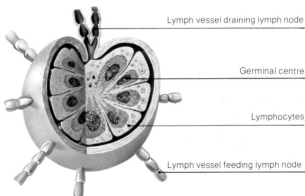

Lymph vessel draining lymph node

Germinal centre

Lymphocytes

Lymph vessel feeding lymph node

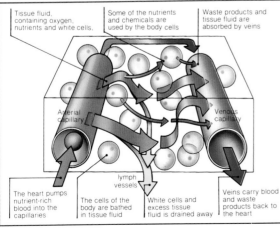

Tissue fluid, containing oxygen, nutrients and white cells.

Some of the nutrients and chemicals are used by the body cells

Waste products and tissue fluid are absorbed by veins

Arterial capillary

Venous capillary

lymph vessels

The heart pumps nutrient-rich blood into the capillaries

The cells of the body are bathed in tissue fluid

White cells and excess tissue fluid is drained away

Veins carry blood and waste products back to the heart

How cells absorb food The cells of the body receive nutrients from the arterial (red) end of the capillaries. Oxygen, released from haemoglobin, and food substances, such as glucose, diffuse into the tissue fluid and then into the cells. Carbon dioxide and the waste products of metabolism diffuse out of the cell and are carried away in the vein (blue).

Other constituents of the blood diffuse into the tissue fluid through spaces in the capillary wall. Large molecules, such as plasma proteins, leave the capillaries in this way, but are only lost to the blood temporarily. They drain into the lymph system (yellow), and return to the blood through the large veins in the chest.

The tissue fluid is subject to two opposing forces. Blood pressure pushes fluid out of the capillary into the space between the cells. But, because blood is richer in protein, osmotic pressure tends to draw fluid back into the blood. In the arterial capillaries the blood pressure is the greater force, so fluid moves outwards. But in the venous capillaries the osmotic pressure is the greater, and fluid is drawn back into the bloodstream.

The heartbeat There are four stages to each 'heartbeat' — two passive, in which the chambers fill with blood, and two active, when the muscles contract to move it.

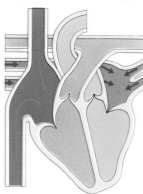

Firstly, the two atria fill up with blood *(above)* — the right with blood from the two vena cavae, the left with blood from the two pairs of pulmonary veins. This stage, in which the atrial muscles are relaxed, is called 'atrial diastole'.

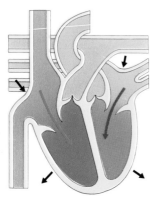

Impulses from the pacemaker trigger contraction of the two atrial muscles (atrial systole). This forces blood into the ventricles, *(above)*. The ventricular muscles have relaxed (ventricular diastole), so that the chambers can fill.

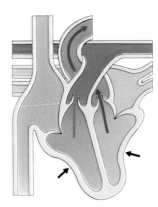

The atrioventricular node stimulates the ventricular muscles to contract (ventricular systole) and pump blood out of the heart *(above)*. As the pulmonary and aortic valves close they make a 'dup' sound.

tissue fluid builds up outside the capillaries causing a puffy, tender swelling.

Back to the heart

The venous system—the network of veins—follows a similar path as the arterial system, only in reverse. Venous capillaries join to form venules, which become small veins and ultimately lead into the main vein of the body, the vena cava. This takes the blood directly into the heart, ready for recirculation.

Blood is forced through the arteries by the tremendous pumping action of the heart. This same pressure helps to push blood through the veins, as does the back pressure that draws blood into the empty pumping-chambers of the heart. But these two pressures are not enough to make blood flow against gravity. In the legs, for example, the construction of the veins is adapted to make the flow of blood to the heart, called 'venous return', easier.

Veins, like arteries, have a muscular wall; in this case it is thin and flexible. The veins of the legs pass through a 'muscle-pump': the muscles contract during physical activity, and as they do so they squeeze the vessels. The flexible walls of the veins are pushed inwards, but expand to allow the resulting surge of blood to move. Blood is forced to move upwards, towards the heart, because simple valves inside the veins allow movement only in this direction. If these valves become incapable of preventing a surge in the wrong direction, blood tends to stagnate, forming distortions of the vessels known as varicose veins.

The lymph system

Not all the tissue fluid that seeps from the arterial capillaries is reabsorbed by the venous capillaries. Some of it enters a coexisting circulation called the lymph system. The lymph vessels start in the spaces between cells. They collect surplus tissue fluid and any excess plasma proteins, and return them to the main veins of the body. The lymph vessels in the intestines also carry globules of fat away from the digestive tract—*see Digestion, p40.* Lymph vessels can rarely be seen unless there is an infection, when they sometimes show as thin red lines. But they form a network throughout the body, which terminates in two large vessels called the thoracic duct and the right lymphatic duct. These join the great veins of the neck.

Scattered throughout the network of lymph vessels are small nodes of lymphatic tissue. These are important sites for manufacture of lymphocytes, one of the five forms of white cell which play a critical role in the defence of the body against disease—*see Natural Defences Against Disease, p52.* Most of the lymph nodes are tiny, but in the thymus, the spleen and the tonsils there are large quantities of lymph tissue. These organs also manufacture lymphocytes, which move freely through the lymph vessels, arteries, veins and tissue fluid to fight infection.

The cardiovascular and lymphatic systems perform a wide variety of essential functions. But none would be possible without the motive force that keeps the various liquids flowing. This force is provided by a remarkable and effective organ—the human heart.

The biological pump

The heart is a superb piece of biological engineering. It beats constantly throughout life, on average 70 times each minute—in a normal life-span over 2,000 million times. But the heart is essentially a very simple pump.

This pump is made up of four chambers, divided vertically by a thick membrane, or septum. Each side has two chambers—the atrium above and the ventricle below. Sir William Harvey, the 17th-century English physician, was the first man to realize that blood does not flow directly from one side of the heart to the other but is pumped out of one side, passes through the lungs and enters the other side. No blood passes across the septum.

Blood flows into the right atrium from the main vein of the body, the vena cava. It passes down into the right ventricle, which contracts to pump the blood to the lungs through the pulmonary artery. Confusingly, this is the only vessel containing de-oxygenated blood that is called an artery; the vessel taking oxygenated blood from the lungs to the left atrium is called the pulmonary vein. Newly oxygenated blood passes into the left ventricle and is pumped into the arteries through the aorta. From there, it begins its return journey around the body.

Valves, nerves and blood

Blood is moved physically by the contractions of the heart muscle, or myocardium. To ensure that it flows in the right direction there are 'flap' valves between each atrium and ventricle. On the right side the valve has three flaps—the tricuspid valve; on the left it has two, which make up the bicuspid, or mitral valve.

The contractions of the heart muscle are initiated by a series of electrical impulses. They must be carefully timed to maintain the natural rhythm of the heart beat. These impulses start from a small bundle of nervous tissue in the right atrium called the sino-atrial node. They spread in waves through the two atria, and then run down a nerve that connects the atria and the ventricles, called the atrio-ventricular node. Doctors can trace the pattern of these electrical impulses, and so monitor the heart's activity, by the use of an electrocardiograph, or ECG machine. Like any other organ or tissue in the body, the heart needs an adequate supply of blood. This comes from the two coronary arteries, which branch off the aorta just after it leaves the heart to form, as the name suggests, a 'corona', or crown, round the surface of the heart muscle. If these arteries are narrowed and obstructed by arterial disease, or blocked by a clot of blood, as in

HOW THE HEART WORKS

The heart is a muscular pump measuring 12cm (4.8in) from top to bottom, 9cm (3.6in) across at its broadest point, and 6cm (2.4in) from front to back. The average heart weighs 310gm (10.9oz) in a man and 255gm (9oz) in a woman.

The pulmonary valve has three flaps, or cusps, which open to let blood flow from the right ventricle and then close to stop it returning.

The pacemaker of the heart, the sinoatrial node, lies beneath these tissues. This is a piece of nerve tissue that sends out electric impulses which stimulate the muscles of the atria to contract.

The atrioventricular node, a nerve which picks up the electric impulse from the pacemaker, is under these tissues. The impulse is conducted down a network of nerves to the ventricles, causing their muscles to contract.

The aortic valve has three cusps which open and close to control the flow of blood from the left ventricle into the aorta.

The tricuspid valve has three cusps which open to let blood from the right atrium flow into the right ventricle. The valve closes at once to prevent any backflow.

The right ventricle receives blood from the right atrium and pumps it into the pulmonary artery.

The right atrium is the chamber of the heart which receives blood from the superior and inferior vena cavae. These two large veins return deoxygenated blood from the body. They enter from above and below and, in doing so, form most of the upper and lower walls of the right atrium.

The aorta is the main artery of the body. It receives oxygenated blood from the left ventricle. The aorta is 3cm (1.2in) wide as it leaves the heart and ascends in an arch behind the pulmonary artery. It branches three times before descending behind the heart and terminating in the abdomen.

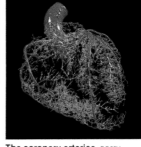

The coronary arteries carry blood to all the muscle cells of the heart and supply them with oxygen and fuel.

Two pulmonary veins return oxygenated blood from the lungs.

The pulmonary artery branches left and right and takes blood to the lungs for oxygenation.

The left atrium receives blood from the four pulmonary veins and pumps it into the left ventricle.

The mitral valve has two cusps which open and close to control the flow of blood from the left atrium to the left ventricle.

The left ventricle is the most muscular of the four chambers because it has to pump blood into the aorta and around the body.

The septum divides the heart into two and is completely impermeable to blood. It stops deoxygenated blood in the right heart from mixing with the oxygenated blood in the left heart.

The aorta descends to the abdomen where it forks into the left and right iliac arteries.

The inferior vena cava conveys blood to the heart from parts of the body below the diaphragm.

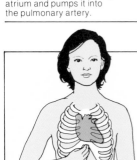

The position of the heart The heart sits at an oblique angle between the lungs, behind the breastbone. One third of it lies to the right of the mid-line of this bone, the other two thirds to the left. The top of the heart lies below the second pair of ribs, and the bottom below the seventh pair.

a coronary thrombosis, an area of heart muscle will die. The result may be a heart attack.

The heart may also be affected by an infection of one of its four layers of tissue. One of these is the heart muscle itself, the myocardium; the outermost layer, the pericardium, is a loose protective sac that is flexible enough to allow the heart to expand and contract during the pumping cycle; the inner layer of this sac, the epicardium, adheres closely to the surface of the heart; while the fourth layer, the endocardium, is a thin membrane lining the inside of the atria and ventricles. Such

an infection is called by the name of the layer involved—pericarditis, for example, if the pericardium is infected.

Pathways for disease

The cardiovascular and lymphatic systems, then, provide the cells of the body with all the essentials for life. But, unfortunately, there are two sides to the coin. Blood and lymph also provide a means for the spread of disease: they act as a transport system for infections, foreign bodies, parasites and malignant cells, as well as for nutrients, oxygen, chemical messengers, wastes and defence mechanisms.

Connections
Anaemia
Anti-histamines
Arteriosclerosis
Atherosclerosis
Christmas disease
Coronary thrombosis
Haemophilia
Heart attack — *see Myocardial infarction*
Hypertension
Oedema
Pericarditis
Varicose veins

The respiratory system

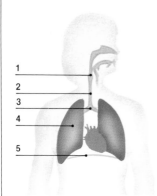

How we breathe Air is taken into the body through the nose or mouth. From there it passes into the larynx, **1**, down the trachea, **2**, which divides into two bronchi, **3**, and into the lungs, **4**. The muscular diaphragm, **5**, contracts, moving down, when air is inhaled and relaxes, moving upwards, when air is exhaled.

A baby takes its first breaths a few seconds after birth. This is the start of a process that will continue until death. Each time the lungs inflate, life-giving oxygen enters the body. When they deflate, waste products such as carbon dioxide are forced out. Breathing is a continuous process, and if the lungs stop working for more than about four minutes, the tissues of the body will die.

Oxygen, a gas, is one of the components of air. It is essential for the release of energy by the cells, and so for all the functions required to maintain life. When oxygen is used to release energy, carbon dioxide is produced—*see Metabolism, p44*. This gas is a waste product, and would eventually poison the body if it were not removed. The respiratory system is designed to exchange the essential oxygen for the waste carbon dioxide by the process called 'respiration'.

Breathing

The lungs are two spongy bags that lie immediately under the ribs, on either side of the backbone. They are connected to the outside of the body by the airway. Each lung sits in a sealed, airtight pleural cavity, sealed in by two membranes called the pleura. The space between the two membranes contains a fluid that helps the pleura slide over each other as the lungs expand and contract.

Directly below the pleural membranes is a dome-shaped muscle called the diaphragm, anchored to the spine at the back and to the breastbone at the front. This muscle plays an important part in the process of breathing, which is divided into two phases—'inspiration', when a breath is drawn in, and 'expiration', when it is released.

To start the phase of breathing called inspiration, the muscle fibres of the diaphragm contract to flatten the dome downwards. At the same time, the muscles of the chest wall contract, swinging the ribs upwards and outwards. Both actions increase the volume of the pleural cavities, reducing the air pressure inside the lungs. As a result, air from outside the body is drawn into the lungs to equalize the pressure, and a breath is taken.

Expiration, or breathing out, is a much simpler process. When the muscles of inspiration relax, the elastic tissue of the lungs recoils, forcing air out of the body.

The airway

The top part of the airway, known as the 'upper respiratory tract', consists of the ▷

HOW THE VOICE WORKS

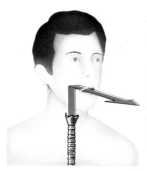

The vocal cords are two membranes which lie across the windpipe and form part of the larynx in the throat *(left)*. Muscles in the larynx, viewed from behind *(below)*, move the two arytenoid cartilages and, as a result, either bring the vocal cords together or alter their tension. Sounds are produced by the vibration of the cords as air passes between them, but this is only possible when the cords are held together.

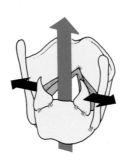

When the voice is not in use *(left)*, the air *(blue arrow)* passes freely through the space between the vocal cords. The two arytenoid cartilages are in their normal position *(black arrow)*, because the laryngeal muscles are relaxed; no sounds can be produced because the air does not vibrate the vocal cords.

The thyroid cartilage forms the front of the larynx.

The two vocal cords can be stretched or relaxed by the arytenoid cartilages and vibrated by the air passing through them.

The vestibular folds lie either side of the vocal cords.

The two arytenoid cartilages control the position and tension of the two vocal cords.

The cricoid cartilage.

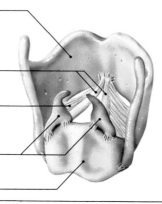

The pitch of the voice is governed by the tension of the cords. When the arytenoid cartilages are brought together and pulled back *(top right)*, the exhaled air vibrates the cords which, because of their tautness, vibrate the air *(blue arrow)* at a high frequency. The pitch of a note produced by a plucked guitar string is determined in the same way. The voice becomes low when the cartilages are moved inward *(below right)* and the cords are loosened.

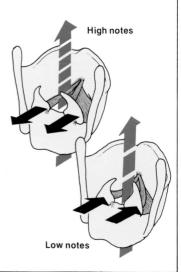

High notes

Low notes

THE FUNCTION OF THE LUNGS

The two lungs have the vital task of extracting oxygen from the air and removing carbon dioxide and water from the blood. In the pair of lungs (below), the left lung is exposed to show the bronchial tree of blood vessels and air passages.

The epiglottis is a small piece of cartilage which closes the windpipe during swallowing.

The Adam's apple is a projection of the thyroid cartilage, the largest cartilage of the larynx.

The larynx, the voice box, lies above the trachea and is made up of nine cartilages.

Each lung is made up of a number of self-contained units, called broncho-pulmonary segments.

The aorta carries oxygenated blood from the heart to the rest of the body.

The heart receives newly oxygenated blood from each lung through the two pulmonary veins and pumps it into the body through the aorta.

The trachea divides into the left and right bronchi. Each bronchus is made of cartilage and muscle and lined with mucus glands.

Each lung contains a huge number of air passages. The main bronchus divides again and again into successively smaller bronchi, so forming the bronchial tree.

The pulmonary artery takes blood to the lungs where it is oxygenated.

The pulmonary artery is the only artery in the body to contain deoxygenated blood. It branches over and over again into a mass of fine capillaries that surround each alveolus.

The network of veins running through the lungs collects the blood that has been oxygenated in the alveoli, and carries it to the two pulmonary veins. These take the blood to the left atrium.

All the bronchi divide into fine bronchioles and each of these leads into an alveolar duct, which opens out into about 30 alveoli. The wall of an alveolus is only one cell thick, so the blood capillaries which surround it are in close contact with the air. As a result, oxygen, carbon dioxide and water can be exchanged across the barrier.

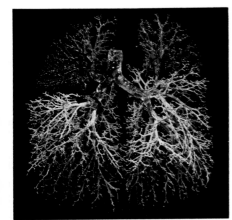

The bronchial tree is divided into self-contained, independently functioning units called broncho-pulmonary segments, which have their own blood supply and bronchi, and can be removed without impairing the function of the others.

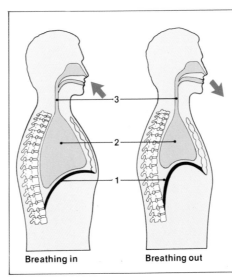

Breathing consists of a two-part cycle, in which air is taken into the lungs, and then released. Inhalation, or inspiration, starts when the muscles of the diaphragm, **1**, contract, together with some of the muscles between the ribs. The diaphragm is pulled down, while the rib-cage moves up and outwards. As a result, the chest cavity enlarges. Like a bellows, air is drawn into the lungs, **2**, through the nose or mouth and trachea, **3**. When the muscles relax, the elastic tissue of the lungs recoils, forcing the air out of the body. This is expiration, or exhalation. The diaphragm then ascends, the rib-cage moves down and inwards and the cycle begins all over again.

Breathing in　　　**Breathing out**

Breathing is regulated by the respiratory centre, a group of nerve cells in the medulla at the base of the brain. Several factors excite or inhibit the centre, increasing the rate of breathing, or returning it to normal.

Two types of cells, sited in the walls of the carotid arteries, **1**, and the aorta, **2**, monitor oxygen and carbon dioxide levels in the blood and its pressure. These cells report any changes to the respiratory centre, **3**.

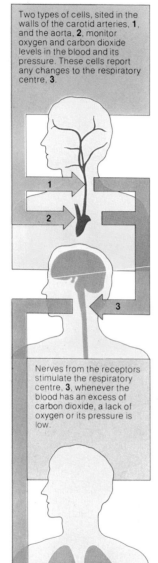

Nerves from the receptors stimulate the respiratory centre, **3**, whenever the blood has an excess of carbon dioxide, a lack of oxygen or its pressure is low.

The respiratory centre sends impulses through the spinal cord to regulate the activity of the diaphragm, **4**, and intercostal muscles, **5**. As the blood pressure and level of oxygen increase, and the carbon dioxide level reduces, the centre slows down the rate of breathing and relaxes the diaphragm and rib muscles after each inhalation.

nose, mouth, pharynx and larynx. Illnesses such as colds and laryngitis are often medically termed 'upper respiratory tract infections'.

As air enters the body through the nose and mouth it is filtered and purified—*see Natural Defences Against Disease, p52.* Thick hairs in the nostrils filter out large particles, while smaller particles and bacteria are trapped in the filmy mucous membranes of the mouth and nose. White cells from the lymph tissue of the tonsils and adenoids attack and deal with the bacteria. Dust is swept towards the throat by a mass of tiny hairs, called cilia, and then swallowed.

Both food and air enter the pharynx, the space behind the mouth and nose, but only air can enter the larynx, the first part of the windpipe. The act of swallowing swings a thin flap of cartilage, called the epiglottis, across the laryngeal entrance, blocking it completely. The larynx is a short, wide tube, formed of cartilage, which, particularly in men, may protrude at the front of the throat as an 'Adam's apple'. It contains the vocal cords, which are manipulated by the laryngeal muscles to produce sounds.

The lower respiratory tract begins just below the Adam's apple, where the larynx is joined by the trachea, or windpipe. This organ is a tube about 25cm (10in) long, held open by rings of cartilage. Just below the second rib, counting down from the notch of the breastbone, the trachea divides into two branches, the left and right main bronchi. The right bronchus is wider, and more vertical than the left. Foreign bodies, such as peanuts, often become lodged here when they have been inhaled, or 'gone down the wrong way'.

Tiny pouches

Inside the lungs the main bronchi divide over and over again, becoming smaller each time. This gives blood and air the opportunity to mix over as wide an area as possible so that the blood can take in oxygen and give up carbon dioxide. The smallest branches of the bronchi are only 0.2mm (0.008in) in diameter, and are called bronchioles.

At the end of each bronchiole, like a bubble of glass on the end of a glassblower's tube, is an alveolar sac. The wall of this sac is made up of tiny pouches, or alveoli, which contain air. There are millions of alveoli in the lungs, giving a surface area for the exchange of gases of more than 50 square metres (538 sq ft)—about the size of the floor of a large garage.

Watery film

Contrary to popular belief, the lungs are never completely emptied of air when breathing is normal. After breathing out, they still contain about 3 litres (5.28 pints) of air. This is called the 'resting respiratory level'.

When a normal, resting, breath is taken, a further 400ml (0.7 pint) of air, known as the 'tidal volume', is drawn in, but only

250ml (0.4 pint) reaches the alveoli, where it mixes with the air already present. The remainder is known as 'dead space air', and fills up the airway. If the length of the airway is increased artificially—for example, by the use of a snorkel tube when swimming underwater—less air will reach the alveoli, so the swimmer will have to breathe more deeply to achieve the same result.

The air that reaches the alveoli is composed of around 21 per cent oxygen and 0.03 per cent carbon dioxide (the rest is nitrogen, which plays no part in respiration). The inspired air mixes with the air already present in the alveoli—which contains around 14 per cent oxygen and six per cent carbon dioxide—increasing the oxygen content. The oxygen dissolves into a watery film that covers the inner surface of the alveolar wall. This is very thin—it is only one thousandth of a millimetre (0.000039in) thick. On the other side is a network of minute blood vessels.

Blood which is high in carbon dioxide but low in oxygen, is pumped towards the lungs by the heart *(p26)*. When it comes into contact with the wall of the alveolus, carbon dioxide diffuses across the thin barrier and dissolves in the watery film on the inner surface. At the same time, oxygen diffuses across the barrier in the opposite direction. It joins up with the dark blue pigment haemoglobin in the red blood cells *(p22)* to form the bright red chemical oxyhaemoglobin. The oxygenated blood is taken to the heart, which pumps it around the body to supply the tissues.

The control centre

The muscles of the diaphragm and chest wall that contract during inspiration are 'involuntary'—they are stimulated without the conscious intervention of the brain. The control centre for these stimuli is a small bundle of nervous tissue in the medulla of the brain. This is called the respiratory centre.

Information from many sources is analyzed here. The carbon dioxide and oxygen level in the blood is monitored by specialised nerves called chemoreceptors in the aortic and carotid arteries; the blood pressure by other nerves called baroreceptors; the degree of expansion of the lungs by stretch receptors. Sometimes the respiratory centre also receives signals from the conscious brain—for example, when a person needs to pant.

During exercise, oxygen is burnt up to provide energy. Carbon dioxide is produced and its level in the blood increases. The chemoreceptors pick up this rise, and the respiratory centre stimulates the muscles to increase how fast the oxygen is taken in to the body and carbon dioxide expelled. The muscles contract and relax more quickly, so that the rate of breathing speeds up, and also contract more strongly, so that more air is drawn in. In this way the 'inspiratory reserve volume' is used—this is the maximum amount of air that the

STRUCTURE OF THE LUNGS

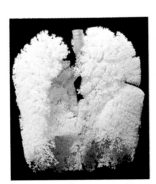

The bronchial tree is a system of tubes, which carry air from the trachea, or windpipe, to the tiny alveoli, which get smaller and smaller (left). The tubes are made up of muscle and cartilage, and lined with mucus glands and tiny hairs called cilia. The trachea, 15mm (0.6in) wide, forms the trunk of the tree and divides into two large tubes called bronchi. At the division, each bronchus is 8mm (0.32in) wide, but then it tapers to 2mm (0.08in) before dividing into smaller bronchi. Each of these branches to form a mass of even smaller bronchioles, without cartilage and only 0.5mm (0.02in) wide. The smallest bronchioles, called respiratory bronchioles, lead into an alveoli duct, which opens out into around 30 blind-ended sacs — the alveoli, shown (right) magnified 480 times.

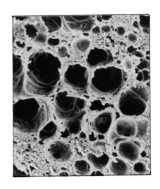

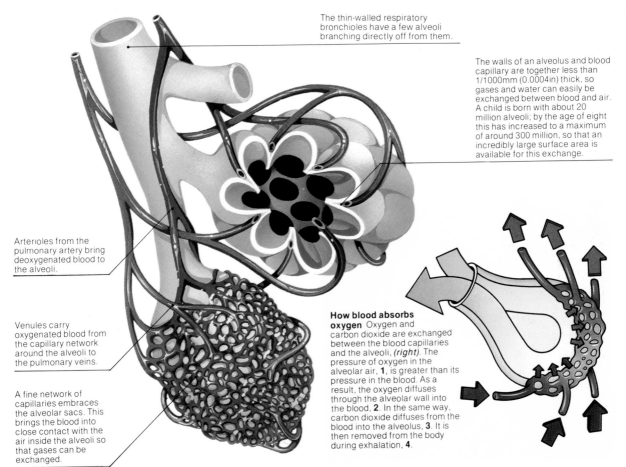

The thin-walled respiratory bronchioles have a few alveoli branching directly off from them.

The walls of an alveolus and blood capillary are together less than 1/1000mm (0.0004in) thick, so gases and water can easily be exchanged between blood and air. A child is born with about 20 million alveoli; by the age of eight this has increased to a maximum of around 300 million, so that an incredibly large surface area is available for this exchange.

Arterioles from the pulmonary artery bring deoxygenated blood to the alveoli.

Venules carry oxygenated blood from the capillary network around the alveoli to the pulmonary veins.

A fine network of capillaries embraces the alveolar sacs. This brings the blood into close contact with the air inside the alveoli so that gases can be exchanged.

How blood absorbs oxygen Oxygen and carbon dioxide are exchanged between the blood capillaries and the alveoli, (right). The pressure of oxygen in the alveolar air, **1**, is greater than its pressure in the blood. As a result, the oxygen diffuses through the alveolar wall into the blood, **2**. In the same way, carbon dioxide diffuses from the blood into the alveolus, **3**. It is then removed from the body during exhalation, **4**.

lungs can hold, over and above the tidal volume. In a healthy young man the lungs can hold as much as 6 litres (10.5 pints) of air.

By contrast, during sleep, when little energy is required, only small amounts of carbon dioxide are produced. The respiratory centre depresses the activity of the muscles, and breathing is slow and shallow.

Sophisticated design

The airway and the lungs are a sophisticated system designed purely to exchange oxygen for carbon dioxide. But like all sophisticated systems, the respiratory system is delicate and sensitive. Its success depends on having a large surface area for the exchange of gases and a free flow of air. Chest diseases such as pneumonia reduce this surface area: the pus produced by white cells (p23) as they attack the bacteria clogs up the alveoli, and large sections of the lung collapse.

But many of the diseases that reduce the efficiency of the respiratory system are self-inflicted—their cause is cigarette smoking. This habit inevitably causes bronchitis, a crippling inflammation of the bronchi and bronchioles, and emphysema, a loss of the lungs' elastic recoil at some stage of life. It also causes that most fatal of all the diseases of the respiratory system— lung cancer.

Connections
Bronchitis
Cold
Emphysema
Laryngitis
Lung Cancer
Pneumonia
Upper respiratory tract infection

The nervous system

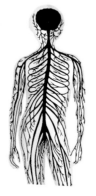

The nerves of the body are organized into the two main systems **(above)**. These are the central nervous system, made up of the brain and spinal cord, and the peripheral nervous system, whose impulses travel to and from the spine through 31 pairs of spinal nerves.

The sophisticated network of sensory cells, nerves, spinal cord and brain, known as the nervous system, acts as overall controller and fine-tuner of all bodily functions. The nervous system detects changes outside the body and monitors the delicate balance of the body's chemistry, then initiates the appropriate response. In addition, the human brain, uniquely in the animal kingdom, has a remarkable capacity for abstract thought, logical argument and emotion.

Chain of command

The human nervous system consists of an intelligence network, a decision-making centre and a chain of command—just like a military unit. Millions of specialized sensors, together with the highly-developed organs of sight, hearing, smell and taste, form the intelligence network that detects changes inside and outside the body. The

information provided by the sensors is passed through networks of fibres, called sensory nerves, to the headquarters, the central nervous system. This consists of the brain and spinal cord and contains the decision-making processes.

The system has several ways of dealing with the information provided by the sensors. Some responses occur automatically—digestive juices, for example, are released when there is food in the digestive tract without conscious control or awareness. Other information is passed to the conscious mind, the highest level of the system. When the bladder is full, for instance, the sensory network informs the brain that there is a need to pass water—the conscious mind decides on the appropriate time and place.

Sometimes the conscious mind intervenes to overrule or adjust responses that are usually automatic. The normal reaction to intense heat, for example, is to back

THE PERIPHERAL NERVOUS SYSTEM

The peripheral nervous system starts at the spinal cord and reaches out to every tissue in the body. It consists of three systems of nerves: motor nerves that conduct motor impulses via the spinal and cranial nerves to the voluntary muscles; sensory nerves that conduct sensory impulses from the body, along the same spinal and cranial nerves to the spinal cord; and autonomic nerves that conduct motor impulses from either the sympathetic trunk or the spinal cord to involuntary muscles, glands and tissues.

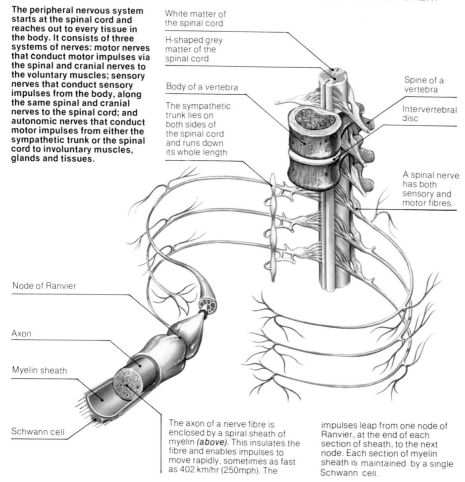

White matter of the spinal cord

H-shaped grey matter of the spinal cord

Body of a vertebra

The sympathetic trunk lies on both sides of the spinal cord and runs down its whole length

Spine of a vertebra

Intervertebral disc

A spinal nerve has both sensory and motor fibres.

Node of Ranvier

Axon

Myelin sheath

Schwann cell

The axon of a nerve fibre is enclosed by a spiral sheath of myelin *(above)*. This insulates the fibre and enables impulses to move rapidly, sometimes as fast as 402 km/hr (250mph). The

impulses leap from one node of Ranvier, at the end of each section of sheath, to the next node. Each section of myelin sheath is maintained by a single Schwann cell.

Each neurone, or nerve cell, has a cell body, branches called dendrites, and an axon *(below)* and is separated from its neighbour by a tiny gap, called a synapse. One neurone contacts the next one in the nerve chain by releasing a chemical called a neurotransmitter from the end of the axon. This crosses the synapse and transmits the electrical impulse carrying the message to the next neurone. The neurotransmitter found at the synapses of most nerves is acetylcholine, though at some autonomic nerve synapses the transmitter is noradrenaline.

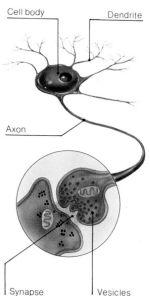

Cell body

Dendrite

Axon

Synapse

Vesicles

SENSORY AND MOTOR NERVES

The senses keep the brain informed about the state of the body, its readiness for action, and about changes in its immediate environment. The brain analyzes this information and initiates an appropriate response. The sudden fear of being run over for example (right) evokes an immediate red alert. The senses inform the brain of the imminent danger, the motor nerves make the correct muscles contract and the autonomic nerves mobilize the body to cope with the necessary evasive action.

All the senses come into play in moments of danger. The eyes and ears of the man (left) warn his brain of the approaching danger by sending impulses down sensory nerves. At the same time, sensors in the muscles and joints alert the brain to the position and preparedness of the body. In a flash, he knows there is no time to lose and decides to run. Motor nerves (far left) stimulate his muscles and autonomic nerves (below) prepare the rest of the body.

The brain sends out nerve impulses (left) which travel down the spinal cord, through the motor nerves to the muscles of the body. Each motor nerve terminates at a large synapse, called a motor end-plate, in the muscle. A chemical neurotransmitter called acetylcholine crosses the plate and stimulates the muscle to contract. The muscles and joints of the body work together as the man runs away from the car, while sympathetic nerves (right) divert blood to these tissues to ensure they receive enough fuel and oxygen.

Brain

Sympathetic trunk

Spinal cord

The sympathetic system
Dilates pupils
Dilates bronchi
Speeds up heartbeat
Inhibits digestion
Dilates blood vessels to muscles
Relaxes bladder

The parasympathetic system
Constricts pupils
Constricts bronchi
Slows down heartbeat
Stimulates digestion
Contracts bladder

away, but the mind of a fireman is trained to consciously override this natural response.

Finally, the conscious mind can initiate actions independently of signals received from the sensors: an everyday instance of this is the decision to bend down and pick up a piece of paper from the ground—an action that does not directly fulfil a physical need.

Once a decision is taken, signals set in motion the various actions necessary to implement it. These are passed down the spinal cord, and sent through another set of fibres, called motor nerves, to the appropriate parts of the body—these may be muscles, glands or the heart. When the decision has been acted on by the body, the sensory network sends another series of messages back to the central nervous system, alerting it to the changes that have occurred.

Thus there are two sets of fibres: the sensory fibres, which carry messages from the tissues and organs of the body to the central nervous system, and the motor fibres, which carry signals of command from the central nervous system to the muscles and glands. Most of these fibres travel in the same nerves to and from the spinal cord, the branching network of nerves being called the peripheral nervous system.

Motor, or command, signals from the brain, reach the tissues of the body by two pathways. One, the somatic system, triggers contractions in the striated muscles that are under the brain's conscious control. The parallel motor, or command, network is called the autonomic nervous system. This triggers glandular secretions and contractions in smooth muscles under involuntary, or subconscious control.

The somatic motor pathways run from the brain, through the spinal cord to a motor end-plate in the muscle. When an impulse arrives at the motor end-plate it makes the muscle contract, and a series of co-ordinated impulses from the brain then enables a series of muscles to act together.

The autonomic nervous system subdivides into the sympathetic and parasym- ▷

The autonomic nervous system consists of two complementary sub-systems — the sympathetic and parasympathetic nerves (above). Most of their fibres conduct motor impulses to parts of the body that are generally under subconscious control, but there are also sensory fibres which feed back information from these areas to the spinal cord. When the man runs away from the car only his sympathetic nerves are stimulated. Various muscles either contract or relax, with the aim of making the man's flight more effective. The pupils of both his eyes dilate; his digestion is inhibited; the blood supply to his skeletal muscles, heart and brain is increased; the blood supply to everywhere else is reduced; his bladder is relaxed; his heart beats faster; and his bronchi dilate, allowing more air to reach the lungs. When the man reaches safety, his body relaxes as the parasympathetic nerves return the body to a normal resting state.

pathetic systems. Fibres of the sympathetic nervous system pass from the brain to the spinal cord and then out to reach the rest of the body. Parasympathetic fibres leave the base of the brain and the lower part of the spinal cord. Most smooth muscle, in the walls of the blood vessels, the bronchi, the digestive tract, the heart and the glands are supplied with both sympathetic and parasympathetic fibres. Depending on the situation and the body's requirements, the signals from the two systems may either balance or complement each other. The activity of the autonomic nervous system is also co-ordinated with the hormonal control of the body's functions.

Sensors

The information-gathering parts of the nervous system provide a huge amount of data about the condition of the body and anything going on about it, and this data is continually updated. Much of this in-

formation is picked up by the four main sense organs—the eyes, ears, nose and tongue. They are in almost constant use, giving the ability to see, hear, smell and taste. In addition, there is one other important sense organ—the skin.

This flexible outer covering of the body contains specialized sensors which can detect touch, temperature, pressure and pain. Some parts of the body are more sensitive than others—the fingers, tongue and lips, for example, are particularly sensitive to touch. During childhood the brain learns to recognize the position of each one of these sensors, for each has its own individual pathway to the central nervous system. Eventually the command centres become able to locate the exact source of any skin sensation and act on it accordingly.

The sense organs give a detailed picture of the outside world, but there are also many sensors within the body itself which

HOW THE EYES WORK

The eyeball, a sphere about 2.5cm (1in) in diameter, acts like a camera and can be moved by a number of muscles. Light reflected from an object enters the eye through the transparent cornea, which focuses the light on to the retina at the back of the eye. The lens helps the cornea to do this and also turns the image upside down. One layer of the retina contains millions of cells called rods and cones which convert the rays of

light into electrical impulses. Other layers contain nerve cells which organize and code the impulses according to the colour, brightness and intensity of the orginal image. The coded impulses are then channelled by the optic nerve to the back of the brain. The impulses are decoded and processed in the visual cortex, where an upright image of the original object is created.

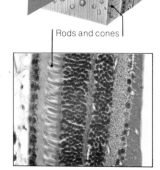

Direction of light

Rods and cones

The different layers of the cells at the back of the eye are shown diagrammatically *(top)* and photographically enlarged *(above)*. The retina contains the light-sensitive rods and cones. The latter are active when there is sufficient light for them to touch on, and detect colour. The rods are responsible for night vision, though they complement the activity of the cones by day, and record the intensity and brightness of light. Both rods and cones contain light-sensitive pigments which are bleached by exposure to light. This causes impulses to travel down adjacent nerve fibres. The sum of the impulses formed by the 120 million rods and six million cones constitute the image relayed to the brain by the optic nerve.

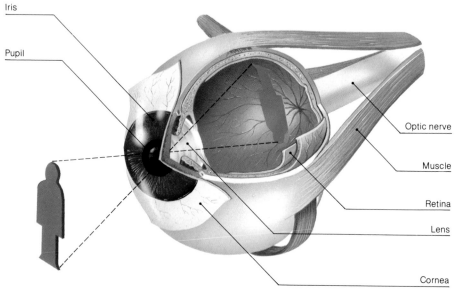

Iris

Pupil

Optic nerve

Muscle

Retina

Lens

Cornea

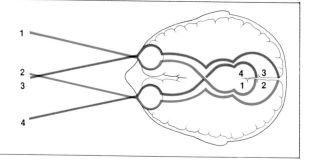

Two visual centres in the brain, one at the back of each cerebral hemisphere, are responsible for sight. Half the optic nerve fibres from each eye cross over to the visual centre on the other side of the brain *(right)*. Thus, the left visual centre 'sees' objects in the right half of the visual field, **1, 2,** and the right centre 'sees' objects in the left half, **3, 4**. This makes stereoscopic vision possible, through which the size, shape and distance of objects can be appreciated.

HOW THE EARS WORK

The ear is divided into three parts: the outer, middle and inner ear. The outer ear (right) funnels sound waves (blue) down to the end of a bony channel where they vibrate the membranous eardrum. These vibrations are transmitted to the three tiny bones — the malleus, incus and stapes — of the middle ear (below). This air-filled chamber is connected to the point where the nose meets the throat by the Eustachian tube. The pressure inside the middle ear may build up, when passing through tunnels or descending from high altitudes, for example, and can be reduced by swallowing or yawning.

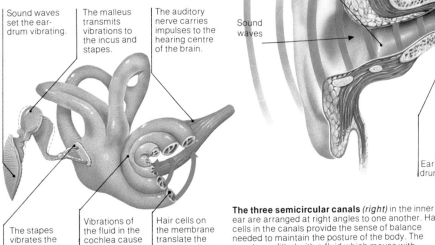

Outer ear | Malleus | Semicircular canals | Cochlea | Auditory nerve

Sound waves

Ear-drum | Incus | Stapes | Eustachian tube

Sound waves set the eardrum vibrating.

The malleus transmits vibrations to the incus and stapes.

The auditory nerve carries impulses to the hearing centre of the brain.

The stapes vibrates the fluid inside the cochlea of the inner ear.

Vibrations of the fluid in the cochlea cause the internal membrane to vibrate.

Hair cells on the membrane translate the vibrations into nerve impulses.

The three semicircular canals *(right)* in the inner ear are arranged at right angles to one another. Hair cells in the canals provide the sense of balance needed to maintain the posture of the body. The canals are filled with a fluid which moves with movements of the head and so triggers the hair cells that send impulses to the brain.

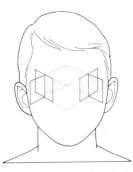

The overall balance of the body is governed by the relationship of the fluid in the semicircular canals of each ear. The semicircular canals on each side are arranged at right angles to the corresponding canal on the other side *(below)*. When the head rotates or moves forwards, backwards or to the side, then the increased activity of one set of hair cells is matched by a decrease in activity of the corresponding set of hair cells on the other side. The difference in this activity is monitored by the brain, together with information from the joint and muscle sensors and the eyes. The brain then makes the necessary adjustments to the posture by stimulating the appropriate muscles.

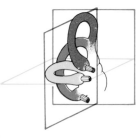

monitor its activity and condition. Some of these, known as proprioceptors, are found in muscles, joints, ligaments and tendons. The proprioceptors tell the central nervous system how much a muscle has contracted, and also register pain. Proprioceptors in the joints keep track of all the movements of the limbs. The brain constantly computes this information, thus achieving a remarkable sense of the position of one part of the body in relation to another. This sense of 'positional awareness' is not dependent on the eyes, and doctors often test it by asking patients to close their eyes and then touch the tip of the nose with one finger.

Other specialized sensors monitor the circulation *(p21)*, respiration *(p28)* and digestion *(p40)*. Baroreceptors measure blood pressure in the great arteries of the body, and chemoreceptors analyze the levels of oxygen and carbon dioxide in the blood. The lungs and airway contain stretch receptors, and the heart's activity is monitored by specialized receptors in the atria and ventricles.

Information channels
The sensors send messages to the central nervous system in the form of tiny electrical impulses. Each sensor is attached to a long fibre called a dendrite, which is, in fact, a long extension of a nerve cell, or axon.

Each single nerve contains literally thousands of dendrites. These are col-

lected together in bundles to make up a single nerve, and the whole complex structure leads from the sensors to the spinal cord.

As the nerves get closer to the spinal cord they join together, becoming larger and larger, often alongside branching arteries and veins. But while the veins and arteries all lead to the heart, the majority of the millions of nerves in the body lead to one of the 62 spinal nerves—two for each spinal bone, or vertebra.

The spinal cord
The spinal cord consists of a column of 33 spiny bones, called vertebrae, which enclose a highly organized mass of nerve fibres and cells. The vertebrae are separated by discs of cartilage—it is these discs which 'slip' in the common problem of a slipped disc—and tied together by ligaments. Though this arrangement allows the bones of the cord a degree of flexibility, it is not designed to cope with the constant jarring and pressure caused by the upright stance that human beings adopted millions of years ago. The inherent incompatibility of the spinal cord with the human posture is the root cause of many back complaints.

The nervous tissue within the vertebrae is covered and protected by three membranes called the meninges, which also form a lining for the tissues of the brain. These membranes—the outer, called the dura mater; the middle, the arachnoid mater; and the inner, the pia mater—may ▷

THE STRUCTURE OF THE BRAIN

The cerebral hemispheres are the largest part of the brain, and contain the highest levels of the decision-making processes. The right hemisphere, identical to the left, is seen from the middle of the brain.

The limbic system links the cortex with the hypothalamus in the centre of the brain.

The hypothalamus contains a number of centres which control functions of the body such as hunger, thirst and temperature.

The optic chiasma is the point at which half the nerve fibres from each eye cross over to the other side of the brain.

The pituitary gland, protruding from the hypothalamus, secretes several hormones which control the function of the body's endocrine glands.

The midbrain has two important relay stations, the substantia nigra and the red nuclei. These organize and dispatch the motor impulses which enter and leave the brain.

The cerebral cortex is a thin layer of grey matter covering the two cerebral hemispheres. Although it is no more than 4mm (0.16in) thick, it makes up 40% of the brain and has about 15 thousand million nerve cells.

The corpus callosum, or white matter of the brain, contains about 300 million nerve fibres which represent the channels of communication between the two cerebral hemispheres.

The two thalami are masses of grey matter lying in the centre of the brain. They receive incoming impulses from all the senses except the nose, and together are thought to be the level at which sensations first register in consciousness. One thalamus is associated with each hemisphere.

The pineal gland, the so-called 'mystery gland' of the body, is thought to be involved in sexual development and the rhythms of sleep and wakefulness.

The cerebellum has two hemispheres, composed like the cerebral cortex, of grey and white matter. While it never initiates movement, the cerebellum is the point of origin for the nervous impulses which are concerned with balance, muscle tone and coordination of movement.

The pons is a relay station in the brainstem whose nerves link the cortex, the cerebellum and the spinal cord. Cranial nerves from the pons also provide conscious control of the jaws, eyeballs, tongue and larynx.

The medulla is the gateway for nerve impulses travelling to and from the brain. It also houses the centres which regulate the heartbeat, respiration, swallowing and salivation.

The spinal cord is a multi-channel communications system that conducts messages to and from the brain. If a sensory signal requires an immediate response, however, an on-the-spot decision, called a reflex, is made in the spinal cord itself.

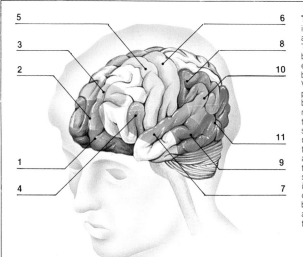

The cerebral cortex is divided into different areas, each having a specific role to play The front lobe controls behaviour, **1**, intellect, **2**, and emotion, **3**. Talking is controlled by the motor speech area, **4**. Voluntary muscles in different parts of the body are controlled by corresponding sections of the motor area, **5**. Sensations from the body are monitored by the sensory area, **6**, and sounds are registered and interpreted by the hearing centre, **7**. The bodily awareness centre, **8**, integrates the information gathered by the sensory area. The ability to read is coordinated by the reading centre, **9**, and the ability to write by the writing centre, **10**. Images are perceived and interpreted by the visual centre, **11**.

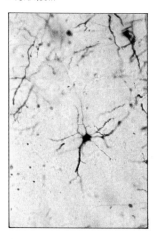

The brain is composed of many millions of nerves, each an extension of a nerve cell, shown *(above)* magnified 400 times. Its axons branch in several directions to link up with other nerve cells, so making up a complex network extending through the body.

become infected in a very serious illness called meningitis. The space between the arachnoid and pia mater, called the sub-arachnoid space, contains a clear, watery fluid called the cerebrospinal fluid, or CSF. Doctors can take a sample of CSF, to test it for the presence of bacteria or viruses when they suspect a disease such as meningitis. This is done by a technique called a lumbar puncture, in which a syringe is passed between the lower, or lumbar, vertebrae, and CSF is drawn off.

Grey and white matter

A cross-section of the spinal cord shows the complexity of its structure. It reveals an H-shaped grey area in the middle of an oval white mass. The grey matter consists of nerve cells and their connections, and the white matter contains nerve fibres. Many of the nerve fibres of the white matter are collected together in columns called tracts, each of which has its own specific destination in the brain. Some of the tracts carry motor, or command signals; others sensory, or information signals.

The grey matter is also divided into sensory and motor areas, and each cell and fibre is connected by a tangle of tiny dendrites to thousands of other pieces of nervous tissue.

In general, the grey matter acts as a clearing house for impulses. It receives information from the nerves and routes it through tracts in the white matter to the brain. It also takes the brain's command impulses from the tracts and routes them to the muscles. But the grey matter is also where the lowest level of decision-making—the spinal reflex—occurs.

The spinal reflex

Some of the simpler responses to sensory information are controlled only by the spinal cord and do not involve the brain. These are called spinal reflexes.

One spinal reflex is tested nearly every time that a doctor gives a patient a thorough physical examination. This is the knee jerk. To test this reflex, the doctor taps the tendon that connects the patella, or kneecap, to the shin bone. Stretch receptors in the tendon send a message along sensory pathways to the grey matter of the spinal cord, where the message is transmitted to a motor nerve cell. A signal is generated immediately. It passes down motor fibres to the quadriceps muscle at the front of the thigh, which contracts, straightening the knee and kicking the leg upwards.

The knee jerk is an extremely simple type of reflex, but there are many others. The contraction of the pupil of the eye in response to a bright light is one—in this case the reflex pathway is not confined to the spinal cord but runs through the lower levels of the brain. More complicated reflexes, involving other parts of the spinal cord and the lower levels of the brain, are conditioned—that is, they develop as a result of training and experience. Driving, for instance, is an acquired skill, consisting, to a large extent, of a complex set of conditioned reflexes.

The command centres

Information gathered by the body's sensors passes into the grey matter in the spinal cord. It is then organized according to type and relayed through the tracts of nerve fibres in the white matter to the command centres of the central nervous system in the brain.

The brain of an adult human being is a complex mass of nervous tissue about the size of two clenched fists. Despite its small size, it is more sophisticated than any computer ever made, as is the system to which it is linked. On average, the male brain weighs around 1,300gm (3lb) and the female brain slightly less, because the brain normally represents about 2% of ▷

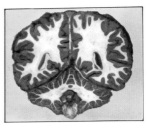

A cross-section of the brain from above shows the hemispheres and the cerebellum. The grey matter of the cortex is stained blue, showing how the folds enlarge the area and so the capacity of the brain.

THE SENSE OF TASTE

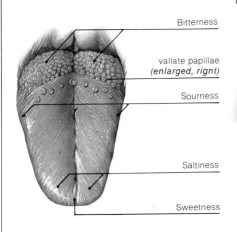

Bitterness

vallate papillae *(enlarged, right)*

Sourness

Saltiness

Sweetness

The four basic taste sensations are localized in specific areas of the tongue *(above)*. 'Sweet' and 'salty' are tasted at the front, 'sour' at the sides and 'bitter' at the back.

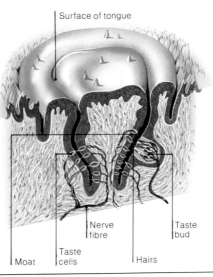

Surface of tongue

Nerve fibre

Taste bud

Moat

Taste cells

Hairs

Around 9,000 taste buds lie within the four kinds of papillae that cover the surface of the adult tongue. The vallate papillae are the largest of the four. They contain a moat in which food dissolved in saliva comes into contact with the taste buds. Between eight and ten vallate papillae form a V-shape at the back of the tongue; their taste buds detect the bitter content of food. Hairs from the cells of each taste bud project into the moat, where their receptors respond to the chemicals in the food. Messages about bitterness are sent, together with impulses from all the other papillae, to the brain where the total taste of a particular food is determined.

THE SENSE OF SMELL

The sense of smell depends on the presence of tiny particles in the air that is inhaled into the nose. These chemical particles, often as small as individual molecules, are carried by the air to the roof of the nasal cavity, where there are millions of receptors called olfactory hairs. These respond to the chemicals by sending impulses through the olfactory nerve for analysis in the olfactory centre of the brain. How this centre distinguishes one smell from another is unknown. The thousands of odours detectable by the human nose can be subdivided into spicy, fetid, fragrant, fruity, resinous and tarry.

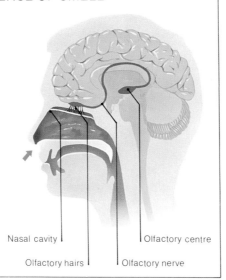

Nasal cavity

Olfactory hairs

Olfactory centre

Olfactory nerve

body weight, and, in general, women weigh less than men. Like the spinal cord, the brain contains grey matter: nerve cells and connections; and white matter: tracts of nerve fibres. The CSF is secreted in, and flows through, a series of four cavities called the ventricles. Finally, the brain has a complicated blood supply, provided by a network of arteries and veins. Any interruption to this blood supply—by a blood clot, say, as in atherosclerosis—may damage nervous tissue: the interruption is known as a stroke.

The brainstem
The first part of the brain, the brainstem, is really an extension of the spinal cord into the skull. It has three parts: the medulla oblongata, the pons and the midbrain. Like the spinal cord, it contains both grey and white matter. Two large tracts of white matter cross from one side of the medulla to the other, carrying motor fibres from the brain to the spinal cord. Just above this, the sensory fibres also cross from one side to the other, with the result that each side of the brain controls the functions of the opposite side of the body.

The medulla contains a number of nerve cell masses, called nuclei. These have a number of functions: they act as relay stations for nerve impulses; as the points of origin for some of the cranial nerves; and they control, through the autonomic nervous system, the activity of the heart, blood vessels, salivary glands and the respiratory system. Decisions made in the medulla are usually automatic, but they can sometimes be influenced by the conscious mind, acting through the millions of tiny connectors that traverse the brain.

Just above the medulla is the pons, which contains yet more interconnecting nerve tracts. The pons acts as a relay station for other parts of the brain, in the same way as the nuclei.

Running through the pons and the medulla is a system of fibres known as the reticular formation. Not much is known about how this works, but it is thought to act as a filter for sensory information, sending some impulses to the conscious mind and rejecting others. By selecting information in this way, it controls the state of consciousness and the rhythms of sleep and waking. Surgical anaesthetics are thought to act directly on the reticular formation, reducing the level of sensory information sent to the conscious mind and causing unconsciousness.

The cerebellum
Just behind the pons and medulla, and linked to the brainstem, is the cerebellum. It is made up of two hemispheres and receives all the information from the proprioceptors—the sensors in joints, ligaments and tendons—as well as sensory and motor information from the higher centres.

The cerebellum acts as a co-ordinator and administrator of the muscles, maintaining a constant tension in the muscles and synchronizing the actions of different muscles. It is linked with the parts of the ear that judge balance and acceleration, and adjusts the actions of the muscles in response to information from them. But the cerebellum cannot initiate movement on its own. It is not part of the conscious mind, and is dependent on the activity of higher centres in the brain in order to fulfil its functions.

The forebrain
More highly developed than in any other animal, the human forebrain is what gives humans their remarkable powers of reasoning and intelligence. In spite of years of research into how it works, very little is known in detail, and as far as scientists can tell, the forebrain is simply a vastly complicated tangle of nerve cells and fibres.

All sensory messages except those from the proprioceptors pass through one of the two egg-shaped masses, called the thalami, above the midbrain. They transmit these messages to the cerebral cortex, the thin outer layer of the cerebral hemispheres.

The cerebral cortex is made up of grey matter, in which a mass of highly evolved and specialized nerve cells analyzes the sensory information sent by the reticular formation and makes the appropriate decision.

The area of the cortex available for this decision-making, the use of intelligence, is huge. In birds and reptiles, the surface of the brain is smooth, but in humans it has developed many folds which increase the surface area available for this function considerably. Specific areas of the cerebral cortex control the sensory information from individual parts of the body, and other parts control the specific motor functions.

A number of other structures and systems lie within the cerebral hemispheres.

CRANIAL NERVES AND BLOOD VESSELS

The 12 pairs of cranial nerves leave the underside of the brain and travel to various parts of the body. The carotid arteries carry blood to the circle of Willis. There, the three cerebral arteries, which take blood to the brain, are linked together with two communicating arteries. This arrangement helps to reduce the chances of a stroke if there is a blockage in only one of the cerebral arteries. In such a case blood can often still reach the brain through the other two arteries.

The brain's two cerebral hemispheres viewed from above. The longitudinal fissure separating the two hemispheres is clearly seen, together with the dense network of veins that carry blood around the brain to enable it to function.

The anterior cerebral artery supplies the top and front of the cerebral cortex with blood.

The anterior communicating artery links the two anterior cerebral arteries and forms part of the circle of Willis.

The olfactory nerve (1) runs from the nose to the brain.

The optic chiasma, where the optic nerves (2) cross over on their way to the brain.

The oculomotor nerve (3) helps to control the muscles in and around the eye.

The trochlear nerve (4) runs to the eye and helps to rotate it.

The trigeminal nerve (5) monitors touch, pain and temperature in the face and also controls chewing.

The abducens nerve (6) helps to turn the eyeball to one side.

The facial nerve (7) controls facial expressions, the tear glands and the salivary glands under the tongue. It also relays information from the taste buds in the front of the tongue to the brain.

The middle cerebral artery carries blood to both sides of the cerebral cortex.

The internal carotid artery carries blood from the aorta to the circle of Willis.

The posterior cerebral artery supplies the back and bottom of the cerebral cortex with blood.

The large basilar artery branches off the circle of Willis, and divides into three pairs of arteries that serve the cerebellum and the medulla oblongata.

The auditory nerve (8) relays messages from the inner ear about sound and balance.

The glossopharyngeal nerve (9) controls the salivary glands in the cheeks and the muscles of the pharynx; it also monitors the taste buds at the back of the tongue. The vagus nerve (10) controls swallowing, the heartbeat, breathing and digestion. The accessory nerve (11) controls muscles inside the larynx, and the trapezius and sternomastoid muscles in the back.

The hypoglossal nerve (12) runs to the muscles of the tongue and helps to control articulation and swallowing.

The nerves leaving the motor area of each cerebral cortex cross over to the other side when they reach the medulla in the brain stem *(right)*. All motor nerves cross over, or 'decussate', in this way. Thus, the result of a serious stroke in an artery of the left cerebral hemisphere would be paralysis of the right side of the body.

One, for example, called the extrapyramidal system, is thought to damp down reflex muscle movements. Damage to this system, as a result of Parkinson's Disease, for example, may give rise to uncontrollable tremors and spasms in muscles and limbs.

Another system that runs through the cerebrum represents the closest science has come to defining the seat of the 'soul' or 'personality'. This is the limbic system. It generates a variety of impulses that control behaviour concerned with self-preservation, fighting and feeding; sex, reproduction and parenthood; fear, rage and pleasure; memory and instinct. The limbic system also acts as a control centre for the autonomic nervous system.

The hypothalamus, just in front of and below the thalamus, translates many of the impulses from the limbic system into bodily actions and functions. By controlling the hormonal secretions of the pituitary gland—*see The Endocrine System, p48*—the hypothalamus in turn controls hunger, thirst, body temperature and sexuality. In this way, hormonal control of the body's systems is integrated with the activity of the autonomic nervous system.

Connections
Anaesthesia
Atherosclerosis
Bacteria
Meningitis
Parkinson's disease
Slipped disc —*see Prolapsed intervertebral disc*
Stroke — *see Cerebrovascular accident*
Virus

The digestive system

Why we need food Everyone must eat to maintain the health of his or her body. Protein, carbohydrate and fat are the three basic ingredients of food. These supply energy and heat, and, together with vitamins and minerals, provide the raw materials for the growth and repair of cells and tissues.

Food is chewed and swallowed.

The stomach mixes the food with acid and enzymes.

Juice from the pancreas and bile from the liver digest the large molecules in the food and break them down into smaller units.

Sugars, vitamins, amino acids, fat, water and minerals are all absorbed from the small intestine and ferried to the liver by the blood.

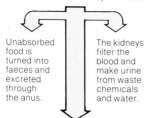

Unabsorbed food is turned into faeces and excreted through the anus.	The kidneys filter the blood and make urine from waste chemicals and water.

The liver controls the use of all the raw materials that are absorbed by the intestine but not immediately used by the tissues. They are released into the blood or stored according to the demands of the body. Sugars are converted into glucose or glycogen, fats are broken down and stored, while surplus amino acids are turned into urea for excretion.

The blood carries the nutrients derived from food to all the cells of the body.

The nutrients diffuse into the cells from the blood. Once there, they are used according to their nutritional value. Sugars are the primary source of energy and heat. Amino acids are used for growth, to repair any damaged tissue or in the production of enzymes.

For the body to stay alive it needs a constant supply of energy. This energy comes from food, which must be broken down into small molecules before it can be absorbed into the body. Only then can it be converted into fuel and used as energy for all the essential functions.

Digestion starts as soon as a mouthful of food is eaten. From the mouth, it passes down a narrow tube about 11 metres (36ft) long, that terminates at the anus. This is the alimentary canal, or the gastro-intestinal tract. It is wider in some places than others—the stomach and the colon, for example—but, nevertheless, forms a continuous tube right through the body. Within the alimentary canal, food is first broken down into smaller particles. These are then absorbed through the wall of the tube, into the bloodstream, to be carried to the cells of the body.

The first phase

The three main constituents of food are carbohydrate (sugar and starch), fat, and protein. The importance of these different types of chemical is discussed in *Metabolism, p44*, while the digestion and absorption of vitamins and minerals, also essential for life, is described in *Diet, p322*. Before carbohydrates, fats and proteins can enter the bloodstream and be used by the body, they must be broken down into their simplest forms—a process that starts in the mouth. Here the salivary glands begin to secrete a fluid called saliva as soon as food is seen, smelt, or even thought of. The saliva lubricates the food and the mouth, making it easier to swallow. It also contains an enzyme, or biological catalyst (a substance helping a chemical reaction to take place) called ptyalin, or salivary amylase, that starts the breakdown of starches. The body produces as much as 2 litres (3.5pts) of saliva each day, but only a little of this is actually used, because the enzyme ceases to act as soon as the food is swallowed.

While the saliva starts to act, the food is broken down into a number of small lumps by the grinding and cutting action of the teeth. It is a fallacy that chewing aids digestion. In fact, its only purpose is to break the food into lumps which can be rolled by the tongue into a bolus—a pellet of food that can easily be swallowed.

Swallowing is the last part of the digestive process that is initiated consciously until the food reaches the end of the digestive tube at the anus. From this point on, every process that food undergoes as it passes along the tube is automatic—it is involuntary and controlled by the parasympathetic nervous system *(p32)*. Even swallowing, once started, is involuntary:

the epiglottis swings across the pharynx to cover the entrance to the airway, and the bolus is forced by the muscles of the throat into a narrow muscular tube called the oesophagus. Here, smooth, or involuntary, muscles contract and relax rhythmically in a wave-like motion called peristalsis, forcing the bolus down the tube. About two seconds later, the pellet of food reaches the stomach.

Breakdown

Just beneath the diaphragm, the digestive tube widens out to form the stomach—a bulbous sac, in the shape of a flattened 'J', which is actually much higher up in the body than most people are aware. The stomach has two functions. Firstly, it stores food, releasing it slowly into the next part of the digestive tube, the intestines, gradually after each meal. If the stomach was not present, small meals would have to be eaten throughout the day, which indeed happens if the organ is removed in a gastrectomy. Secondly, the stomach releases several enzymes that break down food.

The presence of food in the mouth and the action of swallowing stimulates the vagus nerves, producing a reflex action in specialized cells in the stomach wall that secrete hydrochloric acid. The acid is strong, so other cells in the stomach wall secrete mucus that protects the tissues. Acid is also produced in response to anger and stress, and when this state is long-lasting or continual the acid may be too strong for the protective mucus—it eats through the wall of the stomach, forming a gastric ulcer.

The acid has little or no digestive function of its own. Its main action is to kill off bacteria or foreign organisms. But it also converts a precursor of the enzyme pepsin, secreted by the gastric glands in the stomach wall, into its active form. Pepsin is the most important enzyme that the stomach produces, since it splits protein into long chains of its constituent amino acids—*see Metabolism, p44*.

Apart from the release of pepsin, the stomach plays little direct part in the process of digestion, though alcohol and a small amount of water are absorbed into the bloodstream through the stomach wall. But its muscles are constantly active, gently churning and mixing the food into a porridge-like mass called chyme. This is moved slowly towards the pylorus, at the base of the stomach, where a sphincter, or muscular ring, guards the entrance to the small intestine. Only a small portion of chyme is allowed through the pyloric sphincter at a time, and different types of food pass through at different speeds. The

THE DIGESTIVE SYSTEM

Digestion starts as soon as food enters the mouth and continues as it passes through the digestive system. At each stage, food is broken down into its various constituent elements, which can be converted into a form the body can use for energy.

1. The teeth break up food while the tongue mixes in saliva, turns the food into a bolus and pushes it to the throat where it is swallowed.

2. Three pairs of salivary glands release saliva into the mouth when food is present or anticipated.

3. The oesophagus is a muscular tube which contracts in a wave of peristalsis that pushes the bolus from the throat to the stomach.

5. The duodenum releases hormones into the blood when food arrives from the stomach. These stimulate the pancreas to secrete an alkaline juice, rich in enzymes, into the duodenum. The alkali neutralizes any stomach acid and the enzymes break down the food.
Protein is chopped into even shorter amino acid chains by trypsin and chymotrypsin.
Carbohydrates are broken down into small sugar molecules by the enzyme amylase.
Fats are turned into small globules by the detergent action of bile and are then split by the enzyme lipase.

6. The liver secretes a fluid called bile, which helps to break down fats.

7. The gall-bladder, concealed by the liver, stores and concentrates bile. When food enters the duodenum a hormone causes the gall-bladder to contract and release bile into the intestine.

8. The pancreas secretes the hormones insulin and glucagon into the blood, as well as pumping its juice into the duodenum. The two hormones control the level of glucose in the blood, and come into action once glucose has been absorbed by the small intestine.

10. The caecum is a pouch situated at the point where the small intestine meets the colon.

11. The colon, which starts at the caecum, plays no part in digestion. It absorbs considerable quantities of water, however, and electrolytes, such as sodium. Residual faeces are moved into the rectum by the muscular contractions of peristalsis.

4. The stomach mixes the food with gastric juice. The food is churned around, turned into chyme and, little by little, moves into the duodenum over the next four hours after a meal.
Protein The main digestive function of the stomach is to partially break down protein. A protein is a long sequence of amino acids which, by the action of the enzyme pepsin, is chopped into smaller sequences.
Carbohydrate is not digested in the stomach because it is too acidic for the necessary enzymes to work.
Fat Very little fat is broken down by the stomach's juices.

9. The small intestine, divided into the duodenum, jejunum and ileum, is the site of both digestion and absorption. Once food has been broken down by digestion, it is absorbed into the bloodstream. This takes place through millions of tiny villi which line the intestinal wall.
Proteins are absorbed from the intestine in the form of amino acids, their constituent units. Cells needing proteins for growth or repair remove the necessary amino acids from the blood. The surplus is converted into urea by the liver.
Carbohydrates are absorbed as glucose, fructose and galactose. Glucose is used directly by all cells for energy, while fructose and galactose are converted to glucose in the liver.
Fat is absorbed as droplets by lymph vessels called lacteals in the villi. These carry fat to the thoracic duct of the lymphatic system which feeds it into the large vein above the heart. It is then stored in the body.

12. The rectum, the second part of the large intestine, is usually empty. As it fills with faeces, a reflex triggers its muscles to contract and expel them through the anus.

carbohydrate foods may leave the stomach after two hours, while protein takes three hours, and fat as long as four hours. This control is achieved by a chemical called enterogastrone, secreted by the stomach and small intestine when protein or fat is detected in the chyme. It inhibits the nerves that control the actions of the stomach, and so delays the progress of the appropriate foods through it.

Digestion
After leaving the stomach, chyme passes into the duodenum—the part of the alimentary canal where the major part of digestion and absorption take place. The duodenum is the first part of the small intestine—the other parts being the jejunum and ileum.

To start with, specialized cells in the wall of the duodenum analyze the composition of the chyme, and stimulate the secretion of chemicals that will process it. The first of these to be produced is a group of enzymes known collectively as erepsin, which break proteins down further into their constituent amino acids. A hormone called enterokinase is also released, which triggers the preparatory secretion of the protein-splitting enzyme trypsin by the pancreas.

The presence of acid in the duodenum triggers the release of another hormone called secretin, which stimulates the pancreas to produce a secretion rich in the alkali sodium bicarbonate, which neutralizes the acid. In cases of overacidity, there may not be enough alkali to neutralize the ▷

acid, and a duodenal ulcer may form. Food also stimulates the release of yet another hormone, pancreozymin, which stimulates the secretion of a pancreatic juice that is rich in enzymes—amylase, maltase and lipase. Amylase and maltase break carbohydrates down to the simple sugars, called monosaccharides, from which they are constructed.

Fats in the chyme also cause a hormonal response. A chemical called cholecystokinin is released into the blood stream. When it reaches the gall bladder, bile, a thick, greenish alkaline liquid produced by the liver, is forced down the bile duct and into the duodenum. With the help of lipase, bile splits fats into tiny particles called micelles, in the same way as detergent breaks up a scummy layer of fat in a washing-up bowl.

Absorption

The process of digestion continues in the two parts of the small intestine that follow the duodenum—the jejunum and ileum. But following the completion of digestion,

the process of breaking down foods to their constituent parts, another complicated process—absorption—takes place. The constituents cross the intestinal wall and enter the transport system of the body.

Absorption takes place through million upon million of tiny projections of the intestinal wall, called villi, which themselves are covered with yet smaller projections called microvilli. The small intestine is around 3 metres (10ft) long, but the folds of the intestinal wall, the villi and the microvilli increase the surface area available for absorption to as much as 40 square metres (430sq ft)—the size of a large room.

Each villus contains a network of arteries and veins and a branch of the lymph system called a lacteal. The blood vessels are part of the portal circulation, which links the intestines and the liver—*see Metabolism, p45*. Small molecules of sugar and amino acids cross the wall of the villi and enter the portal blood vessels, to be carried to the liver, while tiny globules of fat enter the lacteals.

As well as the fluid that is drunk, the intestine has to cope with the large amount of water produced as part of the digestive secretions. Almost 5 litres (8.8pts) of these secretions are produced by the glands and organs of the digestive tract, and all but 500ml (1pt) are reabsorbed by the small intestine. The balance of fluid in the body is maintained by the kidneys which, in the healthy body, filter the blood and excrete surplus fluid as urine.

The large intestine

The residue of food that has been digested but not absorbed is forced through the small intestine by the impetus of peristalsis until it leaves the ileum by the ileo-caecal valve and enters the large intestine. Just below this valve is the blind sac of the caecum, and the short, worm-like appendix. This is an evolutionary relic from the time when humans ate grass. It has no useful function today, but is prone to an infection called appendicitis.

Around 400g (14oz) of food residue passes into the caecum every 24 hours. As more water is reabsorbed during the passage through the colon, the bulk of this surplus is reduced considerably. To some extent, however, this is compensated by the addition of dead cells from the lining of the intestines, cholesterol, mucus, the broken down products of dead blood cells and dead bacteria. These bacteria make up nearly half the weight of the faeces, and are beneficial, because the toxins they produce help to defend the body against other harmful organisms. They also play a part in the synthesis of the vitamins the body utilizes.

Excretion

The quantity of faeces that reaches the rectum, at the end of the large intestine, depends very much on the type of food that is eaten. A diet high in fibre—*see Diet, p322*—has considerably more bulk than a

The wall of the small intestine contains two layers of smooth muscle *(below)*. Its inner surface is folded, to give a greater surface area for the absorption of food. The muscles contract rhythmically, churning up food and pushing it towards the large intestine. On the folds *(right)*, magnified 240 times, are millions of tiny projections called villi. Each villus has blood and lymph vessels *(below right)* which absorb the carbohydrate, protein and fat in the food.

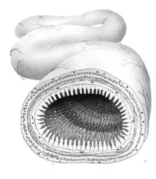

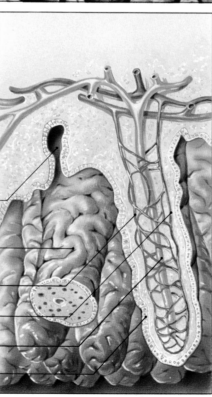

Glands in the wall of the villi secrete 2 litres of salty mucus each day to protect the tissues from stomach acid.

Each villus sticks out into the intestine, bringing blood and lymph as close as possible to the food.

Arterioles carry blood from the arteries to the villi.

Venules carry nutrient-rich blood from the villi to the portal vein.

The lacteals contain lymph, which absorbs the fat from food.

The thin lining of each villus is renewed every 36 hours.

HOW THE KIDNEYS WORK

The kidneys lie at the back of the abdomen, just below the diaphragm and on either side of the spine. Each kidney, 1, is about 11cm (4.4in) long and weighs around 140gm (5oz). It is supplied with blood from the aorta, 2, through the renal artery, 3. The blood from each kidney drains into the inferior vena cava, 4, through one of the two renal veins, 5. The urine from each kidney flows down a ureter, 6, into the bladder, 7. There are around a million nephrons inside the kidney, and each nephron has two parts — a glomerulus, in which arterial blood is filtered, and a convoluted tubule, in which urine collects.

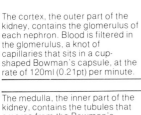

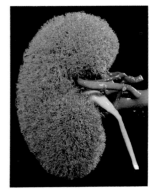

The kidney receives its blood from the renal artery *(red)*, drains it into the renal vein *(blue)* and passes urine into the ureter *(yellow)* as shown in this cast *(above)*.

The cortex, the outer part of the kidney, contains the glomerulus of each nephron. Blood is filtered in the glomerulus, a knot of capillaries that sits in a cup-shaped Bowman's capsule, at the rate of 120ml (0.21pt) per minute.

The medulla, the inner part of the kidney, contains the tubules that emerge from the Bowman's capsules. Organized into pyramids, these collect and concentrate 1.5 litres (0.88pt) of urine each day. Every minute 1.2 litres (0.7pt) of blood are pumped by the heart through the renal artery into the fine glomerular capillaries.

The renal vein collects the blood after the nephrons have removed water, urea and electrolytes.

The renal pelvis collects the urine from every tubule and funnels it into the ureter.

The ureter, 30cm (12in), long carries the urine to the bladder.

The nephrons of the kidney regulate the volume and acidity of the blood, and filter out waste products. Blood is carried to each kidney by the renal artery, **1**, and enters the glomerulus, **2**, of each nephron *(far left)*. The filtration process starts in the glomerulus, (magnified 240 times) where water, salts, glucose, amino acids and urea are removed from the blood *(near left)*. These enter the proximal tubule, **3**, where all the glucose, amino acids and most of the salts and water are reabsorbed into the blood. The fine tuning of the balance of water, salts and acid in the blood is achieved in the loop of Henle, **4**, the distal tubule, **5** and the collecting duct, **6**. These reabsorb small, but vitally important, quantities of water and salt, and return them to the bloodstream through the renal vein, **7**. The urine passing into the ureter each day is, on average, made up of 1.5 litres (0.88pt) of water, 30gm (1.06oz) urea, and 15gm (0.53oz) of salt, surplus vitamins, electrolytes and breakdown products of metabolism.

normal Western diet, and the food residues move through the intestines much more quickly and easily. Low-fibre diets have been shown conclusively to increase the risk of conditions such as diverticular disease, as well as haemorrhoids, or 'piles'.

When there is a sufficient bulk of faeces in the rectum to distend the intestinal wall, sensors indicate to the brain that defaecation, the expulsion of faeces via the anus, may be necessary. In a newborn baby, the sensors trigger a reflex, involuntary action, so that the anal sphincter, a tight ring of muscle, opens automatically. After a few years, however, this reflex is brought under conscious control, so that normally the sphincter can only be opened deliberately.

Faeces are expelled by contracting the muscles of the abdomen and tightening the diaphragm with the breath held. This reduces the space inside the abdomen, and so increases the air pressure, forcing faeces outwards through the anus.

Normally, when a sensible, high-fibre diet is eaten, defaecation is an easy and painless procedure. When faeces are hard and impacted, however, as in constipation, the increase in the pressure necessary to expel them may cause damage to the tissues, or haemorrhoids.

Connections
Appendicitis
Constipation
Duodenal ulcer
Faeces
Gastrectomy
Gastric ulcer — *see Ulcer*
Haemorrhoids
Vitamins — *see Diet, p322*

Metabolism

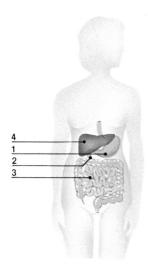

The raw materials needed by the body come from food which is digested in the stomach, **1**, and the duodenum, **2**. Digested food is absorbed through the walls of the small intestine, **3**, and passes into the blood. Broken down into carbohydate, protein and fat, the food is carried by the blood to the liver, **4**, and there processed or stored.

Like any engine, the body needs fuel. The raw ingredients of this fuel are food and air, but they must be processed before they can be used for building tissues, maintaining the body and enabling it to function. The chemical changes that food and air undergo take place on a production line known as metabolism, the chemistry of the body.

The purpose of metabolism

Metabolism is a complex but a vital process. It is the fundamental chemical expression of life itself. The process cannot be seen, but nevertheless takes place in each one of the millions of cells that make up the human body, supplying building blocks for new tissue and repair materials for old. Most important of all, metabolism is the means by which food is converted to energy, essential for maintaining the body, even at rest. We need to breathe and eat to live—without fuel the body cannot function. If the raw ingredients cannot be processed, the tissues, and eventually the whole body, will die.

Fuel for the body

In a car engine, petrol is ignited in the presence of oxygen to provide energy. The human body runs on a slightly different type of fuel. Petrol is made up of tiny particles, or atoms, of carbon and hydrogen—so is food, though it also contains oxygen. In the first stage of the metabolic process, food is broken down into easily manageable units, or molecules, of these constituents and carried by the blood to the sites of energy production throughout the body.

In the process of digestion *(p40)*, food is broken down and sorted into its three main constituents—carbohydrates, proteins and fats. Each of these constituents is made up of a different group of chemicals with certain basic similarities: they all contain atoms of carbon, hydrogen and oxygen. After digestion, each group of chemicals enters the bloodstream in a different form.

All carbohydrates pass through the wall of the bowel and enter the circulation through blood vessels called the portal veins in the form of simple sugars, of which glucose is the most common. Each unit, or molecule, of glucose contains four atoms of carbon, five of oxygen and ten of hydrogen.

Proteins are complex chemicals, each composed of different combinations of smaller chemicals called amino acids. There are about 20 different amino acids, and they each contain atoms of nitrogen as well as carbon, hydrogen and oxygen. Like carbohydrates, proteins enter the circula-

tion through the portal blood vessels in their simplified form, in this case as amino acids.

Fats enter the circulation in a different way. They are absorbed into the lymphatic system through the villi, the tiny projections of the wall of the gut, and pass through the lymph vessels into the main veins of the body. Fats differ from carbohydrates and proteins in that they are not at first broken down into their components within the blood, but carried as minute globules. After a fatty meal, the blood is actually clouded by millions of tiny, milky fat globules.

Chemical soup

The blood can be thought of as a kind of chemical soup in which carbon, hydrogen and oxygen atoms—all the basic requirements for the release of energy—are transported round the body in different forms. The main supply of oxygen is carried in the red blood cells, and comes from the air that is breathed into the lungs—*see Respiration, p28*. Carbon, hydrogen and more oxygen, which comes from carbohydrate molecules, are carried in the form of glucose; from fat as globules that are broken down to chemicals called glycerol and fatty acids; and from protein (with the addition of nitrogen) as amino acids.

As with any manufacturing process, the levels of these basic ingredients are controlled. A control system is especially important in the human body, because unrestricted quantities of glucose can have harmful effects, as in the case of diabetes. The level of glucose in the blood is controlled by the liver, under the direction of the two controlling hormones insulin and glycogen.

The portal vessels carry glucose and amino acids directly to the liver. Here the level of glucose in the blood is assessed, and any surplus is changed to the chemical glycogen, a form of glucose that can be stored in the muscles and the liver until it is required. Controlled amounts of glucose and a mass of amino acids then join the main circulatory systems, so that with the fats already present the basic components of food can be carried to the cells.

The smallest living unit

Every tissue and organ of the body is made up of cells, the smallest independent units of life. Cells vary in size, but all are microscopically small—to be seen they must be magnified between 500 and 3,500 times. Nevertheless, blood flows to and around each cell of the body, carrying amino acids, fats and glucose. It also carries oxygen, the other main requirement for the release of energy, because it is

THE LIVER AND METABOLISM

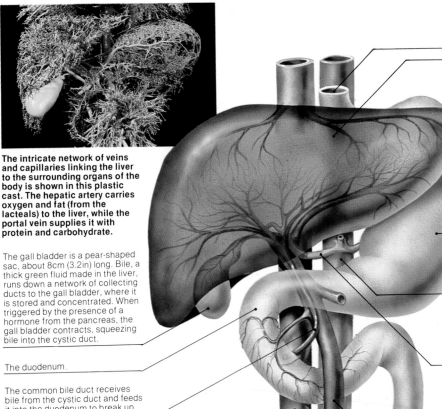

The intricate network of veins and capillaries linking the liver to the surrounding organs of the body is shown in this plastic cast. The hepatic artery carries oxygen and fat (from the lacteals) to the liver, while the portal vein supplies it with protein and carbohydrate.

The gall bladder is a pear-shaped sac, about 8cm (3.2in) long. Bile, a thick green fluid made in the liver, runs down a network of collecting ducts to the gall bladder, where it is stored and concentrated. When triggered by the presence of a hormone from the pancreas, the gall bladder contracts, squeezing bile into the cystic duct.

The duodenum.

The common bile duct receives bile from the cystic duct and feeds it into the duodenum to break up globules of fat.

The inferior vena cava receives blood from the hepatic vein and takes it to the heart.

The oesophagus passes food to the stomach by waves of peristalsis.

The liver has four lobes, organised into many tiny lobules, which contain about half a litre of blood. In the centre of each hexagonally-shaped lobule there is a central vein, around which the liver cells are arranged. This vein collects the products of the cells' metabolism and takes them to the hepatic vein. This relays them to the heart.

The stomach.

The aorta brings oxygenated blood direct from the heart and feeds it into the hepatic artery.

The hepatic artery branches off the aorta to supply the liver cells with blood rich in oxygen and digested fat. This arterial blood makes up a fifth of the liver's total blood supply.

The portal vein collects blood from the stomach, pancreas, spleen, small intestine and colon. This blood, which represents four-fifths of the liver's blood supply, contains all the carbohydrates and protein absorbed by the digestive system.

What the liver does The liver is the key to the metabolism of the body. It controls more than 500 reactions, in which chemicals are manufactured, stored, broken down, recycled or converted to other chemicals. The eight main functions of the liver are listed here.
1. The liver stores glucose in the form of glycogen. The glycogen is broken down to glucose when the level of sugar in the blood falls, or when there is an increased demand for energy.
2. The liver dismantles surplus amino acids, the constituents of protein, releasing toxic ammonia, which it then turns to urea, a constituent of urine.
3. The liver manufactures bile salts, which are essential for the breakdown of fats and the absorption of vitamin K from the intestine.
4. When a diet is low in energy-giving carbohydrate, the liver turns fat into ketone bodies. The cells of the body use these as a source of energy and heat.
5. The liver makes cholesterol. This chemical plays an important part in the manufacture of bile salts and of steroid hormones, such as cortisol and progesterone, elsewhere in the body.
6. Harmful chemicals and drugs, such as barbiturates and alcohol, are broken down and detoxified by the liver. Some of the body's own chemicals, such as adrenaline, are also dismantled, but then recycled.
7. The liver stores minerals, such as iron and copper, and the vitamins A, B12 and D to satisfy the body's needs for over a year.
8. The liver forms new red blood cells, destroys old red cells and removes their breakdown products from the blood. It also makes most of the proteins in blood plasma. It produces fibrinogen and prothrombin, the first two blood-clotting factors.

The hepatic artery supplies the liver with newly-oxygenated blood which contains fat globules. The liver processes these into glycerol and fatty acids.

The portal vein supplies the liver with blood which is rich in nutrients. Proteins, in the form of amino acids, and carbohydrates, such as glucose, are delivered to the liver for storage, breakdown or redistribution.

The bile, which the liver secretes , is carried to the gall bladder and passed to the duodenum.

Fats, amino acids and glucose leave the liver and pass through the hepatic vein to enter the inferior vena cava. They are then taken to the heart, which pumps them around the whole body, where the glucose and amino acids are used as fuel and the fats are stored. Glucose and fats, like fuel oil, are composed of three types of atom — carbon, hydrogen and oxygen. They differ only in the way in which the atoms are linked together. Amino acids, in addition to carbon, hydrogen and oxygen, also contain at least one atom of nitrogen. Because of this essential similarity, enzymes in the liver are able to convert one food product to another.

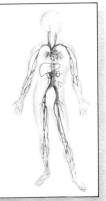

HOW A CELL PRODUCES ENERGY

Every cell in the body needs energy to carry out its functions and to generate sufficient heat to keep the body at a temperature of 37°C (98.6°F). This is the optimum temperature for many of the chemical reactions that take place inside the cells. The fuel for this energy comes from the breakdown products of food — glucose, fat and amino acids. Glucose is the primary source of energy, though fat can also be used. Amino acids, however, are so important for growth and repair of tissues that they are only used for energy-production in an emergency.

Fat The body keeps a store of fat in the adipose tissue which lies below the skin and in the abdomen. When there is not enough glucose to meet the body's demands for energy and heat, fat is sent to the liver where it is broken down to glycerol and fatty acids. The carbon and hydrogen atoms of the fatty acids are burned in the body's cells, producing carbon dioxide and water. The combustion of 1gm (0.035oz) of fat generates 9 calories of heat and energy, more than twice that generated by carbohydrate.

Glucose The blood normally contains 5gm (0.18oz) of glucose, but this level rises sharply after a meal high in carbohydrates. The atoms of carbon and hydrogen of which glucose is made are burned up in the cells of the body, producing heat and energy. Any surplus glucose is either stored in the muscles and liver as glycogen, or converted to fat by the liver and stored in fatty tissue. When the demand for energy increases, the stores of glycogen and, eventually, of fat are mobilized so that more fuel can be pumped to the cells.

Protein All proteins are composed of varying combinations of about 20 amino acids. These are so important for the repair and growth of tissues that they are used as fuel only as a last resort — in starvation, for example. When no food is eaten, the body starts to consume itself. The liver's store of glucose is depleted within 24 hours. As fat is mobilized from its stores around the body, the liver begins to convert its own proteins into glucose. The combustion of 1gm (0.035oz) of this protein generates 4 calories of heat and energy.

The cell is a complex and sophisticated mechanism which needs food and water to live. It contains a number of structures suspended in a water solution, each of which has a specific role.

A membrane of protein and fat surrounds each cell and controls the movement of chemicals in and out of it. Some hormones work by changing the permeability of this membrane in such a way that it becomes easier for glucose to enter the cell.

The Golgi apparatus is a series of flattened sacs and vesicles which store and release protein. Cells which mass-produce complex proteins, such as hormones like insulin, have a large and extensive Golgi apparatus.

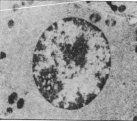

The nucleus of a cell *(above)*, magnified 18,000 times, contains 23 pairs of chromosomes. The countless genes on each chromosome together organize and control all the chemical reactions of the cell.

The mitochondria are where 'cellular respiration' takes place. In this, as in the lungs, oxygen is taken up and carbon dioxide is released. The mitochondria are the powerhouses of the cell. They produce all the energy needed for the cell to perform its role in the body.

The final conversion of food to energy is performed by the cylindrical mitochondria *(right)*, magnified 45,000 times, which generate the energy for the body's cells. Their numbers vary according to the energy needs of an individual cell: liver cells each contain around 200 mitochondria, while sperm have about 20. The ridges inside the mitochondria carry enzymes, specialized proteins that trigger and take part in the final reactions in the breakdown of glucose. These enzymes come into play after other chemicals in the fluid of the cell have broken glucose down to a substance called pyruvic acid. In the mitochondria, this is converted to Acetyl CoA, the raw material for the Krebs cycle *(far right)*. This cycle is the final part of the metabolic process, where energy and heat are released from the food the body absorbs. It is also the point at which the two processes of digestion and respiration link up.

As the carbon and hydrogen

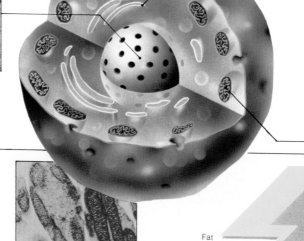

atoms are stripped from Acetyl CoA, heat, carbon dioxide and energy are released. The hydrogen combines with the oxygen, taken into the body in breathing and carried to the cells by the blood, to form water. The carbon dioxide is carried by the blood to the lungs and breathed out.

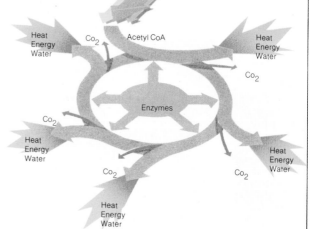

Fat

Glucose

Protein

Heat Energy Water

CO_2

Acetyl CoA

Heat Energy Water

CO_2

CO_2

Enzymes

Heat Energy Water

Heat Energy Water

CO_2

CO_2

Heat Energy Water

inside the cell that energy is made available for the body to function.

The process by which energy is released is often called 'cellular respiration', because it parallels body respiration, in which oxygen is breathed in by the lungs and absorbed, while carbon dioxide is breathed out. Inside the cell, carbon hydrogen and oxygen atoms react together to produce heat, energy, carbon dioxide and water. The release of energy enables the cell to maintain itself and to perform work, while the heat produced by the reaction keeps the body at a constant warm temperature. The waste products, carbon dioxide and water, pass back into the blood and are eventually excreted from the body—carbon dioxide in the air breathed out from the lungs and water in the urine and faeces. This process uses up atoms of carbon, oxygen and hydrogen, so their levels in the blood must be constantly topped up through eating, drinking and breathing.

Inside the cell

Though microscopically tiny, each cell is itself a remarkably complex mechanism. There is a control mechanism (the nucleus), a storage depot (the Golgi Apparatus), and factories (the mitochondria). The release of energy takes place inside the mitochondria.

All the complex chemicals to which food has been reduced pass through the wall of the cell into another soup of chemicals called the cytoplasm. Here they are further simplified to one chemical structure, still made up of carbon, hydrogen and oxygen. This chemical, called acetyl coenzyme A, may be stored until needed, or used directly in the mitochondria as the starting point for the cycle of reactions that produce energy.

The rate at which the energy cycle works is carefully controlled by the brain, acting through the glands of the endocrine system (p48). When extra energy is required, for physical work, or at times of stress, the brain stimulates some of the glands to produce special hormones, or chemical messengers, which act on the cells in the appropriate areas—the legs, for example, when someone is running—to increase energy production.

A certain amount of energy is being used all the time, just to keep the body alive. The heart beats continuously and the muscles of the diaphragm and chest contract to make each breath possible. Both of these functions require energy. The rate at which energy is used for body maintenance varies from person to person, which is why some people can eat large amounts of food without becoming fat, while others put on weight very easily. Generally, however, a woman needs 37 calories per square metre of skin to maintain her body each hour, and a man needs 40 calories per square metre per hour. (As a guide, a 5ft 6in, nine stone woman has 1.7sq metres of skin; a 5ft 11in, 11 stone man has 1.88 sq metres). This rate, called the basal metabolic rate, can be tested and is often a useful indication of diseases of the metabolism or glands.

The cell is like a factory, producing energy and heat from raw materials, creating by-products and making waste. By-products, such as water, and raw materials, such as glucose, are distributed around the body by the blood. The waste products, such as urea from the liver cells and carbon dioxide from all cells, are collected by the blood and removed from the body by the lungs or kidneys.

The blood collects the waste products, by-products and excess raw materials from the cell and delivers them to the liver, lungs or kidneys.

The liver, 1, plays an important part in the removal of waste products from the body. Surplus amino acids, for example, are broken down to form a chemical called urea. The blood carries all these waste products to the kidney, 2, where they are excreted in the urine. As well as urea, the urine contains carbon dioxide in the form of bicarbonate, salt, water and traces of all the substances found in the blood. The yellow colour of urine is brought about by urochrome, a breakdown product of the pigments found in bile. The urine flows down the ureter from each kidney, enters the bladder, 3, and is removed from the body.

Most of the carbon dioxide in the blood is dissolved in the plasma, but some is combined with haemoglobin in the red cells. The blood that reaches the lungs (above) contains a large amount of carbon dioxide, of which only a small amount is removed when breathing out. However, this quantity is the same as that released by the cells in the metabolism of glucose, so the blood level of carbon dioxide remains constant.

Growth and stores

Not all the food products circulating in the blood are used in the release of energy. Glucose, from carbohydrates, is the primary source of energy, though a proportion of both fats and protein are also used. Protein, in the form of amino acids, is also used to build new tissue and to repair old tissues. This is the reason why a high protein diet is especially important for mothers during pregnancy, and for growing children.

Fats that are not required for energy production are stored in special cells in the fatty, or adipose, tissues of the body, while excess glucose is turned into fat and stored in the same way. If the body's energy requirements are more than can be satisfied by the food products in the blood, stored fat is broken down and released for use. A fat person, therefore, will lose weight if he reduces his intake of food, and so the level of food products in the blood.

Connections
Diabetes
Metabolic disorders

The endocrine system

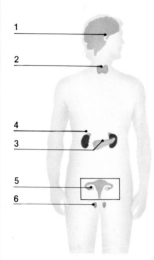

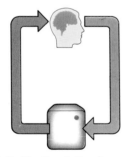

The endocrine glands are the major glands of the body, so-called because they secrete hormones and release them into the blood. They are the pituitary, **1**, the thyroid and parathyroid, **2**, the pancreas, **3**, the adrenals, **4**, the female ovaries, **5**, and the male testes, **6**.

The workings of the human body depend on a whole range of delicate checks and balances. The levels of different chemicals, the fluid volume and the tension of muscles all depend on the body's varying needs at different times and under different circumstances. The requirements of a growing child, for example, are not the same as those of a fully developed adult. The endocrine system detects varying requirements and adjusts the fine-tuning of the body.

The endocrine system is made up of groups of specialized cells that secrete chemicals directly into the bloodstream. These are called the endocrine glands, and consist of the pituitary, the thyroid, the parathyroids, the gonads (ovaries or testes), the adrenal glands, the pancreas, and, in pregnant women, the placenta.

The chemical messengers secreted by the endocrine glands are called hormones, from a Greek word meaning 'to excite'. They link with proteins in the plasma of the blood, and are carried round the body until they reach their target, which may be another gland, a muscle or an organ. There, hormones 'excite' or stimulate the cells of the tissue to action. To ensure that hormone production by the glands, and the action of the target cells, does not continue indefinitely, the endocrine system itself has controls. In some cases, the action triggered by one hormone itself causes the release of another, opposing, hormone; in others a high level of the hormone in the blood automatically inhibits further production of that chemical.

The pituitary

All of the glands of the endocrine system are essential, but none are so important, or secrete so many hormones, as the pituitary gland. This small, reddish-grey bundle of cells is suspended from the base of the skull just behind the cavity of the nose, and secretes eight hormones. It is divided into two parts: the posterior pituitary gland, sometimes called the neurohypophysis, and the anterior pituitary gland, called the adenohypophysis.

The posterior pituitary produces two hormones—the antidiuretic hormone (called ADH, adiuretin or vasopressin) and oxytocin. Both ADH and oxytocin have a very similar chemical structure, and their functions overlap to some extent.

ADH maintains the volume of the plasma, the fluid base of the blood, by increasing the rate at which the kidneys draw water back into the blood from the half-formed urine. When the production of ADH is suppressed, by a disease such as diabetes insipidus, or by the blood alcohol level of a heavy drinker, the rate at which water is reabsorbed from the kidneys slows down. As a result, large quantities of dilute urine are produced. When blood is lost through a serious wound, however, the production of ADH increases: more

THE ROLE OF THE PITUITARY GLAND

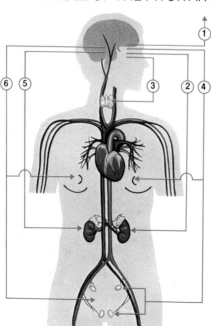

Controlling the pituitary flow
The pituitary gland controls the activity of the other glands by way of a feedback mechanism (above). The pituitary and hypothalamus monitor the blood constantly and check that the hormones of the body are present in sufficient quantities. If one hormone is lacking, the pituitary releases the relevant stimulating hormone, **1**. This travels through the blood to the appropriate gland, **2**, where more of the hormone required is made. The raised level of hormone then feeds back, **3**, to the hypothalamus and pituitary, and production of the stimulating hormone ceases.

The hormones of the pituitary gland regulate the activity of other endocrine glands. This is achieved by a feedback mechanism that involves the hypothalamus in the brain, to which the pituitary is joined. The hypothalamus secretes 'releasing factors' into the blood, which stimulate the pituitary to release its hormones. In addition the brain can affect the output of the pituitary via the hypothalamus as a result of changes of mood, tension and anxiety. These can be caused by the action of blood hormones on the brain through the hypothalamus, as in premenstrual tension, for example.

The anterior pituitary secretes six hormones. Growth hormone (GH), **1**, stimulates the growth of the body's cells. Adrenocorticotrophic hormone (ACTH), **2**, controls the production of steroids by the adrenal glands. Thyrotrophic hormone (TH), **3**, controls the thyroid gland. Three gonadotrophic hormones (GTH), **4**, control the female reproductive organs and the breasts: the follicle stimulating hormone ripens the ovum, the luteinizing hormone controls the corpus luteum, and prolactin stimulates the production of milk by the mammary glands. The posterior pituitary gland secretes two hormones: the antidiuretic hormone (ADH), **5**, controls the reabsorption of water by the kidney, and oxytocin (O), **6**, contracts the uterine muscles and causes the nipples to eject milk.

water is reabsorbed, so that the blood volume can be maintained.

Oxytocin, the second hormone released by the posterior pituitary, is crucial during childbirth *(p60)*. It triggers the contractions of the uterus which force the baby down the birth-canal during labour, and later causes the ejection of milk from the breast during feeding. Oxytocin is sometimes given to induce labour, and also used in the treatment of women who have difficulty in breast-feeding. It is thought that oxytocin may also be active during the muscle contractions of the female orgasm.

Both ADH and oxytocin are produced in response to a demand signalled by nerve sensors and acted on by the brain. Some scientists think that they are actually secreted by nerve fibres running to the gland and just stored in the gland itself.

The growth hormone

The hormones produced by the anterior part of the pituitary gland are called trophic, from the Greek word meaning 'nourishment', because they initiate and regulate growth. All are released under the control of the hypothalamus, a part of the brain that, in response to signals from the nervous system, sends chemical 'releasing-factors' to the pituitary. There is one releasing factor for each hormone. Exactly the right amount of hormone is produced, because its presence in the blood inhibits the production of further releasing factor.

The anterior pituitary secretes six hormones. One of the most important of these is HGH, the human growth hormone. This chemical, released in spurts four times every day, controls the rate of growth of the body. Too little HGH during childhood can cause dwarfism, or stunted growth, while too much can make the child a giant. Overactivity of the gland in later life can cause acromegaly, where the hands, head and feet become huge.

Controlling the metabolism

Shaped like a butterfly, the thyroid gland sits directly over the wind-pipe, just below the Adam's apple. Its main function is the control of the metabolic rate *(p44)*, the speed at which oxygen and food-products are burnt up to produce energy.

When energy is required, during growth, exercise or stress, the hypothalamus stimulates the pituitary gland to produce thyroid stimulating hormone (TSH). In response, the thyroid gland produces two hormones, thyroxine and triiodothyronine. The latter is a less common, but more active, version of the former. Both are formed from compounds of iodine, obtained from food. The hormones are carried to the cells in the blood,

THE THYROID GLAND

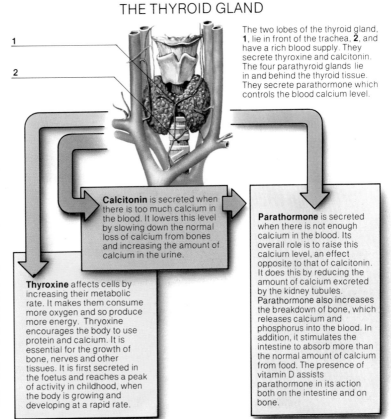

The two lobes of the thyroid gland, **1**, lie in front of the trachea, **2**, and have a rich blood supply. They secrete thyroxine and calcitonin. The four parathyroid glands lie in and behind the thyroid tissue. They secrete parathormone which controls the blood calcium level.

Calcitonin is secreted when there is too much calcium in the blood. It lowers this level by slowing down the normal loss of calcium from bones and increasing the amount of calcium in the urine.

Thyroxine affects cells by increasing their metabolic rate. It makes them consume more oxygen and so produce more energy. Thryoxine encourages the body to use protein and calcium. It is essential for the growth of bone, nerves and other tissues. It is first secreted in the foetus and reaches a peak of activity in childhood, when the body is growing and developing at a rapid rate.

Parathormone is secreted when there is not enough calcium in the blood. Its overall role is to raise this calcium level, an effect opposite to that of calcitonin. It does this by reducing the amount of calcium excreted by the kidney tubules. Parathormone also increases the breakdown of bone, which releases calcium and phosphorus into the blood. In addition, it stimulates the intestine to absorb more than the normal amount of calcium from food. The presence of vitamin D assists parathormone in its action both on the intestine and on bone.

where they increase energy production by speeding up the enzyme reactions of the energy cycle—*see Metabolism, p44.*

Thyroxine is essential for normal development in children, and for normal life in adults, but only in the quantities that the body requires. A deficiency of the hormone in children may lead to cretinism, and in adults to hypothyroidism, or myxoedema. An overactivity of the gland can cause hyperthyroidism, or thyrotoxicosis.

The thyroid also secretes calcitonin, which helps balance parathyroid secretions.

Dissolving bone

The parathyroid glands are four small ovals of endocrine tissue which secrete parathormone, or PTH. This hormone maintains the level of calcium in the blood. This function is essential, because calcium regulates the excitability of the nerves—that is, the ease with which they respond to stimulation. A low level of calcium in the blood can cause nervous and muscular spasms, called tetany, which can be very severe.

Parathormone acts in several ways. It slows down the digestive process *(p40)*, so ▷

that more calcium is absorbed by the body, and less excreted; at the same time, it depresses the activity of the osteoblasts, the cells that form bone by using up blood calcium. Most important of all, it adjusts the action of the kidney, to produce a demand for calcium in the blood. The only store of calcium in the body is bone, so minute amounts of the mineral dissolve from bone into the blood. An over-production of parathormone, however, has serious consequences. In this condition, called hyperparathyroidism, the skeleton literally dissolves into the blood, and is passed out of the body in urine. In normal circumstances, though, the hormone calcitonin, produced by the thyroid gland, counters the action of parathormone by suppressing the dissolution of bone.

Fight or flight

There are two adrenal glands, one just above and in front of each kidney. Each gland is made up of two parts that function independently—the adrenal cortex and the adrenal medulla.

The medulla, or centre, of each adrenal gland makes two vital hormones, adrenaline and noradrenaline (sometimes called by their American names, epinephrine and norepinephrine). Both are produced within a fraction of a second when the brain recognizes danger. Fibres of the sympathetic nervous system (p32), the part of the nervous system that acts independently of the conscious mind, stimulate the adrenal medulla in situations of fear, rage, stress and expectancy; also when the blood pressure is low, or the blood level of sugar or oxygen is low.

The result is the classic 'flight or fight'

reaction. The body is poised for any eventuality: the blood vessels supplying non-essential parts of the body such as the skin and digestive system are narrowed, or vasoconstricted, so that as much oxygen-laden blood as possible is available for the use of the vital organs and muscles. The blood vessels supplying these areas widen, or vasodilate, for the same purpose. The pupils of the eyes dilate to improve vision, and the hairs of the body stand on end to improve physical awareness. The sphincters of the anus and bladder contract, so that complete attention can be given to the task ahead. The muscles of the bronchioles relax, to increase the flow of oxygen to the blood.

Adrenaline also converts glycogen—the form in which glucose is stored in the liver—back to the original glucose. This is the body's primary source of energy, and is carried by the blood to the tissues to provide it—*see Metabolism, p44*. Noradrenaline acts as the chemical transmitter of the sympathetic nervous system.

One property of adrenaline is often used in medicine. An injection of this hormone, often given with a local anaesthetic, constricts the blood vessels near a wound, reducing the loss of blood.

Blood volume

The outer part of each adrenal gland, called the cortex, produces three groups of hormones. One group, the sex hormones androgen, oestrogen and progesterone, is produced in small but significant quantities. Much larger amounts of these hormones, however, are produced by the sex glands—*see Sex and Reproduction, p54*.

The first group of hormones produced by the adrenal medulla are called miner-

THE ROLE OF THE ADRENAL GLANDS

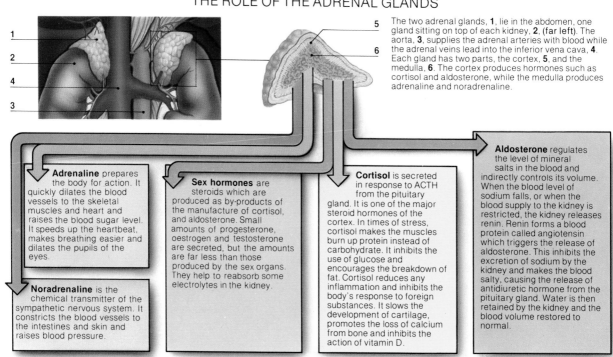

The two adrenal glands, **1**, lie in the abdomen, one gland sitting on top of each kidney, **2**, (far left). The aorta, **3**, supplies the adrenal arteries with blood while the adrenal veins lead into the inferior vena cava, **4**. Each gland has two parts, the cortex, **5**, and the medulla, **6**. The cortex produces hormones such as cortisol and aldosterone, while the medulla produces adrenaline and noradrenaline.

Adrenaline prepares the body for action. It quickly dilates the blood vessels to the skeletal muscles and heart and raises the blood sugar level. It speeds up the heartbeat, makes breathing easier and dilates the pupils of the eyes.

Noradrenaline is the chemical transmitter of the sympathetic nervous system. It constricts the blood vessels to the intestines and skin and raises blood pressure.

Sex hormones are steroids which are produced as by-products of the manufacture of cortisol, and aldosterone. Small amounts of progesterone, oestrogen and testosterone are secreted, but the amounts are far less than those produced by the sex organs. They help to reabsorb some electrolytes in the kidney.

Cortisol is secreted in response to ACTH from the pituitary gland. It is one of the major steroid hormones of the cortex. In times of stress, cortisol makes the muscles burn up protein instead of carbohydrate. It inhibits the use of glucose and encourages the breakdown of fat. Cortisol reduces any inflammation and inhibits the body's response to foreign substances. It slows the development of cartilage, promotes the loss of calcium from bone and inhibits the action of vitamin D.

Aldosterone regulates the level of mineral salts in the blood and indirectly controls its volume. When the blood level of sodium falls, or when the blood supply to the kidney is restricted, the kidney releases renin. Renin forms a blood protein called angiotensin which triggers the release of aldosterone. This inhibits the excretion of sodium by the kidney and makes the blood salty, causing the release of antidiuretic hormone from the pituitary gland. Water is then retained by the kidney and the blood volume restored to normal.

alocorticoids. The most important is aldosterone, but all play a part in the regulation of the volume of the blood. When this decreases, following the loss of blood from a wound, for example, the kidney senses the fall in pressure and releases a chemical called renin into the blood. Renin reacts with proteins in the blood plasma, forming angiotensin.

The adrenal medulla is stimulated by angiotensin to produce aldosterone, which completes the control cycle by acting on the kidneys. The hormone fine-tunes the delicate systems of the kidney so that the amount of sodium reabsorbed from the blood is increased—it also reduces the salt content of sweat. The increased salt content of the blood is sensed by the pituitary gland, and the hormone ADH produced, which increases the amount of water in the circulation.

The second group of hormones produced by the adrenal medulla is called the glucocorticoids, of which the most important is cortisol, sometimes called hydrocortisone. This hormone, whose release is triggered by the production of ACTH by the pituitary gland, has a number of functions. It is an anti-inflammatory agent, reducing inflammation of the tissues, and also reduces the body's response to an allergen, a foreign substance to which the body is sensitive. Preparations based on cortisol are often used to treat conditions that cause inflammation, such as the various types of arthritis.

Cortisol also mobilizes all the body's food stores in times of starvation, or physical or mental stress. It prevents the storage of glucose as glycogen, and breaks down stored fat; cortisol also reduces the protein that forms the tissue of the body to its amino acid components, and converts them to glucose—*see Metabolism, p44*. If there is an excess of cortisol in the blood, as the result of a tumour of the adrenal gland, for example, and the body does not need extra heat and energy, the high level of glucose in the blood may cause the disease diabetes mellitus. Normally, however, the level of cortisol in the blood is monitored and regulated by the hypothalamus and the pituitary gland.

The islets of the pancreas

The blood glucose level is also regulated by another hormone, insulin. This chemical is produced by the pancreas, a gland that secretes digestive enzymes into the intestine, and also passes hormones into the body's bloodstream from small islet cells, called the 'islets of Langerhans' after their discoverer.

Insulin controls the level of the sugar glucose in the blood by making it easier for the chemical to enter the cells. When the level of glucose rises after a meal—*see Metabolism, p44*—insulin either helps to pass it into the cells, if energy is required, or into storage in the liver, if it is not. Insulin also prevents the conversion of glycogen, the storage form of sugar, back to glucose, and slows down the release of

WHAT THE PANCREAS DOES

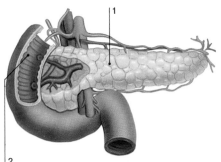

The pancreas, **1**, lies below the stomach and produces four hormones. When food enters the duodenum, **2**, it releases secretin and cholecystikinin into the blood. Specialized cells called the islets of Langerhans secrete insulin and glucagon when the blood sugar level changes. These hormones play crucial and complementary roles in the mobilization and disposal of glucose *(below)*.

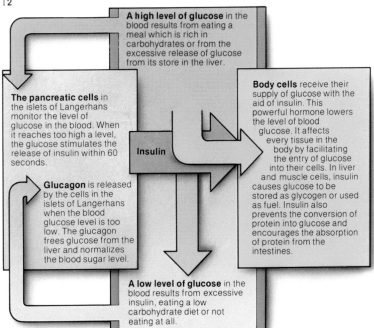

A high level of glucose in the blood results from eating a meal which is rich in carbohydrates or from the excessive release of glucose from its store in the liver.

The pancreatic cells in the islets of Langerhans monitor the level of glucose in the blood. When it reaches too high a level, the glucose stimulates the release of insulin within 60 seconds.

Insulin

Body cells receive their supply of glucose with the aid of insulin. This powerful hormone lowers the level of blood glucose. It affects every tissue in the body by facilitating the entry of glucose into their cells. In liver and muscle cells, insulin causes glucose to be stored as glycogen or used as fuel. Insulin also prevents the conversion of protein into glucose and encourages the absorption of protein from the intestines.

Glucagon is released by the cells in the islets of Langerhans when the blood glucose level is too low. The glucagon frees glucose from the liver and normalizes the blood sugar level.

A low level of glucose in the blood results from excessive insulin, eating a low carbohydrate diet or not eating at all.

other foods from stores in the tissues. If the pancreas produces too little of the hormone, the blood glucose level rises, causing diabetes mellitus. Too much insulin causes a low blood sugar level, which may lead to unconsciousness and hypoglycaemic coma.

Another hormone, called glucagon, is produced by the islets of Langerhans. Glucagon counters the action of insulin by increasing the level of blood sugar. It converts glycogen stored in the liver to glucose, and helps to turn proteins and fats into glycogen to replenish the store. To complete the cycle of controls, glucagon also stimulates the islets to produce insulin, so limiting the scale of its action.

Male and female controls

The endocrine glands, with their variety of hormones and intricate feedback and trigger systems, form a complicated network of controls for every facet of the body's operation. But hormones also control one of the most important parts of our lives—sex, reproduction and birth. These hormones, and the glands that secrete them, are discussed in two later sections—*see Sex and Reproduction p54, and Pregnancy and Birth p60.*

Connections
Acromegaly
Arthritis
Cretinism
Diabetes insipidus
Diabetes mellitus
Dwarfism
Hyperparathyroidism
Hypoglycaemia
Myxoedema
Pre-menstrual tension
Steroids
Tetany
Thyrotoxicosis
Tumour

Defences against disease

We live in a hostile environment. The air that we breathe, the surfaces we touch, the food we eat and the water we drink all carry bacteria, viruses, fungi and parasites that can cause disease—and would inevitably do so, had not the body developed an effective defence system against them. This system ensures our survival. Without it, no one could live for more than a few hours.

There are not one, but several, lines of defence against disease, starting with the skin. A system of barriers and traps protects the openings of the body against the outside world; and killer-cells attack those foreign bodies that succeed in entering the body. The ultimate defence, however, is a complex mechanism known as the immune response.

Barriers and traps

All the openings, or orifices, of the body have hidden barriers and traps, purpose-planned to deal with the particles that cause disease. The nature of these barriers varies widely, depending on the part of the body involved. Wax and coarse hairs trap particles of dust in the ear, for example, while the flow of urine sweeps foreign bodies out of the urethra, and, similarly, the passage of faeces dislodges matter from the anus. The eyes are protected by an antiseptic solution which washes the eyeball. The vagina has two defences: naturally-occurring Doderlein bacteria produce an acid that kills foreign particles, while a sticky lining, called the mucous membrane, traps bacteria so that they can be attacked and destroyed by the body's white cells. If the Doderlein bacteria are themselves killed by vaginal deodorants, or antiseptic douches, the vagina is left open to infection.

The mouth and nose, the largest openings of the body, have four kinds of protection. Thick hairs prevent large particles from entering the nostrils, while smaller particles are trapped in mucous membranes. Here they are attacked and usually destroyed by white cells produced by the lymph tissue (p25) of the tonsils and adenoids.

Killer cells

Debris and dust are propelled towards the throat by a mass of tiny hairs, called cilia, and swallowed. Most foreign bodies that enter the digestive tract (p40) are destroyed by the acid contents, or by the poisons produced by bacteria that live naturally in the intestines and help digestion. If any particles are inhaled, the body's next line of defence—the scavenging white cells—takes up the battle against the invaders.

The white cells that form the body's second line of defence against disease are part of a system known as the reticulo-endothelial system, or the RES. This is not an entity that can be touched or seen, like the respiratory system. Its components are found in nearly all the tissues of the body; they are cells called phagocytes, which engulf and destroy foreign bodies. Many of the phagocytes are lymphocytes, the white cells that circulate in the blood and

THE BODY'S DEFENCES

The human body is the prime target of disease-causing organisms, such as bacteria and viruses. But it has several lines of defence, ranging from simple traps at the entry-points to the elaborate mechanisms of the sophisticated immune system.

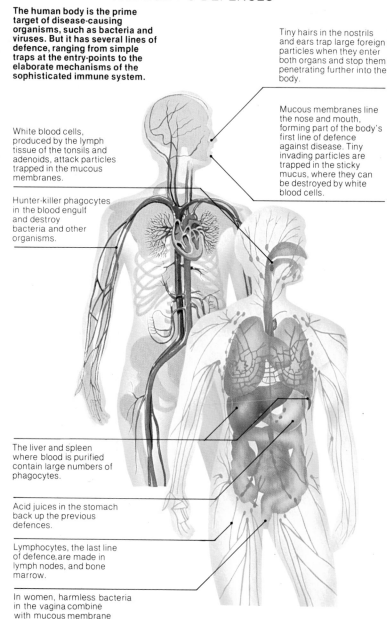

Tiny hairs in the nostrils and ears trap large foreign particles when they enter both organs and stop them penetrating further into the body.

Mucous membranes line the nose and mouth, forming part of the body's first line of defence against disease. Tiny invading particles are trapped in the sticky mucus, where they can be destroyed by white blood cells.

White blood cells, produced by the lymph tissue of the tonsils and adenoids, attack particles trapped in the mucous membranes.

Hunter-killer phagocytes in the blood engulf and destroy bacteria and other organisms.

The liver and spleen where blood is purified contain large numbers of phagocytes.

Acid juices in the stomach back up the previous defences.

Lymphocytes, the last line of defence, are made in lymph nodes, and bone marrow.

In women, harmless bacteria in the vagina combine with mucous membrane to destroy bacteria.

lymph vessels and are manufactured in the bone marrow and lymph organs—*see Blood and Lymph, p37.* Some are macrophages and monocytes, both large cells which are formed by the body in the bone marrow.

While many of the phagocytes roam the body, ready to spring into action when and where they are needed, considerable numbers remain stationary in the spleen and the liver. The reason for this is simple. The spleen acts as a purification plant for the blood. If cut in half, a red, pulpy mass can be seen, studded with patches of white. The white patches produce phagocytic lymphocytes, which attack any foreign bodies that pass through the blood capillaries forming the red pulp. They also engulf worn-out red blood cells, white blood cells and platelets and remove them from the circulation.

Phagocytes in the blood channels of the liver intercept and destroy any foreign bodies that have survived the acid environment and bacterial poisons of the intestine. These enter the circulation through the portal blood vessels, with digested food.

Long-term defence

Despite all these precautions, some disease organisms manage to pass through both liver and spleen and remain unaffected by the vast number of phagocytes in the rest of the body. In these circumstances, one more line of defence is brought into play— the immune system.

This system is a complicated and ingenious process by which the body becomes sensitive to foreign bodies on the first occasion that they invade it and responds by preparing special defences in case they invade the body again. The process forms the basis of vaccination against various types of disease.

The system revolves round the battle between antigens, the name given to all particles that are not natural to the body, and antibodies, the chemicals that the body produces to deal with them. Each type of antigen has a different chemical composition, which can be analyzed by the body—bacteria can be distinguished from viruses, and different types of bacteria from each other.

In response to the presence of an antigen, the body produces antibodies. These are clumps of proteins, called immunoglobulins, which specifically match individual antigens. Antibodies are produced in two different types of lymphocyte: T-lymphocytes and B-lymphocytes. The first type live in the lymph tissue. When an antigen enters the body, the B-lymphocytes produce specific antibodies designed to cope with the problem within

a few hours, and release them into the blood to attack the antigen. The reaction between antibodies and antigens releases histamine, the chemical that causes rashes and inflammation in allergy reactions.

T-lymphocytes act in a different, but equally effective way. When a T-lymphocyte meets an antigen, around 24 hours after the B-lymphocytes have come into play, specific antibodies are produced. These adhere to the lymphocyte's wall. The T-lymphocytes then divide, forming identical clone cells which surround the antigen so that the antibodies can break it down and destroy it.

The level of each specific antibody in the blood reduces gradually over a period of weeks. Both lymphocyte types, however, remember how to recreate the structure of the appropriate antibody required to deal with the particular antigen, if that antigen appears. This gives the body immunity against that specific antigen. The process can be extremely effective; in the case of measles, for example, the antibodies confer immunity for a lifetime.

Vaccination and rejection

Since the principles of the immune system have been understood, doctors have made use of the antibody response not only in the treatment, but also in the prevention of disease. This has been achieved by immunization, more commonly called vaccination. This works in several ways. Dead bacteria or viruses are injected into the body to make it form the appropriate antibodies, as in the case of typhoid fever or diphtheria. Alternatively, a weakened, or related, strain of disease organism may be used to promote the same result. In addition, an extract from the blood of a person who is suffering from a disease may give temporary immunity to another potential victim. This extract, which is rich in antibodies against that disease, is called an immune serum.

The very efficiency of the immune system, however, can cause medical problems. To date, transplant surgery, in which faulty organs are replaced, has not been completely successful because of the problems of tissue rejection. The immune system treats the cells of the replacement tissue as antigens, and destroys them. If the immune reaction is suppressed by the use of drugs, the body is left open to infections that often prove fatal.

Sometimes, too, in otherwise healthy people, the immune system fails to differentiate between antigens and the normal tissue of the body. As a result, it destroys both. Doctors now suspect that many different conditions, called auto-immune diseases, may be caused by this.

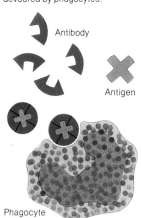

What antibodies do One type of antibody mirrors the structure of the antigen *(below).* The antigen is isolated by antibodies that fit themselves around it to form a chemical jigsaw puzzle. This is devoured by phagocytes.

Antibody

Antigen

Phagocyte

A second type of antibody is able to link together numbers of antigens and neutralize their toxic effects. The phagocytes then engulf this lattice *(below)* and destroy it. In both these antibody mechanisms, the lymphocytes remember the structure of the antigen, and react quickly when it is next encountered to give the body a degree of immunity to it.

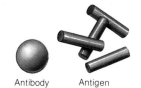

Antibody   Antigen

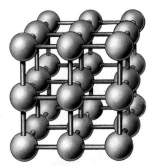

Connections
Allergy
Auto-immune diseases
Bacteria
Diptheria
Histamine
Immunization
Measles
Typhoid fever

Sex and reproduction

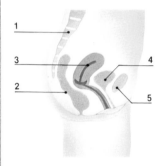

The female reproductive organs are located in the lower abdomen. In front of the tapering backbone, **1**, lies the rectum, **2**. The uterus, **3**, is above and behind the bladder, **4**, while the vagina and urethra run side by side to their respective openings. The pubic bone, **5**, lies in front of the bladder to protect it.

The drive to reproduce and perpetuate the species is shared by all living creatures. In human beings, reproduction has evolved into a complex physiological process that is controlled by a delicate balance of hormones. The reproductive organs are skilfully designed so that a sperm, or male sex cell, has the best possible chance of fertilizing the egg, the female sex cell. Once the egg has been fertilized, the female sex organs provide a protective environment until birth.

Superficially, the sexual anatomy and physiology of men and women appear to be completely different, but in fact there are a number of similarities. Until a foetus is seven weeks old, the male and female organs cannot be told apart without difficulty—*see Embryology, p12*. After that, the differences become pronounced, but some similarities remain. The sex glands—the male testes and the female ovaries—have common origins and work in much the same way, even secreting hormones, or chemical controllers, of the opposite sex.

The female system

A woman's reproductive system is both complex and sensitive. It is designed to place a mature egg, or ovum, in a protected position where it can be reached and fertilized by male sperm.

The opening of the female reproductive tract is called the vulva. Protected by pubic hair, it contains two pairs of lips: the outer and larger labia majora, and the inner labia minora. Both pairs of lips fill with blood and become larger during sexual arousal. The labia minora vary considerably in size. In some women they protrude through the outer lips; in others they can hardly be seen.

Between the lips are two openings. The first is the opening of the urethra, the tube that carries urine from the bladder; the second is the entrance, or vestibule, of the vagina. Also between the labia is the clitoris. Packed with nerve endings, this is a small piece of tissue that, like the male penis, has a sensitive hood, or glans. During sexual excitement, it becomes engorged with blood and erect. Its extreme sensitivity is crucial to sexual pleasure.

The vestibule of the vagina is lined with glands—the greater vestibular glands, or Bartholin's glands, and the lesser vestibular glands. When a woman is sexually aroused, these secrete a lubricating fluid

THE FEMALE REPRODUCTIVE SYSTEM

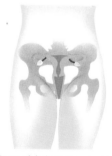

The two pelvic bones protect the female reproductive organs *(above)*. These are shown in detail on the right. The vulva *(below)* is bordered by the labia major, **1**, which covers folds of skin called labia minora, **2**. These protect the clitoris, **3**, the urethral opening, **4**, and the vaginal opening, **5**. Close by is the anus, **6**.

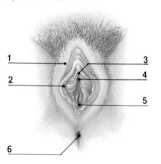

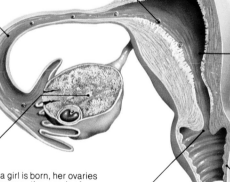

The Fallopian tube, or oviduct, is a muscular channel about 10cm (4in) long. Near the ovary, finger-like projections spread out to direct the egg on release. Each tube is lined with tiny hairs to aid the passage of the egg as it travels down the tube to the uterus. After intercourse, sperm travel up the tube to meet the egg and fertilize it.

A mature egg, or ovum, is released each month from one or other of the ovaries, about two weeks before menstruation.

The uterus, or womb, is a chamber designed especially to receive the fertilized egg and to nourish the developing foetus. It has a lining, or endometrium, which, in response to the monthly cycle of hormones, thickens in preparation for the implantation of the egg. If no egg is implanted, the endometrium breaks down and is shed as the menstrual blood. Beneath this lining is the myometrium, a thick layer of muscle, which contracts strongly during labour to expel the foetus.

When a girl is born, her ovaries contain many thousands of immature eggs. When she reaches puberty, these start to ripen in a monthly cycle and are released. Both ovaries, about the size of walnuts, are attached to the uterus by ligaments. They produce hormones regularly, in direct response to stimulation by the pituitary gland.

The cervix, or neck of the womb is a narrow opening that protrudes into the vagina. Thick mucus deters any sperm from entering the womb when no egg is present, but this thins out during ovulation.

The vagina is muscular and elastic, enabling it to stretch considerably during intercourse and childbirth.

THE MENSTRUAL CYCLE

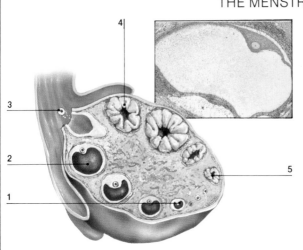

The menstrual cycle is a sequence of events in the female reproductive organs which centres around the life of an egg *(photograph left)*. The follicle of an immature egg, **1**, ripens in one of the ovaries under the influence of the follicle stimulating hormone (FSH). It matures into a Graafian follicle, **2**, which bursts at ovulation in response to the luteinising hormone (LH). The egg is released from the ovary at the same time, **3**, and enters the Fallopian tube. The empty follicle becomes the corpus luteum, **4**, which grows and secretes progesterone. It will degenerate, **5**, 14 days later if the egg has not been fertilized. The start of the period is usually taken as the first day of the cycle. As one cycle ends, another begins because a new egg starts to mature. After five days oestrogen causes the lining of the uterus to grow again. On the fourteenth day ovulation occurs and progesterone is released to aid the oestrogen. The endometrium swells with blood. Its glands widen and become convoluted. The stage is set for fertilization. If this does not occur by day 28, the supply of progesterone stops. This triggers a new period. The endometrial lining is shed and the egg is flushed away in up to 250ml (0.44pt) of blood.

Days of cycle

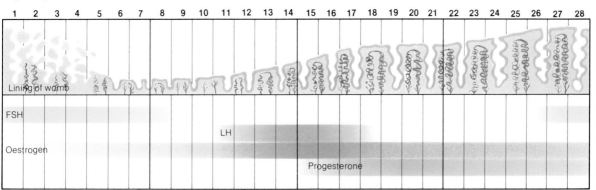

Lining of womb

FSH

LH

Oestrogen

Progesterone

---

that enables the penis to enter the vagina easily.

Just inside the vagina is a thin membrane called the hymen. At puberty, a small opening normally appears in the hymen to allow the flow of menstrual blood. In many girls, exercise ruptures the hymen completely before the first sexual experience. If the hymen is still intact, the first intercourse will break it, with a small amount of pain and a slight loss of blood.

The vagina and the womb

The vagina is a flexible, expandable tube, made up of fibrous connective tissue and smooth muscle. Most of the time it is flat and about 8cm (3.15in) long, running upwards and backwards just in front of the rectum. During intercourse, however, it opens and expands to accommodate the male penis. The vaginal walls are lined with a sticky, protective mucous membrane—see *Natural Defences Against Disease, p52*. Glands in this membrane secrete a fluid that keeps the vagina moist at all times, and their production increases during sexual excitement to help lubricate the entry of the penis.

The upper end of the vagina is connected to the uterus, or womb—the organ that protects the growing embryo for nine months, from conception to birth. The uterus is pear-shaped, about 8cm (3.15in) long and 5cm (1.97in) broad; it has a thick, muscular wall, almost 1cm (0.39in) thick. The neck, or cervix, at the lower end of the uterus bulges downwards into the vagina, with a pouch, or fornix, of the vagina at either side.

Two Fallopian tubes join the uterus— one on either side—towards the top of the pear-shape. Sometimes called by their American name, the oviducts, the Fallopian tubes are about 10cm (4in) long.

The womb is enclosed in a double fold of connective tissue known as the broad ligament. Within this, linked to the womb on each side by the stronger ovarian ligament, are the female sex glands, the ovaries. Each ovary is about 3.5cm (1.4in) long and 2cm (0.8in) wide, and lies close to the funnel-shaped opening of a Fallopian tube. The ovaries have two functions. They release ova, or eggs, and act as endocrine glands *(p48)*, secreting hormones into the bloodstream.

The ripening egg

When a female baby is born, her ovaries contain many thousands of immature ova, called primordial follicles. At puberty, a chemical produced by the pituitary gland *(p48)*, called Follicle Stimulating Hormone (FSH) starts to stimulate these follicles. ▷

Each month several of them start to develop, but usually only one follicle from one ovary becomes fully mature. As it grows, the follicle begins to act as an endocrine gland and secretes the hormone oestrogen. This acts to prime the lining of the womb, or endometrium, for pregnancy, by increasing the supply of blood. It also makes the breasts and vaginal tract more sensitive than usual.

When it is fully mature, the follicle, now called a Graafian follicle, is about a thousand times its original size. It is a hollow ball of cells about 20mm (0.79in) across, and in one wall the mature ovum, which is about the size of a pin-head, can be seen with the naked eye. At this time, the pituitary gland secretes a second hormone—Luteinizing Hormone (LH). This stimulates the follicle to burst and releases the ovum, which is wafted down one of the two Fallopian tubes to the womb by tiny hairs called cilia. This process is called ovulation.

As the ovum travels down the Fallopian tube, ready to be fertilized by a sperm, the follicle that has released it, now called a corpus luteum, secretes yet another hormone: progesterone. This chemical acts on the tissues that have already been primed by oestrogen—the endometrium, vaginal wall and the breasts—increasing their sensitivity even more and preparing them for pregnancy. Progesterone also prevents the release of further eggs; twins, for instance, are produced by the division of one egg, not the release of a second one.

If the egg is fertilized, then the egg itself produces a hormone called Human Chorionic Gonadotrophin (HCG). This maintains the corpus luteum—the follicle that released the egg—and with it, its output of progesterone. If the egg is not fertilized within seven days, the corpus luteum breaks up, the flow of progesterone is reduced, and about 14 days after ovulation the blood-filled lining of the womb is shed, flushing the unfertilized egg out of the uterus and through the vagina. This event is called menstruation. This cycle takes place every month, from the first menstruation, or menarche (at about the age of 12) to the menopause, the end of a woman's reproductive life (at about 48).

The female hormones
Oestrogen is the female sex hormone. The ovary manufactures small quantities of the hormone throughout the menstrual cycle, but its production reaches a peak during the development of the follicle. The adrenal glands also manufacture small quantities of oestrogen all the time.

Apart from its effect on the reproductive organs, oestrogen is responsible for the development of the female 'secondary sexual characteristics'. These are the physical features that distinguish women from men. When oestrogen is first secreted at puberty, stimulated by the hormones of the pituitary gland, it causes changes in the female body. The breasts develop, the internal and external genitals become mature, body hair grows in a female pattern—the upper margin of the pubic hair is concave upwards in women and downwards in men—and fat is laid down under the skin to give the body a gently-curving outline.

After puberty, oestrogen maintains these changes until the menopause. At this time the ovaries stop producing the hormone. This is not a sudden process, but usually takes place gradually over several years. Even though the adrenal glands still produce oestrogen, there is not enough in the body to maintain the sensitivity of the reproductive tract. The vagina, in particular, slowly loses its ability to secrete lubricating fluid.

Many women have been helped to overcome this, and other problems of the menopause by artificial hormone replacement therapy, or HRT. This treatment is not suitable for all women, however, and sometimes causes vaginal bleeding and other problems.

The ovaries and the adrenal glands also produce small quantities of the male sex hormone, androgen. This is quite normal. An excessive production of androgens in a woman, however, may lead to the development of male secondary sexual characteristics such as facial hair, increased muscle bulk and a deep voice. This condition, which is treatable, is called masculinization, or virilism.

The male system
The male reproductive system is much less complicated than that of the female. Unlike the female organs of reproduction, the male organs are mostly external. This is probably because sperm are produced most efficiently at a slightly lower temperature than that of the body.

The external male organs are the penis and the testes, or sex glands. Normally, the penis is a limp, or flaccid, protuberance from the base of the abdomen; an adult's penis measures, on average, between 2.5cm (1in) and 12.5cm (5in) long. The end of the penis, called the glans, is highly sensitive, and is protected by the prepuce, or foreskin. This is sometimes removed just after birth for reasons of hygiene, convention or religion, in a minor operation called a circumcision.

The penis is made up of three columns of spongy tissue that are riddled with blood vessels: the two on the upper surface are called corpora cavernosa, the lowest, which also forms the glans, is the corpus spongiosum. A thin tube running through this tissue, the urethra, carries both urine, from the bladder, and semen, the fluid that contains sperm. When a man is sexually aroused, nerve impulses widen the arteries of the penis, and constrict the veins. Blood is pumped into the corpora cavernosa and spongiosum, but cannot escape. As a result, the penis increases in size and becomes rigid. The erect penis is, on average, between 14cm (5.5in) and 19cm (7.5in) long. Contrary to popular opinion, there is no evidence that the

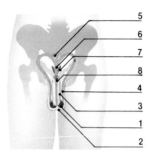

The male reproductive organs are partly external and partly internal *(above)*. The testes, **1**, lie in the scrotal sac, **2**, which hangs behind the penis, **3**. A vas deferens, **4**, runs from each testis and is joined by a seminal vesicle, **5**, just before it enters the urethra, **6**. The prostate gland, **7**, feeds into the urethra just below the point where the two vas deferens join. Below the prostate are the two Cowper's or bulbo-urethral, glands, **8**, which secrete fluid into the urethra before it enters the penis.

length of the erect penis has any physical bearing on a woman's sexual pleasure.

Testes and sperm

The testes are the male equivalents of the female ovaries. They secrete the male sex hormones, the androgens, and produce the male sex cells, or sperm.

The two testes are both egg-shaped, about 4cm (1.5in) long and 2.5cm (1in) thick, and sealed within tough membranes. In the embryo, they occupy a similar position within the body to that of the ovaries in adult women. Around the time of birth, they descend to the scrotum, a bag of skin below the penis, through a channel in the tissues called the inguinal canal. In later life this is a weak area that may give rise to a condition known as an inguinal hernia.

Inside the outer covering of each testis is a tough capsule called the tunica albuginea, from which around 250 spokes project into the heart of the testis, dividing it into compartments like a honeycomb. Each compartment is filled with coils of thin seminiferous tubules, each about 70cm (27.3in) long, where sperm, or spermatozoa, are produced by the division and maturation of germ cells called spermatogonia. Several hundred million sperm are produced every day by the testes, in a ▷

THE MALE REPRODUCTIVE SYSTEM

Sperm from the testes move along the two vas deferens to the urethra. Fluid is added by three glands and the semen ejaculated through the penis.

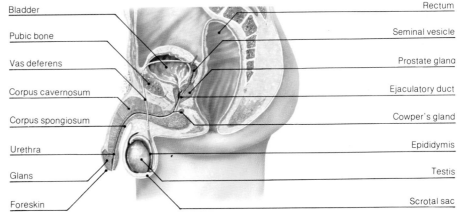

Bladder	Rectum
Pubic bone	Seminal vesicle
Vas deferens	Prostate gland
Corpus cavernosum	Ejaculatory duct
Corpus spongiosum	Cowper's gland
Urethra	Epididymis
Glans	Testis
Foreskin	Scrotal sac

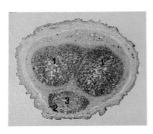

A cross-section through the penis shows that it is composed of three columns of erectile tissue *(above)*. The two upper columns make up the corpus cavernosum, **1**, which is surrounded and separated by a strong envelope of fibres. Running along the base of the penis is the corpus spongiosum, **2**, which expands into the glans, and through which the urethra, **3**, runs. Above the corpus cavernosum lie the arteries and veins which fetch and carry the blood that engorges both the corpora when the penis is erect.

The tunica albuginea surrounds the testis completely with a dense, inelastic capsule. It projects into the body of the testis and creates about 250 lobes in which the seminiferous tubules lie.

The rete testis is a network of tiny tubes which collect the immature sperms from all the seminiferous tubules and conveys them to the epididymis.

Groups of about 500 seminiferous tubules are bunched into each of the 250 lobes of the testis. These tubules are responsible for the manufacture of the 100 million sperm that each testis produces every 24 hours.

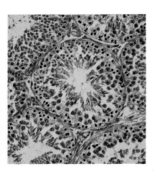

A section of a seminiferous tubule, magnified 200 times, shows the spermatocytes, producing immature sperm, *(above)*. The cells in the spaces between the tubules secrete male hormones.

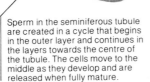

Sperm in the seminiferous tubule are created in a cycle that begins in the outer layer and continues in the layers towards the centre of the tubule. The cells move to the middle as they develop and are released when fully mature.

The scrotal sac is a pouch of skin containing smooth muscle fibres. These contract when the scrotum is exposed to cold or during exercise, wrinkling the skin.

The epididymis a highly convoluted tube which measures about seven metres in length. It connects the network of the rete testis to the vas deferens. The sperms from the testis mature during the few days they take to move along to the lower epididymis, where they are eventually stored prior to ejaculation.

SEX AND INTERCOURSE

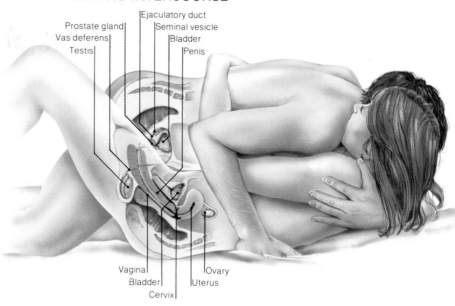

The purpose of sexual intercourse is to allow the male sperm to meet and fertilize a female ovum. Prior to penetration, the genitals of both partners are aroused. The penis is engorged with blood and its muscles contract. The clitoris swells with blood and the exposed vaginal opening is moistened with lubricating fluid and mucus. As the penis penetrates the vagina, the latter expands, allowing the glans of the penis to reach the cervix. The rhythmic thrust of the penis stimulates the sperm to leave the testes. As the sperm reach the ejaculatory duct, the seminal vesicles add a copious sticky secretion and the prostate gland adds a small quantity of milky alkaline fluid. At the moment of orgasm, this semen is ejaculated along the penis and into the vagina.

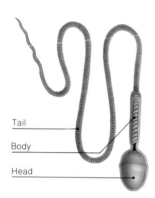

A sperm is a male sex cell. It has a head and a long mobile tail, shown *(above)* magnified 3,600 times. It measures 0.05mm (0.002in) from head to tail. The head is full of chromosomes and the body contains mitochondria that supply energy to the tail. This beats to propel the sperm up to the point where it meets the egg.

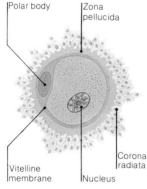

The ovum *(above)*, around 0.12mm (0.048in) across, is the female sex cell. Chromosomes fill the nucleus, which is protected by the vitelline membrane and the zona pellucida. The corona radiata is made up of cells that the ovum takes with it from the ovary.

continuous process that takes more than seven weeks from start to finish. Called spermatogenesis, the process starts at puberty under the stimulus of Follicle Stimulating Hormone (FSH) from the pituitary gland, and continues throughout life. Physiologically, there is no male equivalent of the female menopause, though some men experience a mid-life 'crisis of confidence'.

Storage and semen

As new sperm develop, they force more advanced sperm along the seminiferous tubules into collecting ducts. Tiny hairs in the collecting ducts and contractions of the muscular walls, force the sperm out of the testis into a larger duct called the epididymis, where they are stored for about three weeks. By the end of this period, they are mature, and can move independently.

Mature sperm are forced upwards through the two vas deferens by muscular contractions. Before they can be ejaculated during orgasm, however, they require a fluid transport medium. This is the seminal fluid, or semen.

The two vas deferens run up the body, on either side of the base of the penis, then loop over the bones of the pubis to lie alongside the bladder. Sweeping downwards, they each branch to form a seminal vesicle—a cavity lined with cells that secrete a sticky fluid. Each vesicle holds around 2ml (0.7fl oz) of the fluid, which makes up a part of the semen and acts as a storage medium for some of the sperm.

Below the seminal vesicles, the vas deferens are called the ejaculatory ducts. They run through the prostate gland, between the bladder and the base of the penis, which adds a milky fluid to the mixture of the semen. Within this gland, the two ejaculatory ducts join the urethra, the pathway for both urine and semen. At the base of the penis, the final ingredient is

added. This is a mucous fluid, secreted by the two pea-sized bulbourethral, or Cowper's, glands. About a teaspoonful of semen is produced at each ejaculation, containing as many as 350 million sperm.

The male hormones

Unlike the female hormones, the male sex hormones, called androgens, are produced regularly throughout adult life, the most common being the masculinizing hormone testosterone. All the androgens have similar functions.

As in women, the pituitary gland releases Luteinizing Hormone (LH) at puberty. In men, however, this is usually called Interstitial Cell Stimulating Hormone (ICSH). This is because it stimulates the interstitial cells of the testes to produce testosterone. The adrenal glands also secrete the male hormone, but only in small quantities, because the testes have an inhibiting effect on the glands that is not properly understood. As in the female, both the adrenal glands and the male sex glands produce small quantities of the hormones of the opposite sex—in this case, the oestrogens.

The hormone testosterone stimulates sperm production, the growth of the male genitals and the development of the male 'secondary characteristics'—the male distribution of body hair, facial hair, a deep voice, and an increase in muscle mass. In defects of the testes, such as hypogonadism, synthetic androgens can be given to develop and maintain these characteristics.

Sexual intercourse

Coitus, the sexual act, sexual congress, sexual intercourse—all these expressions mean the same thing. They refer to an act that many people find difficult to discuss, or even imagine. Sexual intercourse is one of the most basic of natural functions, yet one that is inextricably tangled with great emotions, fine sentiments and lust. Only the biological mechanisms of sexual intercourse are described here; other aspects of sex and sexuality are discussed in the third part of this book—*see Sex and Contraception, p338*.

Coitus, the penetration of the vagina by the penis, is preceded by the 'excitement phase', in which the bodies of both men and women are prepared for the act. Sexual excitement is triggered by a wide range of stimuli, which vary from person to person. Physical contact, visual attraction, mental rapport and anticipation all act on the nervous system, which responds by initiating physical changes in the male and female genitals.

In men, the muscles of the blood vessels in the penis expand and contract, filling the organ with blood until it is half-erect, or tumescent. In women, the clitoris fills with blood until it has more than doubled its size, and pushed out of its protective hood. The labia start to open and fill with blood, exposing the entrance of the vagina, where the vestibular glands, like the mucous lining of the vagina, begin to secrete lubricating fluid. The muscles supporting the uterus contract slightly, lifting it and straightening the angle with the vagina. In both sexes, the nipples harden and become sensitive.

During the excitement phase, the sexual partners often move on to activity that is directly physical, but not yet intercourse, called 'foreplay'. This may involve kissing, mutual stimulation of the genitals and erogenous zones—areas of the body that are sexually responsive, such as the breasts—by hand or by mouth, and increased bodily contact. This activity stimulates the sensory nerves until the brain raises the level of excitement to the 'plateau phase'.

The penis becomes engorged with blood and fully erect, and the foreskin is retracted from the glans. The sphincter of the bladder tightens, so that urine cannot be passed spontaneously. In women, the labia expand to their maximum size and open fully, while lubricating fluids are secreted in copious quantities. The uterus reaches its maximum elevation, and the muscles of the thighs relax, parting the legs slightly. Both the male and female bodies are now fully prepared for coitus.

At the start of intercourse, the man and woman take up a position which allows the penis to be placed in the vagina. The number of possible positions is only limited by the ingenuity and athleticism of the partners, but the most common is the 'missionary position'. The woman lies on her back with her legs apart and her knees raised. The man lies on top of the woman, between her legs, and places his penis inside the vagina.

The vagina immediately expands to accommodate the penis, so that the glans is just beneath the neck of the womb. The muscle fibres of the vaginal opening tighten around the base of the penis to hold it

in place. The man then thrusts the penis rhythmically in and out of the vagina, helped by opposing thrusts by the woman. The friction of the penis against the vaginal walls, and the pressure of the base of the penis and lower abdomen against the clitoris, stimulates the mass of sensory nerves in the genitals of both partners. This causes immense pleasure, and leads to the 'orgasmic phase'.

The male orgasm
In the man, orgasm is an intensely pleasurable series of rhythmic contractions of the muscles surrounding the urethra at the base of the penis, and of the urethra itself. These contractions pump about a teaspoonful of semen through the urethra under pressure. The process, called ejaculation, spurts semen containing around 350 million sperm into the upper end of the vagina and the neck of the womb. The sperm swim through the womb under their own power in an attempt to fertilize an egg.

After ejaculation the penis rapidly decreases in size, as blood is allowed to leave the blood vessels. The organ stays tumescent for some time, however, and only returns to its resting state after about 20 minutes. If sexual stimulation continues, some men find it possible to repeat intercourse after the same interval.

The female orgasm
The female orgasm is a much less straightforward process, and is the subject of much discussion and research. It is not essential for reproduction, though obviously desirable for both psychological and physiological reasons. Intercourse nearly always ends in orgasm for a man, but this is not the case for women. The female orgasm is not inevitable: it is bound up with many psychological factors, and experienced in many different degrees.

Full orgasm in the female has many similarities with that of the male, though it normally requires stimulation over a much longer period of time. The muscles in the wall of the vagina contract powerfully several times, then contract in short spasms which gradually die away. The uterus flexes, and the thick muscular walls contract spasmodically. As with the male, there is a great feeling of release and contentment, but the female remains in the plateau phase for much longer. The tissues stay engorged with blood, and there remains a capacity for further orgasms, or for immediate multiple orgasms. Once it was thought that there were two distinct types of female orgasm, vaginal and clitoral. It is now believed that the two are indivisible.

For many women, however, an orgasm is not the cataclysmic event of popular fiction. There is an equally satisfying, prolonged build-up of pleasure, then a slow, gradual release. The genitals gradually pass through the plateau phase and the excitement phase, and eventually return to normal.

The moment of conception A child is conceived the moment a sperm enters and fertilizes the ovum. Of the millions of sperm that enter the vagina, a few hundred reach the ovum and pierce the zona pellucida, but only one penetrates the vitelline membrane.

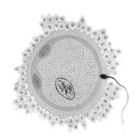

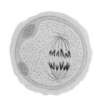

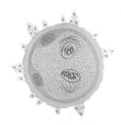

As soon as one sperm has penetrated the membrane of the ovum *(top)*, no other sperm can enter. The sperm loses its body and tail but keeps its head. The nucleus of the ovum divides and produces what are termed polar bodies — there are two of these, neither of which has any known function. The corona radiata begins to break away as the nuclei of the sperm and ovum approach one another *(middle)*. The chromosomes intermingle as each one pairs up with its opposite number. Once this pairing has been achieved, nature's most sophisticated cell has been formed. The pairs of chromosomes then duplicate themselves and begin to draw apart in preparation for the first cell division of the new embryo's life *(bottom)*.

Connections
Circumcision
Hernia
Hormone replacement therapy
Hypogonadism
Menarche
Menopause
Secondary sexual characteristics
Virilism

Pregnancy and birth

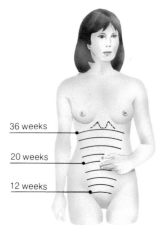

36 weeks
20 weeks
12 weeks

The growth of the foetus The top of the uterus moves up the abdomen as the foetus grows during pregnancy. From the twelfth week, the uterus moves about two fingers' breadth every two weeks. From the twentieth week, by which time it has reached the navel, it moves two fingers' breadth every four weeks.

Milestones in pregnancy The eighth week after fertilization is a milestone in the life of an embryo. All its major organs have been formed. From now on, only their size and the specialization of their cells will increase. The embryo's heartbeat is regular, the kidneys are starting to work and blood is coursing through its body. Its ears, fingers and toes are taking shape. Over the next few weeks the placenta grows considerably to provide the embryo with a totally controlled environment. By the twelfth week, the placenta is about six times heavier than the foetus, as the embryo is now termed. At 16 weeks the foetus weighs the same as the placenta and its sex is distinguishable. About this time, the foetus begins to move, or 'quicken', as its muscles become active. At 28 weeks the baby may move vigorously in the womb and can open its eyes. At 36 weeks the baby is putting on weight rapidly and is ready to be born.

Pregnancy can be one of the most memorable and exciting periods of a woman's life. In a series of subtle and complex physical changes, her body adapts to accommodate and nurture the growing baby. Sometimes these changes can be confusing, or even alarming. But an understanding of the physical and physiological processes of pregnancy and birth will give a woman the confidence to appreciate what should be a fascinating and fulfilling experience.

Signs of pregnancy

Usually, the first sign of pregnancy is a late menstrual period (*p55*), though this is not always the case. A woman may notice some other indications of pregnancy as well: swelling and occasional soreness of the breasts; darkening of the nipples, and the immediate area around them; early morning nausea, or sometimes actual sickness; and, occasionally, the need to pass urine more frequently.

Whether a woman is pregnant or not can be confirmed by a simple test between ten and 14 days from the day on which the final period should have started. A urine sample taken in the early morning is tested for the presence of the chemical HCG (human chorionic gonadotrophin), produced by the developing embryo—*see Embryology, page 13*. Though 'do-it-yourself' pregnancy testing kits are widely available, it is better that the test is

performed by the family doctor. If there is any doubt about the date of the last period, he or she can carry out an internal examination to confirm the diagnosis. If the test is positive, the doctor will also discuss ante-natal care and whether the confinement should take place in hospital or at home.

Hospital or home

Today, most babies are delivered in hospital; it is difficult to find a doctor who is prepared to supervise a home birth. The argument is that a hospital will have expert help and sophisticated equipment on hand if required; it is impossible to be certain that a delivery will be trouble-free, even when the expectant mother has had babies before. Some hospitals have special units in which family doctors can deliver their patients' babies. Many mothers find that such units represent a good compromise between a delivery at hospital and at home—life-saving equipment is on hand, but the mother is attended by a doctor whom she knows and trusts. In the 'domino' scheme, run by an increasing number of hospitals, the mother is attended by a single midwife throughout her pregnancy and at the birth in hospital, and so establishes a similar relationship with her.

There is no doubt that it is much safer to have a baby at hospital than at home; the continuing fall in the mortality rate for babies and mothers can be directly attri-

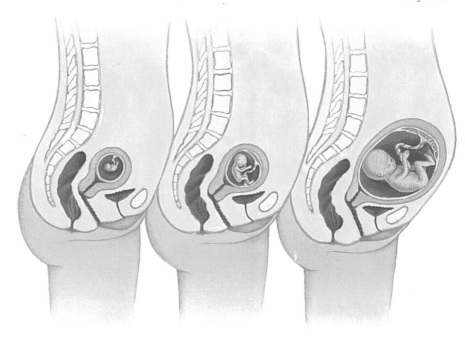

8 WEEKS   12 WEEKS   20 WEEKS

At twelve weeks the head of the foetus *(below)* is still disproportionately large compared with the size of its body, but the nails and external genitals are beginning to appear. Blood flows rhythmically through the lungs at 80 pulses each minute, as if to prepare for regular breathing .

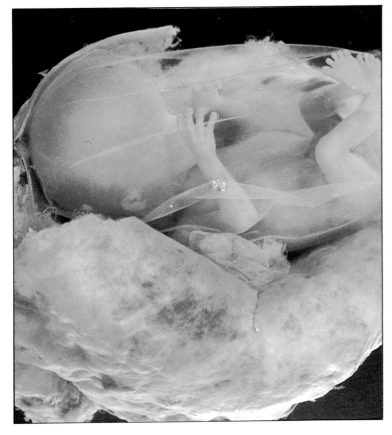

buted to advances in the science of midwifery that depend on the technology available in hospitals.

Nevertheless, hospital delivery has an important limitation. Many women, rightly, have a number of reservations about the traditional methods used to deliver a baby. During recent years, many alternatives have been tested: methods for the relief of pain during labour; different positions for the mother during the delivery; varying approaches to the atmosphere and environment for the birth. Further information on these techniques is available from the National Childbirth Trust.

Doctors should be happy to discuss the various alternatives in detail, stating what they think are the advantages and disadvantages for an individual mother. However, all doctors are limited by the options available at the hospitals in their area; each hospital tends to develop its own methods and to stick to them, so in areas served by only one hospital the prevailing methods will be all that can be offered.

Ante natal care

Wherever the baby is to be delivered, and whatever the method to be used, antenatal care—the education and physical preparation of an expectant mother for the birth of her child—is vitally important. The growing baby is totally dependent on its mother and her lifestyle. Every pregnant ▷

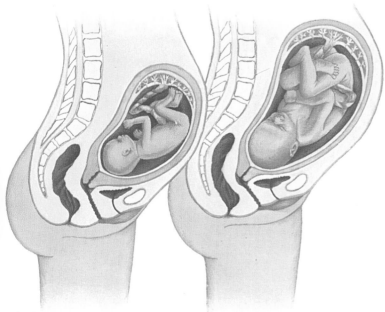

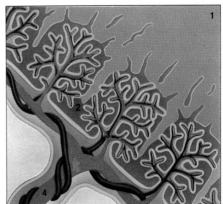

The placenta is a vital link in the uterus lining, **1**, which unites the systems of mother and child. The maternal, **2**, and foetal, **3**, blood vessels are in deliberate close contact so that substances can diffuse from one to another. The umbilical cord, **4**, carries food and oxygen to the foetus while removing its wastes. The placenta also makes three hormones: human chorionic gonadotrophin, progesterone, and oestrogen. Each plays a role in either maintaining the pregnancy or preparing the mother for birth and the production of milk.

28 WEEKS   36 WEEKS

LABOUR AND CHILDBIRTH

The uterus of a pregnant woman becomes more sensitive just before the birth of the baby. The neck of the womb softens, shortens and opens slightly, and the baby's head settles into the pelvis and faces one or other of the hips (right). The scene is set for the three stages of labour.

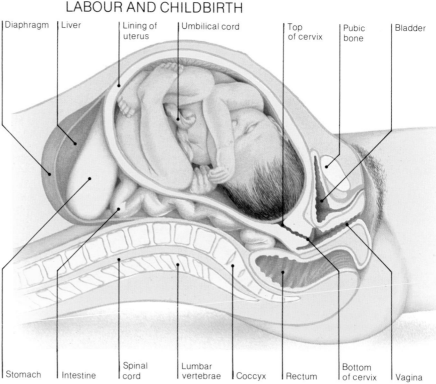

Diaphragm | Liver | Lining of uterus | Umbilical cord | Top of cervix | Pubic bone | Bladder

Stomach | Intestine | Spinal cord | Lumbar vertebrae | Coccyx | Rectum | Bottom of cervix | Vagina

The first stage of labour begins when contractions of the uterus start and ends when the cervix has completely opened. The contractions are gentle at first but rhythmic and intense later. They begin at the top of the uterus and sweep downwards, forcing the cervix to gradually widen. The muscle fibres at the top of the uterus have a unique property: they shorten a little after each contraction and stay shortened while they are relaxed. As a result, the cervix becomes wider and wider as the intensity and frequency of the contractions increase. At the end of the first stage these muscles have widened the cervix enough for the baby to pass through it. This may take as long as 13 hours in a first pregnancy, and up to seven hours in subsequent pregnancies.

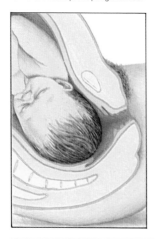

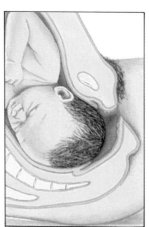

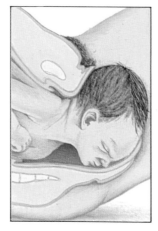

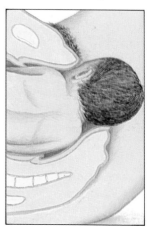

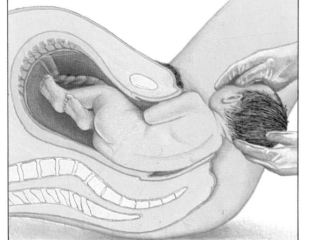

The second stage of labour begins when the cervix is around 10cm (4in) wide and ends, about an hour later, with the delivery of the baby. The mother's abdominal muscles start to contract, pushing the baby downwards and turning its head to face her back *(above)*, while the uterus contracts rhythmically for around a minute every two or three minutes. Following the procedure learnt at ante-natal classes, the mother takes a number of deep breaths, holds them and pushes down, almost as though she was trying to open her bowels. As a result, the baby's head emerges little by little, and once it is free the baby rotates to face the mother's hip again. This makes it easier for the shoulders and the rest of the body to emerge.

The third stage of labour begins after the baby is born and ends when the placenta, or afterbirth, has been expelled. Although the mother's uterus will expel the placenta on its own, midwives usually give an injection of ergometrine to help the process. This powerful drug contracts the uterus for about four minutes, expelling the placenta from the body quickly and so reducing the mother's loss of blood.

mother should attend an ante natal clinic either at a local hospital or at her family doctor's surgery, depending on local practice; generally, she should see the doctor or midwife every four weeks for the first 30 weeks of pregnancy, every fortnight until the 36th week, and then weekly until the baby is born.

On her first visit to the clinic, a complete medical history will be taken. The doctor will want to know whether she has had any illnesses that might affect the confinement, such as hypertension, an increase in blood pressure, or if she has had any previous pregnancies or a miscarriage. A blood sample will be taken—*see Special Tests, p84*—so that blood group and rhesus factors *(p22)* can be checked; this sample will also tell the doctor whether the mother has had rubella, or german measles, an illness that can have serious consequences for the developing embryo if contracted during pregnancy. (Most girls are now encouraged to be vaccinated against rubella in their early teenage years.)

The doctor will also conduct an internal examination and external examination. He or she will assess the size of the uterus, or womb, and check that its appearance corresponds to what is expected. He will also check that the pelvis is sufficiently wide, so allowing the baby a trouble-free exit during labour. The weight and blood pressure will also be checked, to anticipate any problems that may develop during pregnancy. Finally, the urine will also be tested.

This examination gives the expectant mother the opportunity to find out exactly what is going to happen to her, to her body and to her developing baby during pregnancy. All doctors will advise her to give up smoking—there is now conclusive evidence that the substances that enter the blood when a cigarette is smoked can cross the placenta and affect the baby, stunting its growth—*see Abuses of the Body, p328.*

Alcohol should be avoided, or, at the least, drunk in moderation—it, too, can affect the development of the baby. In fact, all drugs should be avoided, unless they are prescribed by a doctor who is aware of the pregnancy. This is especially important in the first four months, when all the major organs and systems of the foetus are formed—*see Embryology, p12.*

There is one exception to this. Occasionally, the vomiting and nausea that some mothers experience during early pregnancy is so severe that a drug has to be prescribed to deal with it. In this case, the risk to the mother and baby brought about by constant vomiting is usually considered to be greater than the risk from drugs.

Diet and exercise

Doctors also emphasize the importance of a well-balanced diet. This should contain sufficient quantities of protein, fresh fruit and vegetables, with high-fibre foods and wholemeal bread. The last two are neces-

sary because constipation is often a problem during pregnancy—*see Diet, p322.* Iron and folic acid may be given as a dietary supplement, though some hospitals now recommend this only if the mother is found to be anaemic. It is important, however, that the pregnant mother does not gain too much weight—this can lead to a serious complication of pregnancy called eclampsia. Though the tendency is to 'eat for two', the average woman should only gain between 8kg and 13kg (17.6lb-28.7lb) during her pregnancy.

The general physical condition of the mother is equally important, so the doctor will suggest that she gets plenty of sleep, and also takes regular exercise. A number of useful exercises to tone the body generally, and help the muscles that will be used during labour in particular, are listed in *Exercise—The Childbearing Year, p320.* As part of this programme, the doctor will recommend that she visits the dentist regularly—dental treatment for expectant mothers is provided free of charge by the National Health Service. Gingivitis, infection and soreness of the gums, is often a problem during pregnancy, but can be treated easily by a dentist.

Throughout the 40 weeks of pregnancy, the health of the mother and baby is constantly monitored at the ante-natal clinic. Weight, blood pressure, urine and the size of the uterus are checked at each visit. At 16 weeks, a blood sample is checked for the presence of a special type of protein *(p44)* called 'alpha foeto protein'—*see Special Tests, p84.* If this is present in an abnormally high quantity, it can be an indication of a congenital abnormality in the baby such as spina bifida.

The diagnosis can be confirmed by another special test called an amniocentesis, when an amniotic fluid sample is taken and analyzed. Amniocentesis can also be used to detect other conditions, such as Down's Syndrome, or mongolism, and is performed as a matter of routine on all mothers who may be at risk—particularly those over 37, or those who have a family history of birth defects. Other suspected inherited defects, such as Rhesus incompatibility, or haemophilia, may be detected by analysis of a sample of blood taken from the umbilical cord.

At the 16-week visit, an 'ultra-sound' examination—*see Special Tests, p84*—will be made of the mother and baby. Harmless sound waves are passed through the mother's body, to give a television picture of the developing foetus. The size of the baby can be checked, and the foetal heart observed while it beats; the doctor will also be able to see if there are twins. Sometimes the sex of the baby can also be established, though not always with certainty. If this ultra-sound scan reveals any potential problems, the test is repeated at intervals.

Ante-natal classes

While the physical well-being of the mother and baby are being monitored at the clinic, the expectant mother, and her ▷

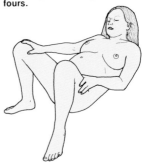

The position a pregnant woman assumes in labour and birth can vary considerably. Alternatives to the conventional lying-down position are standing, squatting or kneeling on all fours.

The lying down or 'stranded beetle' position *(above)* is losing popularity because it means that the mother can only play a passive part in the process of birth. It also reduces the flow of blood to and from the placenta.

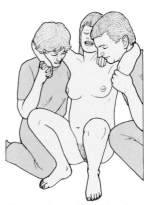

The squatting position *(above)* requires support but does not impair the blood supply to and from the placenta. The position widens the cervix more, reduces the need for muscular effort and gives the mother more control over the birth.

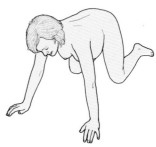

The all-fours position *(above)* has the same advantage as squatting, such as greater comfort and reduced stress. In addition, this kneeling position makes it easier for the baby to rotate as it emerges from the vagina.

Forceps delivery, epidural anaesthesia and episiotomy are all special techniques used by doctors if it becomes necessary to intervene during delivery to ensure the safety of the child or mother.

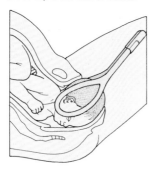

Forceps *(above)* are only used in abnormal deliveries, when, for example, the baby stops descending or is in distress. The mother is given an anaesthetic *(below)*, plus sometimes an episiotomy. The blades of the forceps are fitted firmly round the baby's head and the baby is then carefully manipulated until it emerges. The procedure is safe and painless, but it can be used only when the head has reached the pelvis.

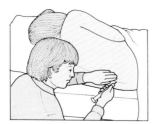

Epidural anaesthesia is given to relieve the pain that many women feel during labour. The woman lies curled up on her side *(above)* to allow the needle to slip between the vertebrae at the base of the spine, so that the anaesthetic numbs the nerves to the lower part of the body. Although the technique is controversial, many women find an epidural essential.

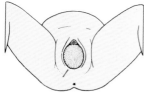

An episiotomy is a surgical incision made to widen the vaginal opening and ease the passage of the baby. The cut is started in the vagina and continued out to one side *(above)*. However, many doctors believe that if an episiotomy is avoided, not only will the mother's tissues recover naturally but will also heal more quickly.

family, are helped to prepare mentally and physically for the actual birth at ante natal classes. These usually begin after the 30th week of pregnancy. Fathers are encouraged to attend the classes, so that they can understand what is happening to the growing baby and the mother, and prepare themselves for an active, supporting role during the birth.

The mother is shown what will happen during her labour, and how to perform some simple exercises that will prepare her muscles. Breathing techniques, which help to control the pain of labour, and reinforce the rhythmic contractions that will push the baby through the birth canal, are also taught. The actual mechanics of the birth are explained, as well as the arguments for and against several controversial medical or surgical interventions in the birth, such as induction of labour, epidural anaesthesia and episiotomy.

Changes in the mother

Physical and physiological changes start in a woman's body from the moment of conception. The hormonal changes of the menstrual cycle are suppressed by the hormones produced by the developing embryo, with the result that menstruation ceases. Thereafter, the hormones circulating in the mother's blood control the growth and nourishment of the embryo. The detailed changes by which the growing baby is nurtured inside the womb are described earlier in this book—*see Embryology, p12.*

By the time the growth of the baby first becomes physically apparent in the twelfth week of pregnancy, all the limbs, organs and systems of the embryo have been formed. The womb may be felt just above the pubic bone. The mother's breasts will have become larger, while her clothes will start to feel tight because of her increased weight. After the first 12 weeks, a period called the 'first trimester', morning sickness usually becomes much less of a problem.

Over the next eight weeks, the womb grows by around two finger-breadths every fortnight, so it reaches the level of the umbilicus, or navel, by the 20th week. Thereafter it increases in size by around one finger-breadth every fortnight, so that it is at its highest point by 36 weeks, just beneath the xiphisternum, at the lower end of the breastbone. From this time, the height of the uterus begins to decrease, as the baby's head slips down into the pelvis. This development, once described as 'lightening', takes place earlier in subsequent pregnancies.

By about the 20th week, most mothers will have felt the baby moving inside them, or 'quickening', as this used to be called. Mothers who have had children before, however, often feel the baby at around the 16th week. Throughout pregnancy, mothers occasionally feel small, painless contractions of the womb. Known as Braxton Hicks contractions, these become more noticeable after the 30th week.

During the second and third trimesters—between the 13th and 36th weeks—many women begin to experience physical problems. Understandably, expectant mothers become tired more easily, while the pressure of the baby on the ligaments of the spine and pelvis and the effect of the hormones of pregnancy may also cause backache. The pregnant uterus sometimes also exerts pressure on a vein called the inferior vena cava, causing the development of varicose veins in the legs. Such problems are annoying and upsetting, but, fortunately, they do not cause any damage to the baby, or permanent damage to the mother.

Changes in the foetus

During the first 12 weeks after conception the embryo grows rapidly, to take the recognizable form of the foetus—*see Embryology, p12.*

Over the next six months, the foetus continues to grow and mature, passing through various distinct stages of development on its way to maturity. During this period, the foetus derives all its nourishment from its mother's blood, which interfaces with that of the foetus in an organ lining the mother's womb, called the placenta.

By 16 weeks, the placenta is fully developed. It has a surface area of approximately 11 square metres (13.2sq yds), and weighs between 500g and 1,000g (1.1-2.2lb) by the time of birth.

Fuel and vital materials for the foetal cells pass through the placenta from the mother's blood. These include oxygen, water, salts, glucose, fats and amino acids—*see Metabolism, p44*—as well as vitamins, and antibodies. Waste products, such as carbon dioxide and water, pass from the foetus to the mother. Unfortunately, viruses and toxic substances such as those produced by cigarette smoke, alcohol and certain types of drugs can also cross the placenta to damage the foetus.

The placenta also secretes three hormones, or chemical messengers: progesterone, which maintains pregnancy; oestrogen, the female sex hormone; and lactogen, which plays a part in the production of milk by the breasts. It is connected to the foetus by the umbilical cord, about 50cm (19.7in) long, consisting of two arteries and one vein.

Labour

It is hard to define precisely the moment at which labour begins. In some women, strong contractions of the womb, recurring every 15 minutes or so, are the first sign of labour. Other women first notice the 'breaking of the waters', the rupture of the amniotic sac that surrounds the baby inside the womb, releasing the amniotic fluid. Another indication that labour has started is the discharge of a red or pink sticky mass—the remains of the plug that seals the cervix, or neck, of the womb.

At this stage, the mother will usually be admitted to hospital, where she will be

CHANGES IN CIRCULATION AT BIRTH

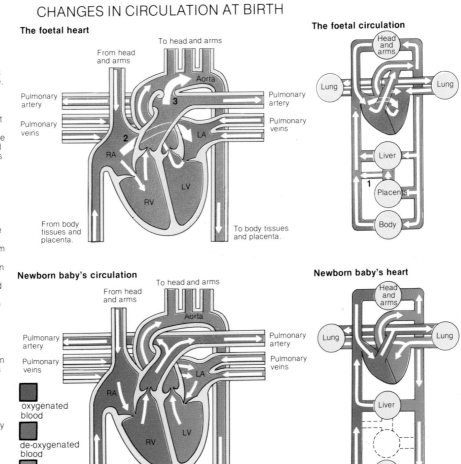

The foetal heart

The foetal circulation

To head and arms
From head and arms
Aorta
Pulmonary artery
Pulmonary artery
Pulmonary veins
Pulmonary veins
RA
LA
RV
LV
From body tissues and placenta.
To body tissues and placenta.

Head and arms
Lung
Lung
Liver
Placenta
Body
1
2
3

Newborn baby's circulation

Newborn baby's heart

To head and arms
From head and arms
Aorta
Pulmonary artery
Pulmonary artery
Pulmonary veins
Pulmonary veins
RA
LA
RV
LV
From body
To body

Head and arms
Lung
Lung
Liver
Body

oxygenated blood

de-oxygenated blood

Maternal and foetal blood

The circulation of the blood in the foetus changes at the moment of birth. In the womb *(far right)*, the foetus receives oxygenated blood from the placenta because both its lungs are collapsed and so ineffective. Most of this blood runs through the liver, while the rest flows through the ductus venosus, **1**, into the inferior vena cava. Most of the blood that reaches the foetal heart *(right)*, flows into the left atrium through a hole called the foramen ovale, **2**. The rest is diverted into the right atrium, where it mixes with blood from the head and arms, and is pumped into the right ventricle. The major part of this blood bypasses the lungs by taking a short cut through the ductus arteriosus, **3**, into the aorta. The rest of the blood supplies the lungs, returning to the left atrium through the pulmonary veins.

At birth, the baby's circulation becomes self-contained. When the cord is cut, the flow of blood from the placenta ceases, making the umbilical vein to the liver and the ductus venosus redundant *(below far right)*. Eventually, they waste away. The foramen ovale and the ductus arteriosus in the heart *(below right)* close off, and from then on the circulation contains blood that is oxygenated solely by the newly-inflated lungs. Sometimes, however, these channels do not close off completely. This is termed a congenital heart defect and may require immediate treatment.

Key

RA Right atrium
RV Right ventricle
LA Left atrium
LV Left ventricle

helped to prepare for the birth. Hospital routines vary, though in all the mother is bathed. In some hospitals the mother's pubic hair is shaved—this is a matter more of tradition than necessity, and many hospitals have discontinued the practice. The majority of doctors, however, still arrange that the mother is given an enema, to move her bowels. The argument for this is that it will remove any possible source of infection, but the procedure is thought to be unnecessary by many doctors unless the mother is constipated.

Normally, labour starts spontaneously. Many factors are involved: among them are the rupture of the amniotic sac by the downward pressure of the foetus, which is thought to trigger contractions of the womb, and the action of the hormone oxytocin, secreted by the posterior part of the pituitary gland, which initiates uterine muscle contractions. Two methods used to start labour artificially, or to 'induce' it, are the rupture of the amniotic sac by the doctor, or an injection of oxytocin. (Recently, the insertion of prostoglandin pessaries high up in the vagina has also proved to be effective).

Doctors may decide to induce labour for several reasons: when pregnancy lasts longer than 42 weeks, because there is evidence that this is harmful for the foetus; and on occasions when a disease that may seriously affect the health of the mother or baby is diagnosed. Such diseases include diabetes, pre-eclampsia, and outbreaks of ante partum haemorrhage, or bleeding from the womb.

During the past decade, however, a tendency to induce labour for convenience's sake has developed in Britain. This has been severely critisized by many people, doctors included, and the trend is now on the decline, though the practice has not, unfortunately, been eradicated.

The stages of labour

In the first stage of labour, the contractions of the uterus increase in strength and frequency, causing the cervix to first shorten and flatten, then to widen, or dilate. During this stage, the mother may rest quietly in bed and chat to her family, or walk around, as she prefers. The first stage can take anything up to 13 hours, though it is generally quicker in the case of a mother who is having a second child. The doctor or midwife will, at intervals, check on the ▷

BREAST FEEDING

Each breast contains a number of ducts that branch throughout the mammary tissue and converge at the nipple. They start in the alveoli where milk — consisting of water, protein, fat and a carbohyrdate called lactose — is produced. During pregnancy, the placenta secretes progesterone and oestrogen, which enlarge the breasts but prevent them from producing milk. Once the placenta is expelled, this inhibition is removed. The pituitary gland then secretes prolactin, a hormone that stimulates the alveoli to secrete milk. When the baby sucks at the breast, or when the baby's cries are heard, the 'nipple reflex' is triggered — nerve impulses travel to the hypothalamus in the brain, which stimulates the production of a hormone called oxytocin. This contracts the alveoli and forces milk along the ducts to the nipple. The process, called 'milk let-down', allows breast feeding *(below)* to begin. When the breast has been emptied, more prolactin is secreted to restart milk production.

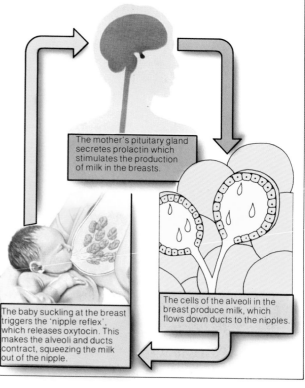

The mother's pituitary gland secretes prolactin which stimulates the production of milk in the breasts.

The cells of the alveoli in the breast produce milk, which flows down ducts to the nipples.

The baby suckling at the breast triggers the 'nipple reflex', which releases oxytocin. This makes the alveoli and ducts contract, squeezing the milk out of the nipple.

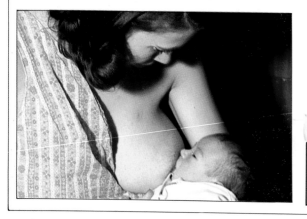

Sex, during and after pregnancy is possible, despite some popular beliefs. Neither intercourse nor orgasms induce labour or a miscarriage, or damage the foetus, in a normal pregnancy. However, women who have had a previous miscarriage are generally recommended not to have intercourse for the first 14 weeks of their pregnancy; those who have a history of miscarriages should not have intercourse during pregnancy unless a gynaecologist has confirmed that there is no risk.

Intercourse may be uncomfortable for a woman, because of her swollen abdomen and tender breasts, and a change in position may be necessary. Many couples find that intercourse is easier if they lie on their sides, face to face. Libido may also suffer, as many women lose their desire for sex, especially during the first 14 and last ten weeks. However, this usually returns soon after the birth.

If the birth has been trouble-free there is no reason why sexual intercourse should not be resumed immediately. However, many women prefer to wait for two or three weeks, until vaginal bleeding ceases and any remaining soreness has disappeared.

extent of dilation of the cervix, and listen to the baby's heart with a special stethoscope. When the cervix is fully dilated to around, 10cm (3.9in), this stage of labour has been completed. The mother is now prepared for the second stage of labour, the delivery of the baby. This usually lasts for around an hour, though it may be shorter for a woman who is having her second baby.

The traditional position for delivery is termed the 'stranded beetle' position. It has many critics, who point out that it is uncomfortable for the mother. The alternative position is the one used by most mammals, in which the mother kneels on all fours. This position is now championed by a number of doctors, who claim good results for it. The method is not yet widespread, however, and it has one considerable disadvantage—it makes the monitoring of the health of both mother and baby during the delivery extremely difficult to achieve.

When the cervix is fully dilated, the mother feels an irresistible desire to push. She is encouraged to do so by the father, if present, helped by the doctor or midwife, who regulates the timing of each effort, and matches it to the contractions. The mother follows the pattern of breathing and exertion that she, and the father, have learned in their ante natal classes. The contractions, and so the pushes, come closer and closer together, and are drawn out more and more.

The effect of these contractions and pushes is to force the baby down the birth canal—normally head first, but bottom first in a 'breech' delivery. Due to the shape of the female pelvis, the baby's head has to rotate, usually through an angle of 90°. The mother is then asked to pant rather than push, so that the head can be delivered slowly and carefully. Once the head has been born, the baby turns back through the same arc, so that the shoulders can emerge. Once this has been achieved, the rest of the baby's body then follows shortly and the birth is complete.

Throughout the delivery, doctors monitor the baby's heartbeat through a stethoscope, but if the doctor suspects that the birth may not be normal an electrode will be attached to the baby's head. In some hospitals, this is done as a matter of routine. The electrode enables the doctor to keep a constant watch on the activity of the baby's heart; the method does not leave a lasting scar.

Though the use of foetal monitoring is very far from the idea of natural childbirth, and may be unnecessary in many cases, it has saved a huge number of lives since its development.

Pain relief and medical intervention
Labour can be extremely painful, especially for a woman who is having her first child. Many mothers hope that they will be able to deliver their child without resorting to artificial pain-killers, but only a few achieve this aim. A number of methods are used to relieve pain in labour, and they should be discussed with the doctor beforehand, so that the mother can make her wishes clear and have them respected. To

an extent, her knowledge of what to expect in labour and her mastery of the breathing exercises taught in ante-natal classes can help the mother to cope with the pain.

Sometimes 'gas and air'—a mixture of nitrous oxide and oxygen—is given by means of a mask which the mother holds to her face. The gas is a mild pain-killer, and does not cause loss of consciousness. Pethidine, a drug similar to morphine, may also be given by injection, and does not harm the baby—it does however, impair the mother's appreciation of her experience. Acupuncture anaesthesia is also occasionally used to relieve pain during childbirth, but its use depends on the availability of suitable trained staff.

The most common method of pain relief is epidural anaesthesia. A local anaesthetic is injected into the epidural space of the spinal cord through a tiny tube, or cannula, placed in the back. This is an extremely effective pain-killer, but does have a number of disadvantages. If the anaesthetic is injected incorrectly, the consequences can be extremely serious; some women find that the anaesthetic has no effect on them. The anaesthetic also relaxes the muscles of the pelvic region, so that the mother has to push harder than normal for a longer period, and has difficulty in feeling the progress that the baby is making. Though some women have strong opinions about epidural anaesthesia, and believe that it is often used unnecessarily, many mothers find the technique very useful, and some find it almost essential.

In some deliveries, the muscles and skin of the mother's perineum, the area around the vulva, are stretched to the point at which a tear in the tissues becomes inevitable. Normally, the doctor or midwife will prevent a tear by making a small cut, about 2.5cm (1in) long, in the perineum, called an episiotomy. This allows the passage of the baby's head, and is easily sewn up afterwards.

Recently, however, studies have shown that such surgical intervention may be unnecessary. It is thought that a tear may heal more quickly than an episiotomy, and may eradicate the risk, small though it is, that a surgical cut may interfere with the mother's future enjoyment of sex. Some doctors also claim that episiotomies are often performed unnecessarily, as a matter of habit and routine. There is considerable discussion about this theory, which is not yet generally accepted. In some hospitals, episiotomies are always performed, in others, a natural tear is permitted. The family doctor will be able to advise on the procedure at the local hospital.

Medical intervention is usually necessary, however, if the second stage of labour is so prolonged that doctors think that the health of the mother and baby will suffer. The delivery of a baby is extremely hard work. If it lasts for too long—over an hour for a first child, and half an hour for a second—the mother will be so exhausted that she is unable to continue. In such cases, the doctor or midwife will normally aid the delivery by the use of obstetric forceps. These are used to grip the baby's head gently, and to ease it out of the birth canal. A 'pudendal nerve block', in which anaesthetic is injected on either side of the vulva, is usually given before this happens. Occasionally, however, even the use of forceps is ineffective. In such cases, more wide-ranging surgical intervention is necessary, in the form of a Caesarian section.

After the birth

As soon as the baby is born, he or she is given to the mother to hold and cuddle. This often happens before the umbilical cord is clamped. At first, the baby is dusky in colour, and often covered with a greasy material called vernix. The doctor quickly calculates the baby's APGAR score—this is a rating system used to assess the breathing, heart rate, musculature, colour and reflexes of the newborn baby. If the score is low, the baby is taken from the mother and given special treatment.

Meanwhile the third stage of labour is under way. In this phase, the placenta, or afterbirth, is delivered quickly and painlessly. Around this time the umbilical cord joining the baby to the placenta is first clamped and then cut, so that the baby becomes completely dependent on his or her own systems—the lungs, for instance, take over the work of respiration.

Immediately after the delivery the mother feels extremely tired, and wants to rest. This is not easy, however, because breast feeding, if this method is to be used, starts almost immediately, as soon as the pituitary gland secretes prolactin. After a few days, the mother will be able to return home, unless there have been any complications. Many mothers feel depressed and unhappy for the first few days. This is quite normal, though often still underestimated, and is known as 'post baby blues'. Some women, however, are affected by serious feelings of depression, known as post partum depression, which can be dangerous and disruptive. The family doctor will be able to give help and advice in such cases.

Some women find that they lose their libido, or desire for sex, for many months after the birth of a baby. The problem is not helped by broken nights, breast feeding and the washing of hundreds of nappies. Libido returns eventually, however, usually when the baby starts to sleep through the night.

Six weeks after the birth, the mother should visit her family doctor. He will check the uterus, to see that it has returned to its former size and shape, and will also discuss contraception. The majority of women do not ovulate or have periods while they are breast feeding, but some do—the widely-held belief that mothers cannot become pregnant while breast feeding is totally incorrect. Mothers who are feeding their babies by bottle must also think about contraception before resuming sexual intercourse.

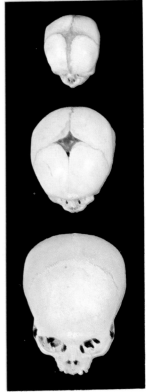

The skull of a newborn baby is made up of five bones that are held together by a flexible membrane *(top)*, allowing a small amount of movement. The six spaces, called fontanelles, where the rounded corners of the bones meet, are only covered by a membrane. The anterior fontanelles can be seen clearly in the front of the skull of an eight-month-old baby *(middle)*. The bones gradually fuse together until the skull becomes rigid at the age of about 18 months. The skull of a five-year-old *(bottom)* shows all six fontanelles closed.

Connections
Anaemia
Ante-partum haemorrhage
Breech presentation
Caesarian section
Congenital heart defect
Diabetes
Down's syndrome
Enema
Eclampsia
Epidural
Episiotomy
German measles — *see Rubella*
Gingivitis
Haemophilia
Hypertension
Placenta praevia
Post-partum depression
Rubella
Spina bifida
Varicose veins
Virus

THE LANGUAGE OF MEDICINE

THIS SECTION OF THE BOOK provides the key to the reader's understanding of medicine and the medical world. It outlines medical procedure and what can happen from the time you first consult your doctor to treatment in hospital. It details the principles of diagnosis, explains both the patient's and doctor's rights and shows how the medical world — from health centre to hospital — is organized to help you. Over 1,000 diseases, medical terms and medical tests are explained in A-Z listings, while, in addition to conventional treatments, there is also a guide to the basic therapies of alternative medicine.

The doctor, the patient and disease

For most people, the first point of contact with the medical world is the family doctor's surgery. The experience is often worrying and confusing. But with an understanding of the nature of disease and the process of diagnosis, a visit to the doctor can be reassuring and even interesting The following pages of this book explain what diseases and symptoms really are, follow the doctor as step-by-step he or she unravels the clues to reach a diagnosis, and show how the doctor and patient can best help each other.

Diseases and symptoms

A disease is normally defined as an abnormal condition of the body that has a specific cause and characteristic outward 'signs' and symptoms. Technically speaking, a 'sign' is considered to be an indication of a disease that is noticed by the doctor but not by the patient, while a symptom is something felt or perceived by the patient himself—but this distinction is often blurred in ordinary conversation.

The symptom with which a patient goes to see the doctor, or 'presents' in medical jargon, is often a pain, or a general feeling of ill-health. This symptom will probably only be one of a number of other indications of an illness that the doctor will discover by questioning his or her patient. At the same time, the doctor will notice any other indications of disease, or signs. When he or she comes to consider the meaning of the patient's signs and symptoms, the doctor has to bear in mind a number of other factors that combine to make the diagnosis of a disease an imprecise and complicated science.

One problem is that very few symptoms automatically indicate a specific disease—a 'tummy-ache', for example, may be a symptom of indigestion, an ulcer, a hiatus hernia, a kidney stone, pancreatitis, period pain or any number of other conditions. A pain in an organ, or particular part of the body, does not necessarily mean that the problem is a disease of that organ. It may be an indirect effect of a disease of another organ, or a whole system. In heart failure ,

a sufferer may visit the doctor complaining of severe shortness of breath—the lungs are congested with fluid because of the weak pumping-action of the heart. But shortness of breath could be the main symptom of a number of other major medical problems, such as asthma, bronchitis and anaemia . Sometimes pain is 'referred' from one part of the body to another, because of the proximity of nerve fibres in the spinal cord—pain from the gall bladder, for example, is occasionally felt in the left shoulder.

Hidden problems

The doctor must also bear in mind that a patient's general feeling of illness may be disguising a condition that does not directly cause pain—often because there is no sensory nerve supply (p32) to the affected area. Cancer of the bowel, for example, can be difficult to detect until its later stages, because there are no sensory nerves inside the bowel. Until the disease affects the lowest part of the bowel a few inches above the anus, where there are sensory nerves, the only outward signs may be weight loss, fatigue and blood in the stools. At the same time, one disease may lower the resistance of the body so that another infection takes hold. The doctor has to consider whether the symptoms caused by this secondary infection are masking the main problem.

Sometimes the patient's pain is not a symptom of a disease or illness at all, but psychosomatic . Many people find an expression of their worries and anxieties in physical pain. The process is not deliberate and the patient's discomfort is no less real for the lack of a physical cause. It does, however, cause difficulties for the doctor, who sometimes cannot rule out physical disease without thorough investigation, but must also be able to recognize patients' emotional problems and give counsel and advice.

Uncertainties

Finally, the doctor has to take into account the many different courses that a disease can take, and often the general lack of any precise scientific knowledge of that particular disease process. Every

person has a different level of resistance to disease, according to age, physique, diet, heredity and previous illnesses, and 'textbook cases' of a disease are not often seen. Even the most common illnesses show a wide variation in course and effect—the incubation period for measles is often said to be 10 days, but it can be anything between 8 and 13 days. Because of these variations it is very difficult, and very unwise, to make any categorical statements about medicine and disease. That is why in this and in other books about medicine the words 'may', 'sometimes', 'occasionally' and 'possibly' are often used. The practice reflects the uncertainty in the science of medicine itself.

Scientists sometimes do not know exactly how diseases work, or occasionally why cures for them work. Medical opinion about diseases is constantly changing, and each change is the result of years of research. Every new experimental result throws a different light on the subject, until eventually a new opinion about an area of medicine comes to be generally held.

With all these complicating factors it is perhaps surprising that doctors are ever able to make a diagnosis. Their ability to unravel the complexities and uncertainties of disease is a skill learned through experience and the many years of intensive training they must undergo before qualification. This is why self-diagnosis, performed by people without a solid background of training and experience, is at best misleading and at worst downright dangerous.

The doctor's diagnosis

Diagnosis—the process by which the doctor identifies the disease or problem that is causing the patient's symptoms—is similar to the art of detection. In a murder story the detective is presented with a number of clues at the outset, and gathers information by questioning suspects and by making his or her own investigations. Once all his information is complete, the detective separates the truth from fiction, discards misleading or irrelevant information and arrests the murderer. The family doctor

PHYSICAL EXAMINATION

During a visit to the doctor's surgery, you will be asked various questions about the symptoms of your complaint. The doctor will then examine you physically, using one or more of the instruments and tests outlined below. The results will help the doctor diagnose your complaint.

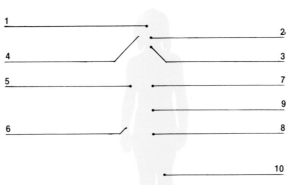
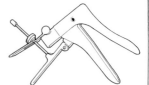
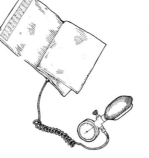

1 An ophthalmoscope enables the doctor to look inside your eyes and detect disorders of the lens and the retina. It shines a beam of light through the pupil and lens to the back of your eye and, at the same time, allows the doctor to see the spot where the light falls. The beam's width and the power of the ophthalmoscope's lens can be altered to suit the doctor's needs.

2 If you are shivery and cold, the doctor may suspect you have an infection and will take your temperature with a thermometer.

3 To examine the tonsils, glands and membranes of your throat, the doctor depresses your tongue with a spatula and shines a light into your mouth.

4 An otoscope or auriscope enables the doctor to examine your eardrum and the outer canal of your ear. The doctor pulls your ear upwards and backwards while shining the light from the otoscope down the canal to the eardrum. In this way, a boil, abscess or some other source of infection can be detected. The doctor may take a swab from your ear while tests may be performed to find out if your hearing is impaired.

5 A sphygmomanometer is an inflatable cuff joined by a tube to a graduated column of mercury or some other means of measuring blood pressure. The cuff is wrapped around your arm and inflated until the pulse ceases in the artery. As the cuff is deflated, the doctor listens with a stethoscope for the pulse. On its return two pressure readings are taken.

6 To measure your pulse rate per minute, the doctor lightly places two fingers on the artery in your wrist and counts the number of pulses he or she feels.

7 A stethoscope enables the doctor to listen to the sounds made by the movement of your heart and lungs. It consists of a diaphragm or an open cone-shaped attachment, through which sounds are relayed via two tubes to the doctor's ears. An alternative method is to use a technique called percussion, in which the doctor taps your chest or your back and senses the tone of the resulting vibrations. By this means, he or she can detect any build-up of fluid in the lungs or abdomen.

8 The doctor uses a speculum to hold open the vagina while he takes a smear from high up in the vagina or from the cervix. He examines the rectum to look for piles or for inflammation of the rectal membrane.

9 Lumps, swellings and cysts are detected by palpation, in which the abdomen and organs are felt with the hands and fingertips. In this way, the doctor can distinguish between a solid and a fluid-filled swelling, and can also feel the foetus in a woman's womb.

10 Symptoms such as double vision may suggest a nervous disorder to your doctor, who will test for this by tapping a tendon below the knee cap with a rubber hammer and seeing if a nervous reflex makes your leg kick.

GENERAL CHECKLIST

Your doctor will check and record other details, such as the shape of your nails, the colour of the inside of your lower eyelid and the condition of your gums. The doctor may check your weight against your height and may test your urine for sugar, protein, blood or other chemicals. A sample of blood may be taken, and sent to a laboratory for tests to see if its haemoglobin and sugar contents are normal. The doctor will look at the condition of your skin and tongue, your posture and for various other things, such as shortness of breath.

---

makes his diagnosis in a less dramatic, but equally effective way.

The doctor's first clue is the symptom with which the patient 'presents'. It is usually a pain, a physical problem or a general feeling of ill-health. The doctor will want to know about the pain in detail—where it is; whether it is constant or comes and goes; if it is related to any activity, such as eating or exercise; when it first came on and what type of pain it is. Pain can take a number of forms, and it is important that the doctor understands its exact nature. It is not enough for a patient to say that he has indigestion—the word means something different to almost everyone. The doctor will probably ask about the character of the pain—whether it is stabbing and severe, a dull ache, vice-like or throbbing.

After the doctor has discussed the patient's symptom, he will probably have a good idea of the general nature of the problem and will start to direct his questions towards the areas of disease that seem most likely. (It may, however, take a some time for this stage to be reached, because many people do not at first admit to their real worry.) The questions will be designed to elicit further symptoms that support the doctor's first impressions, and are likely to be associated with the patient's original complaint. If, for example, he suspects that the problem is in the digestive system *(p40)*, he will probably ask about abdominal pain; the frequency and consistency of

motions; whether there is nausea or vomiting and, if so, the details of the vomit's appearance and character; whether the patient's weight is increasing or decreasing; and many other questions.

Other factors

In the next stage of diagnosis, the doctor tries to relate the patient's symptom to a large number of other factors. He may ask questions that appear to be irrelevant. They are not, and it is important that they are answered truthfully and in full. What the doctor is trying to do is to obtain a clear picture of the patient's life-style, environment and relationships at work and at home. He is likely to ask whether the patient smokes or drinks, and if so how much; whether any patent

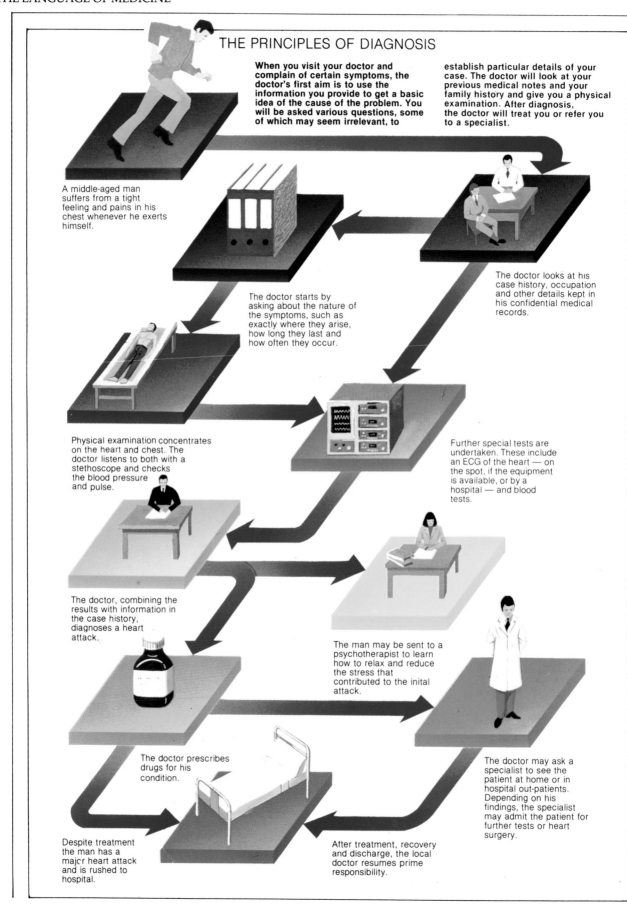

THE PRINCIPLES OF DIAGNOSIS

When you visit your doctor and complain of certain symptoms, the doctor's first aim is to use the information you provide to get a basic idea of the cause of the problem. You will be asked various questions, some of which may seem irrelevant, to establish particular details of your case. The doctor will look at your previous medical notes and your family history and give you a physical examination. After diagnosis, the doctor will treat you or refer you to a specialist.

A middle-aged man suffers from a tight feeling and pains in his chest whenever he exerts himself.

The doctor looks at his case history, occupation and other details kept in his confidential medical records.

The doctor starts by asking about the nature of the symptoms, such as exactly where they arise, how long they last and how often they occur.

Physical examination concentrates on the heart and chest. The doctor listens to both with a stethoscope and checks the blood pressure and pulse.

Further special tests are undertaken. These include an ECG of the heart — on the spot, if the equipment is available, or by a hospital — and blood tests.

The doctor, combining the results with information in the case history, diagnoses a heart attack.

The man may be sent to a psychotherapist to learn how to relax and reduce the stress that contributed to the inital attack.

The doctor prescribes drugs for his condition.

The doctor may ask a specialist to see the patient at home or in hospital out-patients. Depending on his findings, the specialist may admit the patient for further tests or heart surgery.

Despite treatment the man has a major heart attack and is rushed to hospital.

After treatment, recovery and discharge, the local doctor resumes prime responsibility.

THE DOCTOR, THE PATIENT AND DISEASE

medicines are used; if there are any peculiarities of diet. A female patient will be asked about the form of contraception, if any, that she uses, and about periods. If the patient has been attending the same family practice for some years, the doctor will probably have a record of the patient's medical history. If not, he will want to know about previous illnesses and operations—in fact he may ask anyway, to check that his notes are accurate. The medical history of the patient's family may also be discussed, because some diseases are to an extent hereditary.

The answers to all these questions are vitally important. If the doctor finds out that the patient is now or has been a miner, or has worked with asbestos, he may suspect a chest problem such as silicosis that he may otherwise have missed. Similarly, degeneration of the heart valves might be missed in its early stages if the patient does not tell the doctor about an attack of rheumatic fever during childhood.

During the conversation, the doctor will also be trying to assess the patient's state of mind. This is partly in an attempt to identify any mental illness, but more often to gauge the extent to which, in perfectly normal, well-balanced people, the symptoms are psychosomatic. He may ask tactful, but informative questions about work, social and sexual relationships, or use phrases such as 'do you have any special worries?', or 'what made you decide to come and see me at this time?' in an effort to draw the patient out. Often a doctor need go no further in his attempt to make a diagnosis, because the patient requires advice and counselling, not medical treatment.

Physical examination
If the doctor thinks that the patient's symptoms do have a physical cause, he will proceed to the next stage in the diagnostic process, the physical examination. To a certain extent he has been making a rough examination during the preceding conversation. The general appearance will have been noted, as well as the patient's dress, mannerisms, weight, build and state of nutrition; the doctor will also check the colour and texture of the skin and look for any 'facies', the facial expressions that are characteristic of some diseases.

Now the doctor performs a more detailed and specific examination, taking the patient's blood pressure with a pressure cuff, or

sphygmomanometer; taking the pulse and the temperature; listening to the heart and lung sounds with a stethoscope; checking the reflexes with a small rubber hammer; percussing the chest and abdomen by tapping two fingers held against the skin to detect the presence of fluid; palpating, or squeezing and prodding the abdomen and organs to feel for lumps, tenderness or rigidity. All these tests provide vital clues in the diagnosis of disease.

Eyes, ears, the nose and throat and the functions and coordination of individual muscles and joints may also be checked, and if necessary the doctor will perform a rectal or vaginal examination. All the time, he will be watching for any abnormalities of structure or function that may help his diagnosis. Some family doctors now have an electrocardiograph, or ECG machine, in their surgeries, so that the strength and timing of the heartbeat can be checked on the spot. This list of investigations may sound daunting, but it is unusual for them all to be performed on the same patient—normally only those that the doctor considers relevant to the patient's complaint are used.

Interpretation
By now, the doctor has a vast amount of information about the patient and the problem. The next stage of the diagnostic process is interpretation. The doctor must decide how much of the patient's condition can be explained by his environment, how much by mental attitude and how much by disease. There is little that the doctor can do himself about problems whose direct cause is the environment, apart from treating the symptoms and referring the patient to a welfare agency—though counselling may help. A child who continually suffers from wheezy bronchitis because of damp and dusty conditions at home may show a short-term improvement after treatment by a doctor, but in the long term a 'cure' may only be achieved when a family is rehoused. Sometimes the doctor will decide that a patient's condition has a psychological cause, and that the physical symptoms are psychosomatic. It is often difficult for the patient to accept this judgement—to him the pain is real, and there is a natural unwillingness to admit that psychological problems can be responsible. In the past, family doctors took a somewhat stern attitude to patients with such

problems; nowadays there is a general acceptance of the importance of the mind in medicine. Conditions such as depression are regarded as illnesses to be treated by advice, counselling and sometimes a course of drugs, and most doctors are highly trained in these skills. Often it is enough for the doctor to allow himself to be used as a sounding-board by the patient, to encourage him to talk his worries through and reach his own solutions. If the patient's state of mind is less amenable to counselling, and the condition is approaching neurosis or even psychosis, he may be referred to a consultant psychiatrist for specialist treatment such as psychotherapy

Treatment
More usually, the doctor decides that a particular illness is responsible for the patient's symptoms and starts on an appropriate course of treatment. Some people prefer not to know what is wrong with them, so the doctor may not volunteer any information about the nature of the disease, its possible course and the way in which the treatment will work, However, he will usually be only too happy to explain if the patient asks questions. Some diseases will require specialized treatment and nursing care of a type that the family doctor is not able or qualified to give. On these occasions the patient may be sent to to hospital, or to a specialist. Occasionally the doctor will ask for special tests to be made, because even some of the simplest diseases cannot always be diagnosed with certainty without laboratory tests —for some it is necessary to make an appointment at the local hospital, but the family doctor can himself forward samples of blood, urine and faeces to the laboratories *See Special Tests p.84.* Results are returned within a day or so.

This description of the diagnostic process has necessarily been simplified. It is perfectly possible, for example, for environment, psychology and disease to all play a part in the underlying cause of the patient's symptoms. It is quite common for a doctor not to know precisely what is wrong with a patient, but to be certain that the problem is minor and will clear up within a few days of its own accord. There are no rigid rules and no certainties—apart from one. Diagnosis, because of the variable and imprecise nature of diseases, symptoms, individuals and their

The Prescription Your doctor prescribes a drug, by writing a prescription which you then take to a pharmacist or dispensing chemist. You must pay a flat-rate charge unless you are under 16; a woman aged 60 or over; a man aged 65 or over; a holder of a Family Practitioner's Committee certificate, such as a woman with a newborn child; a holder of a prepayment certificate, such as a diabetic or a victim of a long-term illness; a war or service pensioner with an exemption certificate.

A traditional symbol for the word 'Recipe'. It means 'take thou' and is addressed to the pharmacist, but few doctors will write it on prescriptions.

If the patient is under 12, his or her age must be entered here.

The name and address of the patient are entered here by the doctor.

The doctor indicates here for how long the drug should be taken.

After filling a prescription, the pharmacist writes in this column the name and quantity of the drug dispensed. All prescriptions are sent each month to the office of the Pricing Bureau, who work out their cost, deduct the flat-rate charge and reimburse the pharmacist with the difference.

The official stamp gives the name of the Family Practitioners Committee and the name, address and telephone number of the doctor.

NP stands for 'nomen proprium' which is Latin for proper name. This tells the pharmacist to put either the brand name or the chemical name of the drug on the label on the container. If the doctor crosses out the NP, it tells the pharmacist to leave out the name of the drug.

The encircled number tells the pharmacist how many tablets to put into the container.

The Pricing Bureau makes notes in this column about the prescription and its cost once it has been received from the pharmacist.

Prescription form (FP10):

SURNAME Mr/Mrs/Miss — Smith

Age if under 12 years — Initials and one full forename — John R.

yrs mths — Address — 14 Wadsworth Villas, Newtown

Pharmacy Stamp

Pharmacist's pack & quantity endorsement — No. of days treatment NB Ensure dose is stated — NP — Pricing Office use only

Rx
Caps Amoxycillin 250mg Tabs (20)

Tabs Paracetamol
T̄ 4hrly p.r.n. (50)

Codeine Linctus BPC
5mls b.d (300ml)

Signature of Doctor — Date 13.4.83

For pharmacist No. of Prescns. on form — Ealing Hammersmith & Hounslow F.P.C.
106354
Dr J.J.Squires
228 HollyBush Centre
London W12
Tel - 749 1123/4

IMPORTANT: Read notes overleaf before going to pharmacy — Form FP10 (Rev. 81)

COMMONLY-USED ABBREVIATIONS

a.c. (ante cibum)	before food
b.d./b.i.d. (bis in die)	twice a day
o.d. (omni die)	every day
o.n. (omni nocte)	every night
p.c. (post cibum)	after food
p.r.n. (pro re nata)	as required
q.d.s.	four times a day
stat. (statim)	immediately
t.d.s.	three times a day
B.P.	British Pharmacopoeia
B.P.C.	British Pharmaceutical Codex
Tabs	tablets
Caps	capsules

A drug is specified by its generic (chemical) or trade name. Amoxycillin and paracetamol, for example, are generic names, while Amoxil and Panadol are the respective trade names. Each drug has only one generic name, but it may have several trade names since several pharmaceutical companies may manufacture it. If a doctor writes a generic name, he writes BP or BPC after it. This tells the pharmacist to prepare the drug according to the formula in either of these pharmaceutical recipe books. Controlled drugs, such as pethidine, must have their dosage and total quantities written in words and figures to prevent addicts from altering them. A line drawn under such prescriptions prevents the addition of extra items.

circumstances, is a highly skilled art.

Doctor and patient
One of the main problems that a family doctor faces is his lack of time. The Royal College of General Practitioners estimates that the average consultation takes around 5½ to 6 minutes. In this short time, the doctor must get to know the patient, make his diagnosis and consider a form of treatment. Of course most doctors will set aside much longer if a patient needs to talk about emotional problems, but nevertheless anything that helps the doctor to reach a diagnosis more quickly and certainly is of immense value—both to the doctor and the patient. At the same time, the patient must make it clear if he wants a full explanation from the doctor. A few simple rules that help the patient make the most of his visit to the doctor are given below:

1. Come to the point quickly. Do not tell the doctor about one minor symptom when your real worry is different. There is no point in being embarrassed—the doctor sees and hears the most extraordinary things every day. He is bound by confidentiality and is most unlikely to make any moral judgements. His job is to heal, to help and to give advice, not to preach.

2. Always answer the doctor's questions truthfully and fully. Never assume that the doctor already knows about every facet of your life or health—he sees hundreds of people every week and cannot remember everything about everyone. Never decide not to mention something that you think is irrelevant—you may be keeping a vital clue from him.

3. Never have preconceived ideas about the doctor's diagnosis—the innumerable factors to be taken into consideration make it most unlikely that you will be right.

4. Do not feel aggrieved if the treatment that the doctor prescribes is not what you expected. Every case is different, and many commonly held notions about medicine are nonsense. Antibiotics, for example, have absolutely no effect on virus infections, such as influenza. They are only given to people with 'flu if the doctor thinks that a bacterial infection might develop in a patient whose resistance is weakened.

5. If you want an explanation of the doctor's diagnosis and treatment, ask. After all, it is your body and possibly your life that is at stake. If, unusually, the doctor is not forthcoming, it is worth pressing the point.

6. Try to keep in touch with your family doctor. It is a great advantage if he is familiar with your work, environment and family background—besides, one of the great satisfactions in a family doctor's professional life is the health care of a community over the years and the personal relationships that develop.

7. Whenever in doubt, visit the doctor. It is silly, as well as discourteous, to wait until a problem is so bad that the doctor has to make an emergency home visit in the middle of the night. Even though many doctors make their own night calls, some use emergency deputies, who cannot be familiar with the case. Go to the doctor's surgery as soon as symptoms become apparent, or as soon as you have a worry—it is sensible to make a note of your symptoms so that you do not forget to mention one of them during the consultation.

THE DOCTOR'S RIGHTS

In National Health Service general practice, the doctor makes a contract with the government to look after the medical care of patients on his list. He agrees to see them at his surgery when they are ill, and to visit them at home when they are too unwell to come to the surgery. He must also agree to provide a 24-hour emergency service, though this does not always mean that he is on duty personally—a rota is normally agreed between the doctors in the practice, and sometimes a deputizing service is used.

1. The doctor has the right to refuse to sign a new patient onto his list, and is under no obligation to give a reason for his refusal. (In practice it is usually because the patient lives too far from the surgery, because the list is full, or because the patient has a difficult reputation.)

2. He has the right to remove a patient from his list, but must notify the Family Practitioner Committee before doing so, and must continue to treat the patient for 14 days.

3. As an extension of his duty to respect the confidentiality of his patients, the doctor has a duty to refuse to tell the parents of any child aged 16 or over details of the child's medical treatment unless specifically authorized to do so by the child. He also has the right to refuse to inform the parents of a girl under 16 about any contraceptive arrangements she may have made.

4. The doctor is under no obligation to supply medicines or a specific form of treatment that the patient may request—he has the right to do what he thinks is in the patient's best interests. If a patient asks to be referred for an abortion, the doctor has the right to refuse on grounds of conscience, even if there are medical grounds for the operation.

5. A doctor who operates an appointments system at his surgery has the right to refuse to see a patient who goes to the surgery without an appointment, provided that: there are no free appointments during surgery hours; the doctor is satisfied that the patient's health will not be put at risk by the delay; that the patient is offered an appointment within a reasonable time.

6. The doctor has the right to refuse to make a home visit outside normal working hours if he does not consider the situation an emergency—if he is wrong he may have to justify his decision to a disciplinary committee or a court.

7. The doctor has the right to refuse to show any patient the patient's medical records.

THE PATIENT'S RIGHTS

Everyone who lives in the United Kingdom has the right to be registered with a National Health Service general practitioner. (A person temporarily away from home, but within the UK, may register with a doctor in the area in which he or she is staying by visiting a surgery and completing the government form FP19.) If a doctor refuses to sign on a new patient *(see 'The doctor's rights')*, the person may appeal to the local Family Practitioner Committee, who will allocate him to a doctor's practice. Anyone who is not registered with a doctor may nevertheless insist that any doctor within his area treats him in an emergency—this practice is not, however, recommended. It is unfair to the doctor, who is paid according to the number of patients on his list, and unfair to the patient, because the doctor will know nothing about his medical history.

1. The patient has the right to be seen by his doctor without delay in the case of an emergency, and as soon as possible if his problem is not urgent. If the doctor runs an appointments system, the patient may make an appointment by telephoning the surgery; if not he may visit the surgery at any time during normal surgery hours in order to make an appointment.

2. Every patient aged 16 or over has the right to absolute confidentiality about his affairs, his problems and his treatment, unless the doctor is compelled to divulge such information by a court of law. However, in some cases the incidence of infectious or 'notifiable' disease and drug addiction must be notified to the authorities.

3. The patient has the right to consent to the doctor's treatment, except in special cases involving severe mental disturbance.

4. The patient has the right to change his doctor if for any reason he is not satisfied with his treatment. He should ask his doctor to sign his medical card, and then present this card to the new doctor that he has chosen. If the doctor refuses to sign the card, the patient should send it to the local Family Practitioner Committee with a letter of explanation. After a 14-day wait, the patient can then present the card, signed by the FPC, to his new doctor.

5. If a patient believes that a doctor has been incompetent, or has caused damage to his health, he may sue the doctor for damages. It is essential for the patient to obtain professional legal advice before taking this step.

6. The patient may make a written complaint to the Registrar of the General Medical Council if he considers that the doctor is guilty of one of the following forms of serious professional conduct: indecently assaulting a patient; having an 'adulterous or improper' relationship with a patient; showing gross professional negligence; breaching a patient's right to confidentiality; performing illegal abortions; advertising his services; attending a patient while under the influence of alcohol or drugs; or signing a sick-note without satisfying himself that the patient is ill. If the doctor is able to show that a patient has made such an allegation for malicious reasons, he may sue for defamation.

7. If a patient has a less serious complaint about a doctor, he has the right to appeal to the Family Practitioner Committee, who will attempt to resolve the problem.

8. If a patient is not satisfied with the treatment he is receiving from his doctor, he has the right to ask for a second opinion. Usually this will be given by another doctor in the practice, but sometimes a specialist may be consulted.

9. Normally a patient must consult his family doctor in order to obtain any form of medical treatment, but in the case of family planning the patient may go directly to a Family Planning Clinic .
The FP Clinic will not inform the family doctor of a patient's contraceptive arrangements unless the patient gives her permission— but to withhold such permission is unwise.

Surgeries and Health centres

The conventional idea of the doctor's surgery consisting of just a doctor, receptionist and nurse and being held in a private house is rapidly becoming out of date. Many modern practices are centred around purpose-planned health centres, in which the doctor is supported by a team of health care specialists and social workers.

Health centres are normally run by two or more doctors, who have teamed together to form a group practice. The staffing and facilities available obviously vary from example to example — many group practices will not have all the facilities described here available on the spot and will refer patients to the local hospital for some of them. The supporting staff normally include nurses, health visitors, social workers, a chiropodist, speech therapist, dietician, dentist, dental hygienist, educational psychologist and midwife. In both health centres and group practices, there are also special clinics, such as ante-natal, diabetic, family planning and well-baby clinics.

If you need to see a doctor, you should either make an advance appointment with the receptionist, or, as is the case with some doctors, simply walk into the surgery, check in at reception and wait your turn in the waiting room. When you are called, you will have a consultation with the doctor, who, after an initial examination, may send you along to the nurses for some tests. These can include a blood test, blood pressure test and an electrocardiogram (ECG) of the heart. The doctor may later refer you to one of the other specialists in the clinic — one doctor may run the ante-natal classes, for instance — the social worker, the health visitor or to your local hospital.

If you are housebound, or very ill at home, the doctor or health visitor will make a house call. Even when the surgery is closed, the practice, by law, has to offer, or be linked to, an emergency service, so providing 24-hour medical care for its patients. The doctor will also ask the district nurse to visit regularly and help with dressings and bathing. If needed, he or she will also arrange for a home help to do some shopping and cleaning once or twice a week through the social worker.

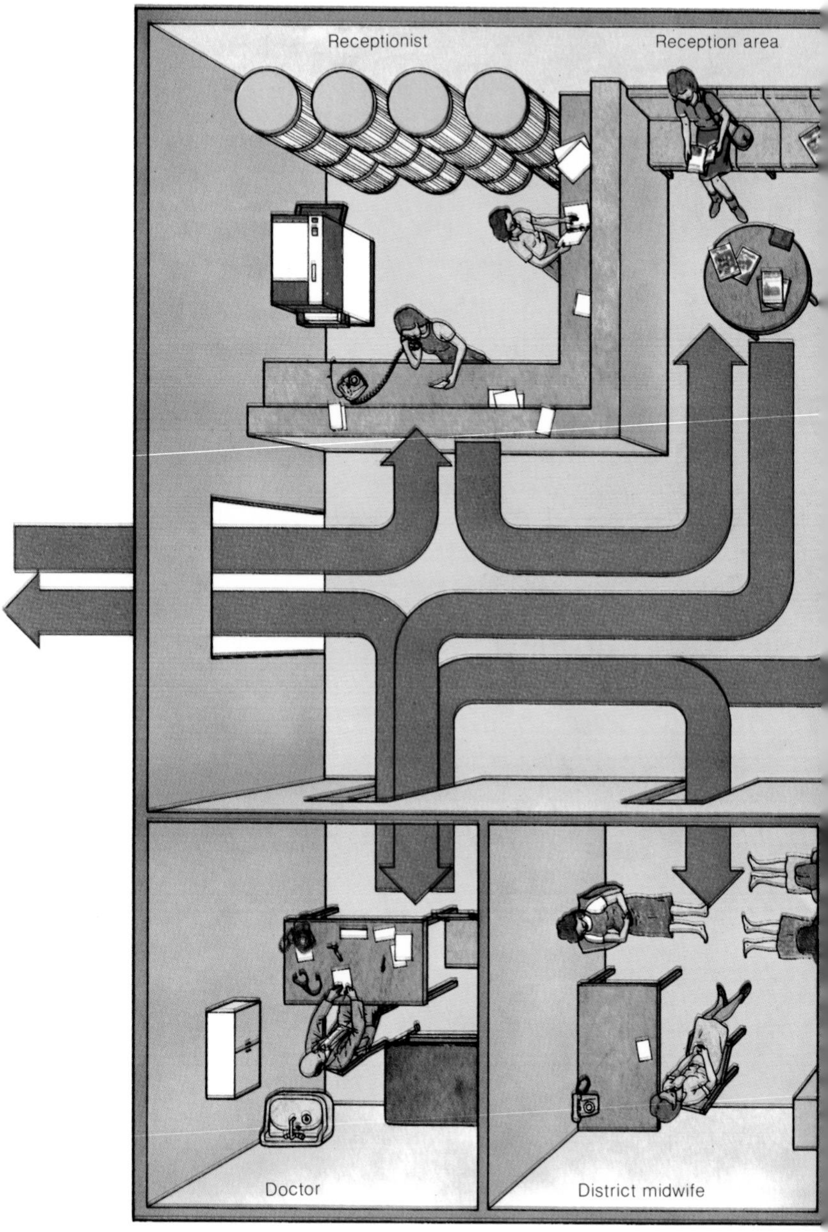

Receptionist Reception area

Doctor District midwife

The first person you see when you walk into the health centre will be the receptionist. Receptionists are responsible for filing your medical records and arranging appointments for you, either over the telephone or on your arrival at the centre. It is best to arrange an appointment in advance, since this will cut down the amount of time you may have to wait. From the reception area, you will be channelled to the doctor, when he or she is free. Doctors are the core of the centre's team. They give advice and treat minor illnesses, such as coughs, colds and 'flu, while their preliminary diagnosis of major problems can be invaluable to the specialist they will refer you to at the local hospital. In addition to their work at the centre, they pay frequent house calls, while they also run special clinics, such as the family planning clinic and the well-baby clinic. Having completed an examination, the doctor will pass you on to the next appropriate member of the centre's health team. Often, this will be the practice nurse, who, among other things, removes stitches,

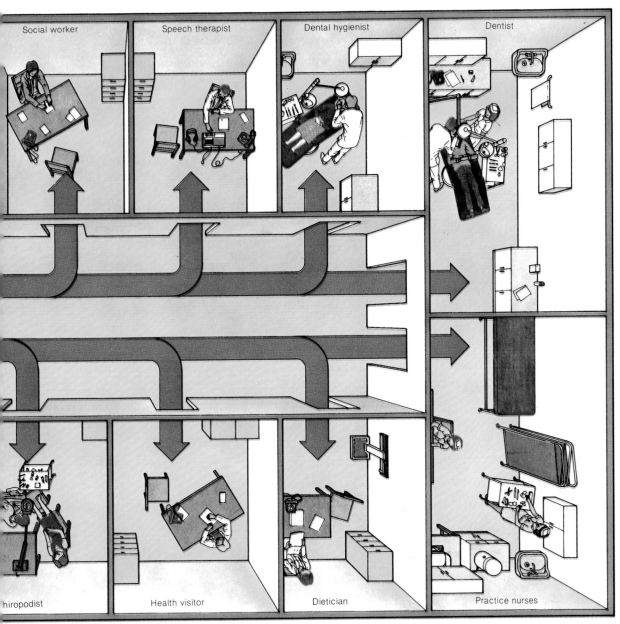

Social worker Speech therapist Dental hygienist Dentist

Chiropodist Health visitor Dietician Practice nurses

changes dressings, takes blood
pressures and gives vaccinations.
She is supported by a health
visitor, a trained nurse who looks
after children up to the age of
five, and a midwife, who cares
for pregnant women. She runs
ante-natal classes and is
responsible for routine medical
checks, such as urine tests and
weight monitoring. Other
supporting specialists include
dentists, dental hygienists,
chiropodists, speech therapists
and dieticians. Dental hygienists
care for teeth and gums by
cleaning and polishing them.

They offer general practical
advice on correct dental hygiene,
showing you how to clean your
teeth properly, and will probably
recommend you use a certain
type of toothbrush, toothpaste
and dental floss. Chiropodists
specialise in the care of feet.
They deal with problems such as
in-growing toe nails, callouses,
verrucas and corns, and provide
special foot care for diabetics
and the elderly. Speech
therapists prescribe and
demonstrate exercises to help
adults and children with speech
impediments, while dieticians are

trained nutritionists, who advise
people with certain diseases,
such as diabetes, on the form of
special diet they require. Social
workers help to deal with welfare
problems, cases of child abuse
and the elderly.

Hospital organization

Hospitals can be frightening places in the abstract. This feature shows what can happen to you when you attend one — either as an in-patient or an out-patient — and how everything is organized to provide the appropriate medical or surgical care.

There are several ways in which you can attend a hospital. One of these — probably the most common — is through a reference from your normal doctor, when he or she requires a specialist opinion on a potential medical or surgical problem. This involves your attendance at the appropriate out-patient clinic, where the specialist will examine you and perhaps send you for special tests, such as X-rays in the radiography department or a blood count in the haematology laboratory. After this, the specialist decides whether to treat you as an out-patient, refer you back to your doctor to continue treatment with the benefit of the specialist's advice, or to arrange for your admission to hospital.

Urgent cases — people injured in an accident, say, or suffering from sudden acute pain — go to the accident and emergency department, or casualty. Again, they can be referred there by their own doctors — in such cases, the result is often an emergency admission — or go there independently. There, you will be examined and either treated and discharged, or admitted.

All hospitals broadly follow this pattern, though they can differ widely in the range of facilities they offer. Some specialist hospitals, for instance, only treat one form of disease, such as cancer. Other, smaller hospitals may not possess an accident and emergency department, or an X-ray unit, of their own. In addition to the strictly medical services mentioned above, many other hospitals have additional facilities, such as physiotherapy departments and various after-care services, such as welfare departments and occupational therapy.

Once you have been admitted to hospital, life follows a fairly set routine in the majority of cases. The specialist you saw in out-patients will normally be in charge of your case, supported by his junior colleagues.

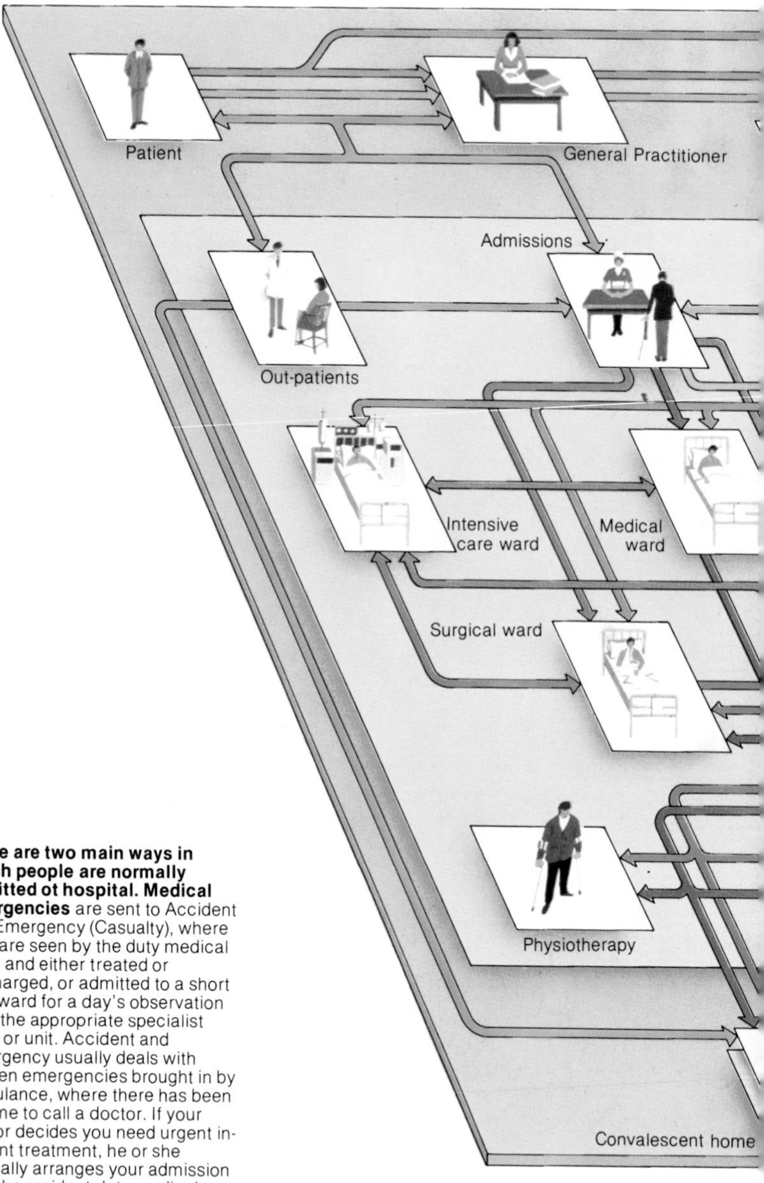

Patient

General Practitioner

Admissions

Out-patients

Intensive care ward

Medical ward

Surgical ward

Physiotherapy

Convalescent home

There are two main ways in which people are normally admitted ot hospital. Medical emergencies are sent to Accident and Emergency (Casualty), where they are seen by the duty medical team and either treated or discharged, or admitted to a short stay ward for a day's observation or to the appropriate specialist ward or unit. Accident and Emergency usually deals with sudden emergencies brought in by ambulance, where there has been no time to call a doctor. If your doctor decides you need urgent in-patient treatment, he or she normally arranges your admission with the resident duty medical or surgical specialists. You will be taken directly to the appropriate ward as a rule, though the specialist may make an initial examination in Accident and Emergency.

Out-patient cases are referred by their own doctors to specialists for advice and further treatment in the appropriate out-patient clinic. Such clinics cover every medical and surgical field; they include clinics devoted to General Medicine, Gynaecology, Chest Clinics, ENT (Ear, Nose and Throat) Clinics, Orthopaedic Clinics and so on. Every specialist examines his or her patients —

often with the back-up of special tests conducted by the hospital laboratories and X-rays — and either treats them on the spot and refers them back to their own doctors for further treatment, or continues treatment in follow-up clinics, or arranges admission to hospital. Normally, such patients are placed on a waiting list until beds are available to them.

Each specialist has a number of beds allocated in the appropriate wards. Surgical wards take in all adult surgical admissions, with the exception of gynaecological cases. The range of surgical problems treated in them can vary

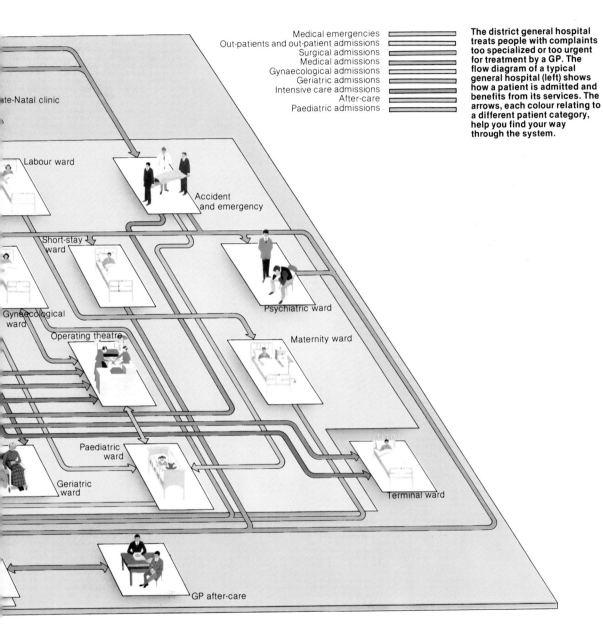

Medical emergencies
Out-patients and out-patient admissions
Surgical admissions
Medical admissions
Gynaecological admissions
Geriatric admissions
Intensive care admissions
After-care
Paediatric admissions

te-Natal clinic

Labour ward

Accident
and emergency

Short-stay
ward

Gynaecological
ward

Psychiatric ward

Operating theatre

Maternity ward

Paediatric
ward

Geriatric
ward

Terminal ward

GP after-care

The district general hospital treats people with complaints too specialized or too urgent for treatment by a GP. The flow diagram of a typical general hospital (left) shows how a patient is admitted and benefits from its services. The arrows, each colour relating to a different patient category, help you find your way through the system.

widely; examples include cases of hernia and varicose veins to orthopaedic conditions.

After treatment, patients are usually discharged as soon as they have sufficiently recovered. After leaving hospital, they are followed up by the specialist who treated them in out-patients, together with their own doctors. Alternatively, especially in cases of major surgery, patients may be transferred to a Convalescent Home. Old people may be moved to a geriatric ward, while people who are fatally ill may be moved to a terminal ward, or, more often, to a separate hospice.

After treatment, the hospital back-up services offer help in recovery, if necessary. These services include physiotherapy, occupational therapy, speech therapy and so on. Often they are concentrated in a rehabilitation centre, which treats both in-patients and out-patients.

Medical admissions follow very much the same route. Like surgical cases, the range of medical problems can vary widely, from heart attacks and strokes to bronchitis, pneumonia and other chest conditions. Heart attack cases are often initially admitted to the Coronary Care Unit, which

provides specialist treatment for heart attack victims and post-operative support for people who have had heart operations. This unit is attached to the Intensive Care Unit, which treats serious accident cases and people recovering from operations

Other important wards include those allocated to psychiatric cases, gynaecology, paediatrics and geriatrics. Gynaecological patients can suffer from diseases ranging from infertility to menstrual problems and uterine cancer; the department usually has obstetric beds attached to it in a labour ward. Paediatrics are

young children under the age of 12 who require surgical or long-term medical treatment. The paediatric wards may have a Special Care Baby Unit attached to them. There, premature babies, or those born with congenital abnormalities, can receive specialist intensive treatment. Geriatric patients, on the other hand, largely consist of people aged 75 or more. They frequently suffer from senile dementia, a chronic incapacitating disease such as arthritis, or are simply incapable of looking after themselves independently.

A hospital who's who

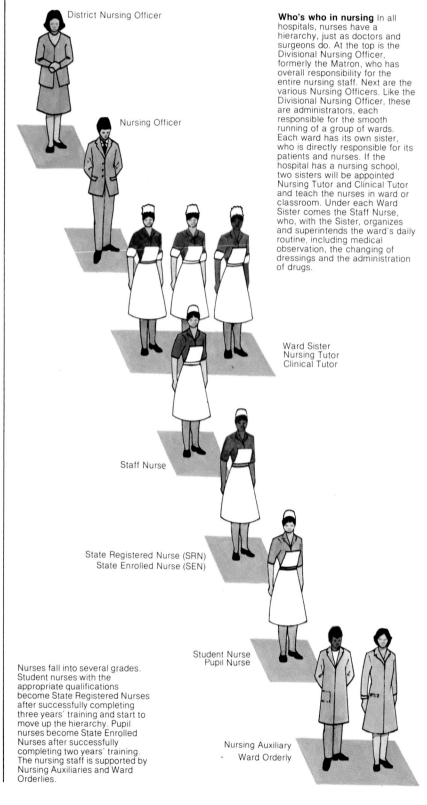

District Nursing Officer

Nursing Officer

Ward Sister
Nursing Tutor
Clinical Tutor

Staff Nurse

State Registered Nurse (SRN)
State Enrolled Nurse (SEN)

Student Nurse
Pupil Nurse

Nursing Auxiliary
Ward Orderly

Nurses fall into several grades. Student nurses with the appropriate qualifications become State Registered Nurses after successfully completing three years' training and start to move up the hierarchy. Pupil nurses become State Enrolled Nurses after successfully completing two years' training. The nursing staff is supported by Nursing Auxiliaries and Ward Orderlies.

Who's who in nursing In all hospitals, nurses have a hierarchy, just as doctors and surgeons do. At the top is the Divisional Nursing Officer, formerly the Matron, who has overall responsibility for the entire nursing staff. Next are the various Nursing Officers. Like the Divisional Nursing Officer, these are administrators, each responsible for the smooth running of a group of wards. Each ward has its own sister, who is directly responsible for its patients and nurses. If the hospital has a nursing school, two sisters will be appointed Nursing Tutor and Clinical Tutor and teach the nurses in ward or classroom. Under each Ward Sister comes the Staff Nurse, who, with the Sister, organizes and superintends the ward's daily routine, including medical observation, the changing of dressings and the administration of drugs.

All hospitals vary in size, in the number and type of their wards and in the kind of service they offer. Every hospital ward, however, has its set routine, carefully planned to give its patients the appropriate medical or surgical care.

If you become an in-patient, remember that the staff of the hospital are there not only to help you, but many other patients as well. Your full co-operation with the hospital staff and observance of the ward routine is therefore essential, even if some aspects of the routine seem fussy, inconvenient or unnecessary. Make sure you bring necessary items, such as nightwear, slippers, dressing gown, flannel, soap, towel, toothbrush, toothpaste and a hairbrush and comb, with you. Bring something to occupy your time, such as a book, though you can also use the hospital library service. Remember to bring some money, too, so that you can buy newspapers, magazines and — if your treatment allows — sweets.

The daily routine varies from ward to ward. Surgical wards generally have a high turn-over of patients, who move to and from the operating theatres and need intensive nursing. On the other hand, patients in a geriatric ward do not have their temperatures, blood pressures and pulses taken regularly. The emphasis is on rehabilitation, occupational therapy and physiotherapy. The children in a paediatric ward spend much of the day with their mothers, or playing under play leaders. There may also be teachers for children.

Whatever its speciality, each ward is usually visited by consultants at least twice a week. These ward rounds are the main medical event of the week. They may be at any time, although they normally follow a fixed routine. The consultant is accompanied by the registrar, the senior house officer, the ward sister and nurses. Together, they examine the medical observation charts, X-rays and other medical notes made on each patient and assess his or her progress. In a teaching hospital, they will be accompanied by medical students, although a patient has the right to refuse student examination.

THE HOSPITAL DAY

Patient Activity	Medical Observations	Food and Drink	Drugs and Medication	Consultant's and Doctor's Rounds
06.30 Patients woken. Routine laboratory samples, such as urines, are collected.				
	06.45 Routine observations, including taking pulse, and temperature made.			
		07.00 Breakfast, except for patients scheduled for surgery under general anaesthetic.		
			07.30 Medication round. This may be before breakfast.	
	08.45 Transfer of patients for routine X-rays starts.			**08.45** Houseman's round. He or she attends the ward as required during the day.
				10.00 Consultant's round. The frequency of this varies, but is at least once a week.
10.30 In surgical wards, transfer of patients to operating theatres in full swing.				
		12.00 Lunch. Normally a choice of menu, except for patients on special diets.		
	12.30 Routine observations, including taking pulse, and temperature made.			
12.45 Patients encouraged to rest after lunch and before afternoon visiting.			**12.45** Second medication round.	
14.00 Afternoon visiting starts. This may be for two hours or continue until early evening.				
14.30 Patients in need of treatment may be transferred to the appropriate department.				
		16.00 Afternoon tea.		
	18.00 Routine observations, including taking pulse, and temperature made.			
			18.15 Third medication round.	
		19.00 Supper. Choice follows the same routine as lunch.		
20.00 Visiting ends. In some wards, this may be earlier; in others later.				
		21.00 Night drink, either hot or cold.		
	21.30 Routine observations, including taking pulse, and temperature made.			
			22.00 Night medication round. Sleeping tablets may be issued.	

The daily hospital routine varies according to the ward and the intensity of the nursing. In a surgical ward, for example, there is a high turn-over of patients, going to and from the operating theatres and physiotherapy. Patients due to have an operation must go without food from midnight on the day before; on returning from theatre, the patient's pulse and blood pressure are taken frequently to make sure there is no blood loss. Surgical paatients have dressings that need changing, drips, naso-gastric tubes or catheters and therefore need considerable nursing.

Who's who in medicine and surgery

The diagrams here show what the main medical personnel of a hospital are called and what they do. Medical students qualify after five years of study. They then spend a year as House Officers, six months on the surgical side and six months on the medical. They then become Senior House Officers and start to specialize. After two or three years, they can either apply for an appointment as a hospital Registrar, or leave the hospital for general practice. After specializing for a few years, a Registrar can apply for a post as Senior Registrar and then for a job as a Consultant in his or her particular field. At each stage, further professional examinations can be taken.

Some of the many different consultant physicians (*top right*) and surgeons (*top left*) are listed here. Each consultant is responsible for diagnosing and treating diseases and disorders of one particular part of the body. The diagram also shows some of the key members of two related branches of medicine, the paramedics and the pathologists.

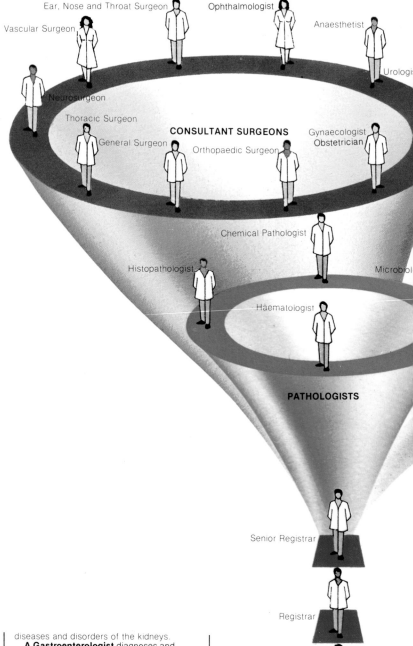

Vascular Surgeon · Ear, Nose and Throat Surgeon · Ophthalmologist · Anaesthetist · Urologi · Neurosurgeon · Thoracic Surgeon · **CONSULTANT SURGEONS** · General Surgeon · Orthopaedic Surgeon · Gynaecologist Obstetrician · Chemical Pathologist · Histopathologist · Microbiol · Haematologist · **PATHOLOGISTS**

Senior Registrar

Registrar

Senior House Officer

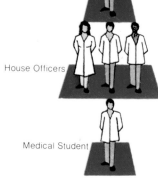

House Officers

Medical Student

CONSULTANT PHYSICIANS

Consultant Physicians are concerned with the medical treatment of disorders and diseases.

A **Chest Physician** diagnoses and treats disorders of the lungs and chest.

A **Neurologist** diagnoses and treats diseases and disorders of the nervous system that have a physical cause.

A **Cardiologist** diagnoses and treats diseases and disorders of the heart.

A **Dermatologist** diagnoses and treats skin diseases and disorders.

A **Venereologist** diagnoses and treats venereal diseases.

An **Ophthalmologist** diagnoses and treats eye diseases and disorders.

An **Endocrinologist** diagnoses and treats diseases and disorders of the endocrine glands and their hormones.

A **Psychiatrist** diagnoses and treats mental and emotional illness.

A **Nephrologist** diagnoses and treats diseases and disorders of the kidneys.

A **Gastroenterologist** diagnoses and treats diseases and disorders of the stomach and intestines.

A **Rheumatologist** diagnoses and treats diseases of the joints.

A **Paediatrician** specializes in the diseases, disorders and development of children.

A **Radiologist** takes X-rays and interprets them for diagnostic and investigative purposes.

A **Geriatrician** specializes in the care of the elderly and their related problems.

CONSULTANT SURGEONS

Consultant Surgeons are concerned with the surgical treatment of disorders and diseases.

An **Obstetrician** specializes in the care of women and babies during pregnancy, birth and post-natally for around six weeks.

An **Anaesthetist** specializes in anaesthetics, the treatment of surgical

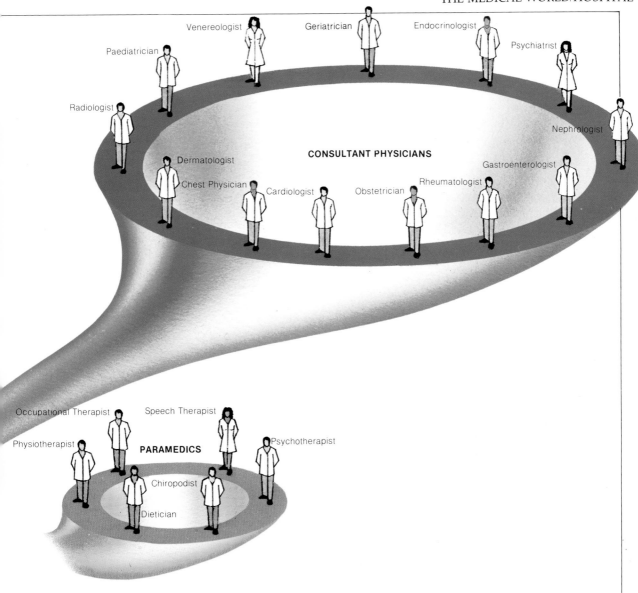

Paediatrician

Venereologist

Geriatrician

Endocrinologist

Psychiatrist

Radiologist

Nephrologist

CONSULTANT PHYSICIANS

Dermatologist

Gastroenterologist

Chest Physician

Cardiologist

Obstetrician

Rheumatologist

Occupational Therapist

Speech Therapist

Physiotherapist

Psychotherapist

PARAMEDICS

Chiropodist

Dietician

shock and the relief of post-operative pain.

A Urologist diagnoses and treats diseases and disorders of the urinary tract.

A Gynaecologist specializes in diseases and disorders of the female reproductive system and family planning.

An Orthopaedic Surgeon specializes in surgical treatment of bone defects and disorders, whether these are caused by disease, injury or age.

A General Surgeon performs operations which lie outside the specialized fields of the other surgeons listed here.

An Thoracic Surgeon is a specialist in chest (thorax) and lung surgery.

A Neurosurgeon specializes in the surgical treatment of diseases of the brain and spinal cord.

A Vascular Surgeon is a specialist in the diseases of the vascular system of the blood vessels, including the arteries and veins.

An Ear, Nose and Throat Surgeon specializes in the diseases and disorders of the ear, nose and throat and of the sinuses and channels which link them together.

PARAMEDICS

Paramedics are not medically qualified, but are trained in specialized fields relating to health care.

A Speech Therapist specializes in the treatment of speech disorders and defects.

A Psychotherapist counsels victims of psychological disorders, helping them to reach an understanding of themselves and come to terms with the problems caused by the disorder.

A Chiropodist diagnoses and treats disorders of the feet, such as corns and in-growing toe-nails. He also gives advice about foot care.

An Occupational Therapist helps to rehabilitate patients with mental and physical disabilities, by taking them through therapeutic courses of work and activity.

A Physiotherapist helps to rehabilitate patients recovering from broken limbs or brain damage by using such techniques as manipulation and movement therapy.

A Dietician specializes in nutrition and organizes a diet to suit special needs, as in the case of a diabetic.

PATHOLOGISTS

Pathologists provide the laboratory back-up to clinical diagnosis and play a vital part in the prevention and detection of disease.

A Microbiologist isolates and identifies the micro-organisms that cause disease.

A Histopathologist analyzes the tissue samples collected in biopsies and performs autopsies. His results help in the diagnosis of a disease.

A Chemical Pathologist analyzes the substances found in the body from samples of blood, urine and faeces. The results are a vital contribution to the diagnosis of disease.

A Haematologist specializes in the study of blood and bone marrow. He establishes the number and character of the different blood cells and helps in the diagnosis of diseases such as anaemia and leukaemia.

Special tests and laboratory investigations

The greatest medical advance in this century has been the development of supporting technology to aid both diagnosis and treatment of disease. The range and variety of special tests is very wide—the number of blood tests alone runs into dozens—all for the purpose of helping the doctor to find out what is wrong with you.

Some tests are used solely to monitor the performance of a particular organ; others are screens, used to eliminate possible problems from consideration; others are used in combination to provide complementary clues to effective diagnosis. The majority of tests are performed in laboratories, on samples of the different types of tissue and body fluids. Generally these can be taken in the family doctor's surgery, but sometimes a visit to hospital is necessary.

Words in *italic* type indicate a cross-reference to another entry within the A-Z of Special Tests, or to the first page of a section within The Systems of the Body or You and Your Health.

ALPHA FOETOPROTEIN—See Blood tests

AMNIOCENTESIS

A method for obtaining a sample of amniotic fluid, which surrounds the foetus in the womb—*see Embryology, p12.* The chemical composition of the fluid is changed by certain diseases of the foetus, such as haemolytic disease of the newborn and spina bifida, and the chromosomal make-up of cells within the fluid is abnormal in conditions such as Down's syndrome. These abnormalities can be detected by chemical analysis of the fluid, and microscopic examination of the cells. Since some disorders are only inherited by men, the sex of the foetus is established during these tests.

The test is not routinely performed on all expectant mothers. Doctors recommend that an amniocentesis is carried out on all expectant mothers who have a high risk of giving birth to an abnormal baby. This group includes women over 37; women who have have previously given birth to an abnormal baby; and women who have a family history of inherited birth defects.

Normally, the test is performed between the 14th and 18th weeks of pregnancy; the exact age of the foetus is determined beforehand, by means of an *ultrasound scan*, because the level of chemicals in the amniotic fluid varies with the age of the foetus. The procedure for an amniocentesis is straightforward, and does not normally involve a stay in hospital. Under local anaesthesia, a needle is pushed through the skin of the abdomen, into the uterus and through the thin membrane of the amniotic sac. The position of the needle is carefully monitored, by means of an ultrasound scan, so that the foetus is not injured. A sample of fluid is drawn off, the needle is withdrawn from the abdomen, and a dressing applied to the skin. Amniocentesis now carries virtually no risk to the mother, and a one per cent risk of damage to the foetus.

The test results do not become available for several days. If any serious abnormalities are discovered, the implications of the disorder, and the possible options, are fully discussed with the parents. In some cases, one option is to terminate the pregnancy by means of an abortion.

See also transcervical aspiration..

ANGIOGRAPHY, AORTOGRAPHY, ARTERIOGRAPHY—see X-rays

AUDIOGRAM—see Hearing test

BENCE-JONES PROTEIN—see Urine tests

BIOPSY

The removal of a small amount of body tissue for laboratory examination.

Different biopsy techniques are used, depending on which part of the body is involved. The tissue sample obtained may also be treated in one of two ways. Generally, it is treated with preservative chemicals and embedded in a wax block. This is then cut into extremely thin slices, called sections. Sections are mounted on a slide, stained, in order to show up the characteristics under investigation, and examined under a microscope by a histopathologist *(p82).*

This procedure takes several days.

On occasions, however, results are needed more quickly. During an operation, for example, the surgeon may need to know whether a tumour contains malignant tissue within a matter of minutes. In such cases, a sample of the tissue is very thinly sliced and frozen—the technique is called frozen section biopsy. The section is immediately examined under a microscope. If malignant cells are detected, the surgeon then removes the cancerous tissue.

Digestive tract biopsy Samples of tissue from the digestive tract may be taken in the investigation of a number of diseases, including ulcers, colonic cancer and colitis. A variety of techniques are used, depending on the portion of the tract that is involved. In all cases, however, the digestive tract must be clear of undigested food and faeces. Patients must fast overnight before the procedure, and their bowels may be emptied by means of an enema. They may be admitted to hospital and placed on a liquid diet. Since there are few pain sensors in the intestinal wall — *see The Nervous System, p32* — the procedure is usually painless. Any discomfort caused by the equipment used can be relieved by mild sedation.

A biopsy of tissue in the upper digestive tract — the oesophagus, the stomach and the duodenum, *see The Digestive System, p40* — is usually carried out in conjunction with gastroscopy — *see endoscopy.* If the doctor sees an area of inflammation or an ulcerous lesion through the gastroscope, he or she pushes a wire down the tube. Two small, shell-shaped cutters at the end of the wire are operated by a lever; they cut off a piece of tissue about the size of a large pin-head.

Biopsies of tissue from the small intestine — the jejunum and ileum, *(p40)* — are carried out by means of a device called a Crosby capsule. This is a small metal capsule attached to a thin tube. The capsule is swallowed and passes through the stomach and duodenum to reach the small intestine, its position being monitored by an X-ray. When the capsule reaches the correct position, suction is applied to the end of the tube. This activates the capsule, which opens up, removing a small piece of tissue from the intestinal lining. The procedure takes around one to one and a half hours.

A biopsy may be performed anywhere in the large intestine by means of a colonoscope, or in the rectum and lower colon *(p40)* by means of a sigmoidoscope — *see endoscopy.* As in an upper digestive tract biopsy, a wire is passed through the fibre-optic instrument. By this means, polyps can be removed without the need for further surgery. This procedure takes around an hour. There may be some discomfort, and afterwards there is sometimes a small quantity of blood in the stools.

Bone biopsy A sample of bone may be taken as part of the investigation of a number of diseases in which the chemical composition of bone or the function of the bone marrow is affected — *see Bone and Muscle, p16.* The substance of bone may be affected, for example, in serious kidney disease and osteomalacia; the marrow is affected in leukaemia and anaemia. Two different procedures are used, depending on whether

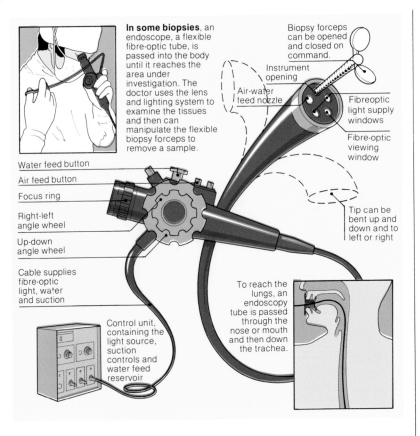

In some biopsies, an endoscope, a flexible fibre-optic tube, is passed into the body until it reaches the area under investigation. The doctor uses the lens and lighting system to examine the tissues and then can manipulate the flexible biopsy forceps to remove a sample.

Biopsy forceps can be opened and closed on command.

Instrument opening

Air-water feed nozzle

Fibreoptic light supply windows

Fibre-optic viewing window

Tip can be bent up and down and to left or right

Water feed button
Air feed button
Focus ring
Right-left angle wheel
Up-down angle wheel
Cable supplies fibre-optic light, water and suction

Control unit, containing the light source, suction controls and water feed reservoir

To reach the lungs, an endoscopy tube is passed through the nose or mouth and then down the trachea.

stained and cultured to discover the precise nature of any infections.

Renal biopsy A sample of kidney tissue is generally taken to discover the precise nature and course of conditions such as nephrotic syndrome, glomerulonephritis and unexplained kidney failure. This is because each of these problems may occur in different ways, requiring different treatment. The patient is admitted to hospital, and the size and condition of the affected kidney is established through *X-rays*. A local anaesthetic is given, and a biopsy needle passed into the kidney through the lower back, guided by X-rays or *ultrasound*. A small piece of tissue is removed, specially stained and examined under a microscope.

Skin and muscle biopsies Samples of skin are taken for staining and microscopic examination in order to determine the precise nature of a rash. The biopsy is taken in an out-patient clinic, under a local anaesthetic. A small piece of the full thickness of skin *(p16)* is taken from the affected site, and the incision closed with a single stitch. Muscle biopsies are more rare, but may be taken to aid in the diagnosis of a muscle-wasting disease, such as muscular dystrophy. A small piece of muscle is taken, usually from a thigh, under local anaesthesia.

Synovial biopsy A sample of synovium, the smooth, moist membrane surrounding a joint — see *Bone and Muscle, p16* — may be taken in cases of severe joint inflammation when the diagnosis is in doubt. Generally, the problem is some form of arthritis, but on rare occasions a synovial tumour or tuberculosis may be responsible. A biopsy needle is pushed into the joint, under local anaesthetic, and a small piece of synovial membrane removed with some synovial fluid. The fluid is *cultured* to detect any signs of infection, and the tissue is stained and examined under a microscope.

BLOOD TESTS

Blood tests play an important part in the diagnosis of many diseases. The sample of blood is taken from a vein—the exception being a test of blood gases, where arterial blood is taken, *see p86*. The most common sites are the front of the elbow—called the antecubital fossa—and the back of the hand. In babies, blood is often taken from veins in the scalp.

The procedure is quick and painless, and can be carried out in the family doctor's surgery. (In hospital, blood samples may be taken by specially trained paramedics called phlebotomists, or venesectionists). A tourniquet is placed on the upper arm to make the veins stand out and the area is cleaned with a small piece of cotton wool soaked in alcohol. A thin, sharp needle is then pushed through the skin and into the vein, and blood is withdrawn through the syringe. Some patients feel slightly faint while blood is being taken, but this soon passes.

The hole in the vein is very small and heals quickly. A plaster is often put over the site of the injection in the skin, but this is not always necessary. The only problems that may arise occur in people who are obese, when it is hard to find a vein, or people who are dehydrated,

the bone or bone marrow is under investigation.

The procedure for a bone biopsy is swift, but can be painful; an overnight stay in hospital is often necessary. A local anaesthetic is injected into the skin over the bone — usually the breastbone or the pelvis — and a piece removed by means of a punch pushed through the skin. Marrow samples are sucked out through a needle passed into the centre of the bone.

Breast biopsy The tissue of a breast lump is examined to determine whether it is malignant before any decision is taken about treatment. There are two methods. In the past, the lump was generally removed in the operating theatre, the patient having been asked beforehand to give her consent to major surgery should this become necessary. A frozen section would be taken, and,if malignant tissue was discovered,a mastectomy would be performed.

Today, many surgeons believe that a mastectomy is unnecessary unless the tumour has spread to involve large areas of tissue. As a result, a different procedure has become accepted practice. In this a sample of the lump's tissue is taken by means of a 'drill biopsy'. The patient is given a local anaesthetic, a hollow needle is passed into the lump and a small piece of tissue extracted. Should this show malignant changes, the woman is asked to return to hospital and the lump is removed.

Liver biopsy Liver tissue may be sampled if the results of liver function tests — see *blood tests* — are abnormal, in order to identify the precise nature of the liver disorder. The biopsy is normally performed in hospital, and involves an overnight stay. A local anaesthetic is injected between the lower ribs on the right side, and the patient is asked to hold his or her breath. The biopsy needle is then pushed into the liver, and a small sample of tissue taken. The procedure usually takes less than five minutes from

beginning to end, the biopsy itself taking less than a second. The biopsy causes discomfort rather than pain, though afterwards some patients experience pain in the right shoulder.

Lung biopsy Samples of lung tissue are most commonly taken by means of special forceps, inserted into the lungs by means of a bronchoscope — see *endoscopy*. Sometimes, however, the tissue under investigation cannot be reached by this means. Since different types of tumour may cause lung cancer, and each requires different treatment, it is therefore essential to identify the tissue precisely. As a result, an 'open biopsy' is often necessary in such cases. The patient is given a general anaesthetic, and the surgeon opens the chest wall to expose the tissue under investigation.

Lymph node biopsy Samples of lymph tissue may be taken to diagnose conditions such as Hodgkin's disease, or to check on the spread of malignant cells from a tumour elsewhere in the body. The procedure is swift, and either performed in an out-patient clinic under local anaesthetic or in an operating theatre under general anaesthesia, depending on how accessible the lymph node is. Lymph nodes near the skin are removed through a small incision — the neck and the groin being common sites. Deeper lymph nodes may require more complex surgical techniques.

Pleural biopsy A sample of tissue from the outer covering of the lung is taken when fluid is detected between the lungs and the pleura, a condition known as pleural effusion. This often has a known cause, such as pneumonia or heart failure, but can also be the result of tuberculosis or a malignant tumour. In order to establish the diagnosis, the patient is admitted to hospital, a local anaesthetic is injected into the skin and a biopsy needle passed into the pleural cavity between the ribs of the back. The sample of pleural tissue is examined to detect any malignant changes, and the effusion is

elderly and have thin veins. In such people the veins sometimes collapse before the sample has been taken. This has no medical significance, but it means that the procedure may take longer than usual and cause some discomfort.

Usually, a blood sample can be taken at any time of day. However, for some tests it is important that blood is taken at a specific time, or that the patient has fasted for 12 hours. This is because the composition of the blood reflects the constituents of any recent meal—*see Metabolism, p44*. As a result, the doctor may ask that you fast overnight before you attend the surgery for a blood sample to be taken.

Depending on the test to be performed, either the whole sample, or its individual constituents are required—*see The Blood and Lymph Systems, p21*. Some of these constituents are unstable, so the blood sample is generally placed in a special bottle, containing preservative and a chemical that prevents the blood from clotting, and refrigerated. Sometimes, however, it is necessary to separate the plasma from the red and white blood cells. This is done by spinning a test tube full of blood in a centrifuge: the cells are deposited at the bottom of the tube and the straw coloured plasma floats at the top.

The blood sample may be analyzed in various different laboratories, according to the test required. Haematology laboratories investigate the functions and characteristics of the constituents of blood, examining, for example, the number and health of red and white cells, the blood group, and speed of clotting. The quantities of chemicals circulating in blood are measured in biochemistry or clinical pathology laboratories; microbiology and bacteriology laboratories test blood for evidence of infection, either looking for the infective agents or for the body's reactions to them—*see Natural Defences Against Disease, p52*. Highly specialized laboratories measure the levels of other chemicals, such as proteins—*see Metabolism, p44*—and hormones—*see The Endocrine System, p48*.

Some tests are still performed individually, but in the majority of cases, machines called autoanalyzers are used. These simultaneously measure a number of different chemical levels in a batch of samples. The results are quickly available, and extremely accurate. As a result, the results are available for most blood tests within 24 hours. In the case of unusual tests,

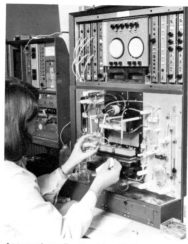

Autoanalyzer Routine blood tests are now performed by auto analyzers, or Coulter counters. These machines can perform several different tests on the same blood sample extremely accurately and their speed makes results quickly available.

however, there may be a longer delay, while technicians wait for a batch to be made up.

The most common blood tests are described below, in alphabetical order.

Albumin A plasma protein, manufactured in the liver, which acts as a carrier for other chemicals in the bloodstream, such as hormones — see *The Blood and Lymph Systems, p21*. The test is performed as part of the investigation of liver function when conditions such as hepatitis and cirrhosis are suspected.

Alpha foetoprotein A protein produced by the human foetus that crosses the placenta to circulate in the mother's blood — see *Pregnancy and Birth, p60*. The level of AFP in the mother's blood is tested during the 16th week of pregnancy, after an *ultrasound scan* has been performed to establish the precise age of the foetus and whether there are twins. This is because the level of AFP increases with the age of the foetus. An unexplained high level of AFP in the mother's blood is an indication that the foetus is suffering from a neural tube defect — see *Embryology, p12* — such as spina bifida. The diagnosis can be confirmed by *amniocentesis*.

Amylase An enzyme, produced by the pancreas and the salivary glands that aids the digestion of carbohydrates — see *The Digestive System, p40*. If any disorder of these glands increases amylase production, the chemical can often be detected in the bloodstream. The test is often performed when a patient complains of an obscure abdominal pain, which may be caused by a disorder affecting the pancreas.

Antinuclear factor An antibody produced in conditions such as rheumatoid arthritis, the collagen vascular diseases and chronic liver disease — see *Natural Defences Against Disease, p52*. Although the test is often useful in diagnosis, it is not conclusive, because antinuclear factor is sometimes found in the blood of perfectly healthy people.

ASO titre An antibody, called ASO or anti-streptolysin-o, a chemical manufactured by Streptococcal bacteria — see *Natural Defences Against Disease, p52*. Streptococcal bacteria are a common cause of sore throats, but may also be implicated in serious disorders of the kidneys and heart. An

ASO titre is performed to establish the precise nature and level of such infections, so that appropriate, specific antibiotics may be prescribed to combat them.

Australia antigen An antigen produced in response to hepatitis virus B, which affects the liver, causing serum hepatitis. Until this test was developed in Australia, hence its name, it was impossible to make a firm diagnosis of serum hepatitis, one of the most common forms of liver disease, and to distinguish it from infectious hepatitis, caused by the A virus. Since the condition is highly infectious, doctors wear rubber gloves when taking blood from patients in whom it is suspected. The test is also performed as a routine screening measure on all expectant mothers and blood donors.

Antibody test Any test designed to establish the presence and number of the specific antibodies produced in response to a type of disease organism — see *Natural Defences Against Disease, p52*. See Blood tests: antinuclear factor, ASO titre, Australia antigen, autoantibodies, Coombs test, Paul-Bunnell test, rheumatoid factor, Widal test; Heaf test; Mantoux Test; STS.

Autoantibodies Antibodies produced to fight the body's own tissues, as a result of an auto-immune disorder. Specific autoantibodies may be produced against different types of tissue, depending on the individual. Common examples include thyroid autoantibodies, mitochondrial autoantibodies — see *Metabolism, p44* — and autoantibodies against DNA, the nucleic acid found in all cells. These may be associated with, respectively, thyroiditis, biliary cirrhosis and rheumatoid arthritis. Autoantibody tests are performed when an auto-immune condition is suspected.

Blood gas analysis A test to measure the concentration of oxygen and carbon dioxide in the blood. This is the only test performed on arterial blood, the reason being that the arterial blood contains the oxygen absorbed from the air in the lungs — see *The Respiratory System, p28*. As a result, a blood gas analysis can give doctors important information about the efficiency of the lungs in conditions such as severe asthma, bronchitis and pneumonia. In these conditions, the concentration of oxygen is likely to be lower than normal, and the carbon dioxide concentration higher.

An arterial blood sample is taken from an artery in the wrist or the groin. No tourniquet is applied, but a local anaesthetic may be given because the procedure is more painful than a venous blood sample. There is also a risk of bruising; this is minimized by applying firm pressure to the site for three minutes after the needle has been removed.

Blood groups See *The Blood and Lymph Systems, p23*.

B12 A test to establish the level of vitamin B12 in the blood — see *Diet, p322*, carried out in cases of anaemia to establish whether the condition is caused by a vitamin B12 deficiency. A *Schilling test*, which measures the body's ability to absorb B12 from the diet, may be performed if the level of the vitamin is abnormally low.

Blood sugar Also known as a blood glucose test, this test establishes the blood level of glucose, the most important source of the body's energy — see *Metabolism, p44*. The level of glucose in the blood temporarily rises after a meal, and is generally higher than normal in obesity. Generally, however, the cause of a permanently high blood level of glucose is diabetes, a condition in which insulin, a hormone vital to the utilization of glucose, is lacking. Levels are also commonly high in people who are overweight. The level is decreased by starvation and fasting, and also falls when an overdose of insulin is taken by a diabetic.

The level of glucose can be tested without any preliminary preparations. Since the blood sugar level changes after eating, however, this is only done in emergencies. When a patient is suspected of having diabetes, a fasting blood sugar is taken — that is, a blood sample is taken after a 12 hour, overnight fast. If this shows a high glucose level, a glucose tolerance test is usually performed. In this, the patient is given a drink containing 50g (around 2oz) of glucose, and blood samples are taken every half-hour for two hours. Urine samples are taken at hourly intervals, to see if any glucose is excreted. This test shows how the body is utilizing glucose, and thus the amount of insulin produced.

Cardiac enzymes Three enzymes released into the blood in a specific order in the days following a heart attack are a result of damage to the heart muscle. The blood level of the different enzymes gives doctors important information about the extent of damage to the muscles; the presence of the enzymes in the blood is often the only way that doctors can be sure that a patient has had a heart attack when the event itself has been minor. Further information about the activity and condition of the heart muscle can be obtained through an *electrocardiogram*.

Clotting time A test to establish how long it takes for blood to clot — *see The Blood and Lymph Systems, p21*. The blood clotting time is increased in certain inherited conditions such as haemophilia, and as a result of treatment with anticoagulants, such as warfarin. The test is commonly used to monitor the effects of anticoagulant treatment, in which a careful balance must be struck between discouraging blood clots, called thrombi, from forming in the vessels, and avoiding spontaneous internal bleeding.

If a blood sample is allowed to stand in a test tube it will clot, or coagulate, of its own accord. The time this takes is called the whole blood clotting time, the normal value being between five and 11 minutes. Since blood clotting is a complex process, however, involving the interaction of 12 factors in the blood, more precise information is often required if the clotting time is abnormally long.

In such cases, two tests can be used to determine which factor is deficient. The first, called the prothrombin time, measures the blood clotting time after tissue has been added to the blood. It can also be used as a test of liver function, because this organ manufactures prothrombin, and is the test used to judge the effect of anticoagulant treatment. The second, known as the kaolin-cephalin test, measures the time it takes for blood to clot after the addition of small quantities of china clay (calcium) and cephalin (an animal fat). This test is used to investigate the cause of excessive bruising, which may be caused by conditions such as haemophilia and Christmas disease. Both are commonly performed as screening procedures before a *biopsy*, because this may cause excessive bleeding if there is a deficiency in the clotting process.

Coombs test A test to detect the presence of autoantibodies — that is, antibodies produced against the body's own tissues as a result of an auto-immune disorder — that cause destruction of the red blood cells in haemolytic anaemia. The test utilizes the fact that some of the autoantibodies are present on the red blood cells in a form that does not have any effect. When such cells are mixed with anti-human-globulin serum, made by injecting rabbits with human serum, the autoantibodies are activated, causing red cells to clump together. The procedure is simple. A blood sample is spun in a centrifuge to separate the red cells. These are washed in a saline solution, mixed with the anti-human-globulin serum, and then examined under a microscope to see how much they have clotted.

Cortisol A test to establish the blood level of the hormone cortisol, also known as hydrocortisone *see The Endocrine System, p48*. Cortisol, a steroid hormone, is produced by the adrenal glands. The test may be performed when an increased level of cortisol is thought to be responsible for problems such as hypertension, diabetes and obesity; the increase may be due to Cushing's disease or, occasionally, to treatment with steroid drugs. Alternatively, the test may be performed as part of the investigation of the symptoms of Addison's disease, in which the level of cortisol is decreased.

The concentration of cortisol in the blood naturally varies between morning and night. As a result, a number of samples may be taken, requiring a stay in hospital.

Creatinine clearance A test of the blood level of creatinine, a by-product of the metabolism of protein in the muscles — *see Metabolism, p44*. Normally, creatine gradually filters out of the muscles and is carried by the blood to the kidneys, where it is excreted in the urine. Therefore, there is a correlation between the level of creatinine in the blood and that in the urine. Both are tested over a 24-hour period that sometimes requires a stay in hospital; a high level in the blood and a low level in the urine is generally an indication of a kidney disorder.

Drug level tests A test of the levels of specific drugs in the blood. All drugs are carried around the body in the bloodstream, broken down by the liver *(p44)* and excreted by the kidneys *(p40)*. However, since patients vary in the efficiency with which their liver and kidneys perform these functions, they may end up with different concentrations in their blood even though the dosage is identical. Since too much of a drug may be harmful, while too little will not have the intended effect, a blood sample may be tested several hours after a drug is administered. Drug tests are also carried out on the blood of overdose victims, to find out which drug was involved and how much of it was taken.

Electrolytes A test to discover the quantities of charged chemical particles, called electrolytes, in the blood. The precise concentration of the main electrolytes sodium, chloride and potassium, is regulated by a variety of hormones which affect the functions of the kidneys. Variations in their level may be an indication of a variety of diseases, ranging from gastroenteritis to kidney failure. Electrolyte levels are measured by means of chemical analysis as part of the diagnosis of such conditions, and may be routinely tested in patients who are taking diuretic drugs. These drugs alter the fluid balance of the body, and so affect the electrolyte concentration.

Electrophoresis A method of identifying and quantifying the various proteins in the blood. Electrophoresis utilizes the principle that chemicals in a solution travel a different distance along a sensitized strip of material according to their electrical charge when an electrical current is applied to the solution. In medicine, the strip used is an electrophoretic protein strip, or EPS. The technique is used when the presence of abnormal proteins is suspected. These may be produced by conditions such as multiple myeloma, a cancer involving the bone marrow.

ESR test A test of the rate at which red blood cells separate from plasma, known as the erythrocyte sedimentation rate, or ESR — *see Blood and Lymph, p21*. A blood sample is placed in a test tube and left to stand, the time it takes the red blood cells to fall to the bottom being monitored. An ESR is performed in conjunction with a *full blood count*, since it gives a rough guide to the health of the patient, and an indication of the presence of infection, inflammation and malignancy.

EPS text *See electrophoresis.*

Folic acid A test to measure the blood level of folic acid, a B-vitamin — *see Diet, p322*. The test is performed as part of the investigation of problems that may be caused by a low folic acid blood level, such as anaemia, or conditions that result in it, such as disorders of the small intestines. The test is routinely performed on expectant mothers, who tend to be deficient in folic acid — they are given supplements for this reason — and on people who are taking drugs to control epilepsy, since these may interfere with absorption of the vitamin.

Full blood count The most common of all blood tests, a full blood count determines numbers of red blood cells, white blood cells and platelets in a small sample. These values are measured by an autoanalyzer, which also establishes the size of the red blood cells and the amount of haemoglobin in them. In addition, the numbers of the five types of white cells are estimated by a technician who examines a stained smear of blood under a microscope — *see The Blood and Lymph Systems, p21*.

The results of a full blood count reflect the general health of the body. Many types of disorder cause characteristic changes in the appearance and numbers of blood constituents. These changes can be confirmed, and a specific diagnosis made, by further, more specific tests.

Gammaglobulins Tests to identify and quantify gammaglobulin proteins in the blood. There are a number of gammaglobulins, but the most important are the immunoglobulins, the antibodies — *see antibody tests*. The different types of protein can be distinguished by a technique called *electrophoresis*.

Haemoglobin An estimate of the amount of haemoglobin in the blood *see The Blood and Lymph Systems, p21* — normally performed as part of a *full blood count*. The amount of haemoglobin is reduced in anaemia, either because there are fewer red blood cells than normal or because each cell contains less haemoglobin than normal. The amount of haemoglobin is naturally more in men than in women, because women have slightly fewer blood cells, and is lower in babies and children than in adults.

Haemoglobin electrophoresis A test to differentiate between different types of globin, the protein constituent of haemoglobin in red blood cells — *see The Blood and Lymph systems, p21*. In certain types of inherited blood disorders, however, such as thalassaemia and sickle-cell anaemia, these globins are abnormal. They can be identified and quantified by a technique known as *electrophoresis*.

Immunoglobulins See *gammaglobulins*.

Iron and iron-binding capacity Tests to measure the quantity of iron carried in the blood plasma and the capacity of the blood to carry iron, which is an essential component of red blood cells — *see The Blood and Lymph Systems, p21*. Iron is transported in the blood by the carrier protein transferrin. A low iron level in the plasma may either be an indication of insufficient iron-binding capacity or of an iron deficiency. The iron-binding capacity test tells doctors which of these is correct. The tests are performed in all cases of anaemia, in an attempt to discover the precise cause of the condition, because if the level of iron is low, insufficient amounts will reach the bone marrow, the site of red cell production.

If the iron-binding capacity is normal, but the anaemia results from an iron deficiency, the problem may result from a disorder of the stomach or small intestine which prevents absorption of iron. In women, a temporary iron deficiency may be caused by heavy menstrual periods or by pregnancy, because the foetus builds up a store of iron. Both problems can be cured by iron tablets.

Lipids A test to determine the level of fats, called lipids, in the blood — *see Metabolism, p44.* Lipid tests are sometimes routinely performed as a screening procedure on people who appear healthy, because abnormally high fat levels increase the risks of atherosclerosis, heart attacks and strokes. Some people have an inherited tendency to high blood levels of lipids; in others the cause is an unbalanced diet — *see Diet, p322* — or conditions such as diabetes and liver and thyroid disorders.

Liver function tests A group of tests that measure the condition and efficiency of the liver. This organ has a number of vital functions — *see Metabolism, p44.* They are performed for two reasons: to distinguish a disorder that directly affects liver tissue from a disorder, such as gallstones, that indirectly affects the liver; and to investigate the cause and extent of a malfunction of the liver, such as that resulting from hepatitis. A number of tests can be used.
Since the liver manufactures plasma proteins — *see The Blood and Lymph Systems, p21* — tests of plasma protein levels, such as the *albumin* test, are included. The blood is also screened for the presence of certain enzymes released when liver tissue is damaged, and the content of bilirubin, a product of the breakdown of red blood cells by the liver, is estimated. Since the liver detoxifies drugs and poisons, some tests involve injecting a chemical into the blood stream, and testing blood samples at intervals to see how quickly the liver breaks the chemical down. Most liver function tests can be performed on blood samples taken at any time of day, without fasting; on occasions, however, the complexity of the tests means that they must be performed in hospital.
See also Coombs test.

Malarial parasites A test to detect to the presence of parasites called Plasmodia, which cause malaria. The parasites can easily be seen when a drop of infected blood is examined under a microscope.

Proteins Tests to establish the level of plasma proteins in the blood — *see The Blood and Lymph Systems, p21.* There are two main types of proteins in the blood, albumin — *see albumin tests* — and globulin. There are several different types of globulin, of which the most common are *gammaglobuins,* the chemicals that form *antibodies.* As a result of disease, new forms of protein may be produced and levels of natural proteins may vary.

Prothrombin time *See clotting time*

Rheumatoid factor A test to detect the presence of specific *autoantibodies* in the blood that may either be associated with rheumatoid arthritis or collagen-vascular disorders.

Sickle-cell test A test used to confirm a diagnosis of sickle-cell anaemia. In this condition, an abnormality of|haemoglobin — *see The Blood and Lymph System* — causes a change in the shape of blood cells when the oxygen content of the blood is low. Characteristic sickle-shaped cells can be seen when a smear of blood is examined under a microscope. The test is routinely performed before a general anaesthetic is given to people whose families come from parts of the world where malaria is common. Though apparently healthy, such people are sometimes mildly affected by sickle-cell anaemia — there is a link between the condition and resistance to malaria — in which case they may be dangerousy sensitive to normal dosages of anaesthetic.

STS (Serological tests for syphilis) A number of tests used in the diagnosis of

syphilis. Previously, the most common test for this disease was the Wasserman reaction; this is no longer used. Instead, a sample of serum, separated from blood, is tested for the presence of an antibody called reagin — *see Natural Defences Against Disease, p52* — which is produced by the body to combat the organism that causes syphilis. Since reagin is also found in auto-immune disorders and collagen vascular diseases, however, a further, more specific test may be necessary if reagin is detected. Several further tests are used, but the most common is called a Reiter protein complement fixation test. Blood tests for syphilis are compulsory before marriage in some countries, notably the United States.

Urea test A test to discover the blood level of urea, a chemical produced by the liver as the last by-product of protein metabolism — *see Metabolism, p44* — and excreted by the kidneys. The test is used as a general screen to detect kidney problems, because a high level of urea in the blood is an indication that the kidney is not excreting urea efficiently.

Uric acid test A test to determine the blood level of uric acid, a waste product produced by the metabolism. A raised level is normally an indication of gout, but|may be a sign of leukaemia, pernicious anaemia, and, in pregnant women, eclampsia.

Viral studies Tests to confirm a viral infection and identify the precise nature of the virus responsible. This is only necessary when precise identification of the virus determines the appropriate treatment, as in infections|of the liver, the heart and the brain, and when the cause of an illness is unknown.
There are two different types of test. Most commonly, the virus is identified by discovering the nature of the antibody produced by the blood to combat the infection — *see Natural Defences Against Disease, p52.* This is done by an *antibody test* in which the protein antibodies are distinguished and identified by *electrophoresis.* Two blood samples are taken. The first, taken at the onset of symptoms, is called the acute serum; the second, taken 10 to 14 days later, is known as the convalescent serum. By plotting the difference between the antibody level in the two samples, doctors can monitor the effectiveness of their treatment and the body's defence systems.
More rarely, the virus is visually identified by means of the huge power of magnification obtainable from an electron microscope. This technique is only available in well-equipped research centres.

Wasserman test *See STS*

Widal test A test to reveal the presence of specific antibodies produced to combat the organisms causing typhoid and paratyphoid fever — *see Natural Defences Against Disease, p52.* A Widal test is routinely performed as a precaution in cases of high fever. The blood sample is taken during the second week of the infection, because the antibodies are produced in large quantities during this period.

CARDIOTOCOGRAPH

An electronic device used to record the contractions of the womb and the heartbeat of the foetus during labour, the most effective guide to foetal health or distress—*see Pregnancy and Birth, p60.* A belt is placed around the mother's abdomen, and a transducer—a device that converts movement to electrical impulses—is attached to it. The impulses are amplified by the cardiotocograph, and either made audible, recorded by a pen on a strip of paper,or viewed on an

oscilloscope screen. The machine can be used to record the mother's heartbeat and respiratory rate as well.

CAT SCAN—see X-rays

CENTRAL VENOUS PRESSURE
A method for establishing the pressure of blood in the central veins of the body, which lead into the right side of the heart—*see The Blood and Lymph System, p21.* It may be necessary to establish the central venous pressure in heart failure, when it increases, or in shock, when the pressure falls and a blood transfusion may be necessary. The procedure carries an element of risk, however, as it involves carefully placing a thin tube, called a catheter, in a vein in the neck. As a result, the test is only used when a patient is seriously ill, and generally only undertaken by experienced staff working in an intensive care unit.

CERVICAL SMEAR/PAP TEST
A test used to detect pre-cancerous changes in the cells lining the cervix of the womb. The procedure for a cervical smear, and its importance, is fully described in section three—*see Routine Health Checks, p346.* The sample of cells is smeared on a slide, stained and examined under the microscope. If abnormal tissue are seen, the test is repeated; if the result is again abnormal, the patient is referred to a gynaecologist, who may take a *biopsy* of the cervical tissue.

CHEST X-RAY—see X-rays

CHOLANGIOGRAM and CHOLECYSTOGRAM—see X-rays

CULTURE AND MICROSCOPY—see MC & S

CYSTOGRAM—see X-rays

DRUG LEVEL TESTS—see Blood tests

ELECTROCARDIOGRAM (ECG)
A device used to monitor the electrical activity of the heart. The contractions of the heart muscle are controlled by a series of electrical impulses which spread through the muscle from the sino-atrial node—*see The Blood and Lymph Systems, p21.* These are detected by electrodes taped to the skin, then amplified and traced on to a moving strip of paper.
An ECG is taken in two stages, so giving a complete picture of the electrical activity. First, an electrode is taped to each wrist and each ankle; a conductive jelly is used to

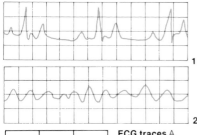

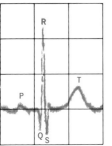

ECG traces A normal ECG trace **1**. The second trace **2**, shows ventricular fibrillation. What happens in each normal beat is shown *(left)*. P — atrial contraction, Q-R-S shows ventricular contraction; T — priming the heart for the next beat.

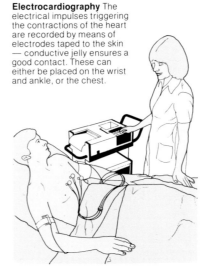

Electrocardiography The electrical impulses triggering the contractions of the heart are recorded by means of electrodes taped to the skin — conductive jelly ensures a good contact. These can either be placed on the wrist and ankle, or the chest.

ensure a good connection: These are then removed, and three electrodes are taped to the chest; one chest electrode may be moved around in order to obtain a satisfactory reading. When an ECG is used to monitor the activity of a patient's heart in hospital, the chest leads alone are used. Many doctors now have an ECG machine in their surgery, and the less complex investigations are routinely performed.

Any deviation from the characteristic PQR ST trace|showing normal heart activity may be an indication of a disorder affecting the heart muscle.

The science of electrocardiography has become extremely sophisticated, and by examining the trace doctors are often able to make a precise diagnosis of conditions such as heart failure, coronary artery disease and valvular heart disorders. Tell-tale signs are also left on an ECG trace when even a minor heart attack has occurred.

In cases of suspected heart disease, doctors may need to know how well the heart responds to an increase in the demand for blood. This is determined by an exercise ECG: typically, the patient steps up and down a pair of steps with electrodes attached to his or her chest.

ELECTROENCEPHALOGRAM (EEG)
A machine used to record electrical activity within the brain. Up to eight electrodes are taped to each side of the brain, and a conductive jelly is applied to ensure a good contact. The electrodes sense the electrical impulses within the brain and convert them into signals. These are amplified and recorded on a moving strip of paper. The test is painless,

and takes between 15 and 45 minutes. It is carried out in hospital as an out-patient procedure.

The signals are divided into four distinct groups on the trace, according to their wavelength: delta, theta, alpha and beta. These are not necessarily present at the same time—the delta wavelength signals, for example, are predominant during sleep, and the beta wavelength signals replace alpha signals during general anaesthesia. Doctors who are experienced in the technique can often interpret variations in an ECG trace with some precision. As a result, the test can be used as an aid to diagnosis of conditions affecting the electrical activity of the brain, such as

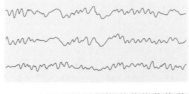

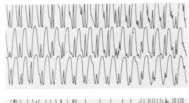

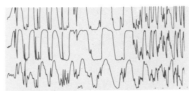

Electroencaphalography The brain's electrical activity is monitored through electrodes taped to the side of the head. The characteristic peaks and troughs of a normal EEG trace *(top)* are altered in conditions such as petit mal epilepsy (middle) and grand mal epilepsy *(bottom)*.

epilepsy, brain tumours and brain abscesses. it can also give important information about the cause and nature of unconsciousness.

See also visual evoked potential.

ELECTROMYOGRAM (EMG) AND NERVE CONDUCTION TEST
Two tests used to record the electrical activity of nerves and muscles—*see The Nervous System, p32.* To produce an electromyograph, a thin needle containing an electrode is passed into the muscle through the skin. The electrode detects electrical signals within the muscle, and the EMG machine amplifies the signals and records them on a moving strip of paper. A nerve conduction test is performed in a similar way, but, in this case, the electrode is taped to the skin above a nerve. By examining the trace, doctors can calculate the speed at which impulses travel along a nerve. The two tests are often performed together, so that doctors can establish whether the cause of a problem affecting movement is a disorder of a nerve or of muscle.

ENDOSCOPY
A technique by which doctors can look inside the body. A number of different devices can be used, each designed to allow a specific organ to be examined; all are generally known as endoscopes. Modern endoscopes are made from flexible fibreoptic cable, which transmits light from one end of the cable to the other without leakage. Two thin cables are used: one to transmit light to the area under examination; the other to transmit an image back to the observer. Generally, endoscopes are gently pushed into the body through an orifice, but in some cases, a special incision must be made. Some types of endoscopy necessitate a general anaesthetic; in others, sedation alone is required.

The wide-spread use of fibreoptic endoscopes has made possible the early diagnosis and effective treatment of a variety of conditions. Biopsies are often performed at the same time as endoscopy—many modern endoscopes are manufactured with in-built biopsy equipment—and harmless growths, such as polyps, can often be removed without the need for more extensive surgery.

Arthroscopy The use of a special type of endoscope to examine the interior of a joint — *see Bone and Muscle, p16.* Since damaged joint tissues may not show up on an X-ray, arthroscopy is sometimes the only effective aid to a diagnosis of the precise injury to a joint. It can also be used to investigate conditions affecting the joints, such as gout and arthritis, and, in association with a synovial *biopsy*, to determine the cause of inflammation in a joint. Patients usually require a general anaesthetic, and have to stay in hospital.

Bronchoscopy Examination of the bronchi of the lungs — *see The Respiratory System, p28* — by means of a flexible endoscope passed into the airway through the mouth or nose. (Some surgeons still use a rigid, non-fibreoptic bronchoscope to examine the vocal cords and the bronchi; in this case, a general anaesthetic is necessary.) Bronchoscopy is used in the investigation of recurring bouts of pneumonia and the early detection of tumours of the lung tissue. The patient fasts overnight and is sedated to minimize discomfort. A short stay in hospital is normally required.

Colonoscopy Examination of the large intestine — *see The Digestive System, p40* — by means of a flexible fibreoptic endoscope, to investigate conditions such as intestinal obstruction, ulcerative colitis, malignant tumours or polyps. The patient is admitted to hospital and given a liquid diet, in order that the bowels are clear; an enema may also be given for this purpose. The procedure can take around an hour, and causes some discomfort, so sedation is used.

Colposcopy Examination of the vagina and the cervix, the neck of the womb. A colposcope, also called a vaginoscope, is a rigid instrument capable of magnification. It is used to examine cells in the vaginal and cervical walls when a *cervical smear* has shown abnormalities. The procedure causes little discomfort, and no anaesthetic is necessary.

Cystoscopy Examination of the urethra and bladder, used to investigate the cause of recurring bladder infections and blood in the urine, and to investigate suspected growths or stones in the bladder. Cystoscopy can be performed in an out-patient clinic, using a local anaesthetic, but many doctors prefer to admit the patient to hospital and use a general anaesthetic. If bladder stones are discovered during cystoscopy, these can usually be removed without the need for further surgery.

Foetoscopy A recently developed technique used to examine the foetus. A thin fibreoptic endoscope is passed through an incision in the mother's abdomen and guided, with the help of an *ultrasound scan*, into the amniotic sac — *see Pregnancy and Birth, p60*. There is no risk to the mother, who is given a local anaesthetic, but a five to ten per cent risk of damage to the foetus. As a result, the procedure is only used when there is a serious possibility that the foetus is suffering from an abnormality, such as spina bifida, or an inherited blood disorder, such as haemophilia. In this case, the foetoscope can be used to take a sample of foetal blood, which can be examined to confirm the diagnosis.
  See also amniocentesis; transcervical aspiration.

Gastroscopy Examination of the stomach and the upper digestive tract — *see The Digestive System, p40* — by means of a fibreoptic endoscope. Gastroscopy is used in the investigation of conditions such as peptic ulcer, oesophagitis and tumour of the digestive tract. It is performed in hospital, after an overnight fast, and sedation is used to minimize any discomfort. Gastroscopy has largely superceded oesophagoscopy, in which a rigid, non-fibreoptic instrument was placed in the patient's mouth to examine the oesophagus.

Laparoscopy Examination of the organs inside the abdomen, such as the intestines, spleen, liver, pancreas and female reproductive organs. A rigid fibreoptic device

is pushed into the abdominal cavity through a small incision just below the navel. Surgical and *biopsy* tools are often built in to the laparoscope, enabling it to be used for minor surgery, such as tubal ligation — female sterilization — the loosening of intestinal adhesions and biopsy of tissue suspected to be malignant. Patients are admitted to hospital and given a general anaesthetic.

Oesophagoscopy See gastroscopy

Proctoscopy See sigmoidoscopy

Sigmoidoscopy Examination of the lower digestive tract, comprising the sigmoid colon, rectum and anal passage — *see The Digestive System, p40*. The sigmoidoscope, a flexible fibreoptic endoscope, is placed in the rectum, while the patient is lying on his or her side; the procedure causes slight discomfort, but no anaesthetic is necessary. About 25cm (nearly 10in) can be examined, to detect areas of ulceration, obstruction, malignant growth or polyps. Sigmoidoscopy is superceding proctoscopy, a procedure in which a rigid device is used to examine the rectum and anus.

EYE TESTS
Methods for examining the eyes and their functions—*see The Nervous System, p32*. Eye tests are performed by ophthalmic opticians—called optometrists in the USA—by family doctors and by medical specialists called ophthalmologists. Ophthalmic opticians are primarily concerned with identifying and correcting defects of vision, while doctors and ophthalmologists diagnose and treat diseases that affect the eyes. However, should an ophthalmic optician detect signs of disease during an examination, he or she will recommend that the patient consults a doctor.

Colour vision tests Tests to determine whether a patient can distinguish certain colours from each other, which may be performed either by an optician, a family doctor or an ophthalmologist. The patient is asked to view specially designed colour plates, called pseudo-isochromatic plates — 'isochromatic' means 'having many colours'; the prefix 'pseudo' means that, in fact, the colours are very similar. On each plate is a pattern, made up of differently coloured dots. There are various different types of colour vision plate, and the patterns on them vary: some show a numeral, for example; others a woman's bikini or a garden tool. People with normal vision can see the pattern; to people with defective colour vision the pattern merges into the background. There are a number of different types of defective colour vision and the precise type of defect that a patient has can only be determined by viewing all the plates in controlled lighting.

Fundoscopy See Ophthamoscopy and retinoscopy

Ophthalmoscopy and retinoscopy
Examination of the eye by means of an ophthalmoscope, a hand-held magnifying device that shines a beam of light into the eye and illuminates the retina — *see The Nervous System, p32*. The retina is sometimes known as the fundus, and the examination as fundoscopy; when the retina is the object of the examination, a more sensitive, highly-powered ophthalmoscope, called a retinoscope, may be used. Eye-drops containing atropine are sometimes given to widen the pupil, allowing the inner eye to be clearly seen. Since atropine causes

drowsiness and disturbance of vision for some time after the examination, however, this practice is becoming less common.
  An ophthalmic optician uses an opthalmoscope to discover how efficiently the cornea and the lens of the eye refract light — that is, how effectively it changes the path of light-rays and focusses them on the retina. This is done by determining the adjustment to the ophthalmoscope lens necessary to focus the beam of light on the retina. If the value obtained is abnormal, the optician will prescribe glasses or contact lens to restore the refracting power of the eye, and thus correct defects in vision. Red and blue filters may be placed in front of the ophthalmoscope to see whether the eyes are more or less efficient at dealing with light of different wavelengths.
  Ophthalmic opticians note any signs of disease during their examination, and, if any are seen, advise the patient to consult a doctor. Family doctors and ophthalmologists use the ophthalmoscope and retinoscope as diagnostic tools.
  Retinoscopy can give vital information about conditions such as a squint — called strabismus — glaucoma, cataracts and keratitis, and can be used to examine the nerves and blood vessels of the retina for signs of disorders affecting the eye, such as papilloedema. However, since the retina is the only part of the body in which nerves and blood vessels can be directly seen in a physical examination, retinoscopy can give vital information about conditions that affect the whole body, such as diabetes and hypertension. For this reason, ophthamoscopy and retinoscopy is an essential part of a physical examination — *see The Doctor, The Patient and Disease, p70*.

Perimetry A test, also known as a visual field test, to establish how much can be seen above and below, and to the sides, when the eyesight has deteriorated. It is also used by doctors as an aid to the diagnosis of disorders involving the nervous system. This is because such disorders may interfere with the nerve signals that pass between the eyes and the brain, cutting off some of them and so reducing the area of vision. Generally, the doctor asks the patient, whose eye is still fixed on the doctor's opposite eye, whether he or she can see the hand move out of the corner of the eye being tested. If not, the doctor moves his hand inwards until the hand can be seen. In this way, the whole visual field can be mapped out, giving the doctor important information about any area in which vision, and possibly nerve function, is absent.

Slit lamp test A test in which a beam of light is played across the front of the eye, directed from the side. The beam of light shows a cross-section of the front of the eye, and allows the doctor or optician to detect any signs of abrasion of the cornea — as may be caused, for example, by dust and dirt under a contact lens.

Visual acuity Tests to establish the extent and nature of a defect in vision, and to determine the appropriate lenses needed to correct the defect.
  Usually, the patient is asked to read a Snellen chart, on which the letters become progressively smaller. People with normal vision — expressed as 6/6 vision in the UK, and 20/20 vision in the USA — should be able read letters 6cm (2.4in) high from a distance of 6 metres (6.6yds). However, a device incorporating a laser has recently been developed to test visual acuity. Its use is likely to become widespread, because the procedure is quick and simple, and no special training is required. The laser beam is directed at a rotating cylindrical screen, on which it produces a speckled image. The patient looks at the screen using one eye at a time; if the image appears to be moving upward, the patient has long-sight — called hypermetropia; if it appears to be moving

downwards, he or she has short-sight — called myopia. If the image appears to move sideways, the patient has astigmatism.

After the patient's visual acuity has been determined, the optician tries out a sequence of lenses, placed in an empty pair of glasses, to correct any defect. When the correct lenses have been found, enabling the patient to read the Snellen chart, or immobilize images on the laser screen, their specifications are recorded. Later, contact lens or glasses are made up to the same specification.

Visual field test *See perimetry.*

FAECAL TESTS

A number of tests to determine the quantity of unabsorbed food residues—*see The Digestive System, p40*—and the presence of blood and disease organisms in the excreta. Generally, faecal tests do not require attendance at hospital. The family doctor provides a receptacle in which the patient places either samples of his or her stools, or the total production of stools over a period. These are delivered to a hospital laboratory for tests.

Faecal fat estimation A test to measure the amount of fat in the faeces. Normally, most of the fat taken into the body in the diet is broken down in the process of digestion and absorbed by the small intestine — *see The Digestive System, p40.* In some conditions, however, such as malabsorption syndrome, insufficient fat is absorbed, and, as a result, the stools are yellowish, greasy and loose — a condition known as steatorrhoea. In order to measure the degree of the deficiency in absorption, the doctor may ask the patient to eat a high fat diet — *see Diet, p322* — for several days, and then to collect two days production of stools. These are chemically analyzed in a biochemistry laboratory.

Faecal occult blood A test to detect the presence of small quantities of blood in the faeces. In this case, only a small sample of faeces is required. This is smeared onto a card impregnated with a chemical that changes colour if blood is present. The test can be performed in the family doctor's surgery, and is extremely sensitive; results may be almost immediate, or delayed for 48 hours, according to the precise nature of the chemical used. The faeces are tested for occult blood whenever the doctor suspects that there may be internal bleeding. This may be the result of a peptic ulcer or polyps, and causes anaemia.

Faecal MC & S The examination of a sample of faeces to detect the presence of disease organisms — *see MC & S* (microscopy, culture and sensitivity).

FOETOSCOPY—see Endoscopy

GASTRIC WASHING—see MC & S

GASTROSCOPY—see Endoscopy

GLUCOSE TOLERANCE TEST— see Blood tests

HEAF TEST

A test to determine whether a person has immunity to tuberculosis (TB). The Heaf test, whose full name is the Heaf multiple-puncture tuberculin test, is simple, quick and painless. It is based on the *Mantoux test*: a small quantity of dead tuberculin bacilli are injected into the skin, and if the body has immunity to TB a small amount of swelling and redness develops at the site within three to seven days. This reaction is caused by the mobilization of antibodies to combat the bacilli; antibodies that have been produced in response to an earlier exposure to the disease—*see Natural Defences Against Disease, p52.*

The injection is normally given at the wrist, by means of a five-pronged punch. A Heaf Test is routinely offered to schoolchildren, at around the age of 13. If the results are negative—that is, the child has now immunity—a BCG immunization is given. The test is also performed on all those who come into contact with TB later in life.

HEARING TEST

A test, also called an audiogram, to determine how well a person can hear. The patient is exposed, one ear at a time, to sounds of varying pitch and volume in a special hospital clinic. The sounds are directed into the patient's ears by means of a pair of headphones, which also block out any extraneous noises. The volume of sound is gradually increased at each pitch, until the patient indicates that the sound can be heard. The results are recorded on a graph, which gives doctors valuable information about the type and cause of any deafness. Hearing tests are routinely performed on people who suffer from deafness, and on schoolchildren in whom hearing difficulties are suspected. They are also given as a safety measure to people who work in noisy surroundings.

HORMONE LEVEL TESTS

A variety of tests to establish the level of certain hormones in the tissues and the blood—*see The Endocrine System, p48.*

Generally, hormone level tests are based on the principles of immunology—*see Natural Defences Against Disease, p52.* Hormones produced by humans are treated as foreign substances by animal tissue, which reacts by producing specific antibodies against them. Once an animal has been sensitized to a hormone, and has produced antibodies against it, an immune reaction will occur when the hormone meets tissue from that animal. As a result, a sample of human tissue or blood containing the hormone causes a reaction when mixed with tissue from the animal; the degree of the reaction shows how much hormone is present in the human sample.

This technique has proved extremely successful at measuring human hormone levels, so much so, in fact, that a number of new hormones have been discovered through its use. Hormone levels in the intestines are commonly tested in the investigation of chronic diarrhoea and gastroenteritis; the sample used being of intestinal secretions taken by a digestive tract *biopsy.* The level of pituitary hormone in blood may also be tested by this means, sometimes after an injection to stimulate the gland, in the investigation of hypopituitarism, and a thyroid deficiency—called myxoedema—or over-activity—called thyrotoxicosis—investigated by measurement of the thyroid hormone, thyroxine. Cortisol and aldosterone levels in blood may be measured in cases of hypertension, and parathormone, produced by the parathyroid glands, measured to determine the cause of a high blood calcium level. The sex hormones, oestrogen and testosterone, may be measured in cases of suspected deficiency, in infertility, and routinely during pregnancy to check on the health of the developing foetus.

HYSTEROSALPINGOGRAM—see X-ray

INFRARED THERMOGRAPHY (IRT)

A method of detecting the pattern of heat radiated from the body. A photograph is taken of the area under investigation in an out-patient clinic, the image being recorded on special, heat-sensitive infrared film. Different colours on the developed film show the different temperatures of various tissues. The technique can give vital information about a number of disorders. Tumours and areas of inflammation, for example, are warmer than their surrounding tissues, and the rate of blood flow through an organ can be measured, because the blood is warmer than the organ.

ISOTOPE SCANS

Methods for monitoring the activity of an organ or area of tissue, by measuring the quantity of radioactive isotopes they take up. An isotope is a radioactive, unstable form of a chemical, which shows up on photographic film. The isotope must be of a chemical that is specifically used by the tissue under investigation. For example, an isotope of iodine is used in investigations of the activity of the thyroid gland, because this chemical is essential to the manufacture of the thyroid hormone, thyroxine—*see The Endocrine System, p48*. A known amount of the isotope is given, in tablet form, by injection or by inhalation. The quantity taken up by the gland and the speed with which the gland uses the isotope is measured at intervals by photographing the gland with a specially sensitive device known as a gamma camera.

Isotope scanning can be used to investigate the activity of a number of other organs and tissues. Radioactive albumin may be injected, for example, or radioactive xenon gas inhaled, to investigate the efficiency of the lungs. The isotopes show up the lung capillaries and outline the air spaces—*see The Respiratory System, p28*—making the technique an important aid in the diagnosis of conditions such as pulmonary embolism. Cysts in the liver can be identified by isotope scans, as can blockages in the vessels of the brain which may indicate the site of a cerebrovascular accident—a stroke—or a tumour. The technique is also used in the investigation of bone disease, the functions of the kidneys and the presence of stones in the ureters, and the structure and pumping efficiency of the heart.

The dosage of radioactivity is less than that received during an *X-ray*, and the isotope is quickly broken down and excreted from the body. Since so little radiation is used, the technique has considerable advantages over conventional X-ray investigations. This, however, must be measured against the complexity of the procedure, and the skill needed to interpret results correctly. Isotope scans are normally performed on an out-patient basis.

IVP (INTRAVENOUS PYELOGRAM)—see X-rays

KVEIM TEST
A test to determine whether a patient has a chronic disorder called sarcoidosis. A solution containing antigens taken from a person who is known to have sarcoidosis is injected into the patient's skin. If the test is positive, a small nodule develops between four and six weeks later. This is *biopsied*, and the tissue examined under a microscope to establish the presence of characteristic sarcoid tissue. The procedure is painless, and is performed in a hospital out-patient clinic.

LAPAROTOMY
An operation to examine the contents of the abdomen. A laparotomy is performed as a last resort when doctors are uncertain of the cause or nature of an abdominal disorder, and other special tests have proved inconclusive. The operation may be performed, for example, in cases of unexplained abdominal swelling, and when there is weight loss of anaemia for no apparent reason; it is also necessary as an emergency procedure when internal bleeding is suspected.

Beforehand, the surgeon asks the patient's permission to carry out any surgery that may prove necessary as a result of the operation. Any diseased tissue will be biopsied, and a frozen section taken—*see biopsy*—so that an on-the-spot diagnosis can be made.

LAPAROSCOPY—see Endoscopy

LUMBAR PUNCTURE
A technique, also called a lumbar tap or a spinal tap, carried out to obtain a sample of the cerebrospinal fluid surrounding the brain and spinal cord—*see The Nervous System, p32*.

A lumbar puncture is only performed when the pressure of CSF is thought to be normal, because the sudden reduction of a high pressure caused by taking a sample is extremely dangerous. For this reason, the optic disc at the back of the eye is usually examined by *ophthalmoscopy* before the test: a swelling of the optic disc is a sign of a raised CSF pressure. A *CAT scan* is sometimes also performed, because this will also show whether the CSF pressure is raised.

There is some discomfort during and after a lumbar puncture, and an overnight stay in hospital is often necessary. For the sample of CSF to be taken, the patient lies on his or her side, curled up in a ball with the knees tucked up under the chin to stretch the back and open the vertebrae—*see Bone and Muscle, p16*. A local anaesthetic is injected into the skin and deeper tissues, and then a thin, sharp needle is either passed between the third and fourth or the fourth and fifth lumbar vertebrae, into the space surrounding the spinal cord. The core of the needle is then withdrawn, allowing CSF to flow up the hollow needle, into a syringe. A pressure-measuring device, called a manometer is often attached to the syringe, to give an instant read-out of CSF pressure.

The sample of CSF is examined in a variety of ways, depending on the nature of the suspected disorder. Most commonly, the fluid is examined under a microscope to see whether red blood cells or white blood cells are present in unusually large numbers, and to detect the presence of micro-organisms. An excess of red blood cells may indicate that there has been bleeding in the brain. This is a sign of a stroke, called a cerebrovascular accident. An excess of white cells or the presence of micro-organisms may indicate an infection involving the brain and spinal cord, such as meningitis or encephalitis.

Other common tests on the sample of CSF include the measurement of sugar levels and of protein. Sugar concentration is determined by chemical analysis, and gives a guide to the nature of any infection; proteins are identified by their levels measured by electrophoresis—*see blood tests*. Disorders such as multiple sclerosis, which are difficult to diagnose by other means, result in characteristic changes to the pattern of proteins in the CSF. The sample of fluid can also be tested for the presence of specific antibodies—*see blood tests*—to identify the precise cause of an infection, and chemically analyzed to establish how much of any drug has reached the CSF.

Patients often experience a severe headache after a lumbar puncture. This can sometimes be avoided if the patient fasts for 24 hours before the test, and lies flat on is or her back for several hours after it. A lumbar puncture may occasionally be used not to test CSF, but to give antibiotics, especially in cases of meningitis.

LUNG FUNCTION TESTS
A series of tests to measure the efficiency of the lungs—*see The Respiratory System, p28*.

The most commonly used lung function test is called peak flow estimation; this is often performed by family doctors as part of a physical examination—*see The Doctor, The Patient and Disease, p70*. The patient is asked to blow as hard and as quickly as he or she can into a small, hand-held device, called a peak flow meter, which records the rate at which air is expelled on a dial. Normally this is between 400 and 500 litres (14-17 cubic feet) of air per minute. The value varies according to the time of day, so several readings may be taken over a period, and averaged. Peak flow is reduced in conditions such as asthma, emphysema and chronic bronchitis, which either reduce the capacity of the lungs or the force with with the lungs can expel air.

If the peak flow meter shows that the efficiency of the lungs has been impaired, more sophisticated tests may be necessary. These necessitate the use of a machine called a vitalograph, or spirometer, usually in a hospital laboratory. The vitalograph, attached to the patient by means of a face mask, measures the amounts of air taken into the lungs and exhaled with each breath, during rest, and, if necessary, during exercise. This allows physiologists to calculate values such as the tidal volume and inspiratory reserve volume—*see The Respiratory System, p28*—and, together with blood gas tests—*see blood tests*—gives doctors important information about the progress and most appropriate way of treating disorders of the lungs.

LYMPHANGIOGRAM—see X-rays

MAMMOGRAPHY—see X-rays

MANTOUX TEST

A test to establish whether a person has immunity to tuberculosis (TB). A solution containing dead TB bacilli is injected to the skin, usually on the forearm. If the person is immune to TB, a reaction appears within one or two days. At its most extreme, this takes the form of a warm, raised, red swelling at the site, between one and two centimetres (0.4-0.8in) across.

A Mantoux test is given to people who have come into contact with a case of TB, and sometimes used to confirm an uncertain diagnosis of the disease. A simplified form of the test, called the *Heaf test*, is routinely given to schoolchildren.

MICROSCOPY, CULTURE AND SENSITIVITY (MC & S)

The examination of fluid and tissue samples to detect the presence of bacteria and to identify the antibiotics that most effectively combat them.

Generally samples are taken by means of swabs: the mucous membranes in the area where infection is suspected are gently wiped with a pad of sterile cotton wool. The smear of fluid and cells so obtained is transferred to a special jar and cultured—that is, it is placed in a nutrient jelly and kept warm to promote bacterial growth. The bacteria that grow can be identified by their ability to take up different stains, and by their microscopic appearance. Often, a sample of the bacteria are put through a sensitivity test. In this, drops of a variety of antibiotics are placed on the bacterial mould, and the results observed to establish which antibiotic is the most effective at fighting the bacteria. This can then be prescribed by the doctor.

Swabs may be taken from any of the body orifices which the doctor suspects may be involved in an infection: the nose, the mouth—

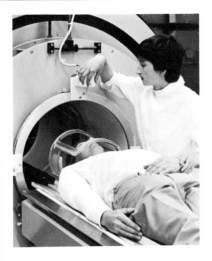

most commonly from the throat, in cases of sore throat—the anus and rectum, the urethra, the vagina, the eyes and the ears. In addition, samples of urine, faeces and sputum can be investigated by MC & S—*see faecal tests; urine tests; sputum tests*.

Stomach fluids and the cells of the stomach lining can be obtained for MC& S testing by means of a process called gastric washing. In this, a tube is passed into the stomach via the oesophagus. Through it, fluid is passed into the stomach, washed round and sucked out again for examination.

MID-STREAM STERILE URINE COLLECTION (MSU)—see Urine tests

MYELOGRAM—see X-rays

NUCLEAR MAGNETIC RESONANCE SCAN (NMR)

A recently devised technique to allow doctors to see through human tissues. The nuclear magnetic resonator produces a strong magnetic field which forces all the differently charged atomic particles in the chemicals that make up the tissues into the same alignment. The NMR then uses a radio pulse to alter their alignment and make the particles move backwards and forwards, emitting electromagnetic signals whose characteristics vary according to the precise nature of the particles, and, therefore, the chemicals comprising the individual tissues. A computer in the NMR analyzes the various electromagnetic signals, and uses them to build up a cross-sectional image of the tissue being scanned.

Though its full potential is still being evaluated, the NMR is thought to be even more effective than the *CAT scan* at providing clear images of tissues deep in the body. Some doctors believe that the

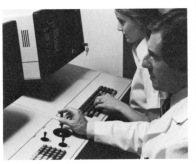

NMR scan NMR allows doctors to scan even the deepest bodily tissues (left) and obtain a detailed visual picture of the effects of disease upon them. The technique works by computer analysis of electro-magnetic signals, which can be seen visually on monitor screens (right) and then stored in a retrieval system.

technique will enable body chemistry to be monitored, and allow a precise assessment of the extent of any damage to tissues, and the ability of tissues to repair themselves. Such information would be of invaluable help to doctors choosing a course of treatment.

The NMR is completely safe, carrying none of the risks of *X-rays*. However, the strong magnetic field it creates may interfere with the operation of metallic implants, such as pacemakers. Unfortunately, cost is a major drawback to the technique. An NMR costs around twice as much as a CAT scanner, and a special, magnetically isolated room must be built to house it.

NUCLEAR SCAN—see Isotope scan

OPHTHALMOSCOPY—see Eye tests

PEAK FLOW MEASUREMENT— see Lung function tests

PERIMETRY—see Eye tests

PROTEINURIA TEST—see Urine tests

PYELOGRAM—see X-rays

SCANS—see Isotope scan; NMR scan; Ultrasound scan; X-rays

SCHICK TEST

A test to establish whether a person is immune to diphtheria. A solution containing a mild solution of the poisonous chemical produced by the bacteria responsible for diphtheria is injected into the skin of the forearm; a control solution, which does not contain the chemical, may be injected into the other forearm for purposes of comparison. If a person has immunity to the disease, antibodies in his or her blood—*see*

Natural Defences Against Disease, p52—will destroy the chemical, and no reaction is seen. In people without sufficient immunity, a red, inflamed area appears at the site of the injection within three or four days. Such people are then immunized against diphtheria. The Shick test is often used to determine which people require immunization in cases of a diphtheria epidemic.

SCHILLING TEST
A test to determine how efficiently the body absorbs vitamin B12—*see Diet, p322*. Poor absorption causes a vitamin B12 deficiency, which can result in anaemia and neurological disorders.

The patient is given two dosages of vitamin B12. The first is an injection, the quantity of vitamin calculated to saturate the proteins which carry it in the blood—*see The Blood and Lymph Systems, p21*. The second dosage is radioactive, and is given in tablet form. Since no more vitamin can be carried by the blood, all of the radioactive vitamin should be absorbed in the intestines and excreted in the urine. The amount in the urine produced for 24 hours after the tablet is taken is measured: if this is less than the radioactive dosage given, there is a deficiency in vitamin B12 absorption. The test is performed in hospital, and, to ensure that all the urine is collected, an overnight stay may be required; since the dosage of radiation is less than that given in an *X-ray*, the procedure is completely safe.

If the Schilling test shows a deficiency in absorption, another test may be performed around two weeks time. The aim is to discover whether the patient is suffering from a type of anaemia known as pernicious anaemia. In this, there is a deficiency of a protein called the intrinsic factor, which is essential to the absorption of vitamin B12. To see if this is the case, the Schilling test is repeated, after the patient has been given tablets containing intrinsic factor. If the test still shows an absorption deficiency, the problem has another cause, such as an intestinal disorder or alcoholism.

SLIT-LAMP TEST—see Eye tests

SPUTUM TESTS
Tests to determine the presence of and identify disease organisms and malignant cells in sputum, the viscous fluid produced in the lungs. The sample is obtained by collecting sputum coughed up by a patient. This is sent to the bacteriology laboratory for *MC & S*—microscopy, culture and sensitivity. A variety of tests are run, but one, in particular,

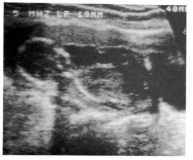

Ultrasound An ultrasound scanner in operation **(right)**. The operator moves the scanning head across the stomach, which has been lubricated with grease to aid its passage. The test is a routine check in pregnancy; **(left)** a typical foetal scan.

is common. This is a test for the presence of the bacilli that cause tuberculosis (TB). A special stain, called a Ziehl Nielsen stain, is used, and the sample is cultured on special plates. A sputum sample may also be examined for the presence of malignant cells in cases of suspected lung cancer.

TRANSCERVICAL ASPIRATION
A recently developed method used to diagnose disease in the foetus while it is still in the womb—*see Pregnancy and Birth, p60*. A thin tube is passed into the womb through the vagina, its precise position monitored by an *ultrasound scan*. When the tube is near the placenta, a small quantity of fluid is sucked out. This contains cells from the foetus, which can be examined for signs of abnormality—*see amniocentesis*.

ULTRASOUND SCANS
Methods of examining the deep tissues of the body by means of high frequency sound waves. Ultrasound waves bounce off the objects at which they are aimed at different rates according to the density of the objects. Dense cartilage, for example, will reflect ultrasound waves at a different rate to loosely packed fibrous tissue. This means that body tissues of different densities can be distinguished from one another.

Ultrasound scans are quick and safe, having no effect on the tissues under examination; scans are performed in hospital out-patient clinics, or in special centres. The sound waves are generated by a hand-held device which is placed above the area to be scanned. The device records the echo of the reflected sound waves, and relays them to a computer. This analyzes the different echoes, and forms an image of the area on a screen. Initially, the use of ultrasound scans was confined to the examination of

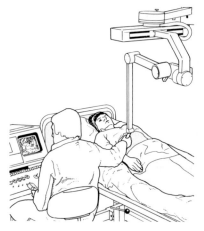

developing foetuses, but now the technique is used as an aid to the diagnosis of disorders in a number of areas.

Abdominal ultrasound The ultrasound investigation of tissues in the abdomen. The technique may be used to guide a *biopsy* needle to the required site, or to make a detailed examination of organs such as the liver, pancreas, kidneys and gall bladder. The gall bladder shows up particularly well, and gallstones, if present, can often be counted. Any enlargement or wasting of the organs can be detected, as can the presence of areas of inflammation, cysts, tumours or a blockage. For this purpose, a special ultrasound technique called B-mode ultrasonography is used.

Heart ultrasound Also known as echocardiography, heart ultrasound can be used to establish the size and shape of the atria, ventricles, valves and aorta — *see The Blood and Lymph Systems, p21*. Recently, a modification of the technique has made it possible to observe the components of the heart during the heartbeat. In this, called real-time echocardiography, the sound beam is directed at the heart in carefully timed bursts, up to 20 times a second. The result is similar to a motion picture, in which a sequence of fixed images run together to give the impression of movement.

Obstetric ultrasound The examination of the foetus inside the womb — *see Pregnancy and Birth, p60*. Ultrasound is used to determine the size and position of the foetus — from this an estimate of foetal age can be calculated — and its rate of growth. Later in pregnancy, the technique is used to detect abnormal presentations of the foetus, such as placenta praevia. If there is any suspicion that the foetus is developing abnormally, specialized ultrasound techniques can give important information about the condition of the foetal heart and kidneys.

Since the procedure is completely safe for both mother and baby, ultrasound scans are routinely given to expectant mothers attending hospital ante-natal clinics. The procedure is also used to guide a needle into the womb in *amniocentesis*, or a tube into the womb in *transcervical aspiration*.

Pelvic ultrasound An ultrasound examination of the pelvic organs, most commonly used to investigate disorders affecting the womb and ovaries, such as fibroids or an ovarian cyst.

URINE TESTS
A variety of tests to examine urine for signs of internal disorders. Depending on the nature of the investigation, a doctor may ask for one of three types of urine sample: a

mid-stream sample, an early morning sample, or a 24-hour collection.

The most common type is the mid-stream urine sample. In this, the patient washes his or her genitals, starts to urinate, stops halfway through emptying the bladder, and directs a small sample of urine into the container provided, before completing urination. The object is to ensure that the sample is uncontaminated by genital micro-organisms, so that doctors can be certain that any such organisms found in the sample come from inside the body. Mid-stream urine samples are usually requested when a doctor suspects that a patient is suffering from a urinary tract infection. The sample is sent to a bacteriology laboratory for *MC & S*—microscopy, culture and sensitivity—to identify any organisms that may be present. If, rarely, a sufficiently uncontaminated urine cannot be obtained by a mid-stream sample, it may be necessary to withdraw urine direct from the bladder. In this procedure, called a suprapubic urine sample, a needle is passed over the pubic bone and into the bladder, under local anaesthetic.

Obtaining an early morning sample of urine is a less complicated procedure. The patient merely has to urinate into the container provided as soon as he or she wakes up in the morning. Early morning samples are requested for *pregnancy testing* and for MC & S to detect the presence of tubercle bacilli, responsible for tuberculosis (TB).

Occasionally, a doctor may ask a patient to collect all the urine passed over a period of 24 hours. Such samples are requested for a *Schilling test*, and in the diagnosis of uncommon conditions such as phaeochromocytoma.

Urine samples are often crudely tested in the doctor's surgery by means of special dipsticks. Various types are available, but those most commonly used contain several strips of paper, sensitized in different ways. One type of dipstick, for example, reacts to the presence of protein, blood, bile pigments, ketones and sugar. In each case, an abnormally high quantity is indicated by a change in colour of one of the sensitized strips; the precise shade is a crude indicator of quantity. Should any dipstick tests prove positive, a urine sample will usually be sent to the appropriate laboratory for a more exact investigation.

Bile Bile pigments, the breakdown products of red blood cells, are found in the urine in conditions such as obstructive jaundice and hepatitis. They are detected by means of a dipstick test, and investigated further by laboratory analysis.

Blood A dipstick test detects the presence of blood in the urine in the first instance, and, if positive, is followed by laboratory investigations of a urine sample. Blood is found in the urine in cases of kidney stones and serious kidney infections, such as pyelonephritis, and in other infections of the urinary tract, such as cystitis and prostatitis. Rarely, blood in the urine is a sign of a tumour in the urinary tract.

Ketones Ketones, the breakdown products of fat metabolism — *see Metabolism, p44* — may be detected in the urine by means of a dipstick test. Their presence is a sign of diabetes, and more rarely, of starvation or a low carbohydrate diet. The exact level of ketones is determined by laboratory analysis.

Proteinuria test A test to determine the amount of protein in the urine. Normally, proteins are filtered from the blood by the kidney, but then reabsorbed into the blood in the same organ — *see The Digestive System, p40*. In cases of kidney disease or infection, such as nephrotic syndrome, proteins tend to be filtered but not reabsorbed, thus appearing in the urine. Proteinuria may also be a sign of pre-eclampsia in pregnant women, and occur harmlessly in young, fit adults — this condition is known as orthostatic proteinuria.

Initially, the protein content of urine is estimated by a dipstick test. Should an abnormal result be obtained, a urine sample may be sent to a biochemistry laboratory in order that the exact quantity and type of protein can be determined. A number of different tests are used, but one — a Bence-Jones protein test — is particularly important. Bence-Jones protein occurs naturally in the body, and is small enough to pass through the kidneys and enter the urine. However, it is produced in abnormally large quantities in conditions such as myeloma, a form of cancer.

Sugar The presence of sugar in the urine is detected by a dipstick test, and further investigated by laboratory analysis. Generally, it is a sign of diabetes, a condition that can be confirmed by a glucose tolerance test — *see blood tests*. However, traces of sugar are sometimes found in the urine of pregnant women. In this case, the condition is normally harmless, but a glucose tolerance test is usually performed to rule out diabetes.

VISUAL EVOKED POTENTIAL

A test carried out by means of an *electroencephalogram* (EEG). The brain waves recorded by an EEG naturally vary according to the sensory stimuli to which the patient is exposed. The visual evoked potential test utilizes this fact by changing the visual stimuli in a fixed manner: light and dark squares, arranged in a chess-board pattern, are rapidly alternated. In healthy subjects this produces characteristic changes to the brain waves. However, in conditions such as multiple sclerosis and epilepsy, these changes are altered in specific ways, making diagnosis possible.

VISUAL FIELD TESTS—see Eye tests

WIDAL TEST—see Blood tests

VITALOGRAPHY—see Lung function tests

X-RAYS

The use of X-ray radiation to obtain an image of the tissues of the body. X-rays are directed on to the area of the body under investigation, and pass through it to record an image on photographic film. The density of the image varies according to the strength of X-rays that reach the film; this, in turn, depends on the density of the tissues through which they pass, because dense tissues such as bone, absorb more X-rays than less dense tissues, such as flesh.

There are two basic types of X-ray: simple, or plain X-rays, and contrast X-rays. Plain X-rays are all taken in a quick, simple procedure—essentially, it is the same as having a photograph taken. Instead of focussing the lens of the camera, the X-ray technician, called a radiographer, asks the patient to stand or lie in a specific position between the machine generating X-rays and the photographic plate. This ensures a clear image of the tissue under investigation.

After the photographic plate has been developed, specialist doctors, called radiologists, can examine the resultant image for evidence of a disorder. Bone fractures show up clearly, as do problems affecting joints and cartilage, such as the damage caused by osteoarthritis and osteoporosis. Chest X-rays are commonly taken, because the size of the heart and lungs can be seen, as well as areas of inflammation, fluid or abnormal growth. The chest is usually X-rayed, therefore, as part of the investigation of conditions such as pneumonia, bronchitis, lung cancer, and heart failure—*see Routine Health Checks, p346*. Low dosage X-rays can used to detect the presence of cysts and tumours in the breasts. This technique, called mammography, is under consideration as a screening technique for the early detection of breast cancer—*see Routine Health Checks, p346*.

Plain X-rays of the abdomen are usually only taken as an emergency measure, because they only show serious problems such as intestinal obstruction. For more detailed information, contrast X-rays must be taken. For these, a special, radio-opaque dye—that is, a dye that absorbs X-rays—is injected into the tissue under investigation to highlight empty spaces and outline soft tissues. A variety of techniques can be used, depending on the area to be examined. Some require special preparations and an overnight stay in hospital; others are performed on an out-patient basis. The various techniques are described on *p96*.

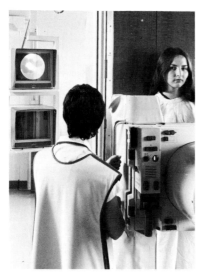

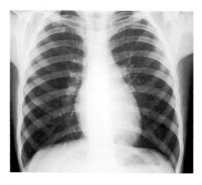

X-rays Radiography is essential in cases of broken bones and in many diseases, since an accurate internal view is a vital aid to diagnosis and treatment. The patient **(left)** is undergoing fluoroscopy after a barium meal; this is a special technique, in which the radiographer can actually see what is happening on a monitor. The chest x-ray **(right)** is on conventional film.

Angiography A contrast X-ray technique, also called arteriography, used in the investigation of blood vessels. Generally, angiograms are taken to establish whether blood vessels are obstructed — for example, by a blood clot or by fatty plaque, caused by atherosclerosis — or unusually narrow, as a result of arteriosclerosis. The technique also shows any increase in blood supply to an area, which may be caused by the extra demands for nutrients made by the quick-growing cells of a tumour.

The exact procedure depends on the site of the blood vessels under examination. In coronary angiography, for example, a thin tube is either placed in the femoral artery in the groin or the brachial artery in the arm, under local anaesthetic and light sedation — *see The Blood and Lymph Systems, p21.* This is carefully pushed through the blood vessels until it reaches the heart; dye is then injected into the coronary arteries, and an X-ray taken. By examining the X-ray plate, doctors can see how much the supply of blood to the heart has been affected by conditions such as coronary artery disease. A similar technique, called renal angiography, can be used to show the presence of a tumour in a kidney.

The arteries of the brain may be examined by carotid, or cerebral, angiography in cases of transient ischaemic attack, or a stroke, called a cerebrovascular accident; it also shows the presence of aneurysms and cerebral tumours. In this case, the dye is injected either through a needle placed in the carotid artery or a tube worked upwards from the femoral artery. The procedure is painful and delicate, and, if a needle is to be placed in the neck, a general anaesthetic is often given.

Barium studies The use of a radio-opaque dye called barium sulphate to obtain X-rays of the digestive tract — *see The Digestive System, p40.* Barium studies are used in the investigation of a number of conditions affecting the digestive system. These include hernias, ulcers, colitis, diverticulitis, and tumours. Barium may be given in a variety of ways, depending on the area under investigation.

A barium swallow and meal is used to obtain an X-ray image of the oesophagus, stomach and duodenum. The patient fasts overnight, and in the morning is given a porridge-like drink containing barium. He or she then lies on a table and several X-rays are taken over a period of about an hour. The table can be tilted, so that the barium coats the entire area under investigation, and air is sometimes pumped into the stomach to distend it to obtain a clearer image. The barium is eventually passed through the intestines and expelled in the faeces, giving

them a whitish appearance. The procedure sometimes causes constipation, which can be relieved by an enema.

The small intestine is examined by means of a barium enema. The patient fasts overnight, and is often given a laxative to empty his or her bowels. An enema containing barium is then placed high in the anal passage, with the help of a tube. After a short interval, X-rays are taken. The procedure lasts for around 30 minutes and may cause uncomfortable muscle spasms. A muscle relaxant may be given by injection to avoid these.

CAT scan A form of contrast X-ray that does not involve the use of a radio-opaque dye. CAT stands for computer axial tomography.

The CAT scan uses a computer to analyze a series of X-rays taken at fractionally different depths of tissue by means of a very thin beam of radiation. The computer interprets the resultant images as a series of cross-section slices through the tissue under examination. Each picture is made up of a large number of dots, shaded to represent different densities of tissue. The procedure is safe and quick, and obviates the need for injection of dyes. Unfortunately, the machine used is not yet widely available

The most common use of the CAT scan is to examine the brain. Unlike conventional X-rays, the CAT scan can differentiate between normal tissues, tumours, abscesses and blood clots. The liver and pancreas show up particularly well on CAT scans, and the technique is sometimes the only way of diagnosing a malignant lung tumour in its early stages.

Cholecystogram and cholangiogram Two tests in which a radio-opaque dye is used to obtain an X-ray of the gall bladder and bile ducts — *see Metabolism, p44.*

A cholecystogram is primarily used to investigate suspected gallstones. The patient swallows tablets containing a dye after his or her evening meal. The dye enters the blood stream at the small intestine and circulates in the blood until it is removed by the liver. By the morning, the dye has accumulated in the gall bladder, and X-rays can be taken. First, however, the patient is given a fatty meal to stimulate the release of bile, so that the common bile duct can also be seen.

This test shows up the gall bladder and common bile duct well, but does not always successfully show the bile ducts in the liver. This may be necessary in cases where it is thought that the bile ducts may be obstructed by a condition such as a tumour. A cholangiogram is performed to investigate this possibility. In the test, a dye is injected into a vein. Within 20 minutes, it reaches the liver and infiltrates the bile ducts, so that

X-rays can be taken. Occasionally, the dye is injected directly into a bile duct. This procedure, called a transhepatic percutaneous cholangiogram, may cause serious complications, however, and is usually only used to confirm the site of an obstruction to bile flow when it has already been decided that surgery is necessary.

Cystogram A test in which a radio-opaque dye is used to obtain X-ray images of the bladder and urethra. The dye is introduced into the bladder by means of a thin tube which is placed in the urethra. The procedure causes some discomfort, but this can be relieved by the use of a lubricating anaesthetic jelly. The patient is asked to urinate — the test is often known as a micturating cystogram — and a series of X-rays are taken. These show whether the urine has a tendency to flow backwards up the ureters towards the kidneys — a condition known as reflux of urine — and demonstrate any obstruction to the normal flow of urine, as may be caused, for example, by prostatic enlargement. The test, which is often performed at the same time as an intravenous pyelogram — *see below* — may also reveal any areas of inflammation caused by a urinary tract infection.

Hysterosalpingogram A test in which a radio-opaque dye is used to obtain an X-ray image of the uterus and Fallopian tubes — *see Sex and Reproduction, p54.* A hysterosalpingogram is commonly used to see whether the Fallopian tubes are blocked in the investigation of infertility. The dye is squirted into the womb through a thin tube placed in the cervix.

Lymphangiogram A test in which a radio-opaque dye is used to obtain an X-ray image of the lymph system — *see The Blood and Lymph Systems, p21.* The dye is injected into one of the lymph vessels, usually at the top of the foot. This spreads throughout the lymph network, outlining the nodes, glands and channels on X-ray. The test gives valuable information on the diagnosis and progress of disorders primarily affecting the lymph system, such as Hodgkin's disease and lymphoma.

Myelogram A test in which a radio-opaque dye is used to obtain an X-ray image of the space surrounding the spinal cord within the vertebral column — *see The Nervous System, p32.* The dye is injected into the space by means of a *lumbar puncture*, while the patient lies on a table that can be tipped to ensure that the dye travels the full length of the spinal cord. The test is used in the investigation of disorders affecting the spine and intervertebral discs, such as spinal tumours.

Pyelogram A test in which a radio-opaque dye is used to obtain X-ray images of the kidneys. The patient is usually asked to fast overnight to dehydrate the kidneys and the dye is injected into a vein, usually at the elbow. It travels through the blood to the kidneys, and outlines their size and shape on X-ray. Any obstruction caused by a kidney stone or a tumour can be seen, and the speed with which the dye reaches the ureters and bladder can be recorded as a measure of the kidneys' efficiency. The test is therefore used in the investigation of a wide variety of disorders and infections affecting the kidneys.

Venogram A test in which a radio-opaque dye is used to obtain an X-ray image of a vein. The test is usually performed in the investigation of a suspected blood clot, most commonly a deep vein thrombosis. The dye is injected into a vein in the hand or the foot, depending on the site at which a clot is suspected.

VENOGRAM—see X-rays

VIRAL TESTS—see Blood tests

THE A-Z OF MEDICINE

THIS SECTION is not only the longest in this book, but is the key to your understanding of the medical problems that can affect us all from even before birth to old age and death.

Over 1,000 diseases and conditions are covered and explained, all extensively cross-referenced where appropriate so that you can follow connections and see how, in medicine, one problem is frequently linked to another.

In addition, the A-Z includes explanations of the technical terms doctors often use in explaining what is wrong with you and how they propose to treat the problem.

The whole section is designed as a medical interpreter, removing the mystique from medicine and explaining it clearly and simply in lay terms.

How to use the A-Z of medicine

THE A-Z OF MEDICINE is the core of this book. Not only does it list a wide range of common diseases and conditions; it explains them all clearly and concisely, following a common organizational plan. Any entry always starts by defining its subject in a simple sentence. It then explains how the disease or condition arises, how it affects you, whether or not it is linked to any other diseases or conditions, and whether there is the risk of complications. It tells you how the doctor will make a diagnosis, what aids he or she will use to help in this, and what treatment will be prescribed.

The A-Z does more than this, however. It takes full account of the fact that doctors are sometimes tempted to use technical language in their explanations, which the average patient often finds hard to understand and frequently fails to get clarified through fear of embarrassment. Thus, common medical terms are also listed and explained. In addition, there is also a full cross-reference system to other parts of the book.

Remember, though, that no book can substitute for the expert advice and care the medical profession is there to provide. Always consult your doctor if you feel ill and never be afraid that you are wasting his or her time. What may seem trivial could become something serious, if left untreated. Similarly, never be afraid to ask if something puzzles you or if you feel unsure why a certain treament is being prescribed. At the same time, never adopt your course of treatment on lay advice. The doctor is there to help you, but equally, you must help your doctor.

In common with the rest of this book, the A-Z of Medicine is fully cross-referenced to enable you to use it fully and to best advantage. The cross-references work in two ways, internally and externally.

Related entries within the A-Z are printed in italic type when they occur within the main text.

Related headwords are cross-referenced to the appropriate main entry.

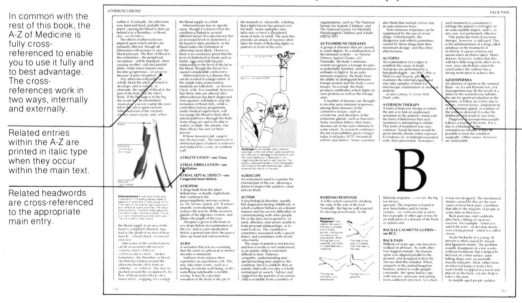

Cross-references also take you to other sections of the book, in which further information is given.

UNDERSTANDING MEDICAL TERMS

In medicine, a large number of terms are derived from Latin and Greek. If you know the meaning of the Latin and Greek components, it will be easy to interpret many medical terms that at first sight seem complex. The ones you will most frequently come across are listed below. The position of the hyphen shows whether the component is placed at the beginning or the end of the term. In the United States the 'a' has been dropped from 'aemia' and 'haem'.

a-, an-: a lack of, an absence of
ab-: away from
ad-: towards, near to
andr-: of the male sex
-anemia: of the blood
anti-: against, opposing
-arch-, -arche-: first
arthr-: of a joint
audio-: of hearing, or sound
aut-, auto-: self
bi-: two
brady-: slowness
-cele: swelling
-centesis: perforation
chron-: time
-cide: destroyer
contra-: against, opposite
cryo-: cold
-cyte: a cell
de-: removal, or loss
derm-: of the skin
dipl-: double
dys-: difficulty, abnormality
ec-, ect-: outside, external
-ectomy: surgical removal
em-, en-: inside, internal
end-: inner, within

enter-: of the intestine
epi-: upon, over
erythr-: red
ex-, exo-: outside of, outer
extra-: outside, beyond
fibr-: of fibrous tissue
-genic: producing
-gram: record, trace
-graph: a device that records
haem-: of the blood
hepat-: of the liver
hetero-: dissimilar
homoeo: alike
hydr-: of water, or fluid
hyp-, hypo-: deficiency in, lack of
hyper-: excess of
-iasis: a disease state
inter-: between
intra-: inside
-itis: inflammation
laparo-: of the abdomen or loins
leuc-, leuk-: white
-lysis: breaking up
macro-: large
mal-: disorder, abnormality
-mania: compulsion, obsession
mast-: of the breast
mega-: abnormally large
-megaly: abnormal enlargement
mes-: middle
met-, meta-: a) change, e.g. metabolism; b) distant, e.g. metastasis
micro-: small
myo-, my-: of the muscles
myelo-: of the spine
nephr-: of the kidneys
neur-: of the nerves
-oma: a tumor
-osis: a disease state
ost-: of bone
-otomy: a surgical cutting
pan-: all
para-: a) near, e.g. paramedian;

b) like, e.g. paratyphoid; c) abnormal, e.g. paraesthesia
path-: of disease
-pathy: disease
-penia: deficiency
peri-: near, around
-philia: craving, love for
phleb-: of the veins
-plasia: formation
-plegia: paralysis
pneu-: of respiration
-poiesis: formation
poly-: many
pre-: a) before, e.g. prenatal; b) in front of, e.g. prevertebral
pro-: before, in front of
proct-: of the anus and rectum
rhin-: of the nose
-stasis: standing still
sub-: below
tox-: poisonous
trans-: through, across
-trophy: growth, development
vas-: a vessel

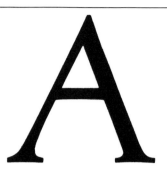

ABORTION

The spontaneous or deliberate termination of pregnancy, in which the foetus *(p60)* is expelled from the womb before the 28th week of gestation. After 28 weeks of intra-uterine life, a foetus is said to be 'viable' and in the eyes of the law has a separate existence from the mother. If pregnancy terminates after this date, the term premature birth is used when the baby survives, and *stillbirth* if the baby is dead at the time of delivery.

Doctors use the term 'abortion' in two different ways. In a spontaneous abortion, or miscarriage, the expectant mother loses her baby against her own wishes. In an induced or therapeutic abortion, however, the termination of pregnancy is a deliberate, considered act and in most countries it is a criminal offence. However, in the UK, in many states in the USA and in several European countries abortions are permitted in certain, specified circumstances, as long as they are performed in approved centres.

About 15% of all pregnancies end in spontaneous abortions or, in lay terms, in miscarriages. The majority of these occur in the first trimester, or three-month period, usually between the sixth and tenth weeks of pregnancy. Three-quarters of all such miscarriages are caused either by a *congenital abnormality*, in which there is some fault in the foetus—in around 40% of cases this is due to a *chromosomal* abnormality—or by defective implantation of the foetus in the womb.

Miscarriages that occur in the later stages of pregnancy are normally caused by illness or abnormalities of the uterus in the mother. In rare cases, *fibroids* may be so large that they distort the uterine cavity and cause abortion, or the womb may be retroverted or bent over backwards, and remain fixed in the pelvis as pregnancy progresses.

Some spontaneous abortions occur because the cervix or neck of the womb gapes and is incapable of staying closed. This is called an incompetent cervix and may be due to an underlying weakness of the cervix or to previous dilatation of the cervix, perhaps at a termination of pregnancy, or to a previous miscarriage.

Cervical incompetence is not particularly common, and is certainly not a normal consequence of termination of pregnancy. It may, however, be a cause of recurrent mid-term abortion and is treated by placing a stitch around the neck of the womb to strengthen it. This stitch is usually removed about a week before the baby is due. Women who have had more than one spontaneous abortion—who are sometimes called habitual aborters—should avoid travel, rest as much as possible and also avoid sexual intercourse during the first three months of pregnancy.

The term 'missed abortion' is sometimes used to describe the situation in which a foetus has died but has not been expelled from the uterus as a spontaneous abortion.

Laws permitting induced or therapeutic abortions differ substantially. For example, in certain states of the USA, liberal laws permit abortion almost on demand, while in others it is permitted only when the continuation of a pregnancy will seriously affect the health of the mother. Under British law, an induced or therapeutic abortion may be carried out only if two doctors state that, having examined the pregnant woman, they feel that continuation of the pregnancy will seriously harm the physical or mental health of the mother or that of her existing children, or that there is a strong risk that if the baby were born it would suffer serious mental or physical handicap.

Over the past few years, the requirements of the law have been more tightly enforced, and in some areas doctors are now obliged to specify in what way the mother's or baby's health will be affected. In some situations, for example when a *congenital abnormality*, such as *Down's syndrome*, has been detected in the foetus, it is not difficult to make such a statement. However, some doctors find, for reasons of conscience and legality, that this becomes more difficult when the decision to recommend an abortion must be based on relieving the mental torment of a woman who suddenly finds that she is accidentally pregnant.

The form recommending an abortion must be signed by two doctors, one of whom is usually the GP and the other the gynaecologist who is going to carry out the operation. After certification, the abortion must be performed either in hospital or in a specially approved and licensed clinic, under local or general anaesthetic—*see anaesthesia*.

An operation before the 14th week of pregnancy may be carried out using a suction curette and the foetus removed by a method known as aspiration. Alternatively, the neck of the womb is gently dilated and the contents of the uterus scraped out in a procedure rather like a *dilatation and curettage (D and C)*. The patient may stay in hospital overnight, but in many places these operations are carried out as day cases.

Termination of pregnancy by either of these methods is safe, with very little danger of *complications* arising. Very rarely, however, a patient develops a temperature after the operation, and continues to lose blood, because she has an *infection* in the uterus. This is easily treated with *antibiotics*. More rarely still, the uterus may be accidentally *ruptured*, or the contents may not all be removed completely. In one or two instances a woman has gone on to deliver a live baby after having an unsuccessful abortion early in the pregnancy.

After about the 14th week of pregnancy, the foetus is too large and well-formed to be removed by the suction method. For this reason, abortion is carried out by injecting *prostaglandins* into the uterine cavity. These cause the uterus to contract and, in effect, to go into premature labour. The developing foetus is expelled vaginally. This is a distressing and painful procedure for the mother, who often has to undergo an operation for removal of retained products of conception.

After a therapeutic abortion, the woman is advised to shower, rather than bath, for the first three days. She should not douche for the first fortnight after what doctors call the TOP (termination of pregnancy). It is also better to use sanitary towels in preference to tampons for the first few days.

The woman will probably not feel like intercourse for the first days after her abortion, though there is no medical reason why it should be avoided, provided that adequate contraception is used. If the pill is the chosen method, it may be started immediately after the operation—or the woman can wait for her next menstrual period. In either case, it is not safe to resume sex immediately without taking additional precautions—*see Sex and Contraception, p338*. Clinics and hospitals usually advise women to have a medical check-up six weeks after an abortion.

The morality of induced abortion is the subject of constant and heated debate. Many people, for moral or religious reasons, reject the legal definition that takes the start of life to be the 28th week after conception, and consider abortion to be equivalent to murder. For this reason, some doctors refuse to refer a patient for a termination for reasons of conscience, as they are perfectly entitled to do—*see The Doctor, The Patient and Disease, p70*. (A patient in this situation, however, has the right to consult another doctor).

They point to the fact that a number of 23 and 24-week-old foetuses have been born prematurely and have survived; a number of doctors believe that the law should be changed to reflect the considerable advances made in the care of premature babies over the last decade. Some people also take the view that methods of contraception, such as the 'morning-after pill' (*p338*), that affect the fertilized egg, are forms of abortion, and therefore reprehensible.

It must be remembered that women have always found ways of dealing with unwanted pregnancies, often at great physical and financial cost. The British Abortion Act of 1967 was introduced to protect women from 'back-street abortionists', and to prevent considerable loss of adult life after criminal abortion.

The subject is one on which various pressure groups have very firm ideas, and several of them are campaigning for a reform of the Act. The Catholic Church condemns all induced abortion, while the Protestant churches have a less rigid approach. Hindu teachings allow abortion only where a pregnancy constitutes a danger to the mother's

life; Islamic law allows abortion up to as late as 120 days and under Jewish law the foetus is regarded as a subsidiary of the mother and abortion is permitted as long as a number of doctors recommend it.

On the whole, it seems that most people now believe that the decision on whether or not to induce an abortion is the sole province of the mother, within whose body the baby is developing.

ABSCESS
A pocket of pus that may arise in any part of the body tissue that has been invaded by *bacteria*.

Pus is the result of a fight against the invading bacteria by the body's defence system (*p52*). This sends large numbers of leucocytes or white blood cells (*p21*) to the site of the infection, and these kill the bacteria by engulfing them.

Pus is a thick, greenish yellow fluid composed of *bacteria*, dead tissue and dead white cells. The continued presence of bacteria in a suppurating infection attracts more

and more white cells to the site and these, unable to kill all the bacteria, die, so creating more pus and enlarging the abscess. The swollen abscess may impinge on other tissues, and this, together with the toxins or poisons produced by the bacteria, causes swelling and pain.

If an abscess does not burst spontaneously, it may be treated with *antibiotics* to kill the bacteria, or lanced, that is, opened with a scalpel and the pus drained out. A *boil*, an abscess close to the surface of the skin, may be lanced under local *anaesthetic*, but abscesses deep in the body may need to be drained in an operation under general anaesthetic. Painful tooth abscesses require special dental surgery.

ACCOMMODATION
The response of the muscles of the eye to changes of focus. The eye muscles contract or relax, so changing the shape of the lens, to adjust focus from a near to a distant object, or vice versa. This response becomes less efficient with age.

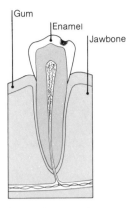 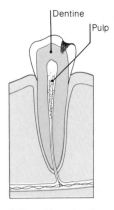 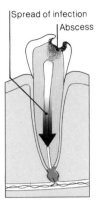

Dental abscesses 1. Bacteria break down sugar to form acid, which attacks tooth enamel.

2. The acid reaches the dentine. Bacteria then pass through to infect the soft tissue of the pulp. This becomes inflamed, causing severe toothache.

3. The infection quickly spreads to the base of the root where, together with poisons from the decaying tooth, it forms a pus-filled abscess. If this is left untreated the tooth will die.

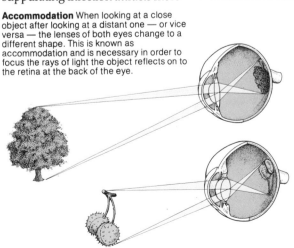

Accommodation When looking at a close object after looking at a distant one — or vice versa — the lenses of both eyes change to a different shape. This is known as accommodation and is necessary in order to focus the rays of light the object reflects on to the retina at the back of the eye.

Looking at a distant horse chestnut is an example of far accommodation. The muscles controlling the shape of the lens are relaxed, making the lens into a flattened disc.

Focusing on the conkers is an example of near accommodation. The same muscles are contracted, causing the lens to bulge and become more spherical.

ACHALASIA

The failure of a muscle to relax after contraction. Achalasia of the muscles in the wall of the intestines is a symptom of *Hirschsprung's Disease* but the term is normally used to denote a constant contraction of the muscles of the lower end, or cardia, of the oesophagus. This condition, which results from damage to the nerves that supply the region, causes difficulty in swallowing, chest pain, and vomiting. The overflow of food from the gullet may pass into the lungs, causing serious *infection*.

Achalasia is treated with muscle-relaxing drugs. Achalasia of the cardia, also called cardiospasm, may also be treated by cutting the affected muscles in a surgical operation. This relieves the *spasm* permanently, but does not interfere with normal swallowing.

ACHONDROPLASIA

An inherited abnormality in which cartilage is not laid down properly at the growing areas, or epiphyses, of the long bones of the limbs *(p16)*. This results in shortened arms and legs, but a normal trunk and skull. The condition, for which there is no treatment, causes a type of *dwarfism*, but does not affect intelligence.

ACIDOSIS

An imbalance in the body's acid-base balance, that is, the relationship between body acids and alkalis. In acidosis there is an increase in the acidity of the body's fluids and tissues. Contrary to popular belief, acidosis is not the same as *dyspepsia*.

Acidosis is caused by a failure of the delicate mechanisms that regulate the acid-base balance, if they become over-burdened with the chemical by-products of metabolism *(p44)*. The over-burdening may be caused by diseases of the lungs, kidneys and the blood, whose interaction maintains the acid-base balance, or by *metabolic disorders*, such as *diabetes mellitus*.

Depending on its severity, the condition may result in an increase in the rate of breathing, tiredness and *nausea*. Sometimes a distinctive aroma of acetone, which smells a little like nail varnish remover, may be smelt on the breath. The treatment of acidosis differs according to its cause.

In the condition known as ketoacidosis, a *complication* of diabetes mellitus, the body becomes *dehydrated* and the patient feels intensely thirsty and suffers from *constipation*, *cramps* and visual disturbances. This condition can lead to diabetic *coma* and is treated as

an emergency. Patients are treated in hospital with insulin to regulate the blood sugar level and large quantities of fluid are given intravenously to correct the dehydration.

ACNE

A common disorder of the skin; there are two types—acne vulgaris and acne rosacea.

Acne vulgaris is generally caused by the hormonal changes of adolescence, and of the *menarche* and *menopause* in women These chemical changes lead to an increase in the activity of the sebaceous glands of the skin of the face, chest and back. The sebum produced becomes trapped beneath the skin, forming a plug called a comedone or blackhead. This becomes infected, causing the skin to become inflamed and covered with red and purplish pimples. They normally disappear spontaneously, but in severe cases they may leave unsightly scars. The condition is often extremely distressing and may aggravate the mental and physical upheavals caused by puberty and the menopause.

There is no completely effective cure for acne, although sunlight, the *antibiotic* oxytetracycline, and

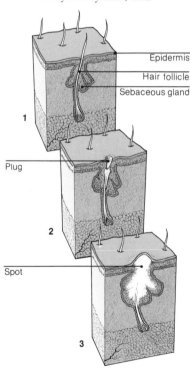

Acne Each hair on the body grows from a follicle and is lubricated by the oily sebum produced by the sebaceous gland, **1.** An excess of sebum from the gland forms a plug or blackhead at the top of the follicle and causes the hair to die, **2.** As sebum continues to be produced, the follicle becomes inflamed and swells into a spot, acne vulgaris, **3.**

medicated lotions may help. The best medicine is preventive, involving meticulous hygiene and frequent washing with soap and water. It is important not to squeeze spots and blackheads, or ugly scars will form. Contrary to popular belief, it has now been shown that there is no relationship between the consumption of sweets and acne, although over-indulgence in such foods is not recommended for other reasons—*see Diet, p322*.

Acne rosacea is a skin disease that affects the face; it is unrelated to acne vulgaris. The first signs of the condition are a rosy glow that follows a hot meal, hot drink or alcohol. As acne rosacea progresses, the blood vessels of the face, nose and cheek become permanently enlarged giving the typical red-faced appearance of the hardened drinker. This is somewhat unfair, because food, hot liquids, and climate, as well as alcohol, may all be responsible. The condition, which is unsightly but not dangerous, affects women more often than men, and is sometimes triggered by the *menopause*.

ACQUIRED IMMUNE DEFICIENCY SYNDROME—see AIDS

ACOUSTIC NEUROMA—see Neuroma

ACROMEGALY

A condition in which the anterior pituitary gland overproduces growth hormone *(p48)*. This is usually caused by a *tumour*, which may be *benign* or *malignant*, within the gland.

The excess growth hormone circulates in the bloodstream, causing the size of the hands, feet and face to increase. If the condition develops during the growing period of adolescence, the result may be gigantism—a grotesque increase in height.

The progress of acromegaly can be halted if the tumour is treated, either by surgery or *radiotherapy*, but any increase in body size that has already taken place cannot be reversed.

ACTINOMYCOSIS

An infection caused by a micro-organism, Actinomyces israelii, that was once thought to be a fungus but is now generally considered to be a *bacteria*. This microbe can cause three different types of the condition.

Actinomycosis is usually found in the gums and jaw. This is because the organism is always present in the mouth. It is usually harmless, but occasionally penetrates the gums to cause a serious infection and swelling of the jaw and the formation of a *boil* that discharges pus through the skin.

If the microbe is swallowed, it may cause an infection of the digestive tract with discharges of pus through the sinuses, which develop between the gut and the skin of the abdominal wall. The disease may later spread to involve the liver and spleen, and, if untreated, may then prove fatal.

Actinomycosis of the lung occurs when the microbe is inhaled. In this form of the disease, the lungs become swamped with pus, which may drain through *sinuses* to the skin, and *pneumonia* often develops.

Actinomycosis is treated with *antibiotics*, although surgery may be necessary to drain the large quantities of accumulated pus.

ACUTE
A term used to describe an illness or condition that has a rapid onset, course and resolution.

ADDICTION
An overwhelming craving for, and habitual usage of a substance—usually a drug, alcohol and to a lesser extent caffeine or nicotine. The addict may be both physically and emotionally dependent on the substance, and often experiences unpleasant mental and physical effects, known as withdrawal symptoms, if it is not taken. Some drugs appear to be more addictive than others, among them *amphetamines*, *barbiturates* and the *opiates*, of which heroin is the most dangerous form. It is also thought that minor tranquillizers of the benzodiazepine family, such as Valium, may cause a degree of addiction. This is thought to stem from what is termed the rebound effect—the original problem recurs when the drugs are stopped and so the patient starts taking them again to relieve it.

The reason why opiates become addictive was discovered in the 1970s by two American scientists, Solomon H. Snyder and Candace Pert. They found, firstly, that opiates bind to special receptors on the surface of the nerve cells in the parts of the brain and spinal cord dealing with the processing of information about pain. These receptors interact with *enkephalins*, chemicals manufactured by the brain which are released when pain impulses pass along the spinal cord to help suppress the sensation of pain before it becomes intolerable.

Normally, enkephalins occupy a certain number of opiate receptors. However, if opiates are taken

habitually, they gradually cause the production of enkephalins to cease. If the supply of opiates is then cut off, pain returns, since there are no enkephalins left to help deal with it. The body craves for more opiates as a result and withdrawal symptoms make their appearance.

Addiction can be treated by gradually withdrawing the drug the addict is dependent on and replacing it with regular dosages of another drug that is less addictive. Heroin addicts are withdrawn on to methadone for example. This withdrawal, although gradual, still causes unpleasant symptoms, but these can be relieved to some extent with the help of *tranquillizers*. The addict, who may be undernourished and suffering from *vitamin deficiencies*, is encouraged to eat and given plenty of rest, and treated for any *infections* and other illnesses resulting from the addiction. He or she will then be gradually withdrawn from the substitute drug.

This treatment may be successful in the short term. However, although many centres include *counselling* or *psychotherapy* in their programme of treatment, a majority of addicts become readdicted within a year of a cure, apparently because their deep-rooted psychological problems are difficult to solve.

In Britain, drug addiction is considered a medical, rather than a criminal, problem. Addicts may be registered by special drug dependency units, and are entitled to receive regular supplies of the drug to which they are addicted and, if they wish, treatment. This policy was introduced some decades ago in an attempt to keep each addict's habit—the quantity of drugs he or she needs every day to stave off withdrawal symptoms—at a constant level, and so prevent the establishment of a flourishing black market in narcotic drugs. It was successful, however, only until the 1960s, when a sudden great increase in drug-taking occurred and the market was flooded with illegal drugs. In the USA and most other countries, drug use by an addict is a criminal offence.

The problems of drug abuse and addiction are discussed in *Abuses of the Body, p384*.

ADDISON'S DISEASE
A condition that occurs when the cortex or outer layer of the adrenal gland above the kidney fails to produce the hormones cortisone and aldosterone—*see The Endocrine System, p42*. This failure is caused by an *autoimmune disease* in 75% of cases, and by *tuberculosis* in 20% of cases. Addison's disease is usually

gradual in onset, but occasionally occurs in an *acute* form.

The reduction in the level of production of the adrenal hormones causes weakness, weight loss, a fall in blood pressure and changes in the colour of the skin. The first signs of the disease, which often precede the appearance of the other symptoms by many years, are a darkening of the mucous membranes of the mouth or vagina, and of those parts of the body, such as the elbows and creases of the palms that are exposed to friction. Areas of *vitiligo*, in which the skin becomes white, may also appear, though this is less common.

The fall in blood pressure, called *hypotension*, may lead to dizziness or fainting attacks, while body hair may be lost, and women may have menstrual disorders. The most important symptom of Addison's disease, however, is tiredness and lethargy.

The condition may prove fatal, unless treated by synthetic hormones. These are taken by mouth, and in most cases restore a normal life expectancy. However, dosages often need to be increased at times of physical stress, such as an illness or operation. Acute Addisonian crises require emergency admission to hospital and treatment with intravenous *steroids* and *saline*.

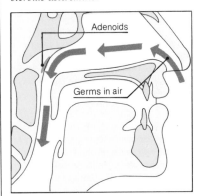

Adenoids When the lymph tissue in the nasopharyngeal recess becomes enlarged in children, the condition is called adenoiditis.

ADENOIDS
Two small masses of lymphatic tissue *(p21)*, similar to the tonsils, that are situated centrally in the nasopharynx at the back of the nose. Unlike the tonsils, they cannot be visually examined unless a special mirror is used.

The adenoids enlarge during childhood and reach a maximum size before the age of 15. After this, they shrink. Their enlargement may be a problem in the first few years of life as they tend to block the nasal passages and cause difficulty in breathing. The child therefore has to breathe through an open mouth and tends to have a heavy lidded, open-mouthed appearance.

Enlarged adenoids may also block the opening of the Eustachian tubes that run from the nasopharynx to the middle ear. This tends to cause recurrent *otitis media*, an infection of the middle ear.

Adenoidectomy, the removal of the adenoids, may be performed before the age of five if there is serious obstruction to the nasal passages or recurrent otitis media. Thereafter, since the tonsils may also cause chronic infection of the throat and upper respiratory tract, the adenoids are usually removed in a combined procedure with the tonsils known as Ts and As or tonsillectomy and adenoidectomy.

See also tonsillitis.

AETIOLOGY
The origin or cause of a disease.

AFFECTIVE DISORDERS
A group of psychiatric illnesses characterized by alterations in *affect* or mood. The two principal affective disorders are mania and psychotic *depression*, which some doctors term the manic reaction and the major depressive reaction respectively. These two illnesses often occur together in an illness known as the manic-depressive reaction.

The movements, speech and, apparently, thought of a patient suffering from an episode of major depressive reaction may slow down to the point of complete apathy and stupor in acute cases. Alternatively, they can become agitated, complaining repetitively. Such patients usually suffer severe *insomnia*, often waking regularly in the early hours of the morning, and may experience physical disorders, such as loss of appetite and weight, and *diarrhoea* or *constipation* and *amenorrhoea* in women.

Patients suffering from major depression usually blame themselves for their problems, yet fail to perceive or admit that they are depressed. The condition may progress to self-destructive behaviour, such as hair-pulling and nail-biting and episodes of *delusion*. Attempts at suicide are common in psychotic depressive states.

Affective illnesses rarely occur in adolescence, but tend to appear between the ages of 20 and 40. Symptoms often arise suddenly and unexpectedly—an apparently normal person may suddenly attempt suicide, for instance.

Several theories attempt to explain the causes of the affective disorders.

Since they tend to run in families there is some evidence that heredity may be a contributory factor. Many psychologists believe that the factors that cause neurotic *depression* may cause major depression in some cases.

Researchers have discovered certain biochemical and physical abnormalities in the brains of patients with affective disorders. There is considerable evidence that depression is linked to a reduction in the level of chemicals called amines in the brain. The tricyclic and monoamine oxidase *antidepressant* drugs are thought to treat depression by restoring amine levels.

Great progress is also being made in another field of research into substances called *endorphins*. These are chemical pain relievers in the brain, which are believed to regulate mood. They are thought to act in times of stress to counteract disappointment and relieve depression. Certain people may lack the requisite endorphins, or perhaps produce too much of some other substance that inhibits their action. However, it has not yet been established whether these biochemical changes are a cause or an effect of depressive illness.

A patient in a manic state will be treated initially with *tranquillizers*, such as chlorpromazine. A depressive patient may be admitted to hospital to deal with the risk of suicide, and treated with *anti-depressants*. If the depressed state is severe and recurrent he or she may be treated with electrotherapy—*see ECT. Lithium* is often used to treat patients suffering from recurrent manic-depressive episodes, since it has been found to be effective in preventing relapse.

See also neurosis.

AGORAPHOBIA
A fear of open spaces, or crowded places, which is so strong that it becomes a phobia—*see neurosis*. Agoraphobia can be a crippling condition; a sufferer may be afraid to leave the house to go shopping, for instance. The condition is often complicated by the fact that many people with agoraphobia are too frightened to seek help. It may be treated with drugs, *behaviour therapy* and relaxation techniques *(p332)*.

AID (ARTIFICIAL INSEMINATION BY DONOR)
A procedure in which a doctor places sperm from an anonymous donor high in the vagina in order to fertilize an ovum—*see Sex and*

Reproduction, p54. AID is used as a last resort in cases of *infertility* caused by a sperm defect .

The sperm is collected from selected donors, coded according to the donor's hair and eye colour, race and other characteristics, and stored in refrigerated sperm banks until required. The donor is never told to whom his sperm has been given, and has no involvement whatsoever with the baby.

The practice of AID still arouses some controversy, though it has been welcomed by many couples who wanted children but had been unable to have their own. Psychological problems have rarely occurred in the parents as a result of artificial insemination, probably because couples are subjected to a lengthy period of *counselling* before being recommended for AID; the effect on the child or young adult who discovers that his or her father is an anonymous donor is less well known, since the practice is fairly modern. However, controversy has recently been caused in the USA by people who discovered in adult life that they were conceived by this method. There is also some dispute about the precise legal relationship between the donor and the child.

See also AIH.

AIDS
The disease now known as AIDS (*Acquired Immune Deficiency Syndrome*) was first identified in the USA in the summer of 1981. Since then, the incidence has increased with frightening rapidity to reach the proportions of a major world health problem by the late 1980s. At first, the condition was thought to be more or less confined to homosexuals and intravenous drug abusers, but now it has become clear that anyone is at risk.

AIDS is caused by a virus, now called HIV (Human Immunodeficiency Virus). A variant form of HIV has recently been found and labelled HIV-II. Where and how HIV originated is unknown. A closely related virus occurs in African green monkeys, which has led many researchers to think that HIV came from that continent. However, there is no agreement about how the virus might have spread to human beings, while some people doubt the theory of the African origin of AIDS.

HIV has been found in many body fluids, including semen, blood, secretions from the neck of the womb, tears, saliva, urine, and breast milk, although only semen, blood, and possibly cervical secretions are likely to transmit the infection. Throughout the world the main method of transmission is sexual intercourse; other methods include the use of contaminated needles and the receipt of infected blood, donated organs, and semen. Pregnant women can infect their unborn children.

Infection is not spread by casual social contacts, and no health care workers have acquired the disease by looking after infected patients, although a few have done so from pricking themselves with needles. The infection is not passed on in saliva or by biting insects. There is no risk in sharing cups, eating or cooking utensils, or toilets with an infected person.

Infection with HIV can give rise to a bewildering range of illnesses. Some are due to infections that occur because the virus damages the immune system, while others—especially those affecting the nervous system—seem to be due to HIV itself. The disease goes through various states. When the virus first gains access to the body there are no symptoms, which is one of the reasons why it spreads so fast: people do not realize that they are potentially infective. At this stage tests for HIV give negative results, but the person concerned can pass on the infection to others.

Blood test results become positive within a year (usually within two or three months). Early symptoms (fever, diarrhoea, night sweats, weight loss, swollen lymph glands, tiredness, persistent cough, loss of appetite) may appear after about a year or after five or more years; these have been called AIDS-related complex (ARC). Finally the full picture of AIDS may develop, with secondary infections leading, for example, to pneumonia. A hitherto rare form of skin cancer (*Kaposi's sarcoma*) is often found. Full-blown AIDS is always fatal.

It has been known for some time that there can be damage to the brain in AIDS, but a worrying recent development has been the discovery that some people who are HIV-positive have symptoms of brain damage, even though they do not suffer from the full-blown AIDS picture. It is still too early to say what this means, but some researchers fear that damage to the brain by HIV may be inevitable in all those infected, and that this aspect of HIV infection will eventually come to outweigh the other effects, serious though these are. Nor is it known, as yet, how many of those who have been infected with the virus will go on to develop overt illnesses. At least one person in three will do so, but the final proportion may well be higher.

There is at present no cure for AIDS, and the medical emphasis is therefore on prevention. The main things to avoid are sexual intercourse with anyone who might be infected and contact with infected blood, especially by sharing needles. If you do have intercourse with anyone who might be liable to be infected, you should use a condom at the very least, though the protection this gives is not complete. Casual sex contacts are naturally the most dangerous; currently, the groups in whom HIV is particularly widespread are homosexual and bisexual men and drug users, but the danger to other groups will increase unless behaviour alters.

A very small number of people have also acquired HIV from blood transfusions. Donated blood is now tested before it is used, so the risk is very much less than it was. (There is no risk at all in giving blood). In the past, some haemophiliacs have acquired HIV from blood products given to stop bleeding, but all blood products are now heat-treated to destroy the virus, so there is no longer any danger in their use.

HIV carriers should take responsible precautions to avoid passing on the virus. They should tell any doctor or dentist who may treat them. They should not share toothbrushes, razors, nail brushes, or anything else that could carry blood, and they should not donate blood, plasma, body organs, or sperm; also, they should not become pregnant. If they cut themselves, they should mop up the blood using household bleach (one part bleach to nine parts water), though the bleach should not be applied to the cut. Fortunately the virus cannot survive for long outside the body.

An enormous amount of work is going on throughout the world to find either a cure for AIDS, or a means of preventing it. Antibiotics can be used to treat the secondary infections that occur, but they do not affect HIV. Anti-viral agents exist, but they have not been very effective against HIV. Moreover, the discovery that HIV affects the brain has complicated matters considerably, both because most of the known anti-viral drugs do not reach the brain cells, and because of the nature of HIV itself.

HIV is what is medically termed a *retrovirus*. This is because it contains an enzyme called *reverse transcriptase*, which causes viral DNA to be produced and incorporated into the nuclei of the patient's cells, which then programme the production of more virus. Consequently HIV is written into the very basis of the patient's life and, so far as is known,

cannot be eliminated without destroying the cells within which it is contained. In the case of the brain this would clearly be undesirable even if it were technically possible.

In spite of these difficulties, a vaccine against AIDS is not out of the question, but it will not be easy to produce; indeed, some pessimistic researchers think it may be impossible. Whether or not a vaccine is eventually found, however, the search for it is likely to have indirect benefits in bringing about a greatly increased understanding of AIDS itself and also of many other viral diseases.

AIH (ARTIFICIAL INSEMINATION BY HUSBAND)
A procedure in which a doctor places sperm from the husband high in the vagina in order to fertilize an ovum—*see Sex and Reproduction, p54.* AIH can be used when a couple find it difficult to conceive because the husband is *impotent*, when there are insufficient sperm in his ejaculate, or when the sperm is of poor quality. In the last two cases, large quantities of sperm are collected from the husband over a period of time and stored until they can be introduced into the cervix in sufficient quantities to make conception likely.
See also AID; infertility.

ALBINISM
A lack of pigment in the skin, hair and eyes caused by an inherited defect of the *chromosomes*. Sufferers from albinism, called albinos, are often extremely sensitive to light because they lack any protective pigment in the choroid coating of the eye.

ALBUMINURIA—see Proteinurea

ALCOHOLIC NEUROPATHY—see Neuropathy

ALCOHOLISM
An illness caused by *dependence* on the excessive consumption of alcoholic drinks, including spirits, wine, beer or methylated spirits. Alcohol abuse may cause a number of physical problems, including *cirrhosis* of the liver, *cardiomyopathy*, peripheral *neuropathy* and some diseases of the brain, as well as physical and psychological *dependence*. There is also a high incidence of gastrointestinal disorders, ranging from alcoholic *gastritis* to ulceration—*see ulcers.* The withdrawal of alcohol from an alcoholic may cause severe *anxiety, tremor, convulsions* and a type of *hallucination* known as *delirium tremens*.

There are great social and

geographical differences in the amount of drinking that is socially acceptable. Consequently, it is extremely difficult to define an alcoholic. Clearly, when the urge to drink is so strong that it adversely affects the life of the drinker, leading to difficulties at home and at work, the diagnosis is obvious.

Alcoholics are often very difficult to treat as they often lack the motivation to attack the problem—even denying it exists. By the time they seek help, their lives may have crumbled around them. They may have lost their jobs, homes, husbands or wives. Rehabilitation therefore becomes a much larger problem than simply stopping drinking. Moreover, they often have other medical problems and may be undernourished.

The large number of alcoholics and dangerously heavy drinkers who maintain an almost normal outward appearance are less obvious, but just as difficult to treat. Alcoholics of this type usually suffer from minor upsets of the digestive tract, such as *diarrhoea* and *gastritis*, and, since alcohol is damaging to the health, they may eventually suffer from serious illness.

Alcoholics may be treated in special centres and private nursing homes. Withdrawal, usually called drying out, takes a long time. During this, the alcoholic is usually given *tranquillizers* to relieve withdrawal symptoms. Drugs such as antabuse, which react with alcohol to cause *vomiting*, may be either taken daily or implanted under the skin to remind the alcoholic not to drink.

Various groups have been set up to help the alcoholic and his or her family. Best known of these is AA (*Alcoholics Anonymous*), an organization whose many branches hold regular meetings to provide information, support and help to alcoholics, whether or not they have given up drinking. A sister organization, Al-Anon, has been formed to help relatives and friends of alcoholics, while Al-Ateen aids young people. 'Accept'is a newer organization that aims to promote education about the harmful effects of alcohol, and to encourage sensible, moderate drinking in the community, as well as to help the alcoholic. By various means, such as group *psychotherapy*, it explores the *personality problems* that cause a person to turn to alcohol

Widespread efforts are also being made through health education in schools, newspapers, magazines and television to explain how normal 'social' drinking can escalate gradually to the point where it becomes a problem that adversely affects life. In the UK and the USA, where excessive drinking damages the health of vast numbers of people every year, organizations interested in health education and in fighting the spread of alcoholism are lobbying for greater government support for this type of publicity.

ALDOSTERONISM

Primary aldosteronism, also called Conn's syndrome, is a condition in which excessive amounts of the hormone aldosterone are secreted by the adrenal cortex of the adrenal glands above the kidney.

Aldosterone regulates the body's salt and water balance.

The condition is usually due to an *adenoma* of the adrenal cortex, or to hyperplasia, the abnormal growth of normal cells in the tissue. It causes the retention of sodium, potassium depletion, and is one of the causes of *hypertension*, or high blood pressure. Potassium deficiency commonly causes physical weakness and excessive thirst or excessive production of urine. Sodium retention leads to water retention and this leads to hypertension.

ALKALOSIS

An imbalance in the relationship between acids and alkalis—called the acid-base balance—in the body, in which the alkalinity of the tissues is increased.

Alkalosis may be caused by an excessive intake of alkaline foods, such as milk and vegetables,and is occasionally seen in vegetarians. It can follow a loss of acid from the body after prolonged *vomiting*, or be caused by a reduction of the level of potassium in the body as a result of the action of *diuretics*. The condition can lead to apathy, weakness, muscular *cramps* and, in extreme cases, *delirium*. It is treated by correcting the biochemical imbalance through a controlled diet, and by removing the primary cause.

Respiratory alkalosis is a variant of this condition, in which the body fluids are highly alkaline and there is an abnormally low level of carbon dioxide in the blood—*see The Respiratory System, p28*. It may be caused by *hyperventilation*, or over-breathing, by high altitude, and aspirin poisoning. It leads to lightheadedness, fainting and tetany, a condition in which there is *spasm* and twitching of the muscles.

ALLERGIC RHINITIS—see Rhinitis

ALLERGY

A hypersensitive reaction of the body to an antibody, a substance that is foreign to it. An allergic reaction is an exaggerated version of the normal response of the body to a foreign substance—*see Natural Defences Against Disease, p52*. However, only certain people have such a hypersensitive response. Antigens that produce allergic reactions are therefore known as allergens.

The body may become sensitive to almost any substance, but the most common allergens are pollen, which causes *hay-fever*, animal hair, dust, fur and foods. The nature of the allergic reaction varies considerably according to the individual affected and the allergen, but it usually causes cell damage and the release of *histamine*: it may involve sneezing, skin rashes and weals, as in *urticaria*, or serious illness. The most extreme form of allergic reaction, called *anaphylaxis*, may prove fatal unless treated.

The symptoms of an allergic reaction can be treated according to their nature, but an allergy can be treated only when the specific allergen responsible for it is identified. This can be done through a process of elimination—in hay fever, for example, different types of pollen may be scratched under the skin of the arm to find out which particular pollen causes a reaction.

Some people can be *desensitized* to an allergen to which they are hypersensitive by the administration of small dosages of it. *Antihistamines* may help relieve the symptoms, but they are unpopular with doctors, since they cause severe drowsiness and other symptoms. For some sufferers, the only treatment is the avoidance of all contact with the substance to which he or she is allergic.

Many scientists think that a wide range of diseases may be caused by allergies of which the sufferer is unaware. So far, the evidence for this belief is inconclusive, though it is generally accepted that many cases of eczema—*see dermatitis and asthma*—are caused by allergy.

There is also considerable debate about the existence of a 'total allergy syndrome'. In this condition, some doctors believe, sufferers have a serious allergic reaction to almost everything around them—often specifically to man-made substances. Such patients have to live in a carefully controlled environment, eating only a small range of foods, some of which may be bizarre. This is expensive and rarely completely successful. Other doctors deny that the condition exists at all. They believe that its symptoms can be accounted for by obsessional *hyperventilation*.

ALOPECIA

The loss of hair from the body. When hair loss occurs in patches it is known as 'alopecia areata'; when all the hair on the head is lost the condition is called 'alopecia totalis'; and when the whole body is involved it is known as 'alopecia universalis'.

The characteristic 'male-pattern' baldness, in which hair recedes from the temples and thins at the crown, is a natural consequence of age, the activity of male sex hormones and *hereditary* factors. Women's hair may also thin temporarily after pregnancy, and permanently during middle to old age, but baldness is rare.

Unnatural causes of serious hair loss may include severe illnesses; endocrine disorders, such as *Cushing's Syndrome—see The Endocrine System, p48*; hypothyroidism—*see myxoedema*; *shock; trauma*; radiation; the intake of poisons, such as arsenic; or adverse reactions to a drug. In these cases, alopecia is treated by removal of its cause.

Patchy hair loss may be due to *fungal* infection, and, in this case, is associated with a scaly scalp and broken hairs. Patchy hair loss is also seen in the second stage of *syphilis*.

There is no specific treatment for patchy hair loss, though *steroid* creams are sometimes used on the scalp. Some doctors treat the condition by manipulating an allergic reaction—the scalp is sensitized to an allergen (often the leaves of the primula plant) and the allergen is then applied to it.

Hair transplantation is practised at some private clinics, but the process is lengthy, painful and costly. In the case of alopecia areata it may also be unnecessary, because the hair often grows back after a few years.

ALVEOLITIS

An inflammation of the walls of the alveoli, the air sacs in the lungs—*see The Respiratory System, p28*. There are two forms of the condition, allergic and fibrosing alveolitis.

Allergic alveolitis is caused by an allergic reaction in the alveolar tissue to particles that are inhaled in breathing. Farmer's lung, for example, is a form of alveolitis caused by inhalation of the spores of mouldy hay, while bird-fancier's lung is caused by sensitivity to pigeon droppings. A few hours after inhalation of the allergen, the sufferer may feel weak, tired and short of breath, and have a cough. Later, breathing may become extremely difficult. In serious cases, treatment with oxygen and *steroids* may be necessary. To avoid a

repetition of the problem, the sufferer must ensure he or she does not inhale the allergen.

Fibrosing alveolitis has no apparent cause, though it may be associated with *rheumatoid arthritis* or *scleroderma*. Here, *inflammation* leads to the formation of fibrous tissue in the alveolar walls; this, in turn, may cause *emphysema* and *bronchiectasis*.

AMBYLOPIA

Any deficiency in vision that cannot be accounted for by a defect in the optical system of the eye. The problem is normally the result of an *inflammation*, or neuritis of the optic nerve. This neuritis may have a variety of causes, including excessive smoking or consumption of alcohol, or *vitamin deficiencies*.

Treatment of the condition depends upon its cause. Vitamin deficiencies can be made good by replacement vitamins, while large dosages of hydroxocobalamine, a derivative of Vitamin B12, help to detoxify cyanide, the agent in tobacco smoke that is largely responsible for neuritis.

AMENORRHOEA

The absence of normal menstrual periods in women after puberty and before the *menopause*.

If periods have not started by the age of 18, the condition is called primary amenorrhoea. It has a number of possible causes. These include a physical deformity of the uterus or vagina, *Turner's syndrome* and, very occasionally, an imperforate *hymen*. It may also be due to disorders of the endocrine system, such as chronic *adrenal hyperplasia*, a *tumour* of the pituitary gland, or thyroid disease. All of these delay maturity.

In secondary amenorrhoea, periods cease. The most common causes of this condition are pregnancy and breast-feeding, but it is often seen in women who have stopped taking the contraceptive pill. In this case, periods may not become regular for up to a year—*see Sex and Contraception, p338*.

Secondary amenorrhoea may also be caused by starvation and weight loss, as in *anorexia nervosa*; by abnormalities of the adrenal and thyroid glands; and by a deficiency of ovarian hormones. It also inevitably follows a *hysterectomy* or *oophrectomy*.

AMNESIA

A partial or total loss of memory. Amnesia may follow physical *trauma*, such as a blow on the head or a fractured skull, or serious physical or mental illness. It may also occur as a consequence of senile

dementia. Amnesia is also commonly a complication of *hysteria* and *alcoholism*. Sometimes the mind blocks out memories of the events that led up to an accident or traumatic event. In this case the condition is retrograde amnesia.

AMOEBIASIS

An infection caused by a micro-organism known as Entamoeba histolica. Amoebiasis is a severe form of *dysentery*. The organism enters the body in contaminated food and drink, and forms infected ulcers in the wall of the colon. Occasionally, an abscess may form in the liver; in rare instances, this penetrates the diaphragm so that pus is coughed up. Treatment is with *antibiotics*, although an abscess in the liver may need to be drained.

AMPHETAMINE

A potentially addictive drug—*see addiction*—that stimulates the nervous system. It acts specifically upon the sympathetic nervous system to increase the heart rate and the rate at which the body uses up its fuel. Amphetamines produce a feeling of well-being and give an impression of alert intelligence, so are especially open to abuse—*see Abuses of the Body, p328*.

Because of their effect on metabolism—*see Metabolism, p44*—amphetamines are prescribed by some doctors as a treatment for *obesity*, but because they are addictive, many doctors believe this to be irresponsible and dangerous. However, they are prescribed in the treatment of *narcolepsy*.

AMYLOID DISEASE

A disease in which amyloid, an abnormal protein, is deposited in organs such as the kidneys, liver and spleen, adversely affecting their functions. Amyloid disease, also called amyloidosis, is usually a complication of other diseases, such as *rheumatoid arthritis, tuberculosis* or *Hodgkin's Disease*. In some patients, however, it develops without any apparent cause, affecting the tongue and heart and giving rise to *cardiomyopathy*. This condition is thought to be caused by a malfunction of the body's natural defences against disease, and is known as primary amyloidosis.

There is no cure for amyloidosis, although in the early stages it may be affected by *steroids*. Treatment is aimed at the underlying disease. Rheumatoid arthritis and tuberculosis are treated with the appropriate drugs. Where amyloidosis has affected the kidneys and caused renal failure, the patient may eventually need *dialysis*.

ANAEMIA

A deficiency of haemoglobin, the chemical that carries oxygen, in the red cells of the blood—*see the Blood and Lymph Systems, p21*. Anaemia causes tiredness, pallor, weakness and a feeling of general *malaise*.

There are many causes of anaemia. These can be divided into four main groups: a deficiency in the production of red cells by the bone marrow; an excessive destruction of red cells by the body; a loss of blood from the body; and other causes.

A shortfall in the production of red blood cells is usually due to a lack of one of the chemicals—most commonly iron—essential to the process. Iron deficiency may be caused by inadequate intake, absorption or utilization of the mineral. As a result, the red blood cells are pale and small.

Two other chemicals essential for red cell production are vitamin B12 and folic acid. A deficiency of either gives rise to a condition known as macrocytic anaemia, in which the red blood cells are abnormally large. A deficiency of vitamin B12 is normally caused by a total *gastrectomy*—removal of the stomach—or by *pernicious anaemia*.

Folic acid deficiency often occurs in pregnancy. It is caused by a combination of an inadequate diet and the demands of the growing foetus. To prevent this deficiency, expectant mothers are often given a a pill in which folic acid and iron are combined—*see Diet p322*. Folic acid deficiency can also occur in alcoholism.

Vitamin C and the hormone thyroxine are also essential to the production of red blood cells. A deficiency of the former, as in *scurvy*, or the latter, as in *myxoedema*, may lead to anaemia.

Anaemia caused by excessive destruction of red blood cells is known as haemolytic anaemia. Red cells may be destroyed by the body either because they have an abnormal shape, as in hereditary *spherocytosis*, or an abnormal constituent, as in *thalassaemia* or *sickle cell disease*. Haemolytic anaemia may also be caused by the action of poisons, and by the antigen-antibody reaction—*see Natural Defences Against Disease p52*—that occurs in *haemolytic disease of the newborn*.

Anaemia may also be caused by a loss of blood. If this occurs during an operation, or as a result of a wound, it can be replaced by blood *transfusion*. Blood may be lost more gradually, however, over a number of years, through heavy periods or *menorrhagia*, or through diseases of the digestive tract. In these cases the anaemia is often more difficult to detect.

A variety of other problems and conditions may cause anaemia. Pancytopaenia is a general reduction in the number of red and white cells in the blood. It may be *idiopathic*, or the result of treatment by *radiotherapy* or certain drugs, or of disease of the bone marrow. The resulting anaemia is called aplastic anaemia, and is often fatal. Anaemia may also be associated with *rheumatoid arthritis, cancer, kidney failure* and *cirrhosis* of the liver.

Anaemia is treated according to its cause. Missing factors in the production of blood cells are replaced where possible, blood loss is stopped, and any treatments thought to cause the destruction of blood cells are halted.

ANAESTHESIA

A loss of conscious bodily sensation. In general anaesthesia, total unconsciousness is induced, whereas in local anaesthesia a particular part of the body is numbed, so that pain cannot be felt, by the use of a local anaesthetic.

General and local anaesthetics utilize two different processes. General anaesthetics are thought to depress consciousness by their action on the reticular formation of the brain—*see The Nervous System, p32*—while local anaesthetics paralyse the sensory nerves in the area they affect.

General anaesthetics should not be used unless a doctor considers them absolutely necessary. This is because they may cause unforeseen reactions in the patient; repeated anaesthesia may strain a weak heart and damage the liver, for instance.

ANALGESIC

A pain-relieving drug that may be taken in the form of a tablet, injection or inhaled gas. The best known analgesic is *aspirin*, or acetylsalicylic acid, but many other compounds of varying strengths can be used. Such preparations may cause damage to the lining of the stomach, and should, if possible, be taken dissolved in water.

The strongest and most dangerous pain-killers are derivatives of opium. The most effective and most addictive of these are, in ascending order of strength, codeine, morphine and heroin. Acupuncture—*see Alternative Medicine, p305*—is another form of analgesia.

ANALYSIS - see Psychoanalysis

ANAPHYLAXIS

A severe allergic reaction. An *allergy* usually produces a mild and localized reaction, but is sometimes widespread and catastrophic. When this happens, the sufferer is said to be in a state of anaphylactic shock. Unless treated, this may be fatal, since there may be a sudden collapse of both the respiratory and circulatory systems.

ANCYSTOMIASIS—see Worms

ANENCEPHALY

A defect in the development of the neural tube—*see Embryology, p12*—in which the uppermost part of the brain and skull of the foetus are either missing or incorrectly formed. Anencephalic babies are normally so badly deformed that they die at, or shortly after, birth. The defect can be detected before birth by

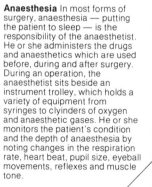
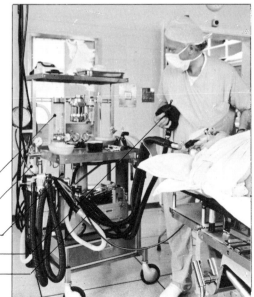

Anaesthesia In most forms of surgery, anaesthesia — putting the patient to sleep — is the responsibility of the anaesthetist. He or she administers the drugs and anaesthetics which are used before, during and after surgery. During an operation, the anaesthetist sits beside an instrument trolley, which holds a variety of equipment from syringes to cylinders of oxygen and anaesthetic gases. He or she monitors the patient's condition and the depth of anaesthesia by noting changes in the respiration rate, heart beat, pupil size, eyeball movements, reflexes and muscle tone.

Flow meter

Cylinders of oxygen

Instrument trolley

Breathing bag

Bellows

Aneurysm An aneurysm is a swelling of an artery which develops because of a weakness in the arterial wall. Aneurysms are defined in various ways. They may be defined according to shape, or where they occur in the body. A dissecting aneurysm, for instance, develops when the inner and outer layers of the wall are separated by blood pushing through a tear in the inner layer. An aortic aneurysm, as the name implies, develops in the aorta, where it forms a balloon-shaped swelling.

Dissecting aneurysm Blood cuts through a tear in the inner layer of the wall and 'dissects' the inner from the outer layer.

Blood vessel

If a blood clot forms in a dissecting aneurysm, it can have the effect of limiting any further dissection.

Aortic aneurysm The pressure of the blood pushes the inner arterial layer through the ruptured elastic and muscular fibres of the middle wall.

Saccular aneurysm

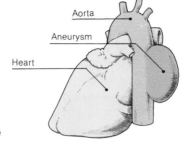

Aorta
Aneurysm
Heart

Aneurysms can develop in any artery of the body. However, they usually affect the aorta and arteries of the brain. Dissecting aneurysms appear only in the part of the aorta nearest the heart; if they burst they are likely to prove rapidly fatal. Aortic aneurysms may develop at any point along the aorta. The two kinds are saccular and fusiform. A saccular aneurysm swells up at a weak patch on one side of the aorta or artery *(above left)*. A fusiform aneurysm is a tubular swelling

Fusiform aneurysm

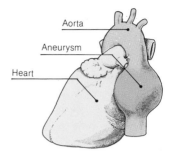

Aorta
Aneurysm
Heart

which develops when the middle layer of the wall is equally weakened all the way around.

A saccular aneurysm may also develop where an artery branches, particularly in the arteries supplying the brain. It is usually congenital and, because of its shape, is called a 'berry' aneurysm. It exhibits none of the warning symptoms of other aneurysms and if it ruptures it may haemorrhage so severely as to be fatal.

Blood vessel

Outer layer
Muscle layer
Inner layer

Berry aneurysm

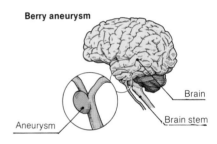

Brain
Brain stem
Aneurysm

amniocentesis—*see Special Tests p84*. This shows up the increased level of alphafoetoprotein, a protein produced in the liver of the foetus, which is present in the amniotic fluid in this condition.

ANEURYSM

A bulge in the wall of an artery, which may vary in shape, size, position and cause.

Aneurysms may sometimes occur in the aorta, the main artery of the body, where they are the result of a weakness of the muscular wall. This may be *congenital*, or caused by *atherosclerosis* or *syphilis*. The condition is extremely dangerous, since the aneurysm may rupture and cause fatal internal bleeding, or compress nearby blood vessels so that tissues are starved of oxygen and die. Sometimes, however, aneurysms can be repaired surgically.

Another dangerous form of aneurysm may develop in the left ventricle of the heart, following a heart attack or *myocardial infarction*. The scar tissue that replaces dead heart muscle sometimes bulges out to form a ventricular aneurysm. This may lead to *heart failure*, because it does not contract efficiently, or the formation of an *embolism*.

The blood vessels of the brain are also sometimes affected by aneurysms. These are normally congenital, but may be a result of old age or *hypertension*. If aneurysms in the brain rupture, they may cause a *subarachnoid haemorrhage*, or intracerebral haemorrhage. Both of these are *cerebrovascular accidents* or strokes and may lead to death or *paralysis*.

ANGINA PECTORIS

A severe pain or tightness in the centre of the chest that may be experienced during exercise or after meals and is usually relieved by rest. The pain, which may spread up to the jaw or down into the left arm, is like someone sitting on the chest, or a tight band around it. It usually lasts only for a few minutes.

Angina occurs when the blood supply reaching the heart muscle through the coronary arteries is insufficient to meet the heart's demands for oxygen and nutrients. It is a sign of *coronary artery disease*, and a warning that a *myocardial infarction* or heart attack may occur. Anyone who experiences angina should consult his or her doctor as soon as possible.

The pain can be relieved by drugs that dilate the coronary arteries and

reduce the amount of work done by the heart. A programme of rest, relaxation and moderate, controlled exercise may also be helpful. In severe cases, however, the coronary arteries may become blocked. If this happens, surgery can create alternative pathways, so that the blood by-passes the diseased arteries, reaches the heart tissue and the angina is relieved.

ANKYLOSING SPONDYLITIS

A *chronic* and progressive disease that causes degenerative changes in the joints of the spine. Ankylosing spondylitis tends to affect more men than women and generally occurs between the ages of 20 and 40. It may be associated with *Crohn's disease* or *ulcerative colitis*.

The first sign of the disease is early morning *back pain* and stiffness; as it progresses the joints of the spinal vertebrae become fused, and the vertebral ligaments become bony until the spine is rigid, a condition often called bamboo spine.

If ankylosing spondylitis is detected early in its course, the condition can be treated successfully by *radiotherapy*. This treatment, however, may give rise to unpleasant, and sometimes dangerous, side-effects. Later, *anti-*

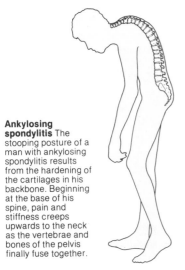

Ankylosing spondylitis The stooping posture of a man with ankylosing spondylitis results from the hardening of the cartilages in his backbone. Beginning at the base of his spine, pain and stiffness creeps upwards to the neck as the vertebrae and bones of the pelvis finally fuse together.

inflammatory drugs, such as phenylbutazone, and *analgesics* may relieve the symptoms.

ANOREXIA NERVOSA

A complex illness, characterized by an overwhelming fear and loathing of body fat, that leads to extreme dieting and, often, self-induced *vomiting* and purging.

Anorexia nervosa usually develops in young women, and is thought to affect around one in 100,000 of the female population, and between one and two per cent of young girls. The condition was first described in the 19th century, when it was thought, incorrectly, to be a disorder of the pituitary gland.

The causes of anorexia nervosa are varied and complex, but many are rooted in unacknowledged family problems. The condition is often seen in girls whose families stress material and academic achievement, but undervalue emotional development. Social pressures and fashions, which equate slimness with attractiveness, also play an important part in the development of the illness.

Anorexics often have an almost absurdly distorted image of their own bodies. They reject the evidence of their own eyes and the reassurances offered by their friends and families, refusing to believe that they are thin and expressing disgust at their fatness. As a result they diet so much that they are in danger of starvation. Sometimes, too, they induce vomiting, or use laxatives, after swallowing the little that they do eat—*see also bulimia nervosa*—in an obsessional, unnecessary attempt to become thin.

Anorexia nervosa is sometimes difficult to detect, and is always hard to treat. This is especially true if the sufferer has a difficult relationship with her parents. Hospital treatment is necessary to restore physical health, but the psychological problems behind the illness require lengthy *counselling* or *psychotherapy*.

Self-help groups for anorexics have recently been set up throughout the UK. They are called Anorexics Aid.

ANOSMIA

A loss of the sense of smell, that may occur temporarily during a cold, or permanently when the olfactory nerves are disrupted by disease or injury.

ANOXIA—see Hypoxia

ANTACID

An alkaline drug taken to relieve discomfort caused by an increase in the acid content of the stomach in *dyspepsia*.

ANTE-PARTUM HAEMORRHAGE

A loss of blood from the vagina in the late stages of pregnancy, prior to the onset of labour—*see Pregnancy and Birth, p60*. If much blood is lost, the condition is serious, and immediate hospital treatment is necessary. An ante-partum haemorrhage is sometimes the result of a *placenta praevia*, in which the placenta partly overlaps the cervix.

ANTHRAX

A serious infection caused by the bacterium Bacillus anthracis, which may be picked up from the carcases or skins of infected animals. Anthrax is therefore a particular hazard for farmers, butchers and woolsorters. The last-named run the risk of inhaling the organism, which can lead to a severe, fatal *bronchopneumonia*. The incidence of the disease has been successfully limited by livestock controls, but isolated outbreaks still occur.

After a short *incubation* period of one to three days, an unpleasant pustule or spot appears on the skin at the point of contact with the bacterium—if, for example, infected meat is eaten, an infected ulcer forms in the mouth or throat. More commonly, the *lesion* occurs on the face or neck, where it appears as a blister surrounded by red, inflamed skin. Later this dries out to form a characteristic black scab. A high fever develops, causing prostration. If untreated, the condition may lead to a fatal *bacteraemia*.

Anthrax can be treated successfully by large dosages of *antibiotics*. There is also an *antiserum*, which can be used in cases of serious illness. A *vaccine* is available to prevent workers at risk from contracting the disease.

ANTIBIOTIC

A drug that fights *bacterial* infection. There are many different types of antibiotic, and they vary in their methods of action and their targets. Bactericidal antibiotics act by killing bacteria, while bacteriostatic types stop the bacteria from reproducing. Broad-spectrum antibiotics are active against a variety of bacteria, while others are active only against specific species or strains. For each different type of bacterial infection, therefore, there is a specific type of antibiotic.

Antibiotics are not active against viruses, and so are not effective in the treatment of viral infections, such as *influenza* or the common cold. On occasions, however, doctors may prescribe antibiotics for patients suffering from viral infections, if they suspect bacterial infection has superseded the initial viral illness. Generally, doctors tend to avoid prescribing antibiotics unless absolutely necessary. There are several reasons for this. Antibiotics may kill the beneficial bacteria that live naturally in the body—those aiding digestion in the intestines, for example, and the Doderlein bacteria of the vagina. Some patients have an *allergy* to certain antibiotics; there is also a danger that bacteria will develop a resistance to an antibiotic, so that the drug will be ineffective when it is needed in the future.

When taking antibiotics, it is important that patients always follow instructions. The full course of drugs must always be taken,

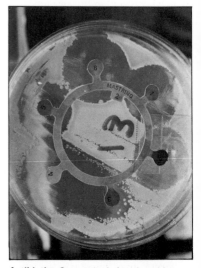

Antibiotics One method of testing which antibiotics are effective in killing specific bacteria is shown *(above)*. Bacteria are left to grow for a few days on a glass dish containing agar, a nutrient-rich substance. A circle of six different antibiotics is then placed on top of the bacterial culture. These are left to seep on to the agar for a couple of days. Those antibiotics that kill the bacteria leave a circle of clear agar; in this case, all six antibiotics were effective.

whether the symptoms clear up during the course or not. If the treatment is stopped before all the micro-organisms have been killed, a relapse may occur. Interrupting a course also brings the risk of micro-organisms developing which are resistant to the antibiotic that has been prescribed. Some antibiotics should be taken on an empty stomach to ensure adequate absorption, and alcohol should not be taken during the course.

ANTICOAGULANT

A drug that prevents blood from clotting—see *The Blood and Lymph Systems, p21*. The most effective anticoagulant is heparin, a substance found naturally in the body. Heparin extracts may be given by injection in the case of deep venous *thrombosis* to prevent further clot formation. However, because heparin extract has to be administered by injection—and also because it is extremely expensive—slower-acting synthetic substitutes, such as warfarin, are prescribed for long-term conditions, such as *atherosclerosis* and deep vein *thrombosis*, and after transient ischaemic attacks, or surgery on the coronary arteries. Warfarin, however, may have serious effects if taken with alcohol, *barbiturates*, aspirin and a number of other drugs. These can interact with warfarin to dangerously stimulate its anti-coagulant action.

The correct dosage of anticoagulants is very closely judged, because an overdose may cause internal bleeding. The effect is monitored by regular blood tests—see *Special Tests p84*.

ANTICONVULSANT

A drug given to prevent, or reduce the severity of, *convulsions* in *epilepsy*. A variety of different anticonvulsants may be given, depending on whether the patient suffers from petit mal or grand mal epilepsy, but the dosage of all of them must be carefully judged to avoid side-effects. The most commonly given anticonvulsants are phenytoin and the *barbiturate* drug phenobarbitone.

ANTIDEPRESSANT

A drug that relieves the symptoms of *depression*. Antidepressants are given only in certain cases of serious depression, as they tend to have a number of unpleasant side-effects. They differ from tranquillizers both in action and use.

There are two groups of antidepressants—the tricyclic drugs, which include imipramine, and the monoamine oxidase inhibitors, such as phenelzine. The former may cause *constipation*, blurred vision, drowsiness and a dry mouth; the latter may have a serious interaction—see *drug interactions*—with a number of products, among them cheese and chianti. People taking antidepressants usually do not notice beneficial effects for several weeks.

ANTI-EMETIC

A drug that prevents *vomiting*, and reduces *nausea*. Anti-emetics are used to prevent *travel sickness* and the nausea and vomiting associated with *migraine*; they are also given to control the nausea and vomiting that may follow general *anaesthesia*.

Unless they have been prescribed by a doctor, anti-emetics should not be used to control *hyperemesis gravidarum*, or morning sickness, during the first few months of pregnancy, because their effect on the developing foetus is not fully known.

ANTI-FUNGAL AGENTS—see fungus

ANTIHISTAMINE

A drug that counters the effect of *histamine* in the body. Histamine is produced as part of the immune response to cell damage—see *Natural Defences Against Disease, p52*.

Antihistamines may be given in the treatment of *allergies*, and insect bites and stings. Because of their *anti-emetic* properties, they are also used in the control of *nausea* and *vomiting*. Unfortunately, they sometimes have a number of side-effects, including drowsiness, and dizziness, and should only be taken on the advice of a doctor, although they can be bought from a chemist without a prescription.

Because they cause drowsiness, antihistamines are sometimes given to children as pre-medication before an operation.

ANTI-INFLAMMATORY DRUG

A drug used to control *inflammation*, especially in the joints. Anti-inflammatory drugs are therefore frequently used in the treatment of conditions such as *rheumatoid arthritis* and *osteoarthritis*—they can help to control the pain, stiffness and swelling of joints that is a feature of these diseases. Some doctors believe that anti-inflammatory drugs can also speed the healing process in injuries of the soft tissues, such as a sprained ankle, but this claim has been disputed.

The most potent drugs of this type are the *steroids*. Unfortunately, these may sometimes cause serious side-effects. Large dosages of aspirin are also effective in the control of inflammation, but such dosages may damage the lining of the digestive tract. There is also a whole range of non-steroid anti-inflammatory drugs, including phenylbutazone, indomethacin, and ibuprofen.

ANTISERUM

A substance derived from blood, which contains antibodies—see *Natural Defences Against Disease, p52*—against a specific disease. Antiserum prepared from the blood of laboratory animals can be used to give a patient with a serious *infection*, such as *tetanus*, a degree of immunity against the disease. The patient then has an immediate supply of antibodies to fight the infection, when there may be insufficient time to wait for the body to form them naturally.

The use of animal blood, however, brings with it the risk of an allergic reaction—see *allergy*—that may be serious enough to cause *anaphylactic shock*. Today, this risk is lessened because antiserums are usually prepared from the blood of a patient recovering from the same disease, who thus has a high level of the required antibodies.

ANURIA

A reduction in the quantity of urine produced by the body, which is usually a serious symptom of *kidney disease*. Medically, the term is not usually used to describe the condition in which urination is impossible because of an obstruction to the ureter. This problem is known as *retention of urine*.

ANXIETY

A state of fear and apprehension that may be accompanied by physical signs, such as a dry mouth, sweaty palms, a fast heart beat and *palpitations*.

Anxiety is a normal response to a number of situations—when confronted by a large, snarling dog, for example, or when a woman finds a lump in her breast. It is, in fact, a beneficial reaction, because the body is preparing itself, through the action of the hormone adrenaline, for fighting, or for running away from danger—see *The Endocrine System, p48*.

Sometimes, however, anxiety takes over a person's life. This condition is called an anxiety *neurosis*, and a sufferer is said to be in an anxiety state. Some anxiety neuroses are focused on particular objects or activities, in which case they are called *phobias*. At other times the neurosis may be general, and have no apparent cause. This condition is termed free-floating anxiety.

The neurosis may be *chronic*, where there is a constant, low-grade anxiety that flares up at times of stress and is often associated with *depression*. In *acute* anxiety, however, the sufferer may suddenly become consumed by fear and dread, and develop a rapid heart beat, trembling hands, sweaty palms and a dry mouth. He or she will be unable to concentrate on anything, but will rush about, flitting from one unnecessary activity to the next. This is a panic attack.

Women tend to be affected more often than men and the condition is frequently linked to a feeling of insecurity during childhood, whether real or imagined. This feeling may not become apparent until it is reawakened by a setback in adult life. The condition also tends to run in families.

Anxiety neurosis is a complicated disorder, and therefore difficult to treat. Mild *tranquillizers* may be prescribed. In more serious cases involving depression, *antidepressants* may be necessary, and *beta-blockers* may also be given to control the physical symptoms. In addition, the patient will need a lengthy course of *counselling* or *psychotherapy* to help come to terms with the underlying problem and so prevent the illness from recurring.

AORTIC INCOMPETENCE
A condition also known as aortic regurgitation, in which the aortic valve of the heart fails to close completely. This allows the blood to regurgitate, or flow back, in the wrong direction. Aortic incompetence is usually either the result of a congenital abnormality in which the valve only has two cusps instead of three, or of damage to the valve caused by *rheumatic fever*.

The effect of the leak from the valve is to increase the amount of blood in the left ventricle, which therefore has to work harder to eject it. The output of the heart is thus increased and the muscle of the left ventricle hypertrophies or enlarges to cope with the added strain. Eventually the left ventricle can no longer cope with this, and begins to fail, causing *pulmonary oedema* and breathlessness—*see heart failure*. In valves damaged by rheumatic fever, *stenosis*—narrowing— and regurgitation of the aortic valve may exist together. This gives rise to two heart murmurs and increases the strain on the heart even further.

Diagnosis is made physically. On listening to the heart with a stethoscope, a typical murmur is often heard. In cases of gross regurgitation, the faulty valve is replaced surgically, though in less severe cases the condition does not stop people leading normal lives— *see valvular heart disorders*.

AORTIC STENOSIS
A thickening of the aortic valve of the heart. On rare occasions, this may occur as a *congenital abnormality*, but is more commonly due to damage caused by *rheumatic fever*. The thickened valve obstructs the outflow of blood from the left ventricle of the heart and may cause the blood pressure to fall. To avoid this, the muscle of the left ventricle enlarges—a condition known as *hypertrophy*—so that it can pump more forcefully. In turn, the blood supply via the coronary arteries may not be sufficient to meet the demands of this enlarged muscle and *angina* may result. Another symptom of aortic stenosis is fainting or *syncope*, because of the restricted cardiac output.

In advanced severe aortic stenosis, the left ventricle is unable to compensate for the reduction in cardiac output in spite of enlarging itself, and eventually fails. This left ventricular failure causes *dyspnoea*, shortness of breath.

Treatment is by surgical replacement.

AORTITIS
An *inflammation* of the aorta, the largest artery in the body. The inflammation normally affects the first part of the aorta, called the ascending aorta, as it travels from the left ventricle of the heart upwards towards the neck before forming an arch. Aortitis is a *complication* of *syphilis*, although it does not occur until 15 years or so after the initial infection—and only then if the syphilis has not been treated at an early stage with antibiotics. It is thus a fairly rare disease.

Diagnosis is difficult because there are few symptoms. Occasionally, however, there may be *angina* and a heart *murmur* as the inflammation can affect the bases of the coronary arteries where they leave the aorta. A chest X-ray may also show the aorta to be dilated and calcified.

APGAR SCORE
A rating system by which five functions of a newborn baby are assessed in a quick examination carried out by a midwife or doctor within the first few minutes of birth. Heart rate, muscle tone, breathing, reflex activity and skin colour—to check for problems such as *cyanosis* or *jaundice*—are each rated either nought, one or two. If the total score is less than seven, intensive care may be necessary. If it is between eight and ten, the baby is normal and healthy and is given routine care.

APHASIA
A condition in which a person finds it difficult or impossible to express him or herself in speech, or to understand fully the meaning of words that are addressed to him or her. Aphasia is caused by a disease that affects the speech centres of the brain, such as a *cardiovascular accident* or stroke.

APHONIA
The loss of the ability to speak as a result of a defect of the larynx, or an illness such as *laryngitis*—*see also aphasia*.

APICECTOMY
A dental operation in which the bottom part, or apex, of the root of a tooth is removed, so that a dental, or apical, *abscess* can be drained.

APNOEA
A pause in breathing that sometimes occurs in conditions such as *hypoventilation* due to a lack of stimulation by the respiratory control centres—*see The Respiratory System, p28*. Sometimes, however, it is a symptom of serious conditions such as *meningitis*, *coma* and heart and kidney disease—*see Cheyne-Stokes respiration*. In these cases it is usually relieved when the underlying disease is treated.

Apnoea is sometimes seen in small children and babies who are perfectly healthy; it may also be a feature of deep sleep in the elderly. In such cases, the patient is observed closely in case the condition is a symptom of serious illness, but this is rare.

APOPLEXY—see Cerebrovascular accident

APPENDICITIS
The vermiform appendix is a worm-shaped projection from the junction between the ileum of the small intestine and the caecum of the large intestine—*see The Digestive System, p40*. It is about 8.3cm (3in) long.

The appendix once played an important part in the digestion of the fibrous cellulose found in grasses. Nowadays, it has no function, but sometimes acts as a trap for hard fragments of waste material, such as a grape pip, or a finger nail. These may block the blind-ended tube, allowing infection to set in. As a result, the wall of the appendix becomes inflamed and swollen. This

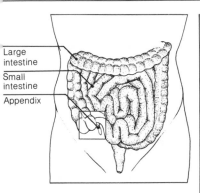

Large intestine
Small intestine
Appendix

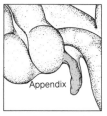

Appendix

The worm-shaped appendix is situated at the point where the ileum of the small intestine leads into the caecum of the large intestine. When the appendix becomes infected or inflamed, it is removed in an appendicectomy by cutting it off at its base and stitching up the hole left in the intestine.

is the condition known as *acute* appendicitis.

The first signs of appendicitis are normally pain and tenderness in the centre of the abdomen, though this may vary from case to case. The pain moves to the right of the abdomen, near the groin. Pressure on this point causes pain, but this is more intense when the pressure is released. As the inflammation becomes more severe, there may be *nausea, vomiting* and a *fever*. Unless the appendix is surgically removed, the inflamed walls of the tube may burst, causing *peritonitis* and infection within the abdomen, which may occasionally prove fatal. The sudden easing of the severe pain of appendicitis is a sign that this may have happened.

Appendicitis tends to affect young people more than the old, and men more than women. Many doctors now consider that *chronic* appendicitis—the once-popular diagnosis of a 'grumbling appendix'—is extremely rare, or even that such a condition does not exist. They believe that recurrent abdominal pains are more likely to have some other cause.

APRAXIA
A loss of the ability to organize and co-ordinate movements, making accurate movements difficult to execute. It is caused by disease of the parietal lobes of the brain—*see The Nervous System, p32.*

ARRHYTHMIA
A disorder in the normal rhythm of the heartbeat—*see The Blood and*

Lymph Systems, p21—that is caused by a defect in the sino-atrial node, the heart's natural *pacemaker*, or an interruption to the impulses that it generates.

There are several different types of arrhythmia, the commonest of which is *ectopic beat*. Others are atrial or ventricular *fibrillation*, the spasmodic contractions of heart muscle, and *heart block*, in which the impulses are either slowed or blocked completely.

Arrhythmias can be caused by almost any condition that affects the heart, although they sometimes have no apparent cause. Most commonly, the nerve impulses are interrupted by an area of dead heart muscle—the result of a heart attack or *myocardial infarction*.

An arrhythmia may be diagnosed by the use of an electrocardiogram (ECG)—*see Special Tests, p84.* It can usually be corrected by drug therapy, or occasionally by the surgical implantation of an artificial pacemaker.

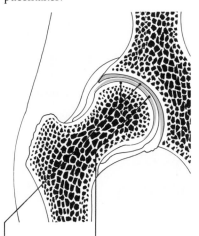

Articulating cartilage covers the bone of the ball of the femur and the socket of the pelvis.

The synovial membrane and its associated fluid fill the space between articulating cartilages.

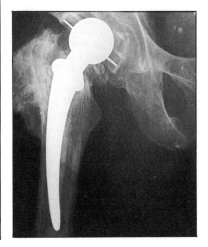

ARTERIOSCLEROSIS
An imprecise term that is frequently used, incorrectly, to describe *atherosclerosis*.

Arteriosclerosis, or hardening of the arteries, is a normal part of the gradual process of ageing, in which degenerative changes occur in the arteries. The arterial walls become hardened by the deposition of calcium, and thickened as a result of the long-term effects of raised blood pressure *(p21)*. There is no treatment for arteriosclerosis.

ARTERITIS—see Polyarteritis nodosa (PAN)

ARTHRITIS
An inflammation of the tissues of one or more joints, usually accompanied by pain and swelling. Arthritis has a number of different causes, and may develop at any age.

Osteoarthritis, the most common form of the disease, mainly affects the hips, knees and shoulders, and is to some extent a result of the

Arthritis Arthritis distorts the joints of the body in two main ways, either as a result of the inflammation of the synovial membrane, or because the cartilage on the articulating surfaces between two bones is worn away. The first condition is called rheumatoid arthritis and the second osteoarthritis *(left)*. Osteoarthritis is common in the weight-bearing joints, such as the hip, knee, spine, and the hands *(below)*.

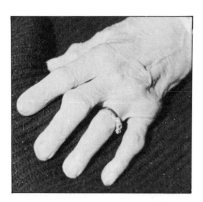

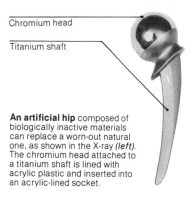

Chromium head

Titanium shaft

An artificial hip composed of biologically inactive materials can replace a worn-out natural one, as shown in the X-ray *(left)*. The chromium head attached to a titanium shaft is lined with acrylic plastic and inserted into an acrylic-lined socket.

natural processes of ageing. *Gout*, a form of arthritis in which crystals form in the joints, is also common in old age; *rheumatoid arthritis* is a disease of the connective tissue and may occur in the young, when it is called *Still's disease*. Arthritis may be a symptom of a large number of infections, such as *rubella* and *tuberculosis*, and is a common feature of fever, or *pyrexia*. In these cases it is called infective arthritis.

The nature of any arthritic disease can often be deduced from the sufferer's medical history and the results of a physical examination. This may include X-rays, blood tests and sometimes the analysis of a sample of fluid from an affected joint—*see Special Tests, p84*.

The treatment of arthritis varies according to its cause. Infective arthritis normally clears up as the infection subsides, but osteoarthritis and rheumatoid arthritis are generally treated with *analgesics* and *anti-inflammatory* drugs. Sufferers are advised to watch their weight, since *obesity* makes their problems worse, while some remedial exercises may be useful in cases of osteoarthritis. Joints which have been extremely severely damaged are sometimes replaced by artificial or prosthetic ones.

ARTIFICIAL INSEMINATION—see AID (Artificial insemination by donor); AIH (Artificial insemination by husband)

ASBESTOSIS
An industrial lung disease, or *pneumoconiosis*, caused by the inhalation of fine particles of asbestos. This substance is fire-resistant, and is used as an insulation material in the construction industry and in ships and brake linings.

As a result of the inhalation of asbestos particles, the tissues of the lungs become fibrosed—that is, they become fibrous and inflexible. The result is a progressive reduction in the efficiency of the lungs, causing shortness of breath, a predisposition to *bronchitis*, and *emphysema*, which eventually leads to *heart failure* and death. The disease may take anything from ten to 20 years to run its course.

Asbestosis may also cause *cancer*. This may be in the form of carcinoma of the bronchus, or a *mesothelioma*, or *malignant tumour*, of the pleura. The likelihood of asbestosis causing cancer is greatly increased if the victim is a heavy smoker.

Asbestosis cannot be cured, though its symptoms can be relieved to a certain extent. It is a serious and potentially lethal hazard for all those who work with asbestos. For this reason, stringent safety precautions should be observed by all those who handle the material—*see industrial diseases*.

ASCARIASIS—see Worms

ASCITES
A form of *oedema*, or swelling, in which fluid collects in the cavities of the abdomen. Ascites is a common feature of *cirrhosis* of the liver, but it also may be caused by *heart failure*, serious infections, such as *tuberculosis*, or *cancer* of the liver or ovaries.

Ascites is treated according to its cause, but may sometimes be controlled by the use of *diuretic* drugs. In some cases, the fluid may be drained by means of a procedure known as paracentesis, in which the fluid is withdrawn or 'tapped', using a hollow needle.

ASPERGILLOSIS
A condition that results from an infection of the body by the *fungus* Aspergillus fumigatus, one of the pulmonary *mycoses*.

Spores of the fungus enter the body in the air that is breathed, and lodge in the lungs. The sites chosen are often dilated bronchi, or may be healed *tuberculosis* scars.

Usually, aspergillosis is symptomless, though the efficiency of breathing may be impaired, and blood is sometimes coughed up. It is treated with fungicides—*see fungus*.

ASPHYXIA
Suffocation caused by an obstruction, or damage, to the respiratory system (*p28*). The resulting decrease in the level of oxygen in the blood, and increase in the level of carbon dioxide, is likely to cause brain damage within a few minutes and death rapidly thereafter.

The only treatment for asphyxia outside a hospital is to remove the cause of any obstruction to breathing and start artificial respiration immediately—*see First Aid, p369*. In a hospital, the life of an asphyxiated patient may be saved if he or she is given oxygen, and artificially respirated, or connected to a ventilator—*see cardiopulmonary bypass*.

ASPIRIN
A drug widely used to relieve pain and reduce *inflammation*, as in *osteoarthritis*. It is also used to reduce the temperature in a *fever* as it has an anti-pyretic action. Aspirin is so useful for treating minor ailments, such as headaches, that it may be used in large amounts. An aspirin overdose causes perspiration, *hyperventilation* and *vomiting*. Small dosages of aspirin have the side effect of causing bleeding from the stomach, which, in some people, may be severe. Aspirin may also very rarely cause an allergic reaction—*see allergy*.

ASTHMA
A condition in which the smooth muscles of the walls of the bronchi of the lungs contract in *spasm*, narrowing the airway and causing shortness of breath and wheezing.

Asthma may be caused by an *allergy*. In this case the condition is known as atopic, or allergic, asthma, and is usually first seen during childhood. It may be caused by a reaction to a number of allergens, such as feathers, the house dust *mite* and animal dander present in the air.

Atopic asthma often accompanies other allergic disorders, such as *dermatitis*, *urticaria* and *rhinitis*. It is thought that the condition may also be caused by a reaction to allergens in food. A sufferer from atopic asthma tends to experience sudden paroxysmal attacks of wheezing and *dyspnoea*. Expiration, or breathing out, is particularly difficult, because the constriction of the bronchi traps air in the lungs. The respiratory rate rises, as does the pulse rate, and the sufferer is sometimes so short of breath that he or she cannot speak. The level of oxygen in the blood falls, and *cyanosis* may develop. If the attack does not end, the sufferer is said to be in status asthmaticus. If untreated, this condition may prove fatal.

When asthma develops later in life it does not normally involve an allergic response. This condition, known as intrinsic asthma, tends to affect more women than men, and is *chronic*. There may be wheezing and shortness of breath on exertion, and occasional *acute* asthmatic attacks. These may be exacerbated by *infections* and by psychological upsets, and this is the reason why asthma is often described, incorrectly, as a nervous disease.

Asthmatic attacks are treated by *bronchodilators*, drugs that widen or dilate the bronchi. These may be given by injection or by mouth, or taken from an inhaler. *Steroids* may be given to subdue the allergic reaction in atopic asthma, and *antibiotics* to cure any infection that may be responsible for an attack in intrinsic asthma.

During a serious attack, or when a sufferer is in status asthmaticus, oxygen and chest *physiotherapy* may be necessary to make breathing

Asthma Asthma attacks can range from mild to severe. While they cannot be prevented, they can be eased or reduced. A breathless child can quickly become exhausted and so should be placed in a comfortable position *(below)*. Keeping an asthma diary *(right)*, in which a full account of each attack is recorded, may identify the factors which precipitate an attack and may help the doctor in deciding appropriate treatment.

Day		1	2	3	4	5	6	7	8	9
Number of Spincaps taken that day—		3	3	3	3	3	3	3		
COUGH	None	0	0	0	0	0	0	0	0	0
	Occasional	1	1	1	1	1	1	1	1	1
	Often	2	2	2	2	2	2	2	2	2
WHEEZE	None	0	0	0	0	0	0	0	0	0
	Occasional	1	1	1	1	1	1	1	1	1
	Often	2	2	2	2	2	2	2	2	2
ENERGY	Usual self	0	0	0	0	0	0	0	0	0
	Easily tired	1	1	1	1	1	1	1	1	1
	Mostly inactive	2	2	2	2	2	2	2	2	2
PLAY/GAMES	Normal	0	0	0	0	0	0	0	0	0
	Slight cough and/or wheeze	1	1	1	1	1	1	1		
	Severe cough and/or wheeze	2	2	2	2	2	2	2	2	
MEALS	Usual self	0	0	0	0	0	0	0	0	
	Some interest	1	1	1	1	1	1	1	1	
	No interest	2	2	2	2	2	2	2	2	
SLEEP	Normal	0	0	0	0	0	0	0	0	
	Mildly disturbed	1	1	1	1	1	1	1	1	
	Poor night	2	2	2	2	2	2	2	2	
	TOTAL SCORE	0	0	0	3	6	2	0	0	
REMARKS										

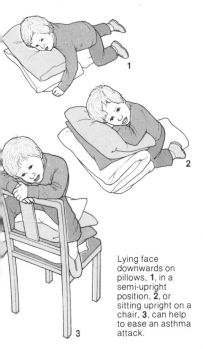

Lying face downwards on pillows, **1**, in a semi-upright position, **2**, or sitting upright on a chair, **3**, can help to ease an asthma attack.

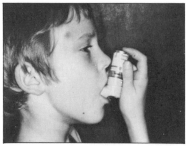

The aerosol spray must be pressed at the start of breathing in to ensure that the drug reaches the lungs. To achieve this, the patient first breathes out, places the mouth around the mouthpiece and then inhales.

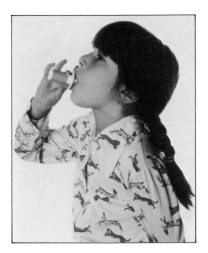

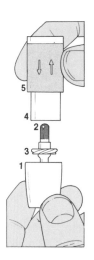

A spinhaler produces a fine spray of the drug with which it is charged and propels it into the lungs as the patient, whose head is tilted back, breathes in *(left)*. To reload, the spinhaler is held upside down by the mouthpiece, **1**, while a new capsule, **2**, is inserted into the propeller, **3** The inside of the body, **4**, is screwed back on and the outside of the body, **5**, is moved down, so piercing the capsule.

easier, in addition to steroids and bronchodilator drugs. Once the allergen that causes atopic asthma in a sufferer has been identified, that person should make every attempt to avoid it.

Treatment enables many asthma sufferers to live perfectly normal lives—some, in fact, to overcome their problems to become famous in fields as diverse as sport and opera.

See also cardiac asthma.

ASTIGMATISM
A defect of vision in which the image appears to be horizontally or vertically distorted. Astigmatism is normally the result of an abnormal curvature of one of the surfaces of the eye. The condition can be corrected if cylindrical glasses are worn—these produce an opposite distortion to that produced by the abnormal curve, and the two distortions cancel each other out.

ATAXIA
An unsteadiness when making voluntary movements—that is, movements carried out under the conscious control of the brain. The condition is caused by disturbance or degeneration of the cerebellum, the unsteadiness resulting from an inability to co-ordinate the actions of the muscles involved in movement. Patients with ataxia may stagger when walking or have difficulty in pronouncing words properly.

Ataxia is a common problem after certain types of *cerebrovascular accident*, or stroke, and may occur in *alcoholism*. It is also one of the symptoms of long-standing syphilis affecting the nervous system. Certain forms of the disease are inherited, as in the case of Friedrich's ataxia, which first appears in adolescence, and causes spasticity of the limbs. These severe types are fairly rare.

Ataxia is a progressive disease for which there is no cure. Patients have a normal lifespan, although they become gradually more disabled.

ATHEROSCLEROSIS
A disease in which there is a degeneration of the walls of large and medium-sized arteries, as well as the coronary and cerebral arteries. Unlike *arteriosclerosis*, this disease cannot be accounted for solely by the normal processes of ageing.

In the first stage of atherosclerosis a fatty patch or plaque, called an atheroma, builds up to form on the wall of an artery. This is made up of the fats that circulate normally in the blood—*see Metabolism, p44*—with cholesterol in particular making up the bulk of the contents. Elements of fibrin and blood cells combine with the lump, binding it still more strongly to the arterial wall. Then, calcium is laid down

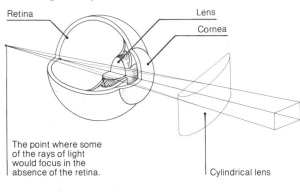

Retina · Lens · Cornea

The point where some of the rays of light would focus in the absence of the retina.

Cylindrical lens

Astigmatism In astigmatism, some of the rays of light reflected from an object do not focus on the retina at the back of the eye. The condition is caused by an abnormal curvature of the cornea or the lens and the distortion it produces of the resulting image can be corrected by wearing special glasses with cylindrical lenses

within it. Eventually, the atheroma, now hard and fixed, partially blocks the artery, causing the blood to dam up behind it in a thrombus, or blood clot—*see thrombosis*.

The effects of atherosclerosis depend upon which arteries are primarily affected, though all atheromas will increase or raise the blood pressure. The flow of blood to the extremities—the peripheral circulation—will be impaired, often causing swollen, cold and painful limbs, while minor injuries may become gangrenous—*see gangrene*—because of poor circulation.

Any atheroma will partly or wholly block the artery in which it develops, and so reduce, or eliminate, the supply of blood to the part of the body that the artery feeds. If the blockage is in the leg, the result may be intermittent *claudication*, a severe cramp-like pain felt in the calves upon exercise. Atherosclerosis of the coronary arteries causes *angina*, and, when

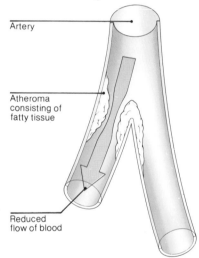

Atherosclerosis A high level of fats and cholesterol in the body gradually leads to deposits of atheroma, or fatty tissue, on the inner walls of the arteries, particularly at the point where an artery branches. The result is atherosclerosis. The diminished space within the artery hinders the flow of blood. This leads to a rise in blood pressure and, eventually, the risk of a stroke or heart attack.

the blood supply to an area of the heart is completely blocked, may lead to the death of an area of heart muscle—a heart attack, or *myocardial infarction*.

Atheromas in the cerebral arteries can be associated with *transient ischaemic attacks* (TIAs) or *cerebrovascular accidents*—strokes. Sometimes, the thrombus or blood clot that has formed around the atheroma breaks off to form an embolus—*see embolism*. This may be pushed around the circulation by the flow of blood until it blocks off a major artery, stopping, for example,

the blood supply to a limb.

Atherosclerosis has no specific cause, though it is known that the condition is linked to several different factors. It is also known that an increased level of cholesterol, a fat found in dairy products, in the blood makes the formation of atheromas more likely. However, there is no conclusive proof that the level of cholesterol in foods such as butter, eggs and milk has any relationship to the level of the fat in the blood, though the theory has caused considerable controversy.

Atherosclerosis is a disease that can be avoided to a large extent, if the simple rules of preventive medicine are followed— *see Routine Checks, p346*. It is essential, however, that these rules are obeyed after atherosclerosis has been diagnosed. *Anticoagulants* will help to stop the formation of blood clots, while a controlled exercise programme, under medical supervision, will encourage the blood to find other arterial pathways through the body. Some drugs are said to be able to widen, or dilate, the arteries, but their efficacy has not yet been proven.

If these measures fail, surgery may be necessary. The narrowed or obstructed piece of artery is removed and replaced by a vein, or synthetic *graft*.

ATHLETE'S FOOT—see Tinea

ATRIAL FIBRILLATION—see Fibrillation

ATRIAL SEPTAL DEFECT—see Congenital heart defects

ATROPINE
A drug made from the plant belladonna, or deadly nightshade, that counteracts the parasympathetic nervous system— *see The Nervous System, p32*. It relaxes smooth, or involuntary, muscles, reduces the activity of the secretory glands of the digestive system, and dilates the pupils of the eyes.

Atropine is given in the form of eye drops before an examination of the eye, and as a pre-medication before a general *anaesthetic* because it dries up nasal and oral secretions.

AURA
A sensation that acts as a warning that the onset of a physical or mental disorder is imminent.

Sufferers from *epilepsy* often experience an aura before a fit. This may take many forms, such as a feeling of extreme well-being, or that something indefinable is terribly wrong. It may be a peculiar sensation in the head or the pit of

the stomach or, classically, a feeling that a light breeze has passed over the body. Some epileptics may *hallucinate* or have a disordered sense of taste or smell. The aura that precedes an attack of *migraine* often takes the form of flickering lights or patterns in front of the eyes.

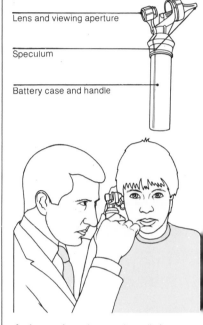

Lens and viewing aperture

Speculum

Battery case and handle

Auriscope An auriscope, also called an otoscope, is the instrument used to examine any infection or damage to the eardrum and the canal leading to it. Basically it is a magnifying device with a light source. The battery case and handle is interchangeable with those of the ophthalmoscope, used to examine the interior of the eye.

AURISCOPE
An instrument used to examine the external part of the ear, allowing a doctor to inspect the auditory canal and eardrum.

AUTISM
A psychological disorder, usually first diagnosed during childhood, in which a sufferer behaves in a distant manner and has severe difficulties in communicating with other people. He or she does not respond to, or need, affection, and seems unable to form personal relationships, or to want to do so. The condition is sometimes associated with a speech defect, and sometimes with *mental subnormality*.

The cause of autism is not known, and how it works is not understood, so an autistic child is extremely difficult to treat. Patience, sympathy, understanding and special teaching may improve the condition, but it is unlikely that an autistic child will ever play a wholly normal part in society. Advice and support for the parents of an autistic child is available from a number of organizations, such as The National Society for Autistic Children, and The National Society for Mentally Handicapped Children and Adults (MENCAP).

AUTO-IMMUNE DISEASES
A group of diseases that are caused, to some degree, by a malfunction of the immune system— *see Natural Defences Against Disease, p52.* Normally, the body's immune system recognizes a foreign invader as potentially harmful, and produces *antibodies* to fight it. In an auto-immune response, the body loses the ability to distinguish between foreign protein and the body's own tissues. As a result, the body produces antibodies which fight its own proteins as well as the foreign ones.

A number of diseases are thought to involve auto-immune responses, among them diseases of the connective tissues, such as *scleroderma*, and disorders of the endocrine glands, such as *thyroiditis*. Some scientists believe that many diseases are in fact auto-immune to some extent. As research continues, the list of possibilities grows longer; today it includes *AIDS*, *rheumatoid arthritis* and *diabetes*. Some scientists

also think that *multiple sclerosis* has an auto-immune basis.

Auto-immune responses can be suppressed by the use of *steroid* drugs. Unfortunately, the dangerous side-effects sometimes caused by these drugs limit their maximum dosage, and thus their effectiveness.

AUTOPSY
An examination of a corpse to establish the cause of death. Autopsies are performed by a histopathologist—see *Who's Who in Medicine and Surgery, p82*—who examines the internal organs and may take samples of them for microscopic examination or chemical analysis.

See also Coming To Terms With Death, p366.

AVERSION THERAPY
A form of *behaviour therapy* in which the aim is to link an unpleasant sensation in the patient's mind with the form of behaviour that such treatment is attempting to inhibit. This form of treatment was once common. Social deviants would be given electric shocks when exposed to evidence of, or material associated with, their perversion. Nowadays,

such treatment is considered to infringe the patient's civil rights to an unacceptable degree, and is, in any case, not particularly effective.

One particular form of aversion therapy, however, is still used. This is the administration of a drug called antabuse in the treatment of *alcoholism*: it causes *vomiting and nausea* when alcohol is taken. Many doctors, however, realize that this will have little long-term effect on its own, since alcoholism cannot be cured unless the sufferer has a strong motivation to achieve this.

AZOOSPERMIA
An absence of sperm in the seminal fluid—see *Sex and Reproduction, p54*. Azoospermia may be the result of a defect in the seminiferous tubules, the site for sperm production in the testicles, or follow *orchitis* due to *mumps, venereal disease*, underactivity of the pituitary gland, or a failure of the testes to descend.It is also the deliberate end result in *vasectomy*.

Diagnosis of azoospermia usually follows a *biopsy* of the testis. If it is due to a blockage in the seminiferous tubules, it may be possible to treat the condition surgically. Other causes, however, are untreatable.

B

BABINSKI RESPONSE
A reflex action caused by stroking the side of the sole of the foot. Normally, the big toe will respond by moving downwards.

Babinski Response If the side of the sole of the foot is stroked with a sharp pointer, the big toe normally turns downwards. When the big toe curls upwards, the reflex is called the Babinski response

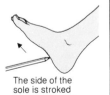

The side of the sole is stroked from the heel to the toes.

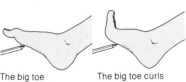

The big toe normally curls downwards.

The big toe curls upwards.

In the Babinski response, however, the big toe moves upward. The response is found in new-born babies and in stroke victims—*see cerebrovascular accident*—but in people of other ages it may be an indication of a disease of the brain or spinal cord.

BACILLE CALMETTE-GUÉRIN— see BCG

BACK PAIN
Millions of years ago, our ancestors walked on all fours. As with other four-legged animals, the human spine was aligned parallel to the ground, and designed to bear the stresses that this entailed. When, uniquely in the animal kingdom, humans started to walk upright constantly, the spine had to cope with stresses, pressure and jarring from a different direction, for which

it was not designed. The mechanical strains caused by this are the root cause of most back pain, a problem that affects the majority of people at some time in their lives.

Back pain may start suddenly, after heavy lifting or vigorous exercise, for example—when it is said to be *acute*—or develop slowly over a long period—when it is called *chronic*.

Acute backache in a young, fit person is often caused by muscle and ligament strains. The problem usually disappears in a few weeks without treatment, but is helped by bed rest on a firm surface, pain-killing drugs and, occasionally, muscle-relaxants. Heat, either from an infra-red lamp or from a hot-water bottle wrapped in a towel and placed on the back, can also help to relieve the pain.

In middle-aged people sudden,

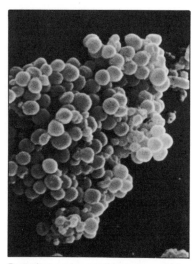

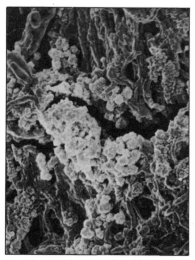

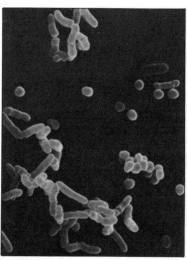

Bacteria are microscopic organisms which generally range in size between 1/50,000 to 1/5,000 inch (1/500 to 1/5,000 millimetre). Many bacteria are harmless or even beneficial to humans, but there are a number which cause disease. Colonies of spherical

Staphylococcus aureus *(above left)* are responsible for infection in wounds, septicaemia and boil. The spherical bacterium called Beta Haemolytic Streptococcus *(above middle)* causes tonsillitis and scarlet fever. The spherical Streptococcus mutans

(above right) forms part of the plaque found on teeth. It turns sugar into an acid and so causes dental caries, one of the commonest diseases known to man.

severe back pain is often caused by a 'slipped disc'—*see prolapsed intervertebral disc*—especially after an attempt to lift a heavy weight incorrectly.

Sudden back pain may also be due to the collapse of a vertebra: the bone becomes compressed into wedge shape, sometimes trapping whole nerves. In young people this is sometimes the result of a severe trauma, such as jumping on to a hard surface from a great height. In older people, however, a vertebra may collapse spontaneously as a result of *osteoporosis*. In this condition, which is a natural consequence of ageing to some extent, the bone substance becomes less dense. In women this may be caused by a fall in the level of hormone secretions after the *menopause*. In both men and women, collapsed vertebrae may be caused by *tuberculosis* of the spine, or by secondary deposits in the bones from a *cancer* elsewhere in the body. These secondary deposits are called *metastases*.

The collapsed vertebra will show up on an X-ray of the spine. In uncomplicated cases, in which the spinal cord is intact and has not been compressed or damaged, treatment with *analgesics* is all that is necessary. In a fit young patient a plaster of Paris jacket may be applied to try and reduce the fracture and prevent deformity. The jacket has to be worn for three months, during which time the person leads an active life. In the elderly, however, it is important to establish whether osteoporosis or an underlying disease has caused the problem, as well as to treat the back pain directly with analgesics.

When the spinal cord has been injured, and there is danger of *paraplegia*, a loss of nerve supply to the limbs, an operation called a *laminectomy* may be necessary to try to limit the damage.

Chronic backache is an entirely different problem, usually associated with poor posture. In women, the pain may become worse during pregnancy or before a period. In young men, morning backache and stiffness is, very occasionally, a sign of *ankylosing spondylitis*.

Remedial exercises to improve the posture may relieve the symptoms of backache. Sufferers may also obtain relief from pain by acupuncture treatment, or by following the principles of the Alexander technique—*see Alternative medicine p305*. Some people find that manipulation of the vertebrae by an osteopath—*see Alternative Medicine, p305*—is effective, but it is important to consult your doctor, who will normally suggest that you have a spinal X-ray before undertaking such treatment.

As with acute back pain, heat applied to the back and pain-killers often give immediate relief, while support from a firm mattress at night may solve the problem in the long term. *Obesity* is a major cause of back pain, because the spine cannot support the extra strains that are put upon it. If you are overweight and have back pain, the most effective cure is to lose weight—*see Diet, p322*.

Occasionally, backache is a symptom of serious disease. The list of possible causes is long, but it includes *cancer*, *kidney failure*, *heart disease*, *duodenal ulcers* and *pneumonia*. For this reason, a doctor

should be consulted if back pain is severe, or lasts for more than a few days. However, in the vast majority of cases, backache is caused by mechanical stresses and strains. These can be avoided, to an extent, if a few simple rules are followed. If you are overweight, lose weight, develop the habit of standing and sitting correctly, and learn how to lift heavy objects without straining yourself.

BACTERAEMIA—see Septicaemia

BACTERIA

A group of microscopic organisms, most of which have only one cell. Together with *viruses*, they are popularly known as 'germs' and live in the air, the soil, in water or in any environment that provides them with their nutritional needs.

Not all bacteria cause disease in humans. Some live harmlessly inside the body, and are beneficial— bacteria called *Escherichia coli*, for instance, aid digestion in the intestines, while the *Doderlein bacteria* help to keep the vagina free of infection. Other bacteria, however, invade the body and cause disease in a variety of ways. They excrete poisonous waste-products which destroy the body's own cells; the inflammation they cause may block blood and lymph ducts and endocrine glands; and they appropriate the body's chemical fuels for themselves.

Some of the bacteria that cause disease infect the body only when its defences are lowered, while others are so virulent that even the healthiest individual is unprotected unless he or she has been *immunized* against them. Fortunately, however, drugs called *antibiotics* can kill bacteria. Depending on the type of antibiotic, they can either break down the cell walls of bacteria, so killing them, or stop them reproducing. Most bacterial infections can be cured by antibiotics, therefore, as long as treatment is given before serious damage is caused.

Bacteria are classified according to their shape. They may be spherical, rod-like, spiral, comma-shaped or corkscrew-shaped. Spherical bacteria have the suffix '-coccus' attached to their names; a rod-like bacterium is a bacillus. Another general classification is derived from the way bacteria react to a coloured stain called Gram's stain. Those that take up the stain are called Gram positive; those that do not are Gram negative. Bacteria are also classified according to whether they need oxygen: those that do are said to be aerobic, and those that do not are called anaerobic.

These classifications are important in the treatment of disease, because some types of antibiotics are more efficient at killing or controlling certain bacteria than others.

If a doctor suspects that bacteria are responsible for a patient's infection he or she may take a sample of the pus at the site of the infection. Pus forms as a result of the fight by the body's white cells against infection, and contains both living and dead bacteria. This sample—a 'swab' from the throat in cases of an upper respiratory tract infection, such as *tonsillitis*, for example—is examined in a laboratory. The bacteria found are classified according to their shape, oxygen needs and staining properties, so that the doctor can prescribe the most appropriate antibiotic to deal with the infection.

BALANITIS
An inflammation of the glans, or head of the penis. The condition may take a number of forms, and has a variety of causes, but is usually associated with a condition called *phimosis*, in which the foreskin is tight. The foreskin can only be retracted with difficulty, making it hard to clean the glans. This provides an environment in which the organisms which cause the disease can multiply.

When the glans is only slightly red and sore, the condition is most likely to be the result of a bacterial infection. This can be cured easily by the application of an *antibiotic* cream. If the infection is allowed to develop untreated, antibiotic tablets may be needed. Occasionally it may be

necessary to make a cut in the foreskin to allow the pus to drain away.

If the tip of the penis is sore and red, and there is a discharge from the urethra, the most likely cause is a fungal infection called *candida albicans*. This causes 'thrush', and can be transferred during intercourse. The problem can be treated with antifungal creams, but a doctor may also test the urine for the presence of sugar. This predisposes towards candidial infections, and is a symptom of *diabetes*.

Sometimes, balanitis is caused by a sexually transmitted disease, such as *herpes genitalis*, *gonorrhoea*, or *syphilis*. The glans will be red and sore, while the glands in the groin may also be enlarged. In the case of herpes and syphilis, there may also be small ulcers on the glans. If these are found it is important to visit a doctor without delay, and to stop any sexual activity in the meantime.

BARBITURATES
A group of drugs that depress the activity of the central nervous system. Depending on the particular drug used, barbiturates may have *hypnotic*, *sedative* or *anticonvulsant* effects. Barbitone, the first barbiturate, was introduced in 1903 and its hypnotic effect was used to induce sleep. Since that time, many barbiturates have been manufactured, each with individual properties. They vary in the duration of their action and in their effects, which may range from mild sedation to general *anaesthesia*.

Nowadays, however, most doctors prescribe *benzodiazepines* to induce sleep or to sedate patients, instead of barbiturates. There are several reasons for this: the dangers of possible overdoses; the potentially fatal *drug interactions* between barbiturates and alcohol in the bloodstream; the general abuse of barbiturates and their addictive side-effects—see *Abuses of the Body*, *p328*.

However, two types of barbiturate are still prescribed for specific purposes. Phenobarbitone, a slow-acting barbiturate, is widely used as an anticonvulsant in the control of *epilepsy*. Fast-acting barbiturates, such as thiopentone, are given intravenously as an anaesthetic prior to surgery.

BARTHOLINITIS
A bacterial infection that affects women, in which one or both of the Bartholin's glands in the vulva becomes inflamed. These small, mucus-secreting glands are situated at the base of the labia majora, one on each side of the vaginal opening.

During sexual arousal they secrete the fluid that lubricates the vulva and eases penetration by the penis.

Bartholinitis is by no means rare, and is sometimes associated with *gonorrhoea*. The first signs are discomfort in the vulval area, and a red swelling at the site of the glands as the bacteria multiply. If it is caught in time, the condition can be treated successfully with bed rest, *antibiotics*, pain-killers and hot salt baths. However, when the infection has progressed so that an *abscess* has formed, minor surgery may be necessary. The technique used is called marsupialization—the abscess is opened and cleaned, and its edges are stitched to the skin until it has healed.

Sometimes the infection appears to clear up spontaneously, without surgery. In fact the abscess may have merely sealed off, forming a cyst, which can become infected once more. This is called a Bartholin's cyst, and is normally removed surgically once its presence is discovered.

BASAL CELL CARCINOMA
A form of *cancer* that affects the skin. The condition is often known as a rodent ulcer, but is called a basal cell carcinoma in medical terminology because it arises in the basal cell layer of the epidermis of the skin (*p16*).

Basal cell carcinomas develop more commonly in the elderly than the young, and men are more frequently affected than women. White-skinned people who have spent much of their lives in bright sunshine are especially at risk. Scientists believe this is because of the cumulative effect of the ultra-violet radiation that sunlight contains. The condition is rarely seen, however, in dark-skinned people.

The cancer most commonly affects the face. The first sign is a small painless lump, and this enlarges over about a year to a raised area around 12mm (0.5in) wide. The centre of the lesion ulcerates and often becomes covered by a crust.

As the condition progresses, the cancerous cells grow downwards into the dermis of the skin, and may erode the muscle, cartilage and bone that lie beneath it, causing considerable damage.

However, basal cell carcinomas are distinguished from most other forms of cancer by the fact that they rarely spread, or metastasize, to other parts of the body. If the condition is recognized in sufficient time, therefore, it can be cured by *radiotherapy* or by surgical removal of the cancer.

BATTERED BABY SYNDROME

The deliberate injury of babies or young children. Those affected may be bruised or burnt, have broken bones, be undernourished or mentally under-stimulated, or a combination of these things.

It is likely that, over the centuries, there have always been some children who have suffered from physical or mental cruelty. However, the problem has been highlighted in the last 20 years by a series of tragic cases in which children have died as a result of their treatment. Since battered baby syndrome was recognized, a considerable amount of research has been devoted to it.

From the evidence that has been gathered it appears that most injuries are inflicted on battered children by their parents or by an adult who is living with either parent. Often, one or other of these adults was battered himself as a child. Baby battering is more common when there is bad housing, unemployment, drug addiction or alcoholism, and when the other children in the family are difficult or disturbed.

On occasions, the child may contribute to the problem—when, for example, he or she is difficult to handle, misbehaves to attract attention or does not sleep or feed properly. In a proportion of cases there are difficulties in the birth of the child involved. A mother whose child is taken away at birth, to be nursed in an incubator because of illness, for example, may sometimes be unable to establish a normal mother-child bond with that child. This, of course, is the exception rather than the rule.

If there is gross neglect or serious physical damage, there is little difficulty in deciding that a child has been the victim of battered baby syndrome. However, the situation is rarely as clear-cut as this. Most cases are brought to the attention of the social services by a child's teacher, doctor or neighbour, who has noticed bruises or remarked on the regularity with which the child breaks bones or injures himself. Social workers then have to decide whether these injuries are caused by the child's parents, or are innocent— the result of the boisterous rough and tumble of children's play.

If it is discovered that bruises or minor injuries have been caused by the parents, the social workers, doctors and others who care for the children and the family have a further difficulty. They have to decide where legitimate disciplining of children ends and where 'battering' begins: to judge what is normal and what is harming a child either physically or mentally. There are many different views about corporal punishment, ranging from complete abhorrence of the concept to the more traditional view that a child should be spanked when he or she disobeys the wishes of the parents.

When, however, it is thought that a child may be at risk of further injury—either physical or mental— the social services have a statutory duty to protect that child. An application is made to a magistrate for a 'place of safety' order in the first instance. This allows the baby to be kept in hospital, even against the parents' wishes, while all the health workers concerned, such as the health visitor, family doctor and social worker, meet as a committee to discuss the case and make recommendations.

This step is not taken lightly. Those involved are aware that to break up a family in this way can be extremely distressing, for both parents and children. After a period of discussion by the committee, and *counselling* of the parents, the child may be returned home if it is thought that the danger is over, though the situation is reviewed at intervals. The committee is likely, in any case, to recommend that the child's name be placed on the 'at risk' register, which is circulated to doctors, social workers, and hospitals. If the child is subsequently brought into casualty with bruises and broken bones then the circumstances will be investigated carefully and the social workers informed.

Sometimes, however, the committee may decide that the situation is unlikely to improve and that the child should spend more time in care; this means that the social services must make a formal application in the Juvenile court for the child to be taken away from the parents and placed in care. The social services assume parental responsibilities for the child. This does not mean that the child has to spend the rest of his youth in a children's home. Such children often spend some time with foster parents, or return home if social workers are satisfied that conditions there have improved and that there is no risk of further harm for the children.

BCG

A vaccine, known as BCG, or bacille Calmette-Guérin after its inventors, that gives immunity against *tuberculosis*. It contains a strain of the tuberculosis bacterium that is harmless, but it is sufficiently active to prepare the body's defences against related strains—*see Natural Defences Against Disease, p52.* This type of vaccine, containing live bacteria, is said to be 'active', or 'live'.

If a person has had a form of tuberculosis, or has been vaccinated against the disease, he or she will have immunity against a further attack. Whether immunity is present can be discovered by means of a Heaf Test—*see Special Tests, p84.* Children between the ages of 10 and 13 are given a Heaf Test routinely, as are all those who may come into contact with the disease, such as prospective nurses and medical students and the relatives and friends of tuberculosis sufferers. Those who have a negative response to the Heaf Test are given BCG vaccine by injection. The vaccine is 80% successful in preventing tuberculosis, giving protection for up to seven years.

A BCG vaccination should not, however, be given to anyone who has a *fever*, or who has been given a live vaccine, such as an oral *polio* vaccination, within the preceding fortnight. The reason for this is that the body's defences may not be able to cope with two different types of bacteria at the same time, however harmless they may be on their own.

BED SORE

An area of skin damage, and often ulceration, that is caused by constant pressure on the affected parts of the body, and a consequent restriction of the blood supply to the area. Bed sores usually affect patients who are immobile in bed after a stroke, for example, or an operation. They are a particular problem for the elderly, who already have a poor supply of blood to the skin.

Bed sores form on the heels, over the sacrum or base of the spine, and on other areas, such as the buttocks, which take the weight of the body when lying flat in bed. The skin breaks down, or ulcerates, and often becomes infected, especially if the patient is also incontinent. Within a short time large cavities form. These are very difficult to treat.

The problem will not occur, however, if the invalid is turned in bed frequently, so that the body's weight is shared over other areas of skin. Regular washing and massaging the skin to assist circulation also helps, while the areas that take the strain of the body should be kept dry—*see Home Nursing, p352.* In hospital, patients with bed sores are often given water or ripple mattresses since they distribute the weight more evenly than a sprung or foam mattress.

Given proper attention, the ulcer will heal normally. In extreme cases, however, when the cavities formed are very large, surgical debridement, or removal of dead tissue, and skin grafting are necessary.

BED-WETTING—see Nocturnal Enuresis

BEHAVIOUR THERAPY

A form of psychological therapy based on the belief that many symptoms and patterns of disturbed behaviour are acquired early in life as conditioned responses to situations that cause anxiety, and persist long after the anxiety has disappeared. A person who was bitten by a dog as a child, for instance, may develop a *phobia* or exaggerated fear of dogs that may last for the rest of their life.

Behaviour therapy to treat this problem could involve curing the patient's phobia of dogs by *desensitization* methods. The therapist first helps the sufferer to an understanding of the root cause of the phobia by talking through the childhood incident. Next the patient is shown pictures of dogs, and, over a period of some months, encouraged to look at them for longer and longer periods. Eventually, the procedure is repeated with live dogs. At each stage the patient discusses his or her reactions with the therapist, and, by talking through any anxiety, becomes desensitized to the phobia.

This process is usually combined with relaxation therapy. In this, the patient learns to relax by using bio-feedback techniques. These indicate how much the muscles contract and tense in the hands, for example. The patient learns to control this, so that he or she can learn how to monitor their own progress. An alternative method of desensitization involves flooding the patient with the unpleasant stimuli, rather than gradually exposing them to the symptoms.

Another form of behaviour therapy is known as positive conditioning. Its aim is to help patients develop the normal reflexes that they may have failed to develop in early life, such as the ability to retain urine at night, or to achieve an orgasm. The process is similar to that of desensitization, but goes a stage further. Patients are led to understand the reasons behind their problem and then led, by training and encouragement, to overcome their physical inabilities.

Reinforcement therapy, a third type of behaviour therapy, is also known as operant conditioning. It is based on the simple principle of rewarding desirable behaviour. It is used to treat patients who have unacceptable standards of personal hygiene, or behave in a bizarre manner; such patients often have serious *personality problems*. The patient discovers, through trial and error, that the behaviour thought desirable by the therapist brings useful or satisfying rewards. The hope is that the patient will eventually repeat the socially acceptable behaviour until it becomes automatic, and not conditional on a reward.

Perhaps because it set out to treat symptoms rather than causes, much controversy surrounded the introduction of behaviour therapy in the 1960s. However, since it has often proved successful in treating the conditions described above, it is now accepted as a useful psychiatric tool.

BELLADONNA—see Atropine

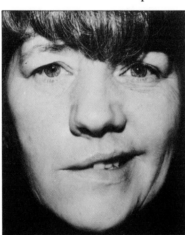

Bell's Palsy is a condition in which fluid accumulates in the facial nerve and, as a result, the nerve may swell into the facial canal. The result of this is the paralysis of the side of the face which is served by the nerve. The woman *(above)* has no control over the muscles on the left side of her face, her tongue has lost some of its ability to taste, the flow of saliva has also been reduced and hearing on the affected side has deteriorated.

BELL'S PALSY

A condition of unknown cause in which one of the two facial, or 7th cranial, nerves swells up within its canal. The wall of the canal constricts the swollen nerve to cause a paralysis of the muscles on the side of the face supplied by the affected nerve. The facial muscles sag, so that the mouth droops open, and it is often impossible to close the eye.

The swelling rarely develops in any part of the nerve containing sensory fibres, but when it does there is a loss of taste in two-thirds of the tongue and a reduction in the flow of saliva. Skin sensation is not reduced, but occasionally hearing on the affected side becomes more acute. Bell's palsy affects both sexes equally and may occur at any age.

Treatment is usually with oral *steroid* tablets, which reduce the swelling and free the nerve with the result that most patients recover completely within a few months. If the eye cannot be closed, it is protected by an eye shield so that the ulcers do not develop on the cornea.

BENDS

A painful condition caused by too rapid a reduction in atmospheric pressure, when, for example, a deep-sea diver surfaces too rapidly, or when an aircraft suddenly becomes depressurized.

Normally, a certain amount of nitrogen, a gas found in the air that we breathe, is dissolved in the blood and tissues. At high pressures—at the bottom of the sea, for example—the quantity is increased. If the pressure suddenly becomes much lower—when a diver surfaces rapidly, or an aircraft climbs quickly to altitude—the nitrogen turns into a gas again and forms bubbles in the blood and tissues. These may cause intense pain, particularly in the joints of the knees and shoulders, within a few hours; they may also block small blood vessels, causing paralysis and damage to the brain and heart. The condition can be treated by returning the affected person to a high-pressure environment as quickly as possible. The nitrogen bubbles then redissolve in the blood, and the patient can be returned to a low pressure in a safe, controlled way. Divers avoid the problem by taking care not to surface too quickly, or by use of a decompression chamber, in which pressure is reduced gradually.

BENIGN

A term that means 'non-malignant', and therefore harmless, when used to describe a *tumour* or disease.

BENZODIAZEPINES

A group of drugs that act as minor tranquillizers and are sometimes used as light sedatives, as a treatment for mild *anxiety*, and as muscle relaxants. The best known of the benzodiazepines are Valium—whose generic name is diazepam—Mogadon—nitrazepam—and Librium—chlordiazepoxide. Valium may also be given by injection to control status epilepticus—*see epilepsy*—and to make people slightly sleepy during uncomfortable procedures such as gastroscopy, in which a tube is passed into the stomach through the mouth.

The benzodiazepines have replaced *barbiturates* as the main drugs used for night sedation. This is partly because they are more selective. While barbiturates depress the whole central nervous system—*see The Nervous System, p28*—benzodiazepines concentrate their effect on the limbic system of the brain, the seat of emotions. They are also less dangerous. It is most unusual for anybody who has taken an overdose of a benzodiazepine drug to die, because the drugs themselves are not sufficiently poisonous. Instead, the person falls into a very deep sleep.

Until recently, benzodiazepines were not thought to be addictive. Scientists now think, however, that the long-term use of drugs such as Valium causes a psychological dependence upon them. This is mainly because a temporary rebound effect can affect patients after completing a course of such drugs. In a case of acute anxiety, for instance, the patient can feel worse than ever after ceasing to take Valium and therefore resorts to more. In the same way, a few sleepless nights can follow after a course of Mogadon. Advance warning of the potential problem can help patients come to terms with it. In addition, many doctors believe that such drugs should only be prescribed for short-term use—*see Abuses of the Body, p328.*

BERIBERI
A nutritional disorder caused by a deficiency of thiamine, or vitamin B1, in the diet—*see Diet, p322.*

Beriberi is a common condition in underdeveloped countries, where polished rice, which contains little or no Vitamin B1, is the staple food. In the West, it is sometimes seen in alcoholics, who tend to suffer from dietary deficiencies—*see Abuses of the Body, p328.*

In the early stages of the disease the symptoms are mild: tiredness, loss of appetite, slight *oedema*, a raised pulse and occasional *palpitations*. Sufferers from beriberi may continue to exhibit these symptoms for many years. Sometimes, however, the condition progresses to one of two more serious forms, called wet beriberi and dry beriberi.

These serious forms of beriberi are the result of different effects of the lack of thiamine on the metabolism of carbohydrates. Its absence has two possible effects: in the first, waste chemicals, intermediate stages in the breakdown of carbohydrate, accumulate in the tissues. This causes the peripheral blood vessels to swell and leak fluid, which causes massive *oedema*. As a result, the heart has to work so hard that it becomes enlarged. This condition is called wet beriberi and is one of the causes of *cardiomyopathy*.

In dry beriberi, thiamine deficiency means that the tissues are unable to use glucose, the normal fuel for the cell, properly. This primarily affects the nervous system, which uses only glucose for energy. The condition causes a peripheral *neuropathy*, the symptoms of which are pins and needles, *paraesthesiae*, and numbness in the legs. The calf muscles waste away and may be tender when squeezed. Walking becomes increasingly difficult and eventually impossible.

In the West, alcoholics and those suffering from malnutrition sometimes develop a brain disorder called Wernicke's encephalopathy. This is thought to be due to thiamine deficiency. The physical symptoms are great mental confusion, disorientation, and *amnesia*. The treatment for all types of beriberi is simple. If the condition is in its early stages, it clears up rapidly with the addition of thiamine to the diet. However, long-standing beriberi may have already caused significant damage to the heart muscle, thus increasing the chances of *heart failure* or a *heart attack*.

BETA BLOCKER
Drugs that block some of the effects that adrenaline would normally have on the heart, lungs and peripheral vessels. The heart is under the control of the autonomic nervous system—*see The Nervous System, p32*—the sympathetic part of which causes it to beat faster and more strongly. When sympathetic impulses are blocked by a beta blocker, such as propranolol, both the pulse rate and blood pressure fall. Thus, these drugs are used to treat high blood pressure, or *hypertension*, and some *tachycardias*, or fast pulse rates.

Unfortunately, beta blockers cannot be used to treat these conditions in all patients, because they may make an existing disease worse. They should not be used, for example, when there is a risk of cardiac failure. In these circumstances, blocking the sympathetic impulses to the heart may precipitate *heart failure*.

The treatment of asthmatics and bronchitics with beta blockers may also cause problems. In both cases, the result may be a dangerous tightening and narrowing of the bronchi, called bronchoconstriction. In insulin-dependent *diabetics*, beta blockers may make it impossible for the patient to feel the shakiness and sweatiness which heralds impending *hypoglycaemia*, a serious reduction in the level of sugar in the blood.

Because beta-blockers slow the pulse, there are also useful in the treatment of *anxiety*. However, they only treat the symptoms of the complaint, not the cause. Research is also in progress to study their effectiveness in the treatment of *schizophrenia*.

BILHARZIA—see Schistosomiasis

BILIARY CIRRHOSIS
Primary biliary cirrhosis is a rare disease in which the bile ducts inside the liver are destroyed by a slow and progressive inflammation. The condition most commonly affects middle-aged women, and its direct cause is unknown. It is thought by many scientists, however, to be an *auto-immune disease*. Secondary, or obstructive, biliary cirrhosis, is a different condition in which the liver becomes damaged as a result of a long-standing blockage of the bile ducts by *gall stones*.

The first symptom of primary biliary cirrhosis is often itching all over the body. Later there may be an enlarged liver and spleen, and a feeling of general tiredness. Because of the interference to the production and circulation of bile, fat is inadequately absorbed during digestion. As a result, the stools are often pale, loose and fatty. There are often fatty deposits, known as *xanthelesma*, around the eyes and in the creases on the palms of the hands. As the disease progresses, *jaundice* develops and the bones become painful and brittle.

Once biliary cirrhosis is suspected, the diagnosis can be confirmed by liver function test, a liver biopsy and a blood test—*see Special Tests, p84*—to detect the presence of antibodies produced by the *auto-immune* reaction. Unfortunately, there is no specific treatment, although the symptoms caused by the inadequate metabolism of fat can be relieved by a low-fat diet—*see Diet, p322*—and pain in the bones relieved by vitamin D supplements. Sufferers may be given immunosuppressive drugs, in an attempt to reverse the condition, but these have not yet proved their efficacy. Some patients recover spontaneously, or go into a period of *remission*, but in the majority the disease becomes progressively worse over five to ten years until there is *liver failure*.

BILIARY COLIC
A severe abdominal pain, lasting for about an hour, that is felt when a *gall stone* blocks the common bile duct or

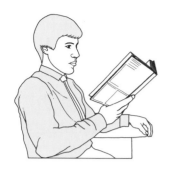

Blind Spot The blind spot lies at the back of the eye where the optic nerve leaves the retina *(right)*. There are no light-sensitive rods and cones at this spot, so any light rays falling here cannot be detected. To demonstrate the presence of this blind spot, hold this book up at arm's length and either close or cover up one eye. With your open eye, focus on the cross to the left and slowly move the book towards you. When the book is about 12 inches (30cms) away, you will find that the round spot on the right has disappeared, leaving that side of the page blank.

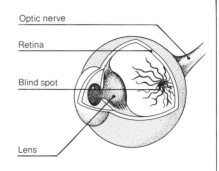

Optic nerve

Retina

Blind spot

Lens

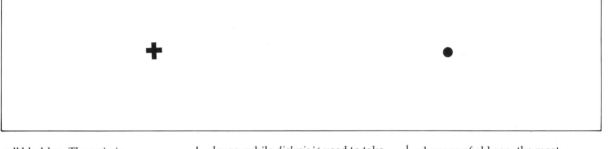

gall bladder. The pain is concentrated in the upper right-hand side of the abdomen, and may spread to the right shoulder and the back.

The pain of biliary colic is so severe that, characteristically, the sufferer draws his or her knee up to the chest in an attempt to relieve it. There may also be nausea and vomiting, and a *fever* if the blockage has led to an infection of the gall bladder. The pain is treated by powerful *analgesics* in the short term. Eventually, however, a *cholecystectomy* is carried out to remove the stones and the gall bladder, to prevent a recurrence of the problem.

BIOPSY—see Special tests

BIRTHMARK—see Naevus

BLACKWATER FEVER
A condition associated with falciparum *malaria*, whose name derives from the sudden passage of quantities of dark red or blackish urine. The urine is coloured by the blood pigments produced as a result of a massive *haemolysis*, or destruction of both normal and infected red blood cells. The precise cause of blackwater fever is not known, but the condition usually occurs in people who have been inadequately treated for malaria, or who have been taking anti-malarial quinine tablets irregularly. The condition may cause a blockage of the kidney tubules, leading to *renal failure*, with vomiting and collapse, and, eventually, death. Blackwater fever may be treated by *steroid*

drugs, while *dialysis* is used to take over the function of the kidneys.

BLEPHARITIS
An inflammation of the eyelids. This is usually caused by an accumulation of *dandruff* in the eyelashes. As a result, a red, scaly rim forms around the edges of the eyelids. The problem can be avoided if the scales of dandruff are removed by washing, and the eyes are kept clean. The eyes may also become inflamed as a result of a bacterial *infection*, in which case the condition is treated with warm salt washes and an *antibiotic* cream.

Sometimes blepharitis is caused by an *allergy* to eye make-up. The obvious treatment is to discontinue the use of the responsible eye-shadow or mascara.

BLIND SPOT
The place at the back of the eye where the optic nerve meets the retina. Since there are no photoreceptors, or light-sensitive cells, on the blind spot, no light is absorbed, and any image focused on that area cannot be seen.

BLINDNESS
The inability to see well enough to perform any task for which eyesight is essential. People whose vision is so poor that optical aids, such as glasses, magnifying lenses and large print books, cannot help them to work are therefore classified, in the terms of the National Assistance Act, 1948, as blind. In the majority of cases in Britain, blindness is caused by degeneration of the eyes with age.

Other than the degenerative

changes of old age, the most common causes of blindness in the West are *glaucoma, cataracts, detached retina,* retinal vein *thrombosis,* accidents and gonococcal ophthalmia. This is a form of *conjunctivitis* caused by the bacterium which is responsible for *gonorrhoea.*

In addition to these major causes, blindness may be the result of a variety of less common conditions. These include xerosis, in which the conjunctiva becomes thickened and dry in the areas where it is exposed to light; *keratosis, xerophthalmia, syphilis* and *lead poisoning.* Blindness is also an occasional complication of two more common problems: *diabetes mellitus* and *toxicariasis,* an infestation of cat and dog roundworms that affects, so researchers believe, around two per cent of the population of Britain each year.

In Britain, those classified as blind are placed on a national register and are entitled to a number of social benefits. These include special training in braille and in the use of a stick or, in some cases, a guide dog. Blind children are able to attend special schools or classes, in which they are shown how they can live a relatively normal life.

Blindness is much less common in the West than in the Third World, where few of these benefits are available. The main causes of blindness in the Third World are different from those in the West. *Trachoma,* an infectious form of *conjunctivitis* caused by a microbe called Chlamydia trachomatis rife in the tropics, is the most common cause of blindness in the world. Next in importance is onchocerciasis, or river blindness, a disease of tropical Africa, southern Arabia and Central America that is caused by Onchocerca volvulus, a worm that is transmitted to humans through fly bites. The worms live in the eye; when they die they cause an *allergic* inflammation, which leads to death of tissue, conjunctivitis, inflammation of the cornea and iris. *Glaucoma, cataracts* and blindness follow. Scientists believe that the onchocerca worm is currently responsible for more than 20,000,000 cases of blindness.

Many millions of people are blinded by vitamin A deficiency—*see vitamin deficiency diseases*—and a further 50,000 to 100,000 children are blinded every year by *keratomalacia*, in which the cornea becomes soft and perforated.

BLOCK—see Heart block; Nerve Block

BLOOD POISONING—see Septicaemia

BLOOD PRESSURE—see Hypertension

BLUE BABY—see Congenital heart defects

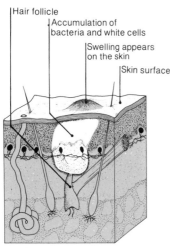

Boil A blocked hair follicle in the skin which becomes infected with Staphylococcus bacteria develops into a boil *(above)*. Both the bacteria and the white blood cells that fight them accumulate in the follicle and form a thick pus-filled swelling.

BOIL
An small area of inflammation caused by *bacteria* that usually develops in a sweat gland or hair follicle in the skin. A boil begins as a painful swelling and after two or three days a core of dead tissue and pus forms; this eventually bursts, expelling bacteria and the white cells that have been fighting them so that

healing can begin. This process can be speeded up by bathing the boil in hot water and applying hot poultices.

Boils should not, however, be squeezed or lanced with unsterilized equipment, since this may spread the infection. A stubborn boil, or one in a particularly uncomfortable place, such as the buttocks, should be lanced by a doctor and covered with a surgical dressing. Boils on the face or neck or in the ears are usually treated with *antibiotics*, taken by mouth, since there is a slight danger that the infection may be carried by the blood to the delicate internal organs.

BORNHOLM DISEASE
A viral infection caused by viruses of the Coxsackie group. These cause *inflammation* and necrosis, or death of muscular tissue. The illness, which is also called pleurodynia and epidemic myalgia, was given its name after a series of outbreaks that occurred on the Danish island of Bornholm during the 1930s. It tends to occur in small *epidemics*.

After an incubation period of anything up to two months, infected patients experience headaches, *fever* and severe pains in the lower chest and abdomen, which give rise to the most colourful name for the condition—Devil's grip. The muscles of the chest wall are tender, but the lungs are not usually affected. There is no specific treatment for Bornholm disease, but rest and pain-killers usually help to relieve the symptoms. Probably the most important therapy is reassurance that the pain is due to a viral illness and will disappear within a few days, since many patients suspect that it may be heart disease.

BOTULISM—see Food-poisoning

BRADYCARDIA
A regular, slow heart beat that gives rise to a pulse rate of under 50 to 60 beats a minute. Bradycardia is a normal state in young, fit athletes, who often have slow pulse rates as a result of their physical training. In those who are not young or fit, however, bradycardia is abnormal. There are two main causes of the condition.

The first, and most common cause of abnormal bradycardia is over-medication with drugs such as digoxin, a refined form of *digitalis*, and *beta blockers*. In these cases the drug is either stopped and another substituted, or the dosage is reduced.

The second main cause of bradycardia is *heart block*. In this

condition, no impulses reach the ventricles from the natural *pacemaker*, the sinoatrial node in the right atrium. The ventricles then beat at their own intrinsic rate, or unstimulated rate, of between 30 and 40 beats a minute. This slow pulse rate often produces symptoms of faintness and dizziness. If the heart block does not clear up on its own, it is treated with drugs or by the insertion of an artificial heart pacemaker to return the heart beat to its normal rate of 60 to 70 beats a minute.

Bradycardia may also be found in cases of *hypothyroidism*, or myxoedema, and in cases of raised inter-cranial pressure.

BRAIN DEATH
With the advent of *transplant* surgery and sophisticated intensive-care equipment, the definition and diagnosis of death has become a complex and emotive subject. Prior to this, people were said to be dead when their heart stopped beating and they ceased to breathe. Death was diagnosed when the patient could not be roused and neither a pulse nor a sign of respiration could be detected; a small mirror would be held in front of the mouth to check that no vapour from expired air formed on it. In addition, the pupils were dilated and failed to change size when a bright light was shone into them. In time, the body stiffened up, in a process known as rigor mortis, and became a waxy, greyish colour. Under these circumstances, it was easy to determine that someone was dead.

However, this commonsense definition of death is based on simple clinical findings that have recently had to be modified. It is now possible for the brain to be so severely damaged that it will never recover and all brain functions have ceased, but for the action of the heart and lungs to be sustained indefinitely by modern technology and drugs. As a result, patients in this condition do not die, in the traditional sense of the word, until their life-support systems have been disconnected.

The problem for doctors is to decide when they should switch the life-support systems off if their patient is being kept alive, in a technical sense only, by artificial means. They have to weigh up their own desire to save and prolong life, the distress that the situation causes to relatives, the shortage of hospital beds and intensive-care equipment and the consequences for another patient whose life may be saved if the person is a potential transplant donor.

To avoid this dilemma, doctors follow a strict set of rules, which state that life-support systems must not be disconnected unless the patient meets all the criteria that satisfy a diagnosis of brain death. The diagnosis is made on the basis of carefully defined clinical tests, evidence from EEG tests and carotid angiography—see Special tests p84. If no cerebral activity whatsoever is found to exist, the diagnosis of brain death is made.

There is rarely any doubt about this diagnosis. If reflex or electrical activity can be demonstrated in the brain by tests, the brain is considered to be alive and functioning at a basic level. The tests are stringently applied, under the supervision of a senior doctor. If any doubt whatsoever exists, the patient is maintained on life-support systems, and his or her case is reviewed periodically. Relatives are usually consulted and informed of the test results and their wishes respected.

BREAKTHROUGH BLEEDING
Bleeding in the middle of the menstrual cycle, which may occur in women who are taking the contraceptive pill—see Sex and Contraception, p338.

The first task for a doctor in cases of inter-menstrual bleeding is to eliminate the other possible causes of the problem. These include cervical erosion, dysfunctional uterine bleeding and cervical or uterine cancer. They are excluded by a detailed pelvic examination and a cervical smear—see Routine Health Checks, p346—before true breakthrough bleeding can be confirmed.

The condition is caused by a breakdown in the hormonal control of menstruation, which causes some of the endometrium, the lining of the uterus, to shed. The mechanism is not completely understood—in some women the cause is a deficiency of the hormone oestrogen, while in others it is a deficiency of the hormone progesterone. As a result, the treatment for breakthrough bleeding may be either a change to a pill with a higher dosage of oestrogen, or one with a higher dosage of progesterone.

Breakthrough bleeding may occur for the first couple of cycles of a new pill, but the problem usually clears up on its own by the third or fourth cycle.

BREAST LUMPS
The presence of one or more hard lumps in the breast. Most women who discover lumps during a regular examination of their breasts—see Routine Health Checks, p346—are terrified that they are caused by breast cancer. However, there are many other causes of breast lumps and one recent study of over 1,200 lumps showed that only a quarter of them were due to cancer. Breast cancer, nevertheless, is a serious and widespread problem—5% of all women develop a cancer of the breast at some stage in their lives. It is therefore essential to consult a doctor as soon as any lump is found in a breast.

The most common cause of breast lumps has a confusing variety of names. The best known of these is fibroadenosis, but the condition may also be called mammary dysplasia or chronic cystic mastitis. This condition, which affects women between the ages of 20 and 50, causes both breasts to become lumpy, painful and tender. The symptoms are usually worse during the latter half of the menstrual cycle—see Sex and Reproduction, p54—and improve once the period starts.

Fibroadenosis is thought to be caused by a hormonal imbalance, in which too much oestrogen and too little progesterone is produced. It is often a part of the pre-menstrual syndrome—see premenstrual tension.

Women who suffer from fibroadenosis are first reassured that their complaint is not caused by breast cancer. They are then advised to wear a well-fitting bra, and treated with pain-killers, and sometimes with diuretics. Progesterone may be prescribed to relieve premenstrual tension. The oral contraceptive pill (p338) has a variable effect on this type of breast disease, sometimes improving it and sometimes making it worse. The condition may clear up if the woman changes to a different type of pill.

A form of mastitis, in which an abscess develops in the breast of a nursing mother whose nipples become cracked and sore, is another common cause of a breast lump. The condition can cause considerable pain when the breast is engorged with milk, but can be treated by antibiotics.

Cysts, or fluid-filled lumps, are also common. They develop because the breast is a gland arranged around a system of ducts, any of which may become blocked. Cysts may be treated by aspiration, that is emptied with a needle and syringe. The fluid is sent to a laboratory for analysis to ensure that it does not contain cancer cells. As long as the breast lump disappears completely after aspiration, and the fluid is not blood-stained, no further treatment is necessary. However, up to half of the patients who are treated for cysts in the breasts develop another cyst at some time in their lives.

A single breast lump in a young woman may be a fibroadenoma, a benign tumour that arises in breast tissue. Fibroadenomas can grow very large; a few have been found weighing over 500 grams (1lb). These lumps are usually removed surgically.

Carcinoma of the breast, which usually first appears as a painless breast lump, most commonly affects women over 30, the peak incidence being between the ages of 40 and 80. Sometimes the lump is tethered to the underlying muscle, or the skin over it is puckered. There may be a discharge from the nipple, and glands can often be felt in the armpits or in the hollow above the collar bone. If the presence of a breast lump is not reported to a doctor, and the cancer is allowed to grow, a small ulcer often appears in the skin overlying the lump. Infection sets in, and sometimes causes an offensive odour.

In many cases, it is difficult for a doctor to be certain of the cause of a breast lump. As a result, he or she will normally refer the woman to a specialist, who will order special tests, such as mammography, a breast X-ray, or a biopsy, in which the lump is removed surgically and examined under a microscope—see Special Tests, p84. This procedure is routine; it does not mean that the patient has breast cancer.

If breast cancer is diagnosed, and the cancer is at an early stage, it is unlikely to have spread, or metastasized to another part of the body, and the treatment has a good chance of success. For this reason, it is vital to examine the breasts regularly, and to consult a doctor immediately, if a lump is discovered. Treatment may involve the removal of all or part of the breast—see mastectomy—and radiotherapy.

BREECH PRESENTATION
The 'bottom down' position of the foetus in pregnancy and labour—see Pregnancy and Birth, p60. The vast majority of babies—some 96 per cent—are 'head down' or cephalic presentations; only three per cent are breech presentation; the remaining one per cent present either shoulder first or in other ways.

Once a breech presentation has been diagnosed by palpation—see The Doctor, Patient and Disease, p70—or ultrasound scan—see Special Tests, p84—an attempt may be made at about the 34th week of pregnancy to turn the foetus so that the head engages in the mother's pelvis,

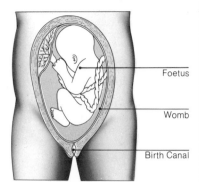

Breech Presentation In a breech presentation *(above)*, the foetus is upright in the womb and presenting its buttocks to the birth canal. This is the opposite of normal presentation, in which the foetus is upside down in the womb, presenting its head.

producing a cephalic presentation.

This gives the baby's head time to 'mould' and accommodate to the shape of the mother's pelvis. When a breech presentation persists, so that at labour the baby's bottom is the first part to be born, the baby's head will not have had time to mould. To protect the head on the last part of the baby's journey down the birth canal, the obstetrician may place forceps gently around it .

Occasionally, when the breech baby is very large indeed, or the mother's pelvis is narrow, it may be necessary to deliver by a *caesarian section*.

BRIGHT'S DISEASE—see Nephritis

BRONCHIAL CARCINOMA—see Lung cancer

BRONCHIECTASIS

A lung disease in which the smaller bronchi, the tubes that carry air through the lungs, are abnormally wide—*see The Respiratory System, p28*.

In rare cases, bronchiectasis is congenital, or present at birth, in which case it is the result of abnormal development of the bronchi in the foetus. More commonly, however, it arises because parts of the bronchial tree— *see The Respiratory System, p28*— become obstructed; by thick mucus, in the case of *cystic fibrosis*; or by pus, in the case of chronic infections, such as pulmonary *tuberculosis*, *bronchitis*, an *abscess* of the lung or *bronchopneumonia*. Occasionally, the obstruction may be due to a *tumour* or a foreign body that has been inhaled.

If it is persistent, an obstruction from any cause will eventually weaken the bronchial wall. This weakness, in turn, causes the bronchi to become distended. Pus

tends to accumulate in the affected bronchi, and causes a chronic cough, in which infected sputum is brought up. Generally, those affected by bronchiectasis do not feel unwell. After a cold, however, or an attack of *influenza*, bouts of tiredness, *fever* and night sweats may continue for several weeks, with a persistent cough and the production of large quantities of infected sputum. This may be streaked with blood, and sometimes blood itself is coughed up. This problem is known as *haemoptysis*, and is caused by bleeding of the blood vessels in the distended bronchioles.

Doctors usually suspect that bronchiectasis may be present in patients who have a history of lung infection and complain of a persistent sputum-laden cough. The diagnosis is confirmed, and distinguished from that of chronic bronchitis, by bronchography. In this test, a special dye is used to show up the shape and size of the bronchi on an X-ray.

If the bronchiectasis is confined to one segment of the lungs, the affected tissue may be removed surgically in an operation called a *lobectomy*. If the majority of the lung tissue is affected, this is impossible and *antibiotics* are the only possible form of treatment.

BRONCHITIS

An infection of the bronchi of the lungs—*see The Respiratory System, p28*. The condition may be acute, or of sudden onset, or chronic, long-standing and progressive.

An attack of acute bronchitis often follows a viral illness of the upper respiratory tract, such as *influenza*, or a cold. This lowers the resistance of the body to the invading bacteria. The trachea and bronchi become inflamed as a result of a bacterial infection. In response, the production of sputum increases and itself becomes infected with bacteria. This causes a cough and the production of quantities of greenish-yellow infected sputum. Sometimes, there is a pain in the chest, as well as *fever*, *dyspnoea*, or shortness of breath, and wheeziness. After treatment with *antibiotics*, the symptoms usually clear up within a few days. Occasionally, however, an attack of acute bronchitis may develop into bronchiolitis, in which the infection spreads to the bronchioles, or into lobar *pneumonia*.

Cigarette-smoking and a cold, damp, dusty, smoky or foggy atmosphere, all predispose people to chronic bronchitis, because the disease is caused by long-standing irritation of the lining of the bronchi. The mucus-producing glands in the

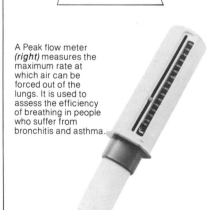

Bronchitis exists in two forms. Acute bronchitis, in which mucus infected with bacteria is expelled from the lungs, follows a viral illness of the upper respiratory tract. The trachea and, in some cases, even the tiny bronchioles, become inflamed *(left)*. Chronic bronchitis develops as a result of frequent irritation of the air passages. Large quantities of uninfected mucus which narrow the tube are produced.

Trachea

Lung

Bronchus

Bronchioles

Inflamed bronchioles restrict the passage of air.

A Peak flow meter *(right)* measures the maximum rate at which air can be forced out of the lungs. It is used to assess the efficiency of breathing in people who suffer from bronchitis and asthma.

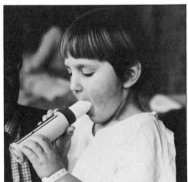

bronchi secrete abnormally large quantities of mucus in an attempt to soothe the irritation. This sticks to the bronchial walls, and even blocks the smaller air passages, the bronchioles. The membrane lining the bronchi swells, obstructing the airway and reducing the space available for the passage of air even further. Chronic bronchitis is thus also known as chronic obstructive airways disease, or COAD.

Chronic bronchitis cannot be cured, and unless its cause, which is most commonly cigarette-smoking, is removed, the disease becomes progressively worse until there is respiratory failure. Eventually, chronic bronchitis is fatal, but it takes many years for the disease to develop to this stage. Up to the final few years, the damage to the lung tissues of smokers can be halted, but not completely reversed, by giving up smoking—*see Abuses of the Body, p328.*

The first signs of chronic bronchitis are shortness of breath and a cough with sputum during the winter months. Later on, these symptoms persist throughout the year, and become more noticeable after physical activity, such as a brisk walk. The symptoms can be relieved to a degree by *bronchodilator* drugs, taken either as tablets or by means of an inhaler. These drugs work by widening the bronchioles and increasing the air space in the lungs.

From time to time, the condition is made worse by attacks of acute bronchitis, and this combination can cause serious problems. *Antibiotics* are given to treat these attacks.

BRONCHODILATOR
A drug that dilates, or widens, the bronchi of the lungs—*see The Respiratory System, p28.* Bronchodilators are therefore used in the treatment of *asthma*, in which the muscles of the bronchial walls contract in a spasm, and *bronchitis*, in which the walls of the bronchi become swollen and their apertures blocked by mucus. They may be taken in tablet form, inhaled from aerosol sprays, taken rectally in the form of suppositories, or given by an injection into a vein. Two of the most common types of bronchodilators are called salbutamol and aminophylline.

BRONCHOPNEUMONIA
A serious, and potentially fatal, infection of a segment of lung tissue—*see The Respiratory System, p28.* It is a special hazard for children and old people. This type of pneumonia, which is also known as acute lobular pneumonia, occasionally affects children after an attack of *measles* or *whooping cough*, and the elderly after an attack of acute *bronchitis*. Scientists believe that bronchopneumonia is caused by the inhalation of the disease-producing organisms that cause such infections, and those responsible for other infections that affect the upper respiratory tract, such as *influenza*.

Bronchopneumonia causes the bronchi in the affected segment to become clogged with pus, the result being the collapse of the lung tissue served by these tubes. The patient does not recover from the upper respiratory tract infection as expected. Instead, a high *fever* develops and the pulse starts to race. There is a cough, by which infected, greenish sputum is produced, as well as shortness of breath and fast breathing.

The illness generally lasts for several weeks, and is treated with *antibiotics*. Because of the danger that bronchopneumonia may be fatal, it is especially important that the diseases and upper respiratory tract infections that cause it should be promptly treated in old people and children, the groups most susceptible.

BRONCHOSPASM
A spasmodic constriction of the bronchi—*see The Respiratory System, p28*—which may be caused by an *asthmatic* attack, an *allergy*, such as *hay fever*, or a serious bacterial infection, such as acute *bronchitis*. When the bronchi are constricted, the flow of air to the lungs is reduced and the tissues suffer from a shortage of oxygen. The seriousness of this is determined by the severity of the bronchospasm: in some cases the spasm is hardly noticeable; in others, the sufferer is prostrated, dyspnoeic, or short of breath, and becomes *cyanosed*, through lack of oxygen.

Bronchospasm is treated by *bronchodilator* drugs, and, if the cause of an attack is a bacterial infection, *antibiotics* are also given. People who suffer from asthma, hay fever or acute bronchitis often carry an inhaler through which they take a bronchodilator when they become aware that a bronchospasm is imminent.

BRONZED DIABETES—see Haemochromatosis

BRUCELLOSIS
A bacterial infection, also called undulant fever, Malta fever and abortus fever, that is caught from close contact with animals infected with the bacterium—for this reason it is an occupational hazard for farmers, abattoir workers and veterinary surgeons—and by drinking unpasteurized milk that has been produced by infected animals.

The precise type of the bacterium, and the type of animal from which it is caught, varies from country to country. In Britain, the bacterium is Brucellosis abortus—so-called because it causes cattle to miscarry. In America and the Far East, the organism is B. suis, which is caught from pigs; in Malta, B. mellitensis is caught from goats.

The incubation period of brucellosis is about three weeks, after which symptoms similar to those caused by *influenza* appear. These include sweating, weakness, loss of appetite, headache, pains in the joints and limbs, a cough and a sore throat.

A provisional diagnosis can be made from the history and occupation of the sufferer; it is confirmed by special blood tests—*see Special tests, p84.* The disease is treated initially with the *antibiotic* tetracycline, but other antibiotics may be needed if the symptoms persist or become worse. Brucellosis may be prevented however if unpasteurized milk is avoided, or boiled before it is drunk.

BRUISE—see Ecchymosis

BUBONIC PLAGUE—see Pasteurella pestis

BUERGER'S DISEASE
An uncommon disease of unknown cause that affects the blood vessels. Buerger's disease, also called thromboangiitis obliterans, occurs in men, and very occasionally in women, who are between 25 and 40 years old and smoke cigarettes.

In Buerger's disease, the arteries, normally those in the legs, become inflamed. Clots may form as a result, and these impair the supply of blood to the legs. In the early stages, this makes the feet cold and painful and causes *intermittent claudication*, in which the calves become painful after light exercise, such as a brisk walk. The toes may turn a dusky blue colour as a result of *cyanosis*, a shortage of oxygen.

There is no specific treatment for the condition, though any injury to the feet, however minor, should always be treated promptly, in order to prevent an infection. However, the progress of the disease is often arrested if the sufferer stops smoking immediately. If he or she continues to smoke it is likely that *gangrene* will develop in one or both of the legs, and that clots will start to form in arteries throughout the body, making a heart attack likely. Eventually, it may become necessary to amputate the affected limb.

BULIMIA NERVOSA

A condition commonly known as 'gorge-purge' syndrome, which is closely related to *anorexia nervosa*. The sufferers are usually young women, who make themselves vomit after eating a meal in an attempt to lose weight. Some girls eat normal quantities of food before vomiting; others starve for several days and then gorge themselves, eating excessive amounts of food, before vomiting.

Sufferers from anorexia nervosa are normally emaciated and show the symptoms of *malnutrition*. In contrast, girls who suffer from bulimia nervosa usually find that the gorge-purge technique is a way of keeping their weight stable, rather than losing weight. The practice often has dangerous consequences, however. Stomach acids enter the mouth and throat each time that a person vomits, so frequent vomiting can cause *ulceration* and, eventually, perforation of the oesophagus and infections of the teeth and gums. Treatment of the condition itself is similar to that for anorexia nervosa.

BUNDLE BRANCH BLOCK—see Heart block

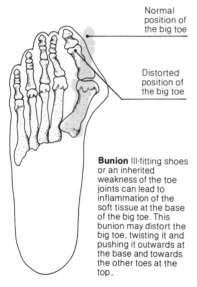

Normal position of the big toe

Distorted position of the big toe

Bunion Ill-fitting shoes or an inherited weakness of the toe joints can lead to inflammation of the soft tissue at the base of the big toe. This bunion may distort the big toe, twisting it and pushing it outwards at the base and towards the other toes at the top.

BUNION

A painful inflammation of the soft tissues around the joint between the big toe and the foot. The direct cause of a bunion is rubbing from ill-fitting shoes. However, underlying this, sufferers from a bunion often have an abnormality of the foot, in which the big toe tends to bend over towards the other toes. This

abnormality tends to run in families and is called hallux vulgus.

The inflammation can be reduced if sufferers from a bunion remove its cause by wearing good-quality, well-fitting shoes. Sometimes, a pad placed under the front of the foot, or between the big toe and the next toe, may help to ease the discomfort.

The bunion can be removed by surgery, in a procedure known as Keller's operation. In this, a piece of bone is removed from the base of the big toe, and the toe is straightened out. However, recovery from the operation is long, painful and tedious. The patient has to wear plaster clogs for several weeks after surgery, and may not be able to return to work for almost a month. As a result, Keller's operation is rarely performed unless the patient finds that the pain caused by the bunion has become excruciating, and that walking is difficult.

BURKITT'S LYMPHOMA

A disease commonly found in African children, in which a malignant *tumour* forms in lymph tissue. Burkitt's lymphoma is thought by doctors to be caused by a virus known as the Epstein Barr virus.

The most common site for the tumour is the lymph tissue around the jaw. In its early stages, the tumour loosens the teeth, which eventually fall out. As the tumour grows, it often spreads up the cheek bone and invades the eye socket, first making the eye bulge, and eventually destroying the eye completely.

The tumour may also, less commonly, arise in one of the abdominal organs, such as the kidneys, liver or adrenal glands. Wherever the tumour arises, however, it will spread, or metastasize, throughout the body if it is not treated, causing death. The treatment usually begins with the surgical removal of the primary tumour, and continues with the use of *cytotoxic*, or cancer-killing, drugs and *radiotherapy*. Burkitt's lymphoma is particularly sensitive to such treatment, and there is a good prospect that patients will survive for up to six years.

Symptoms similar to those caused by Burkitt's lymphoma have recently been recorded in an unusually high number of male homosexuals in America. As a result, this group is being monitored in an attempt to establish whether there is any link between Burkitt's lymphoma and male homosexuality. The provisional theory is that the Epstein Barr virus, which causes the disease, may be linked to the auto-immune

disorders to which male homosexuals appear to be particularly susceptible—*see auto-immune deficiency disease*.

BURNS—see First Aid, p369

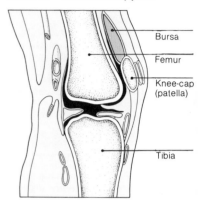

Bursa
Femur
Knee-cap (patella)

Tibia

Bursitis is an inflammatory condition, which affects the bursae, fluid-filled pouches which reduce friction between the bones, muscles and ligaments where they meet in a joint. The condition can be caused by injury, infection or simply by pressure. In response to these, the membrane producing the fluid steps up production, with swelling as the result. The commonest form is housemaid's knee, in which the pre-patellar bursa beside the knee-cap becomes inflamed, so causing the knee to swell.

BURSITIS

An inflammation of a bursa, a small, fluid-filled pouch that acts as a shock absorber in a joint and reduces friction between bones, muscles and ligaments. In response to an injury, an infection, or, most commonly, to unusual pressure, the membrane lining the pouch increases its production of fluid. As a result, the bursa swells up, restricting the movement of the joint and causing pain and tenderness.

Bursitis may develop in any of the large joints of the body, such as the ankle and the elbow, and is often associated with the presence of a *bunion* at the joint between the big toe and the foot. The most common form of bursitis, however, affects the pre-patellar bursa in front of the knee. This condition, called housemaid's knee, is caused by constant kneeling.

The treatment for bursitis is simple. The excess fluid is removed from the affected bursa by means of a needle and a syringe, and the joint is bandaged tightly until the pain and tenderness disappear. *Antibiotics* may be given to prevent any infection. In the case of housemaid's knee, the sufferer should avoid kneeling until the bandages have been removed, and thereafter should protect the knees with cushions when kneeling. If bursitis recurs, however, it may be necessary to remove the affected bursa by operation.

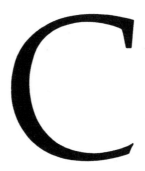

CAESARIAN SECTION

A surgical operation in which a baby is delivered through an incision made in the abdominal wall and the lower part of the uterus—*see Pregnancy and Birth, p60*. The amniotic fluid is drained, the baby lifted out and the cord is cut. Then the placenta is drawn out and the layers of the incision are stitched. The operation may be conducted under general *anaesthesia*, or the mother may be given an *epidural* to relieve pain, so that she remains conscious during the delivery.

The incision used to be made vertically—from just below the navel to the pubic hair—but is now usually made horizontally, along the 'bikini line' where the scar is less visible. This is called a lower segment caesarian section.

The operation may be performed for a number of reasons: when the health of the mother or child would suffer from prolonged labour because the pelvis is too narrow for the baby's head; in a complicated *breech presentation*, when the baby cannot be turned manually; and in *placenta praevia*, when the placenta lies across the cervix, the entrance to the uterus, and might therefore bleed dangerously during labour. It is also performed if the baby shows signs of oxygen deprivation; when the mother suffers extreme *toxaemia of pregnancy*; when labour does not start, and cannot be induced; or when labour becomes prolonged and ineffectual.

CALCULUS

The deposit, also known as tartar, that forms on the teeth, causing *caries* or *periodontal disease*.

Calculus is also the medical name for a stone, a hard, insoluble mass, that can form in any hollow organ. Stones commonly form in the gall bladder and bile duct—*see gallstones*—or the kidneys, ureters or bladder—*see kidneys*. They are made up of deposits of substances such as bile pigments, or the breakdown products of red blood cells, calcium salts and cholesterol, which are usually dissolved in the fluid inside the organ. Why stones form is not

fully understood, but diet is known to be a contributory factor.

CALLUS

The hardening and thickening of the skin that occurs in parts of the body subject to constant friction. The fingers and toes, and the palms of the hands and the soles of the feet are typical sites. If much hard skin develops, a callus may become painful. In this case, the callus is sometimes called a corn.

The area of hardened skin may be removed by rubbing with a pumice stone or other abrasive, or by treatment with a preparation containing salicylic acid, a chemical often used in the treatment of skin disorders. However, the callus will reform unless the cause is removed. Labourers who handle heavy equipment often develop permanent calluses on their fingers. A callus is also the name for the mass of blood, and tissue containing bone-forming cells, that accumulates around the ends of bones after a *fracture*. Eventually, as calcium salts are deposited in the callus, the fractured bones heal.

CANCER

A *malignant tumour* that arises as a result of the abnormal growth of tissue. While a *benign* tumour continues to grow on the site on which it forms, a malignant tumour tends to spread to other parts of the body.

When a cell undergoes cancerous changes, it divides spontaneously and rapidly forms a colony, an abnormal mass whose cells have no specific function. This continues to grow until the healthy cells in the tissue are outnumbered and the colony begins to spread. It may become large enough to disrupt blood vessels and cause bleeding, or obstruct hollow organs.

When the tumour has become established, cancerous cells begin to slough off into the lymphatic fluid or bloodstream, and a small proportion of these establish new colonies elsewhere in the body. This process is known as *metastasis*. The more malignant the tumour, the more

likely it is to metastasize.

Cancers are of two main types. Carcinomas arise in the epithelial tissue that lines the skin and internal organs of the body. Sarcomas occur in the connective tissue, and the muscle, fat, bone, cartilage, blood and lymph vessels that make up the superstructure of the body. Within these two main groups, tumours are subclassified according to their structure.

Although cancer can develop anywhere in the body, it most commonly affects the lungs, the digestive and excretory systems, the blood, the lymphatic system, the prostate gland in men and the breast and uterus in women. Tumours in other sites, such as the skin, throat and brain, are far less common, although certain types of cancer may be prevalent in certain parts of the world. For example, cancer of the oesophagus is rare in the West, but fairly common in parts of China. The reasons for this are not known.

There is no single cause of cancer. Many different factors lead cells to change their behaviour, and only a few are known. However, many carcinogens, or substances known to cause cancer when exposed to living tissue, have now been isolated. Coal-tar derivatives and other products used in the synthesis of dyes have been shown to contain carcinogens, as have arsenic, asbestos and cigarette smoke. The US Government has banned the use of certain food additives, especially colorants, because of their carcinogenic properties. Exposure to excessive radiation of any kind, even to the sun, can also cause cancer.

Although there is as yet no evidence that *viruses* can cause cancer in humans, they are clearly involved in some way in the development of certain tumours. *Burkitt's lymphoma* is one example. Since several tumours that arise in animals are known to be caused by viral infection, it is possible that researchers may yet discover a close link between viral infection and cancer. Some kind of genetic exchange may take place between

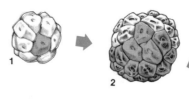

Cancer Tissue becomes cancerous when its cells start to divide uncontrollably. In the nucleus of every cell, the genes on the chromosomes control when and how often the cell divides. This control may be lost when the genes transmit confused messages to the rest of the cell. The loss of control may be triggered by chemicals called carcinogens, such as the tar in cigarettes, by certain viruses — though this is not yet proven — stress and other unknown factors. The cells in a particular tissue normally divide at set times and at regular intervals. A carcinogen, virus, stress or an unknown factor disrupts the genetic mechanism which controls cell division, **1**. The cells divide quickly and randomly, **2**. The cells merely divide and grow, playing no role in the maintenance and function of the tissue, **3**. One of two things can then occur. Either the tissue may mysteriously revert to its normal pre-

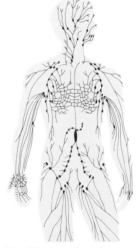

cancerous state, or it may develop into a malignant tumour. The malignant tumour grows rapidly, eventually shedding cells into the bloodstream and lymph vessels, **4**. This is called metastasis and is how cancer spreads to other parts of the body, where it can trigger other cells to become cancerous, forming secondary tumours.

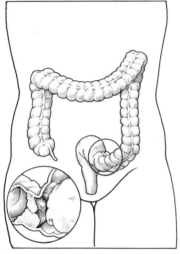

Cancer of the large intestine *(above)* develops slowly and may be completely cured if treated early enough. An area of the intestine *(inset)* obstructs the passage of faeces, bleeds easily and may be ulcerated. There may be no symptoms at all until the intestine finally ruptures.

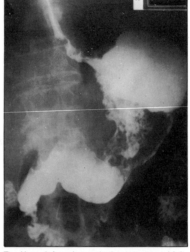

The X-ray *(above)* reveals the extent to which a stomach cancer has spread. Stomach cancer, which sometimes develops from an ulcer, affects twice as many men as women and may be cured if the tumour is removed at an early stage. The initial symptoms may be indigestion, loss of appetite and occasional

vomiting. When a malignant tumour breaks up and metastasizes, cancerous cells enter the lymph system **(above)** and the bloodstream. In this way, a tumour spreads to other parts of the body where it causes secondary tumours. When this happens, the cancer becomes very hard to cure and eventually may be fatal.

the DNA, or the genetic material of a virus, and that of a human cell, that might cause a cancerous mutation.

There may be some truth in the old idea that chronic irritation—or repeated injury to certain tissues—may be the underlying cause of cancer. For instance, since chafing causes the skin cells to multiply, chronic irritation may be responsible for some cancers of the skin. It is also possible that injuries may affect the genetic make-up of a cell and bring about mutations.

Hereditary cancers are very rare, but they do exist. Certain *congenital* tumours appear at birth or shortly afterwards, and a small number of human cancers that occur later in life show a predictable pattern of inheritance. The reason may be that people inherit a predisposition to develop the disease. Psychologists see a link between anxious, over-conscientious, introverted people and the likelihood of developing cancer in later life, and believe that

there may be a cancer-prone type of personality, who may be taught to alter his or her outlook and lifestyle in such a way as to prevent the development of the disease—*see Stress, p332.*

There is an interval of one to ten days between the time a cancer cell first appears and its division into two cells known as 'daughter' cells. This means that if a tumour continues to grow at this rate, its volume should double every five days on average.

However, only the fastest-growing childhood tumours double in volume so quickly. It has been established that the rate of growth of a malignant tumour decreases with time, and that after about the first 30 doublings, most double in size at a rate that varies from ten to 400 days. Since the interval between the origin of a tumour and the time when it becomes apparent may be several years, it follows that, if pre-cancerous cells can be discovered by

screening, they may be stopped from developing further by simple surgery.

Screening, by means of manual examination of the breast—*see Routine Health Checks, p346*— cervical smears—*see Special Tests, p84*—and even by microscopic examination of the sputum coughed up by smokers in the morning, may represent the beginning of a revolution in the diagnosis and treatment of cancer.

Self-screening is the second most effective early-warning system. There are eight important signs of cancer; anyone who notices one of them should see a doctor immediately:
* Unusual bleeding or discharge, especially from any body orifice, such as the vagina or rectum
* A lump or thickening in the breast or elsewhere in the body
* A sore that does not heal
* Any persistent change in bowel habits, especially alternating *constipation* or *diarrhoea*

* Persistent hoarseness or coughing
* Persistent *indigestion* or difficulty in swallowing
* Any change in the size, shape or appearance of a wart, or mole.
* An unexplained loss of weight.

Cancer, however, is a clever mimic of other ailments, and a doctor presented with such symptoms will carry out various further tests. Modern technology has put a vast range of diagnostic techniques at the doctor's disposal. Using an endoscope, for instance— *see Special Tests, p84*—it is possible to look inside hollow organs, such as the oesophagus, bronchi, stomach, bladder and rectum.

X-rays are very helpful in diagnosing carcinoma of the lung— *see lung cancer*—and, with the aid of a barium *enema*, a tumour in the large bowel may show up on X-ray as well. Disturbances in the pattern of blood vessels can be detected by injecting an artery or arterial network with a 'contrast medium', such as a dye, and scrutinizing the pattern produced by an X-ray of the affected part. This process, known as arteriography, is an accurate method of detecting tumours of the brain, liver, kidney and bowel.

Medical researchers have recently discovered that certain tumours of the brain, liver, spleen and pancreas absorb certain isotopes, radioactive forms of some elements. Small, harmless dosages of these are injected into the veins, and the radiation emitted by the tumour is recorded. This method has been very useful for detecting metastases.

X-rays also show up cancers of the lymphatic glands if 'contrast medium' is injected into the system. The spectacular CAT scan (Computerized Axial Tomography) is a method of measuring the rate at which X-rays are absorbed by tissues. Since tumours absorb different amounts of radiation from healthy tissues, their location and structure can be mapped using this technique. Scientists believe that a new technique, called nuclear magnetic resonance, or NMR, will map tumours even more effectively.

If any of these tests prove positive, a biopsy is usually carried out to identify the tumour, so that the appropriate course of treatment can be decided.

Different cancers require different treatments according to their type, their site and whether or not they have metastasized. Some, such as cancers of the skin or the lymph glands, may be treated by *radiotherapy* or removed surgically. Complex techniques have been developed to ensure that the correct dosage of radiation is delivered only to the tumour, and not to surrounding tissues and organs.

Chemotherapy or drug therapy as a form of cancer treatment began more than 100 years ago, when arsenic was used to treat *Hodgkin's disease*. Now more than 30 chemicals, known as *cytotoxic drugs*, are available to treat and cure cancers. Since these drugs are highly toxic to healthy as well as cancerous tissue, they are usually administered by what is known as a 'pulse-type' routine: a two-week period of treatment may be followed by a treatment-free week to allow the healthy cells time to recover. *Antibiotics* that prevent bacteria from multiplying are also sometimes effective against certain cancer cells.

It is unusual for a patient to receive only one form of treatment; a combination of methods is more effective. Surgery to remove the primary cancer will be followed by chemotherapy or radiotherapy to kill any stray cells and so reduce the possibility of metastasis. However, both techniques are uncomfortable and may cause dizziness, vomiting, and temporary loss of hair.

Cancers of the sex organs, some of which are believed to grow when stimulated by hormones, often respond to hormone therapy. For example, ovarian tumours in pre-menopausal women are thought to be dependent on oestrogen, the female hormone, and are treated with a drug that is antagonistic to it. However, this may cause *virilism*, the appearance in women of male *secondary sexual characteristics*, such as increased body hair. Similarly, cancer of the prostate gland in men may be treated with stilboestrol, an oestrogen.

Success may depend on whether the cancer is fast- or slow-growing. Certain stomach cancers and brain tumours may grow so quickly that they are fatal before treatment can take effect. Inevitably, some cancers cannot be cured. The reasons why they kill, however, are not entirely understood. Some tumours surround and block blood vessels in the area in which they form, thus starving other tissues and organs of their essential blood supply. Others compress vital organs such as the air passages, blood vessels or nerves, or obstruct hollow tubes, such as the digestive or urinary tracts, so that essential body functions are affected and eventually cease.

Some cancers, such as breast cancer, tend to *ulcerate*, leading to infection and bleeding, while others, in the endocrine glands, for example, sometimes cause abnormal hormone secretion. Many tumours cause biochemical changes in the body: some activate the immune response—*see Natural Defences Against Disease, p52*—causing the tissues in which they are growing to release *antigens*. The body reacts by producing antibodies which destroy the antigens and the tissues that manufacture them.

Treatment given to patients with incurable cancers is aimed at relieving the symptoms and keeping the tumour at bay. This is called palliative therapy. It includes radiotherapy, chemotherapy, and also surgery. It can be surprisingly successful: an American, Mrs Winona Melick, born in California in 1876, had four cancer operations between 1918 and 1968, yet in 1980 she celebrated her 104th birthday. Much of the fear of cancer is based on memories of the sufferings of friends and relatives who may have died in pain. However, advances in the understanding and treatment of cancer, and research into the nature and relief of pain, mean that people with terminal cancer should experience little or no pain.

Relatives of a cancer patient can now call on a range of medical and social services, including help with nursing at home. They can also draw upon professional *counselling* to help them deal with the psychological problems that they and the patient will inevitably have to confront. People who treat cancer patients feel that the greatest challenge families now face is not whether to tell a person that he or she has cancer, but how to find the best way of helping him or her to come to terms with the disease. The medical profession correctly places emphasis on how to help the patient enjoy what might be many years of remaining life.

Hospices and homes are also available, where dying patients may spend their remaining days with sympathetic nursing and medical care, which is aimed mainly at preventing physical pain and relieving psychological stress—*see Coming to Terms with Death, p366*.

Nowadays there is always hope. Attempts to understand why some cancers simply shrink and disappear without trace have led to investigation of the ways in which the body fights invasion by foreign bodies—*see interferon*—and of how to make a tumour channel its energy into something it does quite naturally—slough off more and more cells until there are no more left to grow. Recent studies into the possible links between *carotene* and cancer have also raised hopes that it may, eventually, be possible to prevent the development of cancers by dietary means.

**CANCER OF THE CERVIX—see
Uterine cancer**

**CANCER OF THE COLON—see
Colonic cancer**

**CANCER OF THE KIDNEY—see
Kidney disorders**

**CANCER OF THE LIVER—see
Hepatoma**

**CANCER OF THE LUNGS—see
Lung cancer**

**CANCER OF THE OVARIES—see
Ovarian tumours**

**CANCER OF THE SKIN—see Basal
cell carcinoma; Melanoma**

**CANCER OF THE STOMACH—
see Stomach cancer**

**CANCER OF THE TESTICLES—
see Testicular tumours**

CANDIDIASIS
An *infection*, also called moniliasis or
thrush, caused by a yeast-like
fungus, Candida albicans. This is
usually found in the intestine, the
vagina, the mouth and on areas of
sore skin. A number of factors may
cause chemical changes in the body
that destroy the body's immunity to
candidiasis and encourage the
fungus to grow. These include
treatment for some other condition
with *antibiotics* or corticosteroid
drugs; a change in the level of
hormones in the body as a result of
pregnancy or the use of oral
contraceptives—*see Sex and
Contraception, p338*; and conditions
such as *diabetes mellitus* and
leukaemia. The vagina is the most
common site of the infection in
women; symptoms include itching,
inflammation (often caused by
scratching) and a thick, milky white
discharge.
In general, candidiasis affects the
warm, moist parts of the body, such
as the folds of the skin—the groin
and anus, under the arms or
beneath the breasts—and is often
present, together with *napkin rash*, in
babies. It can affect the nail folds of
people whose hands are frequently
in hot water, and can invade the
lungs, the intestine and the urinary
tract. Candidiasis may invade the
bloodstream of people with
debilitating diseases, such as
leukaemia, and those on
immunosuppressive drugs—drugs
that suppress the natural defences of
the body against infection. Babies
sometimes contract candidiasis of
the mouth while passing along the
vagina during birth.
Candidiasis is infectious. When

thrush is sexually transmitted from
women to men it causes *balanitis*, an
inflammation of the end of the
penis. Such infections are usually
treated with a fungicide, nystatin, in
the form of a cream, lotion or
pessaries. Internal infections require
treatment with fungicidal drugs. The
complaint often recurs, occasionally
in conjunction with other vaginal
infections such as *Trichonomas
vaginalis*, which then requires
specific treatment of both the patient
and her partner.
Some people are more prone to
infection than others. Careful
attention to personal hygiene—*see
Health and Hygiene, p334*— and
avoiding wearing nylon underwear
and tight trousers, may help to keep
the condition at bay. Anyone who
suffers from recurrent thrush should
not use bubble bath or add other
similar products to the bathwater,
and should never wash the genitals
with antiseptics or household
disinfectants, since this may damage
the skin and aggravate the problem.

**CAPD (CONSTANT
AMBULATORY PERITONEAL
DIALYSIS)—see Dialysis**

CARBUNCLE
A collection of *boils* in the skin and
underlying tissue. A carbuncle
results from a *bacterial* infection that
affects several sweat glands or hair
follicles at the same time. It begins as
a tender, inflamed area of skin, but
grows larger and deeper than a boil.
Eventually pus is discharged.
Men and *diabetics* tend to be more
susceptible to carbuncles than
women and children. The back of
the neck, the upper back and the
buttocks are the most common sites.
Bathing with hot water and
applying warm compresses while
the carbuncle is developing help to
maintain the blood supply to the
area and so aid the body to fight the
infection—*see Natural Defences
Against Disease, p52*. *Antibiotics* are
usually prescribed, but a deep
carbuncle may have to be lanced and
drained by a doctor. A carbuncle
should always be covered with a
clean dressing while it is healing.

CARCINOGEN—see Cancer

CARCINOID
A *tumour*, also called an
argentaffinoma, that affects the
argentaffian cells in the glands of the
intestine. Carcinoids may be *benign*
or *malignant* and most commonly
attack the tip of the appendix and
the small intestine. They may also
occur in the rectum, the bile ducts,
the pancreas, the bronchi and the
ovaries.

Carcinoid tumours often produce
serotonin, a neurotransmitter
chemical—*see The Nervous System,
p32*—usually found in the brain.
This, when circulating in the blood
in abnormal quantities, gives rise to
a set of symptoms known as the
carcinoid syndrome. These include
flushing, *tachycardia* or increased
heart rate, swelling of the face, low
blood pressure, or *hypotension*,
stomach pains with *diarrhoea* and
symptoms of *malnutrition*. The latter
are caused by incomplete absorption
of food from the diet—*see
malabsorption syndrome*.
These symptoms usually appear
only when the tumour is
established. The tumour is usually
removed surgically, and appropriate
treatment given to suppress further
growth—*see cancer*.

CARCINOMA—see Cancer

CARCINOMATOSIS
A carcinoma that has metastasized
or spread widely over the body—*see
cancer*.

**CARDIAC ARREST—see
Myocardial infarction**

CARDIAC ASTHMA
The wheeziness and shortness of
breath experienced by people with
heart failure. It is caused by a build-
up of fluid, or *oedema*, in the lungs.
The wheeziness becomes more
pronounced when the patient lies
down, usually when they go to sleep
at night. There are three reasons for
this. First, the position makes
depressing the diaphragm more
difficult; second, it increases the flow
of blood back to the heart from the
legs; third and last, there is a
redistribution of body fluid, as the
oedema which has collected around
the ankles is reabsorbed on lying
down.
Sufferers wake up very short of
breath and often sit up and struggle
to a window to try to breathe more
easily. This change of position helps
breathing, and the symptoms may
subside.
Treatment of cardiac asthma is the
same as that for *heart failure*. Diuretics
are prescribed to reduce the volume
of fluid in the body, and the patient
may be advised to sleep in an
upright position.

**CARDIAC TAMPONADE—see
Tamponade**

CARDIOMYOPATHY
A general term used to describe
damage to the heart muscle that may
gradually lead to a number of
serious problems. These include
enlargement of the heart;

palpitations, or irregular heartbeats; *embolism*, the obstruction of an artery by a clot; or *heart failure*.

It is often difficult to determine the cause of cardiomyopathy, but *viral infection*, *amyloid disease*, *beriberi* and *alcoholism* and *hereditary* factors may all predispose to the condition. There is no specific treatment for cardiomyopathy, but the disorder sometimes clears up when treated.

CARDIOPULMONARY BYPASS
A method of maintaining the circulation of blood while the heart is temporarily stopped for surgery. The blood is directed through an external heart-lung machine. Tubes are inserted into the superior and inferior vena cava, the principal veins of the heart, and into a large artery, such as the femoral artery in the leg. The tubes from the veins are connected to a pump-oxygenator, a machine that takes over the pumping action of the heart, and replaces the lungs by oxygenating the blood. This is returned, under pressure, to the femoral artery. Meanwhile, the operation can be carried out on a heart that is empty of blood and has ceased to beat.

CARDIOSPASM—see Achalasia

CARDIOVERSION—see Defibrillation

CARIES
Decay of the enamel and dentine of the teeth. Caries is a particular hazard to people who eat sweets or sugary foods, to people who do not clean their teeth regularly or efficiently, and, for an unknown reason, to those under 30.

Caries results from the presence of *plaque* on the teeth. Plaque contains *bacteria*, and residual carbohydrates from food. The bacteria attack the carbohydrate, which, as a result, forms an acid. This eats away at the enamel of the teeth, and opens the pulpy interior of the tooth to infection by the bacteria, which causes inflammation.

The first areas to be attacked are those that are difficult to clean: the biting surfaces of the molars; the crevices between the teeth and the border between teeth and gums. If the inflammation is not treated, an *abscess* can form.

A tooth with a developing cavity caused by decay may be sensitive to cold or sweet substances. As the cavity enlarges, this sensitivity becomes gradually more acute until, as the dentine is eaten away, the nerves become irritated and toothache begins. A small cavity may be repaired by a dentist, who will drill away the decayed part of

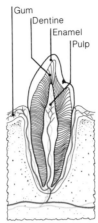 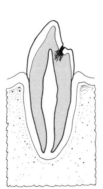 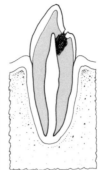 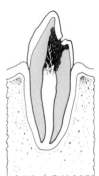

Gum
Dentine
Enamel
Pulp

Caries 1. Bacteria in the pits and fissures of the teeth produce an acid from the sugar in the food. The acid eats into the enamel covering of the tooth.

2. The acid erodes the enamel, the hardest substance in the body, and creates a cavity. Eventually, it reaches the softer layer of dentine.

3. The dental decay spreads rapidly through the dentine. Bacteria pass along the dentine's minute canals and infect the pulp at the heart of the tooth.

4. An increased blood supply, bringing extra white cells to fight the infection, inflames the pulp. This presses on the nerves and causes toothache.

the tooth and replace it with a filling. However, a tooth in an advanced state of decay must be extracted.

If the teeth are regularly cleaned and disinfected with toothpaste or antiseptic mouthwash, caries is much less likely to develop—*see Health and Hygiene, p334*. Decay begins only if *bacteria* are given time to act on the surface of the teeth, and if there is residual carbohydrate on which they can feed—a diet low in carbohydrates—*see Diet, p322*—has been shown to reduce the incidence of caries. Saliva is known to play an important role in preventing tooth decay, and eating sweets between meals when saliva production is low is particularly bad for the teeth.

Fluorine, an element necessary for the formation of the bones and teeth, is now known to be an important agent in the prevention of tooth decay; experiments in adding fluorine to water supplies have had the effect of reducing the occurrence of dental decay in whole populations. There is some controversy about the fluoridization of water supplies, however. Toothpastes containing fluoride, the same chemical in a different form, can help prevent caries in areas where it has not been added to the drinking water, and many people feel that they should be able to decide for themselves whether to use fluoride toothpaste to prevent caries, rather than have the preventive measure imposed upon them.

CAROTENE
The natural chemical that gives plants and many animals their red, orange, brown and yellow colouring. In nature, carotene exists in three forms: alpha, beta and

gamma. Only beta carotene is used by the human body. It is found in milk and in certain vegetables—carrots, broccoli and tomatoes, for example—and is converted into vitamin A in the liver.

Recent studies in America, Britain, Japan and Norway have indicated that not only is there a link between the level of carotene in the blood and the incidence of *cancer*, but that people with high carotene levels are less likely to contract the disease. So far, the results of these studies have been impressive, but not conclusive—it is not clear whether carotene or vitamin A is the protective factor, or whether cancer, once established, uses up large quantities of the vitamin. Research into the connection between carotene and cancer continues, and scientists hope for a breakthrough in the near future.

At the least, the studies add to the argument for a diet rich in fruit and vegetables—*see Diet, p322*. It is important that vitamin A supplements are not taken in more than the dosage recommended by a doctor, because vitamin A is a potentially fatal poison if taken in excess.

CARPAL TUNNEL SYNDROME
A condition in which pressure on the median nerve, as it passes into the palm of the hand through the wrist, causes pain and weakness in the fingers and thumb. The syndrome occurs most frequently in middle-aged women, and also may be a *complication* of pregnancy, or of conditions such as *rheumatoid arthritis*, *myxoedema*, or underactivity of the thyroid gland, or *acromegaly*.

The thumb and the index and middle fingers on one or both hands

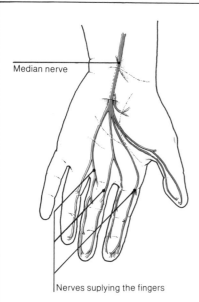

Median nerve

Nerves suplying the fingers

Carpal Tunnel Syndrome A cross-section through a wrist *(below)* shows the median nerve lying among the tendons. between the carpal bones and a tough membrane that lines the carpal tunnel. When the tissue swells around the nerve and the tendons, the result is a constriction of the nerves leading to the fingers *(left)*. The initial consequence is pins and needles and the long-term result the wasting of the muscles supplied by the nerves.

Section through a wrist

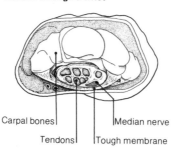

Carpal bones | Median nerve

Tendons | Tough membrane

may feel numb, tingling or painful, especially after use, or in bed at night. Rest, or splinting the hand, may be all the treatment needed. If the condition persists, *steroid* injections, or surgery to release the pressure, may be tried. *Hormone replacement therapy* with thyroxine relieves the symptoms in people suffering from *myxoedema*.

CARRIER
A person harbouring micro-organisms or *genes* responsible for a disease, but who has none of the disease's symptoms.

An insect or animal may also be a carrier of an infectious micro-organism or other substance to another insect or animal, or to man, and is called a vector. A prime example is the female Anopheles mosquito, which transmits the *malaria* protozoa from person to person.

A person who bears a gene for an abnormal trait, but who does not suffer from the disorder, is said to be a carrier of that gene. A well-known example is *haemophilia*, a disorder in which wounds will not heal because the blood fails to clot. The gene is carried by the female members of a family, but only the males suffer from the disorder.

CATARACT
The clouding of the lens of the eye. Some degree of clouding of the edges of the lens is common among elderly people, but when the opacity spreads inwards to reach the part of the lens that lies directly behind the pupil of the eye, it impairs vision and is called a cataract.

The clouding is caused by a thickening or coagulation of the proteins of which the lens is made. This may be an inherited disorder,

or it may happen as part of the ageing process, when it is called a senile cataract. It may also be the result of disease or injury to the lens. People with *diabetes*, certain *metabolic disorders*, and *vitamin deficiency diseases* often develop cataracts. Babies whose mothers contracted German measles—*see rubella*—in the early stages of pregnancy may be born with cataracts. People such as glassblowers, who are constantly exposed to infra-red or other forms of radiation, also tend to develop cataracts.

A fully formed cataract impairs vision to the extent that the affected eye can distinguish only the presence of light and the direction from which it is coming. By shining a light sideways across the eyeball and examining the shadow cast by the iris, the degree of development of the cataract can be estimated. A very narrow shadow will indicate a mature, or advanced, cataract.

When the cataract is mature, it is treated by removal of the opaque lens. This may be done with a scalpel or by disrupting the lens with high-frequency sound waves, and then extracting it by suction through a tiny incision. The surgeon has to ensure that all of the affected lens fibres are removed.

The lens is not essential to sight, so when it has begun to obstruct the entry of light, removing it may restore vision. Without a lens the eye accommodates automatically to distance, but corrective spectacles, contact lenses or a lens implant are necessary for reading and other close work. Unfortunately, however, the operation is not always successful, although an operation that fails to restore vision is unlikely to cause further damage to the patient's already impaired eyesight.

CATARRH
A term used to describe the excessive secretion of thick phlegm by the mucous membranes of the air passages to the lungs, the larynx, the nose and the sinuses.

Catarrh is generally caused by the common cold, and is exacerbated by smoking. A series of colds in close succession may cause *chronic* catarrh. This may be relieved with *decongestants*, but if the sinuses become infected, treatment with *antibiotics* is necessary—*see sinusitis*.

CATECHOLAMINES
A group of naturally occurring chemicals, which are important in the functioning of the nervous systems—*see The Nervous System, p32*. Most of them act as neurotransmitters, or carriers of nervous impulses, across the synapses between nerve endings. They are derived from an amino acid, tyrosine, and adrenaline is probably the most important.

CATHETER
A tube designed to be inserted into an opening in the body in order to inject or remove fluids. The tube is normally made of a plastic or rubber substance; a plastic catheter is likely to be used if it is to be left in place for a long time.

There are many catheters, designed to penetrate different openings. The commonest is the urinary catheter, used to drain the bladder. Catheters are also designed to be inserted into the body's internal organs during surgery. The cardiac catheter is used to pass along a blood vessel into the chambers of the heart, and the Karman catheter, used for *abortion* by suction curettage, is designed to pass through the cervix into the uterus.

CAUTERY
A cautery is a surgical instrument, which uses electricity or corrosive chemicals to destroy abnormal tissue growths, such as warts, or *verrucas*. A type of cautery, known as diathermy, is often used to seal off small blood vessels during an operation.

CELLULITIS
An *inflammation* of the connective tissue—*see Bone and Muscle, p16*—usually caused by *streptococcal infection*. Streptococcal *bacteria* enter the skin through a superficial wound—for example, a small cut near the toe nails caused by bad chiropody, or foot care. Infection spreads along the connective tissue and may become widespread, depending on the resistance and state of health of the patient. The

skin over the affected part appears red and shiny, and may itch. There may also be some swelling and a feeling of heat in the affected limb.

Treatment consists of rest in bed with the affected limb raised, and a course of *antibiotics* to kill off the bacterial infection.

CEREBRAL PALSY

A general term used to describe the presence of brain damage from birth. The causes of the brain damage, and the time at which it occurs, are very variable and often completely unknown. Viral infections of the foetus, *hypoglycaemia* and *metabolic disorders* during pregnancy are all possible causes. Severe rhesus incompatibility—*see haemolytic disease of the newborn*—may also be a factor. This may lead to *kernicterus*, a condition in which bile pigments are deposited in the brain and cause permanent damage after birth.

Many cases of cerebral palsy are caused by brain injuries which occur during labour and delivery—*see Pregnancy and Birth, p60*—when the baby may become anoxic, or short of oxygen. During the first few weeks of life, serious *infections*, such as *meningitis*, may also cause permanent brain damage.

Whatever the cause of cerebral palsy, the resulting brain damage affects the child's intellect and development, although it is not progressive. Children who have suffered brain damage are divided into two main groups, depending on the part of the brain affected. One group is said to be spastic—*see spastic paralysis*—and the second suffer from athetosis, a tendency to make slow, writhing movements.

The spastics, the largest group, generally have stiff limbs and over-emphasized tendon reflexes that cause jerky movements, and rigidity of the muscles. The spasticity usually affects half the body—either the arm and leg on one side, or both legs. Sometimes all four limbs are affected, the legs more than the arms. Spastics have a tendency to *convulsions*. However, their intelligence is usually normal.

Children with athetosis differ from spastics in that their limbs are less rigid, and they make odd, irregular, twisting movements. These do not occur during sleep. A baby with this type of cerebral palsy usually appears floppy with poor muscle tone and control of the head. Speech may also be affected, but, again, the child often possesses normal intelligence.

It is most important that cerebral palsy is diagnosed at an early stage, so that special treatment may begin at once. This is why developmental checks are carried out on babies from six weeks after birth—*see Health and Your Child, p348*. Babies are observed closely to check whether primitive responses are persisting for an abnormally long time, as this is an indication that normal development is not taking place. If a parent is worried about the development of their child, they should always tell the doctor about their suspicions. These are the most valuable aids to the diagnosis of cerebral palsy in an infant, and should be fully investigated.

Treatment is aimed at overcoming the disability as far as is possible, and at preventing deformity. The parents of the affected child can help a great deal by participating in the therapy: he or she can turn feeding, dressing and nappy-changing into exercises to overcome the spasticity or increased muscular tone, and help the child to relax. This postural *physiotherapy*, as it is called, has superseded the old-fashioned practice of correcting the position of the limbs by splinting and the use of surgical appliances. Drugs have little place in the treatment of cerebral palsy.

Throughout the child's life, the parents need support, encouragement and practical help to ease the burden. Apart from the welfare agencies—*see Looking After Disabled People, p358*—help is available from a number of voluntary organizations and charities.

CEREBRAL HAEMORRHAGE— see Cerebrovascular accident

CEREBROVASCULAR ACCIDENT (CVA)

The term used to describe the interruption of the blood supply to any part of the brain, which triggers a series of events that may culminate in a stroke. When the blood circulation to any part of the brain is disturbed, the cells in that area die and that part of the brain ceases to operate. The result is a deterioration of the mental or physical functions controlled by the affected part of the brain.

Such an accident can be caused by any of three blood vessel disorders. A cerebral *thrombosis* is a clot that forms and partially or totally blocks an artery that may have already been narrowed by *atherosclerosis*. A cerebral *embolism* is a small blood clot formed elsewhere in the bloodstream that is carried along by the blood until it similarly obstructs an artery leading to the brain.

In a cerebral *haemorrhage*, the affected artery bursts. The escaping blood seeps into the surrounding cerebral tissue, where it eventually clots. This form of stroke is one of the risks associated with *hypertension* and is therefore one of the reasons why excessively high blood pressure should be treated promptly.

Whatever the cause, the results of a stroke vary, depending on which part of the brain is involved, and the severity of the original accident. The effects are often confined to one side of the body, because damage is usually limited to one side of the brain. The side of the body affected is the opposite one to the damaged area of the brain—that is, if the right side of the brain is damaged, the left side of the body is affected, and vice versa. In the case of an accident involving the middle cerebral artery, for instance, the physical results are *paralysis* of half the face, the arm and the leg on the opposite side of the body to the artery involved.

Among the many other possible effects are visual disturbances, *incontinence* and weakness of the affected parts of the body. When the brain stem is involved, there may be severe *vertigo, vomiting*, double vision or *nystagmus*.

Strokes can happen suddenly—in the case of a massive cerebral haemorrhage, unconsciousness is quickly followed by *coma* and, in many cases, death—or the symptoms can develop over a period of a days or more.

The type of stroke is diagnosed according to the speed of onset of its symptoms and the disabilities it causes. In the case of cerebral haemorrhage, a lumbar puncture—*see Special Tests, p84*—may be necessary to confirm the diagnosis, while a CAT scan—*see Special Tests, p84*—may be necessary to pinpoint the exact location of the leakage. In cases of cerebral embolism, special X-rays called carotid arteriograms—*see Special Tests, p84*—can determine whether or not it is possible to operate and remove the clot. However, this is possible only if the artery involved is large and accessible, and effective only if the operation is performed quickly.

The first medical priority is to preserve life, particularly if the patient is unconscious. In such a case, careful nursing is needed to keep the patient's airways clear and functioning, to give nourishment and to maintain the circulation.

However, there is no cure for a stroke. The main aim is to limit the degree of disability as much as possible and to help the patient come to terms with the limitations this imposes. Here, *physiotherapy* has a vital role to play, the aim being to encourage an unaffected area of the brain to take over the functions of the part that has been irreversibly damaged. *Speech therapy*, for instance, will be suggested if the patient suffers from *dysarthria*, or impairment of speech, while later in the recovery process *occupational therapy* can help the patient establish a new routine of performing everyday tasks, such as dressing. *Steroids* may be given to limit the amount of swelling in the brain in certain cases.

The chief factor in recovery, however, is the degree of determination to get well the patient possesses, and here the support of doctor, family and friends can be vital.

See also Looking After Disabled People, p358.

CERUMEN

The earwax lining the ear canal, or the external auditory meatus. It helps to prevent the dust and dirt that enters the ear from reaching the ear drum. Cerumen is produced by glands in the outer ear canal; if too much is secreted, it may cause partial *deafness*.

Before the wax can be removed, it is softened with ear drops. The ears are then syringed with warm water and the wax washed out.

CERVICAL CANCER—see Uterine cancer

CERVICAL EROSION

A condition that occurs when some of the cells forming the delicate lining of the neck of the womb spread to cover the tip of the cervix. This extension of the cervical lining normally causes the discharge of a small amount of mucus and may result in bleeding after sexual intercourse. The condition is not a disease and carries no serious risks. The area is so delicate, however, that it is susceptible to *infection*.

Cervical erosion is a fairly common problem. Some women seem to have a tendency to develop it, while others face the problem for the first time during or after pregnancy, or when they begin taking the oral contraceptive pill— *see Sex and Contraception, p338.*

In most cases no treatment is necessary. However, many patients are given a regular vaginal examination and cervical smear—*see Routine Health Checks, p346 and Special tests, p84*—in case there are other, more serious problems. In the few cases where the *discharge* and bleeding are very severe, the cells can be destroyed by *cautery*. The operation is painless, and is often performed in hospital out-patients, or during a 24-hour stay in hospital.

CERVICAL SMEAR—see Special tests, p84; Routine Health Checks, p346

CERVICAL SPONDYLOSIS—see Spondylosis

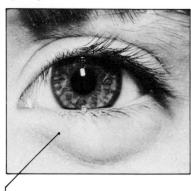
Swelling on eyelid

Chalazion A chalazion is a painless swelling on one of the eyelids, which may grow as large as a pea and become infected. If it fails to disappear, it should be removed.

CHALAZION

A painless swelling on the eyelid, also called a meibomian *cyst*, caused by blockage and *inflammation* of one of the sebaceous glands along the edge of the eyelid. Small chalazions usually disappear within a month or two without medical treatment. However, larger chalazions, which may be the size of a small pea, often persist. If bacterial *infection* sets in the eyelid becomes swollen and painful, and there may be a discharge of pus.

A chalazion can be treated with *antibiotic* ointment, or removed surgically under local anaesthesia in the outpatient department of a hospital.

CHANCRE

A painless *ulcer* that usually appears on the genitals during the first stage of *syphilis*. It may develop anything from nine to 90 days after infection, though the most common interval is four weeks. It usually occurs on the vulva in women, and the glans or body of the penis in men. However, it may appear on the vagina or cervix, where it cannot be seen, or on the lips of both sexes if there has been oral sex, where it may not be diagnosed as a symptom of *venereal disease*.

The chancre is highly infectious, though the symptoms are often so slight that it is not even noticed by the patient, or else it is dismissed as a small sore. It will usually disappear after about three weeks. If syphilis is not treated at this early stage, it will progress to a second, more serious, stage, at which a cure is considerably more difficult.

CHANCROID

A painless, soft sore, similar to a syphilitic *chancre*, that forms on the genitals of both men and women. Chancroids are transmitted by sexual contact, and are common in many parts of the world, especially in the Far East. However, they are rare in Britain. Chancroids are caused by a variety of *haemophilus* bacteria, called Haemophilus ducreyi, and can be treated successfully by *sulphonamide* drugs.

CHANGE OF LIFE—see Menopause

CHEMOTHERAPY

The use of drugs to treat disease. The term tends to be used specifically for the treatment of *malignant* disease with *cytotoxic* drugs.

CHEYNE STOKES RESPIRATION

Very uneven breathing that usually accompanies the terminal stages of an illness. The sufferer's breathing slows down until it stops for several seconds, then speeds up to a peak before slowing down again.

Cheyne Stokes respiration may occur in patients in *coma*; in elderly patients with *heart failure*; or in patients with head injuries or a brain *tumour*. It is caused by a decrease in the blood flow and, consequently, the supply of oxygen, to the respiratory centre—*see The Respiratory System, 28*—in the brain. Drugs which stimulate respiration are sometimes used to treat the condition, though the main need is to treat the underlying disease.

CHICKENPOX

An infectious disease caused by a virus of the *herpes* family. It is spread by droplet infection from coughing or sneezing, or by contact with the condition's characteristic spots. The incubation period for chickenpox is 14 to 21 days, after which a mild fever develops. The spots first appear in the mouth on the palate, and are followed on the second day of the illness by a characteristic itchy rash of dark-coloured spots, which spreads from the body to the legs, arms, head and face. These are highly infectious, and appear at intervals over the next three days, the older ones crusting over to form scabs. These disappear after about 12 days, the patient being infectious until all the spots have crusted.

Medical treatment is usually unnecessary, unless the eyes are involved, the fever is exceptionally high, or there is considerable coughing or vomiting. If a doctor is called, he or she will prescribe antibiotics to deal with the possibility of further infection. The rash should be kept clean and dry, while painkillers, plus a soothing calamine lotion, will help relieve the fever and the discomfort caused by the itching spots. The spots should not be picked—if they are, they will scar to leave unsightly pock-marks.

An attack of chickenpox usually confers life-long immunity to the disease. In children under the age of 10, chickenpox is usually mild. In adults, however, it may occur in a more severe form, particularly in people suffering from a blood disorder, or on long-term *steroid* therapy. In such cases, the body's resistance is usually boosted by an injection of *antiserum*.

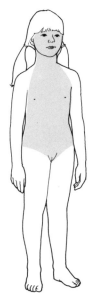

Chickenpox Characteristic signs of chickenpox are the rash of itchy dark red macules, which first appear on the trunk, face and scalp. Over the next few days, the rash spreads to the armpits and the groin. In severe cases, the rash develops on the mucous membranes of the mouth and around the eyes. The macules become blisters and then scabs.

CHLAMYDIA
An infection caused by a micro-organism, Chlamydia trachomatis, that is midway between a *virus* and a *bacterium*. It may be sexually transmitted in humans.

Chlamydia is responsible for a number of genital infections, and the disease may now be more common than *gonorrhoea*, which it tends to mimic. The two diseases often occur together, making diagnosis and treatment of both conditions difficult.

Chlamydia is thought to account for about 40 per cent of all cases of nonspecific urethritis (NSU)—*see urethritis*. It may also cause

epididymitis, an inflammation of the epididymis in the testicles. In women it is a cause of *salpingitis* or *pelvic inflammatory disease*, and cervicitis, an inflammation of the cervix. The infection may produce no symptoms, but in some women it causes vaginal *discharge* and soreness, and pain in the pelvis.

The effect of chlamydia on pregnant women is being studied at present. Reports from the USA suggest that infection acquired between the third and sixth months is associated with an increase in the rate of *stillbirths* and death within the first few weeks of life. Chlamydia infections are also thought to be the commonest cause of severe *ophthalmia neonatorum*, an infection that affects a baby's eyes at birth. The organism may also cause *conjunctivitis* in both babies and adults.

Chlamydia is also responsible for a severe eye disorder known as *trachoma* and a *venereal disease*, Lymphogranuloma inguinale. This disease, which is common in the tropics, causes the enlargement of the lymph nodes in the groin. It can be treated with *antibiotics*, but occasionally the enlarged lymph nodes need to be removed surgically. Patients and, if possible, their sexual partners, are treated with *antibiotic* eye ointments, or tablets, depending on the nature of the infection. The progress of the treatment is usually checked by repeated examinations.

CHOLANGITIS
An *inflammation* of the bile ducts, that causes *fever*, shivering, sweating and *jaundice*. Cholangitis usually results from an obstruction to the bile ducts, or occurs after an operation on them. It is treated initially by *antibiotics*, but, for a permanent cure, the blockage must be removed surgically.

CHOLECYSTECTOMY
The surgical removal of the gall bladder. The operation is usually carried out as a treatment for chronic *cholecystitis*, a bacterial infection of the gall bladder that causes *fever* and acute pain in the upper abdomen. This is often due to cholelithiasis, or the presence of *gallstones*, which blocks the flow of bile from the gall bladder into the intestine.

In a cholecystectomy, the patient is given a general *anaesthetic*, and the gall bladder removed through a small cut just below the ribs of the right side of the chest. The procedure takes around two hours, and the patient normally remains in hospital for about 14 days. He or she is able to resume full activity after

about two months. A normal diet can be followed in the majority of cases, because bile, necessary for the digestion of fats, still reaches the small intestine from the bile ducts in the liver. The only difference is that, after a cholecystectomy, bile cannot be stored.

CHOLECYSTITIS
An *inflammation* of the gall bladder caused by *bacterial infection*. Cholecystitis almost always occurs in association with *gallstones*, a condition that predisposes a patient to infections.

The first symptoms of cholecystitis are *fever*, pain in the upper abdomen, *nausea* and *vomiting*. In some patients the pain is *referred* to the back, or the right shoulder; while others develop *jaundice*. The condition may become chronic, when the symptoms recur time and time again.

Cholecystitis is first treated with antispasmodic drugs, rest, sedation, and, in serious cases, by surgical drainage of the gall bladder. If this treatment is not effective, however, a *cholecystectomy* may have to be performed.

CHOLELITHIASIS—see Cholecystectomy

CHOLERA
A highly infectious disease, caused by *bacteria*, that is usually transmitted by eating food or drinking water contaminated by the *faeces* of an infected person. It can also be contracted by eating shellfish from contaminated water.

The bacteria are strains of Vibrio cholerae, and cause an infection of the small intestine. After an incubation period of between a few hours and several days, severe *diarrhoea* and *vomiting* suddenly occur. The bacteria act on the gut to produce an increase in its secretion of fluid, which is evacuated from the bowel as a watery motion, said to look like ricewater, and causes acute *dehydration* with muscular *cramps*.

In severe attacks, *kidney* and circulatory failure may cause death within 48 hours of the onset of the symptoms. Cholera tends to occur in *epidemics*, especially among undernourished people who live in insanitary conditions, where the death rate can be as high as 50 per cent of the cases contracted. However, the disease can occur in a milder form, especially if it attacks healthy adults.

Since diseases such as *enteritis*, *dysentery*, *malaria* and *food-poisoning* have similar symptoms to those of cholera, diagnosis depends upon bacteriological identification of the cholera bacillus in the faeces—*see Special Tests, p84*. Treatment consists of replacing the lost fluid as quickly as possible—by mouth, intravenous injection, a *drip*, or a tube passed through the nose into the stomach. Once the fluids have been replaced, *antibiotics* can be used to help bring the bacteria under control.

Cholera is a *notifiable disease* under the international health regulations. *Immunizations* are available for people visiting countries in which outbreaks occur, but these are effective only for six months.

CHOLESTEATOMA

A ball of tissue that usually forms in the middle ear, but may occasionally form in the nervous system. Cholesteatomas, so-called because they contain crystals of cholesterol, may become infected and damage surrounding structures, such as the ear drum and the delicate bones of the inner ear.

Slight deafness, ear ache and a *discharge* from the ear are symptoms of a cholesteatoma in the middle ear; there may also be headache, dizziness and weakness of the facial muscles. Diagnosis is by examination of the ear and the hearing.

Cholesteatomas tend to occur in people who have failed to have treatment for minor infections. These may become chronic, and cholesteatomas may form as a result. The blockage must be removed before there can be a permanent cure. A small cholesteatoma may be removed under local *anaesthesia*, but if there is damage to the ear a more complicated operation is usually necessary. Surgery often considerably improves hearing.

CHOREA

Involuntary, spasmodic movements that are due to a disease of the basal ganglia in the brain—*see The Nervous System, p32*. The condition takes two forms—*Sydenham's chorea* and *Huntington's chorea*.

CHRISTMAS DISEASE

A disease, named after the first patient in whom it was diagnosed, with symptoms identical to those of *haemophilia*. Approximately one in ten patients with suspected haemophilia are eventually proved to have Christmas disease. Like haemophilia, Christmas disease is caused by a deficiency of one of the 12 substances essential to the process of blood-clotting—*see The Blood and Lymph Systems, p21*. However, the condition is less serious than haemophilia, as it can be treated with extracts of the missing blood coagulation factor.

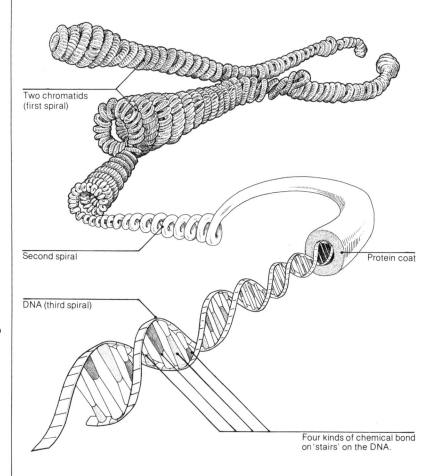

Chromosome The nucleus of every cell, with the exception of the ovum and sperm, contains 46 chromosomes arranged in 23 pairs. One chromosome of each pair comes from the mother and the other from the father. The first 22 pairs are called autosomes, while the twenty-third pair, which determines sex, is made up of the sex chromosomes. Men have a large X and a small Y sex chromosome *(above)*; women have two large X sex chromosomes.

Two chromatids (first spiral)

Second spiral

Protein coat

DNA (third spiral)

Four kinds of chemical bond on 'stairs' on the DNA.

During cell division, each chromosome is duplicated into two identical threads called chromatids *(top)*. Each chromatid consists of deoxyribonucleic acid (DNA) coated with protein and is twisted into spirals, each of which is twisted into still smaller spirals *(middle)*. If a small spiral is unravelled, and the protein removed, the double helix of a DNA molecule is revealed *(bottom)*.

The DNA molecule is like a spiral staircase with four kinds of 'stairs'. These 'stairs' are chemical bonds which can be repeated in any order and in any number, making a string of different combinations. Each combination is a gene and each gene plays a role in the function of the cell. On the 46 chromosomes, there are an estimated total of 50,000 different genes.

CHROMOSOME

Chromosomes are found in all cells and are the means by which genetic information is stored and carried from one generation to the next. They usually exist as pairs that duplicate when the cell divides, and so ensure that the daughter cells are exact replicas of the parent cell.

Each chromosome consists of tiny strands of protein wrapped in spirals of DNA (deoxyribonucleic acid), the nucleic acid on which almost all life is based. The DNA is arranged into a sequence of *genes*.

Almost all cells in the body contain 23 pairs of chromosomes. The sole exceptions are the female egg and the male sperm. These reproductive cells each have 23 single chromosomes which, at the moment of fertilization, form pairs. These pairs possess all the necessary information for the fertilized egg to develop and grow into a human being.

One of these pairs—number 23, the sex chromosomes—determines sex. All females have a matching pair, designated XX; all males have a dissimilar pair, XY. The human egg always has one or other of the mother's X chromosomes, while the father's sperm provides either an X or a Y chromosome. When a sperm with an X fertilizes an egg, the child will be a girl (XX). But when a sperm with a Y fertilizes an egg, the child will be a boy (XY). The father's chromosome contribution therefore determines the sex of a child.

Chromosomes provide the supply of genetic material that governs the development and maintenance of every characteristic of the body. Their existence as pairs—one of each pair from the father and one from the mother—means that two genes control each characteristic.

An abnormal chromosome constitution is usually responsible for *congenital abnormalities*. During the formation of the egg or sperm, a chromosome may be damaged or lost. Damaged chromosomes usually result in faulty genes, and these fail to operate. The loss of an entire chromosome normally results in the death of the foetus, but sometimes females are born without one of their X chromosomes. This gives rise to a condition known as *Turner's Syndrome*. However, children are more often born with one extra chromosome.

People with *Klinefelter's Syndrome* may have three or four sex chromosomes. Those with XXY are basically male with female attributes. Some Russian women athletes, whose physical prowess was far superior to that of their competitors, have been shown by a sex test to have XXY chromosomes. XXYY or XXXY chromosomal constitutions cause *mental subnormality*.

Men with an extra Y chromosome (XYY) are taller than average and may be unusually aggressive. Research has revealed a higher than normal incidence of XYY males among prisoners, especially violent criminals. In the USA, several XYY men have been acquitted of criminal charges in the USA, on the grounds that they were helpless victims of their own genetic inheritance.

People with three chromosomes instead of two in the number 21 pair have *Down's Syndrome*. The extra chromosome comes from the mother when her original pair fail to separate in the egg cell prior to ovulation.

CHRONIC

A chronic or lingering disease is one that develops very gradually and is of long duration. Many chronic diseases, such as chronic *bronchitis*, produce permanent changes in the affected organ or part of the body, so that the disease becomes incurable.

CIRCUMCISION

The removal of the foreskin of the penis, an operation that in some societies is traditionally carried out shortly after birth for religious reasons. Circumcision is commonly believed to reduce the risk of infection of the penis, but so long as the foreskin of uncircumcised men and boys is kept clean, there is no risk to health.

Parents often believe circumcision to be necessary for baby boys whose foreskin cannot be pulled back over the head of the penis. This is, however, quite normal in a very young baby. At birth the foreskin is still joined to the end of the penis, and it begins to separate only after the baby is six months old. It cannot normally be retracted completely until the age of four or five.

The condition in which the foreskin cannot be retracted sufficiently is known as *phimosis*. Circumcision will eliminate the problem. It is a simple, straightforward operation requiring a stay of a day or two in hospital.

CIRRHOSIS

A chronic disease of the liver in which death of liver cells is followed by *fibrosis*, or the deposition of fibrous tissue, and renewal of the remaining liver tissue. Cirrhosis is usually a consequence of longstanding *alcoholism*; in men, any more than six whiskies or three pints of beer a day for between five and 16 years is enough to cause cirrhosis, depending on the individual. In women half this quantity may cause the disease—*see Abuses of the Body, p328*. The reason for this difference between the sexes is not known.

Death of the liver cells may also follow *Wilson's disease*, and *haemochromatosis* or bronzed diabetes. In rare cases, acute *hepatitis* may lead to cirrhosis. Instead of recovering completely as is usual, a patient's condition may progress to chronic active hepatitis and, finally, cirrhosis. Occasionally, cirrhosis develops without any apparent cause, in which case the condition is known as cryptogenic cirrhosis.

Symptoms may be many and varied, or entirely absent, and the presence of cirrhosis is often confirmed only at an *autopsy*. However, there is usually a general feeling of *malaise*, anorexia or loss of appetite, *vomiting*, weight loss and a feeling of discomfort in the upper abdomen. In the early stages the liver may be enlarged, and a doctor will be able to feel it during an examination. As the disease progresses, however, the liver begins to shrink as its volume is decreased by the death of liver cells and *fibrosis*.

Jaundice may occur, although this is usually very mild, as well as high blood pressure in the portal system, the veins that lead to the liver. This is caused by the destruction and distortion of the cells in the blood vessels of the liver, and leads to *ascites*, the collection of fluid in the peritoneal cavity.

The increase in the pressure of blood in the portal veins leads to enlargement of the blood vessels at the points where the portal circulatory system communicates with the vessels of the systemic circulatory system. These are in the lower part of the oesophagus and upper stomach, and are called oesophageal varices when they are engorged with blood. These varices may rupture and bleed; the bleeding may be mild and chronic, but sometimes it is acute, and large quantities of blood are lost. If this happens the patient will require copious blood *transfusions* and intensive care if he or she is to survive.

The liver failure associated with long-standing cirrhosis may lead to hepatic encephalopathy. This is a confused, almost comatose state, caused by the high level of nitrogenous products circulating in the blood. They are produced by the digestion of proteins and would normally be detoxified by a healthy liver. This condition is treated by reducing the amount of protein in the diet.

Gynaecomastia or enlargement of the breasts, wasting away of the testicles and *impotence* are symptoms of cirrhosis in men. In women there may be atrophy of the breasts, and irregular periods or no periods at all, called *amenorrhoea*, due to the failure of the liver to detoxify the male and female hormones.

If, as a result of case history, physical examination and abnormal results from liver function tests—*see Special Tests, p84*—a doctor suspects that a patient has cirrhosis, a biopsy—*see Special Tests, p84*—will be carried out to confirm the diagnosis. There is no specific treatment for the disease, although a number of measures may prove helpful. These include stopping or treating the cause, especially if the cirrhosis is due to alcohol abuse; making sure the patient follows an adequate diet; and treatment of *oedema* and ascites.

Bleeding from oesophageal varices causes a number of other problems. These include haematemesis, or vomiting of blood, and melaena, the passage of black, tarry *faeces* that result from the presence of blood high in the digestive tract. Bleeding varices are treated by compressing the blood vessels by passing a tube with a balloon on its end down the digestive tract and then blowing it up. Alternatively, a sclerosing, or hardening, agent may be injected into the blood vessels. Sometimes an operation known as a porta-caval shunt is carried out. This is a complicated procedure whereby a further connection is made between the portal and systemic circulations. It is only recommended when the patient is thought fit enough to withstand the procedure and its side effects.

Special filters that mimic liver function are sometimes used as a short-term treatment of liver disorders, but perhaps the best hope for the treatment of irreversible cirrhosis in the future lies with liver transplantation. A number of liver transplants have been performed, with varying degrees of success, and research is continuing.

CLAUDICATION—see Intermittent claudication

CLAUSTROPHOBIA
An irrational fear of confined spaces. This *phobia* may make everyday living very difficult since sufferers may be unable to travel in cars, trains or lifts. Severe cases may be treated by a psychologist with *desensitization* therapy.

CLEFT LIP AND PALATE
A *congenital*, or inborn, deformity in which the upper lip and palate fail to fuse during development. It affects around one in every 1,000 babies, in either a major or minor form.

A cleft lip, called a hare lip, is a minor form of the condition, in which there is a vertical split, of variable size and position, in the upper lip. The split is repaired surgically, under general *anaesthesia*, when the child is about three months old.

The deformity is more serious if the split extends back across the palate, when the condition is called a cleft palate, because the baby may be unable to suck, making feeding almost impossible. A special plate can be fitted to the baby's palate at feeding time to overcome this problem. However, a cleft palate is a difficult defect to repair by surgery, and the operation, performed when the baby is about a year old, is not always completely successful. There are often speech defects later in life, but these can be helped by speech therapy.

CLIMACTERIC—see Menopause

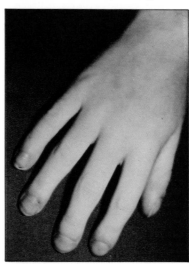

Clubbing Some heart and lung diseases cause the ends of the fingers to become clubbed *(above)*. As the tissue thickens at the base of the nails, they become curved, while the fingertips become rounded and spatula-shaped.

CLINICAL TRIAL
A term used to describe the systematic scientific testing of various kinds of treatment to see whether or not they are effective. In many cases the design of the trial consists in comparing two groups of patients: one receives the treatment to be studied, while the other receives either a different treatment or a *placebo*—a drug or other treatment that has no effect but resembles the treatment being tested. Clinical trials are nearly always at least *single blind*—that is,

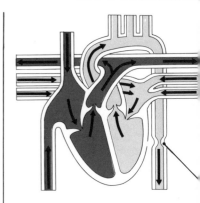

Coarctation

Coarctation of the aorta is a congenital heart defect, in which, in some babies, the aorta is narrowed *(above)* as it descends from the heart towards the lower half of the body. As a result of the constriction, less blood can be pumped to the lower half of the body, causing a delayed, weak femoral pulse, while the upper half of the body, in contrast, suffers from hypertension, or raised blood pressure.

the patients do not know whether they are receiving the active treatment or the placebo—and often they are *double blind*, when the doctors, too, are kept in ignorance about which group has received the active treatment until after the trial. The aim is to eliminate unconscious bias from the results. Sophisticated statistical methods are used to assess the outcome of clinical trials.

CLUBBING
Changes in the nails that occur in certain diseases of the heart and lungs, such as *lung cancer*, bacterial *endocarditis*, cyanotic *congenital heart defect* and *bronchiectasis*. The tissue at the bases of the nails thickens, so that, in extreme cases, the fingers and toes have a club-like appearance. Occasionally, however, clubbing is not a symptom of disease, but a harmless inborn abnormality.

CLUB FOOT—see Talipes

COARCTATION OF THE AORTA
A *congenital heart defect* in which part of the aorta, the body's main artery, is narrowed in one segment, usually where the ductus arteriosus joins the aorta in the foetus. The narrowing causes high blood pressure—*see hypertension*—in the upper half of the body, since it is supplied by large arteries that branch off from the aorta before the narrowing. The lower half of the body, however, may have weak or delayed pulses and there may even be *cramps* in the legs. Treatment is by surgical removal of the narrowed segment.

COELIAC DISEASE

An *allergy* of the small intestine to gluten, a protein found in wheat and rye flour. The disease reduces the ability of the intestines to absorb nutritive substances from the diet, and is therefore a cause of *malabsorption*.

Symptoms usually begin when cereals are first introduced into the diet of babies at about four or five months. They include poor appetite and growth, excessive wind and large, fatty stools that float on the surface of the lavatory water and smell foul. If the disease is not diagnosed and treated early in childhood, the child's growth may be permanently stunted.

Diagnosis is made in hospital, where blood and stool samples are examined—*see Special Tests, p84*. If these show positive results, a biopsy of the small intestine will be carried out. This is done by giving the patient a small capsule to swallow, which, on its way through the digestive tract, extracts a piece of the small intestine and is then excreted in the faeces, from where it is retrieved.

If coeliac disease is diagnosed, a *gluten-free diet* may be recommended. After a few weeks the child's general condition greatly improves, and the symptoms disappear, but the gluten-free diet must be adhered to for life.

COLD

The most common infection of the upper respiratory tract occurring in humans. Its medical name is coryza. It is caused by one or more of a large group of *viruses* that are spread when infected people cough or sneeze.

The incubation period is from one to three days, after which the symptoms of nasal *discharge*, sneezing and mild *fever* occur. These symptoms, which are similar to those of *measles* and *rubella*, or German measles, may last for up to a week, and occasionally progress to *sinusitis* or *bronchitis* as the resulting *catarrh* becomes secondarily infected with *bacteria*.

Although research into the common cold has continued for many years, there is still no cure for the infection. Some scientists, led by Linus Pauling, the American Nobel prize winner, believe that massive dosages of vitamin C help kill the virus and thus cure the cold. Unfortunately this theory has not yet been proven; many scientists, indeed, believe that it is completely without foundation. However, research into the treatment of *cancer* by *interferon* has indicated that this substance may eventually hold the key to treatment of the problem.

Unfortunately, interferon is extremely difficult, and expensive, to produce.

Until progress is made in the search for a cure for the common cold, the only treatment is to relieve the symptoms. The mild fever may be controlled by *aspirin* or paracetamol, while the nasal congestion can be relieved by *antihistamine* preparations. These act as decongestants. A day or so in bed is as helpful in controlling the further spread of germs as in fighting the cold. Contrary to popular belief, *antibiotics* have no effect whatsoever on viruses, and, therefore, on a cold. However, they are sometimes given to sufferers from a cold to prevent secondary infection by bacteria.

COLD SORE—see Herpes

COLECTOMY

An operation to remove all or part of the colon or large intestine, usually as a treatment for *colitis*.

COLIC

A succession of acute abdominal pains caused by spasm in hollow or tubular organs. Colic is a symptom of a number of disorders of the digestive system—*see The Digestive System, p40*—such as constipation. In babies, when it is called infantile colic, the problem is often caused by wind in the intestines.

Renal colic is a symptom of a *calculus* or stone which has moved from the kidney into the urethra— *see kidneys*. It begins as a severe pain in the abdomen, which gradually moves down to the groin, and then subsides, usually within two hours.

COLITIS

An *inflammation* of the colon. The symptoms are usually *diarrhoea*, sometimes with blood and mucus, and pain in the lower abdomen. Colitis may be due to a *bacterial* infection, or to a number of other disorders—*see amoebiasis, Crohn's disease, irritable bowel syndrome, ulcerative colitis*.

A variety of special investigations—*see Special Tests, p84*—may be needed to determine the exact cause of colitis. These may include X-rays, a barium enema, and endoscopy. If colitis is caused by bacterial infection, *antibiotics* will be given. Drugs to stop the diarrhoea may also be needed, as well as anti-spasmodic drugs to relieve the abdominal pain. Since the disease tends to recur, and may become *chronic*, a long-term course of an anti-inflammatory *sulphonamide* drug is usually prescribed once the patient recovers, to prevent this from happening.

Repeated attacks of colitis may

damage the intestines. In patients with chronic colitis a colectomy, an operation to remove the damaged section of the colon, may be performed. This may necessitate a *colostomy* or *ileostomy*.

COLONIC CANCER

The presence of a *malignant tumour* in the large intestine. The condition is one of the more common types of *cancer*, and tends to affect people over 50, men slightly more often than women.

Most commonly, tumours occur at the lower end of the colon, where it runs through the pelvis—*see The Digestive System, p40*—or at the junction of the sigmoid colon and the rectum. Colonic tumours tend to grow in one of two ways: either around the intestinal wall, narrowing the tube and causing an *obstruction*; or through the intestinal wall, spreading inside the tube. Whichever the type of tumour, colonic cancer is extremely difficult to diagnose, because there are often no symptoms until a late stage.

As a result, the first symptoms may be vomiting, loss of appetite, changes in the normal pattern of defaecation—sometimes with alternating diarrhoea and constipation—and the presence of blood in the faeces. Most sufferers also experience some abdominal pain, but this may range from mild to severe.

Diagnosis is by sigmoidoscopy or a barium enema—*see Special Tests, p84*. A proportion of cases, however, are discovered during an operation to treat either an intestinal obstruction, or *peritonitis* resulting from perforation of the intestinal wall. Treatment of colonic tumours generally involves surgery. The affected portion of intestine is *resected*, and, if sufficient healthy bowel remains, the two severed ends are joined together. However, if the tumour has grown sufficiently to affect a large area of intestine, the whole colon may be removed, and a *colostomy* fashioned.

Colonic tumours are generally slow-growing types of cancer, and a large proportion of patients live for many years after a resection.

COLOSTOMY

A surgical procedure in which the large bowel or colon is made to open out on to the surface of the abdomen. The *faeces* it contains are thereby diverted from the rectum and collected in a bag on the skin surface.

A colostomy may be temporary or permanent. A temporary colostomy is made to relieve the lower part of the colon and rectum, often after

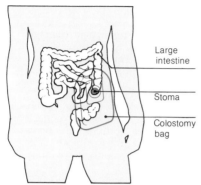

Large
intestine

Stoma

Colostomy
bag

Colostomy A colostomy is an operation in which part of the colon or large intestine is removed. It can be performed in the treatment of cancer, colitis, or diverticulitis and can be either temporary or permanent. A temporary colostomy is often carried out as part of major bowel surgery to give the colon the chance to heal before resuming its normal function. One consequence is that, after the operation, food has to be re-routed via a colostomy bag. This is worn externally around the waist and linked to the healthy tissue through an opening in the abdominal wall

major bowel surgery, so that it has a chance to heal before it once again has to transport faeces.

A permanent colostomy is made when a large amount of the colon is removed, because of *cancer*, for example. At first, the motions are often rather loose and unformed. After a few weeks, however, the colostomy patient learns which foods to avoid and how to cope with the inconvenience of colostomy bags and belts. Generally, the colostomy fills about twice a day, and there are now disposable bags that may be changed after each bowel movement.

A sealing substance, which is applied to the skin so that the disposable bag adheres firmly, occasionally causes irritation of the opening, or stoma—*see stomatitis.* This and any other problems that arise in the management of colostomy equipment may be treated, and advice on how to prevent or minimize them is available from specialist stoma therapists. A voluntary body called The Colostomy Welfare Group can advise colostomy patients on how to contact a therapist, and helps them adjust to their treatment.

COLOSTRUM
A milk-like substance that is secreted from the breast, usually just after, but occasionally just before, childbirth. A rich mixture of protein, lactose or milk sugar, protective *antibodies*, white blood cells and *serum*, it is produced for two or three days after delivery, and is followed by the secretion of breast milk.

COLOUR BLINDNESS—see
Defective colour vision

COMA
A state of unconsciousness so deep that there is no reaction to external stimuli. The sudden, brief losses of consciousness that occur in *syncope*, or fainting, and in *epilepsy*, are not comas. A coma can last anything from a few hours to months, or even years.

More than 50 per cent of coma cases follow a severe blow on the head, or an obstruction to the circulation in the brain caused by *hypertension*, *thrombosis*, a *tumour* or an *abscess*. Coma may also be brought about by *poisoning* from alcohol, narcotic or other drugs or toxic gases and fumes. In *meningitis*, the onset of coma is usually gradual, while in *diabetics* the onset of *hypoglycaemic* coma is usually very rapid.

A patient in a coma will be pale, with dilated pupils, and cannot be roused by external stimulation. He or she should not be moved by anyone other than medical personnel, unless it is essential to save life. Movement could be extremely dangerous, especially if the coma was caused by injury to the spine or head. Any tight clothing should be loosened; the patient should be covered and kept warm, and a doctor or ambulance called—*see First Aid, p369.*

The patient is usually moved to hospital for diagnosis and treatment. Injuries will be treated, or, if the coma is due to poisoning, the stomach will be washed out. Coma in a diabetic may be caused either by a lack or an overdose of insulin, and is treated accordingly.

A patient in a coma may be fed intravenously, by means of a *drip*, while urine is extracted by a *catheter* placed in the urethra. It is necessary to clean the mouth regularly and to treat the areas of skin that come into contact with the bedclothes in order to prevent *bedsores*. An ointment is applied to the eyelids to prevent them from sticking together.

Although patients in coma are not apparently responsive to any outside stimuli, it is believed that certain areas of the brain may be aware of the outside world; a young British girl, who had been in a coma for some weeks following an attack, recovered shortly after her doctors arranged for her favourite music to be played continuously to her, day and night. Doctors believe that this outside stimulus may have penetrated the patient's unconscious and hastened her recovery from the coma.

COMMUNICABLE DISEASE
A *contagious* or infectious disease, that is one that can be passed from one person to another. *Infection* can take place directly, by physical contact, by droplets coughed or exhaled into the air by an infected person, or by using an object that has been handled by an infected person and to which the micro-organisms that carry the infection, such as *bacteria* or *viruses*, are able to adhere—*see Health and Hygiene, p334.*

A disease can also be spread by a *carrier*, a person who, though infected by the disease-carrying organisms, does not show symptoms of the disease.

COMPLICATION
A secondary complaint that arises in a patient who already has a disease or disorder, often as a consequence of the original complaint. For instance, *emphysema* may be a complication of chronic *bronchitis*.

COMPULSION
An irresistible urge to carry out certain acts or rituals. Everyone has persistently recurring thoughts: it is common, for example, to worry that a door may have been left open, or the gas left on, after having left the house. Urges towards ritualistic behaviour, such as touching wood, are also common. However, a person with an obsessive compulsive *neurosis* finds that such thoughts and urges occupy so much time that they seriously interfere with daily life. Moreover, obsessive thoughts may become linked with compulsive acts; for example, thoughts of germs contaminating objects in everyday use leads to a compulsion such as excessive hand-washing.

Compulsive rituals apparently serve two main purposes. They give the person affected a feeling of order and control in a confusing and threatening world. They also serve as a defence against the anxiety caused by obsessive thoughts. Continual activity helps to prevent such thoughts and their accompanying anxieties from intruding into the mind.

Traditionally, long-term *psychoanalysis* has been used to treat patients suffering from obsessive compulsive neurosis; in recent years, however, the use of *tranquillizers*, combined with such psychiatric techniques as *group therapy* and *behaviour therapy*, help to reduce the patient's anxiety while helping him or her probe and come to terms with its underlying cause—*see also obsession, phobia.*

CONCUSSION
Loss of consciousness resulting from a blow to the head. Concussion may last for only a few seconds; if a

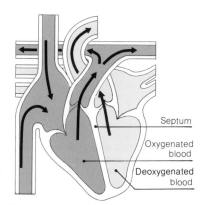 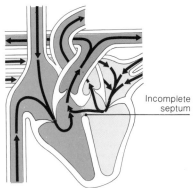 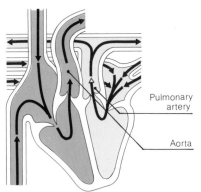

Congenital heart defects The two sides of a normal heart *(left)* are divided by a muscular wall called a septum. This separates the oxygenated blood in the left side from the de-oxygenated blood in the right side. In one of the most common congenital heart defects, the septum is incomplete *(middle)*. This defect, called a 'hole in the heart', allows the two types of blood to mix, so that some of the blood pumped to the body is deoxygenated. In many cases a septal defect is minor, causing few ill-effects. If it is serious, however, surgery may be required. Transposition of the great vessels *(right)*, in which the aorta and pulmonary artery are transposed, is extremely serious, and major surgery is needed to save the baby's life.

person remains concussed for several days or even longer, he or she is said to be in a *coma*.

A patient recovering consciousness after concussion tends to be dazed and confused at first and subsequently often suffers from *diplopia*, or double vision, *headaches*, weakness or a degree of *paralysis*, and even *amnesia*, or loss of memory, as a result of bruising of part of the brain. Normally, these effects gradually disappear as the brain tissue heals; in cases of severe concussion, however, there may be permanent physical or psychological effects, such as persistent irritability and *depression*. Because of this, it is important that any person who has been concussed, but recovers without treatment, should nevertheless have a medical check-up to rule out the possibility of any damage.

A person who appears to be concussed should only be moved by medical personnel, and should be kept warm until help arrives—*see First Aid, p369*. He or she will be taken to hospital, where the cause of the unconsciousness will be investigated. If unconsciousness is prolonged, *steroids* are sometimes used to reduce any *inflammation* of the brain tissue.·

CONFABULATION
The unconscious invention of a memory of events, often with considerable circumstantial detail, in order to fill in a gap in memory. An example of this is *Korsakoff's psychosis*, in which the memory for recent events fails almost completely, often as a result of *alcoholism*. In this, a sufferer may tell a ward nurse or psychiatrist that he met him or her earlier the same day. However convincing the story may seem to both the listener and the patient, it will be completely untrue.

Confabulation may be a symptom of a number of different conditions in which loss of memory occurs.

CONGENITAL
A condition that is inborn, or present from birth. Congenital conditions include all disorders present at birth, whether they are inherited or caused by an environmental factor such as damage in the womb or during birth.

CONGENITAL ABNORMALITY
A malformation which is present from birth and has therefore occurred during the development of the foetus in the womb. The range of congenital abnormalities is almost limitless and depends in part on when the damage occurred and what was responsible for it. Numerous well-defined syndromes exist, while there are often no obvious causes for others.

In congenital *rubella*, for example, the baby may be deaf, and have various heart defects, especially patent ductus arteriosus—*see congenital heart defects*. It may also have cataracts. In this case, the mother's infection with German measles early in pregnancy is known to have affected the baby. In *spina bifida*, however, there are no known causative factors, although research is in progress to establish whether vitamin deficiencies are a possible cause—*see vitamin deficiency diseases*.

It is also thought that the older the mother is, the greater the risk of such an abnormality. The incidence of *Down's syndrome*, for instance, increases with maternal age.

Two other established causes of possible congenital malformation are X-rays and drugs. X-rays during the early months of pregnancy are known to put the developing foetus at risk, possibly by causing mutation of its genetic material. Some drugs can also affect foetal development, so it is very important that medical advice is followed on which, if any, drugs to take during pregnancy.

CONGENITAL HEART DEFECTS
Heart defects are fairly common *congenital* abnormalities—that is, present at birth—affecting one in every 1,000 babies born. They have been found at post-mortem examinations in up to 10% of infants who die in the first few weeks of life, though, depending on their seriousness, congenital heart defects are by no means always fatal or even serious problems.

The reasons why heart defects occur are not fully understood, but some may be due to the effects of drugs taken by the mother, or *viruses* that affect her, during the critical second and third months of intrauterine development—*see The Embryology of the Body, p12*. The virus that causes German measles, or *rubella*, for example, has a well-known association with heart defects, as well as with other congenital abnormalities.

The defects may be minor, and cause no problems. Some are detected only on routine examination of the chest when an abnormal *murmur* is heard. On the other hand, major defects may be incompatible with life, in which case the baby dies shortly after birth; or they may cause *cyanosis*, in which the skin takes on a blue tinge due to a lack of oxygen, shortness of breath and difficulty in feeding, leading to retarded growth.

Heart defects can be broadly subdivided into two groups. First, there are those that do not interfere with the circulation to any great extent and do not cause cyanosis. Two abnormalities of the aorta fall into this category: *coarctation of the aorta* and congenital *aortic stenosis*.

Other congenital abnormalities that do not cause cyanosis include dextrocardia—a rare condition in which the heart is on the right side of the chest rather than the left, and the other major organs are the wrong way round as well.

Pulmonary stenosis—*see valvular heart disease*—is a condition in which there is a narrowing of the pulmonary valve on the right side of the heart. It may occur as a congenital defect, causing *heart failure*. If the symptoms are severe, a valvotomy, an operation to widen the valve, may be needed.

The second group consists of more serious heart defects that cause cyanosis and other distressing symptoms, such as *dyspnoea*, or shortness of breath, and difficulty in feeding. They often require emergency surgery to correct the abnormal circulation.

The most common heart defect that causes cyanosis is Fallot's tetralogy. This is a combination of four separate but interrelated defects. During the development of the foetus, a septum, or partition, normally grows downwards to divide the primitive arterial trunk into two compartments: one is the aorta, which arises from the left ventricle of the embryo's heart; the other, from the right ventricle, is the pulmonary artery. This septum should continue to grow until it meets the septum between the ventricles.

In Fallot's tetralogy, however, the septum deviates to one side, and fails to join the ventricular septum below it—this is called a ventricular septal defect, or a 'hole in the heart'. This means that the aorta overrides both the left and right ventricles. As a result, deoxygenated blood from the right ventricle passes into the aorta to be circulated around the body, instead of travelling to the lungs through the pulmonary artery for re-oxygenation. The resulting shortage of oxygen in the body causes cyanosis.

Pulmonary stenosis causes an enlargement of the right ventricle of the heart, as the body attempts to make up for the deficiency. These two problems, together with the overriding aorta and the ventricular septal defect, are the four abnormalities that make up Fallot's tetralogy.

In serious cases of Fallot's tetralogy, the baby may die within days of birth. Normally, however, the baby becomes cyanosed during the first few months of life. In mild cases, the problem does not become apparent until infancy, when the heart is unable to respond to the increasing physical demands made

on it. As a result, the infant becomes cyanosed after exercise, and, characteristically, squats on his or her heels in an attempt to relieve the symptoms.

In such cases, the defects are corrected by surgery when the child is around seven. If serious problems arise before this, however, a temporary operation called an anastomosis may be performed. In this operation a branch of the aorta is connected to the pulmonary artery, to increase the amount of blood that reaches the lungs.

One heart defect , however, is usually fatal. This is an abnormality known as transposition of the great vessels. In this, the two great arteries, the aorta and pulmonary artery, are mixed up, so that the aorta arises from the right ventricle instead of the left, and the pulmonary artery arises from the left ventricle. Oxygenated blood cannot be pumped around the body, since there are, in effect, two separate circulations—one through the lungs and one around the body. However, if this defect occurs in conjunction with a hole in the heart, or septal defect, the baby can survive, since the septal defect enables the two circulations to mix.

Atrial and ventricular septal defects and *patent ductus arteriosus* are another group of heart defects, which, if severe, may cause cyanosis. These defects allow blood to pass from the left side of the heart to the right, that is they cause a *shunt—see The Blood and Lymph Systems, p21*. If the ductus arteriosus, which connects the aorta and the pulmonary artery in the foetus, is patent—that is, it fails to close shortly after birth—blood from the left ventricle and aorta, where the pressure is higher, is shunted back through the pulmonary artery and around the lungs. This puts an extra strain on the heart and causes high blood pressure in the lungs, a condition known as pulmonary *hypertension*.

If the pressure in the right side of the heart and in the lungs becomes higher than in the left side, the flow of blood is reversed so that it flows from the right side back to the left. This means that deoxygenated blood, which has not been through the lungs, will circulate, and cyanosis will develop. The degree of cyanosis depends on the proportion of deoxygenated blood circulating. If this is about one-third of the total flow, the baby will appear blue or cyanosed.

A patent ductus arteriosus is tied off in a simple surgical operation that is usually carried out around the age of five years.

Septal defects are, as the name suggests, defects or holes in the septum or wall that divides the right and left sides of the heart. The defect may be between the atria, when the condition is known as an ASD or atrial septal defect, or between the ventricles, when it is known as a VSD or ventricular septal defect. The holes may vary in size and in the symptoms they produce. Generally, blood flows through the holes from the left side, where the pressure is higher, to the right side, where it is lower. This places a strain on the right side of the heart, and again leads to an increase in pressure in the pulmonary circulation.

A number of small septal defects have been known to close spontaneously or can often be left alone, with no serious ill effects. Large defects need to be closed surgically to restore a normal circulation and minimize the load on the lungs and right side of the heart.

Cardiac medicine and surgery is now so advanced that the majority of defects may be mended successfully. It is important that the parents and child understand the problem and how to cope with it, and that the parents are not overprotective. The majority of children can live a normal life, go to a normal school and participate in sport .

CONJUNCTIVITIS

An inflammation of the mucous membrane, called the conjunctiva, which covers the outer layer of the eyeball and lines the eyelids. It may be the result of an infection by *bacteria* or a *virus*, or be caused by an *allergy* or reaction to a foreign body, such as an eyelash. In the case of a bacterial infection, both eyes are usually involved, whereas a viral infection often affects only one eye.

Conjunctivitis causes irritation, dryness and grittiness of the eyes, usually with a watery discharge and redness. In severe cases, the eye may become intensely painful, and there may be a sticky yellowish discharge which causes the eyelids to stick together during sleep.

If the infection is minor, bathing the eyes with a lotion will ease the irritation. In more severe cases, eye drops and ointments may be necessary to reduce the inflammation, together with *antibiotics* or *antihistamines* to treat an infection or an allergy respectively.

CONN'S SYNDROME—see Aldosteronism

CONSTIPATION

A condition in which defaecation is infrequent and difficult. Most commonly, constipation results when people ignore the desire to defaecate. However, it may, on occasions, be a symptom of a serious problem, such as a *tumour*, or the contraction of part of the bowel. Both conditions cause constipation by blocking the passage of faeces.

Constipation is a common side-effect of taking *antidepressant* drugs, iron tablets and painkillers. It is an especially distressing problem for the terminally ill, who take high dosages of strong painkillers, and is also a hazard for those who are bedridden—*see Home Nursing, p352*—and for pregnant women. Sometimes the disorder is the result of *anxiety*, or an *obsession* with the frequency of bowel movements.

Many people believe that less than one bowel movement a day indicates constipation, but, in fact, the range of frequency is wide; twice a week may be just as normal as twice a day. A person suffering from constipation, however, may not defaecate for a week or even considerably longer. The pressure from the build-up of faeces in the rectum causes discomfort and tiredness. There may be pain when defaecation eventually occurs, and the stools consist of small, hard pebbly faeces, rather like those of a rabbit.

A diet deficient in roughage is a common cause of constipation, because roughage is needed to allow the faeces to move easily through the intestines. In the affluent countries of the West people consume relatively little roughage, or dietary fibre. This leads to a lower frequency of bowel movement than in countries where a higher proportion of unprocessed food is eaten. The most effective remedy for constipation is, therefore, to ensure that the diet includes plenty of fruit and vegetables, beans, wholemeal bread and cereals containing bran and fibre—*see Diet, p322*.

Constipation during pregnancy may also be caused by a poor diet, but the problem is exacerbated if the pregnant uterus causes the veins in the rectum to become dilated and painful. This condition is known as piles, or *haemorrhoids*.

The occasional use of a mild laxative, preferably a natural one such as prunes or syrup of figs, may help occasional constipation. However, it is not wise to take strong purgatives regularly. They will relieve constipation temporarily, but, unless the underlying cause is treated, it will recur. If recurrent constipation is treated with purgatives the body will become accustomed to its daily dosage and cease to perform naturally without

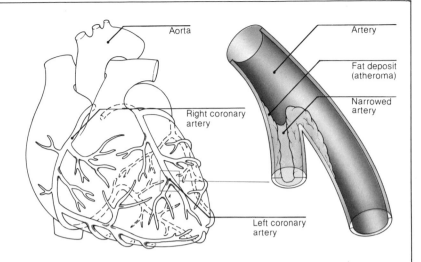

Aorta

Right coronary artery

Left coronary artery

Artery

Fat deposit (atheroma)

Narrowed artery

Coronary Artery Disease The muscles of the heart are supplied with blood by the left and right coronary arteries which branch off the aorta as soon as it leaves the heart *(above left)*. A network of smaller vessels branches off these arteries, spreading over the heart to bring its cells oxygen and fuel. The point where one of these vessels branches into another is where fat deposits called atheroma

can collect *(above right)*. The result of this is that the vessel can become narrowed, so restricting blood flow. This is atherosclerosis. The condition can be dangerous, since, when the heart needs to beat faster, as in exercise, the narrowed arteries cannot bring enough oxygen to the heart muscle. Consequently, the severe heart pain of angina is felt across the chest.

drugs. In this way, self-medication becomes a cause of chronic constipation.

Chronic constipation may be a sign of a serious disorder. If it occurs in a person with previously regular bowel habits, and is interspersed with *diarrhoea*, it may be a symptom of *cancer* of the bowel. For this reason, recurrent constipation should always be reported to a doctor.

CONTAGIOUS DISEASE
Any disease that is transmitted by direct personal contact, that is not communicable by water or air as are infectious diseases. Among the contagious disease are *viral* and *bacterial* diseases, such as genital *herpes*, *hepatitis* and the *venereal diseases*.

CONTUSION
A discoloration of the skin, usually caused by a blow or pressure on the area, in which the tissue may be damaged but the skin is not broken. The discoloration is due to damaged blood vessels; the colour of the contusion changes as the bile pigments, the breakdown products of dead red blood cells, are themselves broken down and absorbed. In some blood disorders, such as *haemophilia*, a contusion may occur spontaneously when there has been no injury.

CONVULSION
A violent muscular spasm caused by a brief disorder of brain function. It is usually accompanied by a brief

loss of consciousness.

Convulsions are also known as fits or seizures. They often occur in childhood, when they tend to be associated with infectious diseases such as *diphtheria*, which cause fever and high temperature, and are known as *febrile* convulsions. However, they can also be due to various metabolic disorders, including lack of oxygen and *epilepsy*.

Febrile convulsions can be treated by sponging the patient with tepid water to lower the temperature, and administering drugs such as aspirin. Convulsions due to *epilepsy*, or metabolic disorders such as *porphyria*, can be prevented by medication with *anticonvulsant* drugs.

It is most important to ensure that a person in a convulsion has an unobstructed airway; the most effective way of doing this is to turn the patient on one side so that he or she will be unable to obstruct the nasal passages with the tongue, or choke on vomit—*see First Aid, p369*.

COOLEY'S ANAEMIA—see Thalassaemia

CORNEAL TRANSPLANT—see Keratoplasty

CORONARY ARTERY DISEASE
The narrowing of the arteries bringing the blood to the heart, so that insufficient blood is supplied to the myocardium, the heart muscle. Coronary artery disease is caused by *atherosclerosis*.

CORONARY ARTERY SURGERY

Surgical treatment of coronary artery narrowing was first introduced in the 1960s, and since then its effects have been studied very intensively, so that a great deal is now known about the outcome. Coronary artery bypass consists, as the name applies, in bypassing the narrowing in the coronary arteries by grafting a vein, usually the long saphenous vein from the leg. One end is joined to the aorta and the other end to the coronary artery below the narrowing.

The operation is very effective in relieving angina, being successful in about 85 per cent of cases. There is a tendency for angina to recur, but 65 per cent of patients are still angina-free after five years. Second and even third operations can be carried out, although these are more difficult technically. Moreover, patients with severe coronary artery disease, in whom there is a high death rate, have improved prospects for survival after surgery.

Another relatively new technique for relieving coronary artery obstruction is transluminal coronary angioplasty. In this procedure a special balloon-tipped tube (a catheter) is passed into an artery in the leg or arm and advanced until it reaches the region of narrowing in the coronary artery. The balloon is then inflated several times for about five seconds in order to break down the narrowing.

CORONARY THROMBOSIS

The formation of a thrombus, or blood clot, on the inner wall of a coronary artery. The blood clot forms round an atheroma, a build-up of fatty plaque in the artery caused by *atherosclerosis*. A coronary thrombosis is the final stage of *coronary artery disease*; reduction or cessation of blood supply to areas of heart muscle supplied by the affected artery causes a heart attack—*see myocardial infarction*.

COR PULMONALE

A *hypertrophy*, or increase in size, of the right ventricle of the heart *(p21)*. It is caused by *congenital heart defects*, especially those that affect the right side of the heart, such as Fallot's tetralogy, and by diseases such as *emphysema*, which reduce the activity of the lungs, making the right ventricle work harder to compensate for them. The strain on the heart tissues resulting from the increased size and activity of the right ventricle may lead to *heart failure* Cor pulmonale is treated according to its cause.

COT DEATH (SIDS or Sudden Infant Death Syndrome)

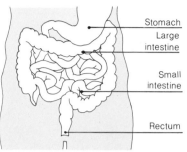

Stomach
Large intestine
Small intestine
Rectum

Crohn's Disease Crohn's disease is an inflammation of the intestinal tract, particularly the last portion of the small intestine *(above)*. The large intestine, and rectum may also be involved. The affected part is swollen and ulcerated, causing the intestinal space to become very narrow and severely hindering the passage of digested food through it. An X-ray *(right)* taken after a barium meal has been swallowed, shows the narrowed transverse section of the large intestine in a patient with Crohn's disease.

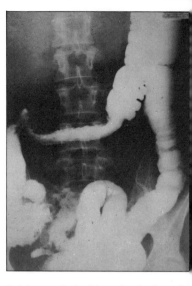

The death of a baby, usually when it is asleep in its cot at night, from an unknown cause. It is now the commonest cause of death between the ages of one and 12 months, but the cause (or probably causes) are still not understood.

There are wide variations across the world in the frequency with which SIDS occurs. In Hong Kong, for example, SIDS is rare, and it is also rare in the children of mothers who come from India, Bangladesh, and Africa. One possible explanation is the position in which babies are put to sleep: babies who lie on their stomachs are more likely to suffer cot death, perhaps because the face is an important site at which cooling may occur, so that lying on the face may lead to overheating. Another idea is that overcrowding, which is common in poorer countries, is beneficial to babies, because it provides them with plenty of stimulation.

In some cases at least, SIDS seems to be due to blockage of the nose and throat; some babies appear to have throats that close easily as they breathe in, and this may cause them to stop breathing at night. Many babies who die suddenly have had a viral infection of their nose – a cold, in fact. This may make obstruction of the nose and throat worse, and may also, if the baby is over-dressed, make it liable to develop a dangerously high temperature.

Some babies who die appear to have had something wrong with their immune systems. They would then be at increased risk of dying from a relatively minor infection.

At present, most specialists believe that the answer to the puzzle of SIDS will probably be found in research directed towards the way the respiratory system works. It is not yet thought advisable to nurse

babies on their side or back, though this is something that will have to be considered.

COUNSELLING

A technique in which a trained therapist or counsellor helps people to sort out their problems themselves. The personal views of the counsellor should not influence the interview. Instead, patients are encouraged to talk about their problems freely and examine the appropriate areas of their lives. The main aim is to help the sufferers to understand why certain problems exist and, through doing so, find a way of coping with them, or prevent their recurrence.

CRAB LOUSE—see Pediculosis

CRACKED NIPPLES—see Mastitis

CRAMP

A sharp pain felt in the muscles, usually occurring after unaccustomed exercise. The pain is due to prolonged muscular contraction and can sometimes be relieved by stretching the muscles and rubbing the affected area. This helps relax the muscle and restore the circulation.

Night cramps are a common problem, especially for elderly people. The exact cause of these cramps is not known, but they often occur in people who have a disease that affects the peripheral blood vessels, and are sometimes made worse by *diuretic* therapy.

Folk remedies for cramp, such as putting magnets in the bed at night, abound, but, unfortunately, they are rarely effective. The only medical treatment is to give the drug quinine. This acts directly on the muscle to increase the refractory period—that is, the period during which the muscle recovers from one contraction and is unable to perform another.

CRETINISM
A congenital disorder of the thyroid gland, caused by a deficiency of thyroid hormones at birth. The symptoms, which include stunted growth, impaired hearing, mental retardation and distorted features and physique, appear at about six months. The delay is because infants are able to benefit for some time after birth from the thyroid hormones that they absorbed from the mother's bloodstream while still in the womb. If the condition is diagnosed early enough at a developmental check—see *Health and Your Child, p348*—thyroid hormone can be given, and there is a good chance that the child will develop normally—see also *myxoedema*.

CROHN'S DISEASE
An inflammatory disease of the bowel, also known as regional enteritis and terminal ileitis. The disease is of unknown cause and usually affects young adults between the ages of 20 and 40 years. Crohn's disease may affect any part of the bowel, but most commonly, the last part of the small intestine, the terminal ileum, is involved.

In the first stage of the disease the mucous membrane lining the bowel becomes *oedematus*, or swollen with retained fluid. As a result, the bowel becomes narrower and narrower, until, eventually, it closes off completely, obstructing the passage of faeces. At the same time, ulcers, or open wounds, and cracks, known as fissures, form in patches on the bowel lining. These patches of diseased bowel are interspersed with patches of healthy bowel. The fissures may be deep enough to penetrate its full thickness and sometimes *fistulas* or new, abnormal openings develop between two adjacent lengths of intestine, or between the intestine and the adjacent bladder or vagina.

The symptoms depend on the site and severity of the disease. When the condition is *acute*, they may mimic those of *appendicitis*. When the disease is *chronic*, the most common feature is pain in the lower abdomen. This is often accompanied by *diarrhoea*, occasionally with pus and blood in the stools. There is also likely to be *malabsorption* and weight loss with general tiredness. The symptoms sometimes abate for as long as a year. Normally, however, they return, and the patient's condition deteriorates gradually.

Crohn's disease is sometimes associated with *arthritis*, although the exact relationship is not clear.

Diagnosis is made through a case history and physical examination. An X-ray, taken after the patient has consumed a barium meal—see *Special Tests, p84*—often shows up the damage to the mucous membranes and sometimes areas of deep ulceration can also be seen.

There is no known cure for Crohn's disease, but a number of general measures may help. These include treatment of the diarrhoea, a low-fibre diet—see *Diet, p322*—to help the colicky pain, treatment of the malabsorption with a low fat diet and iron and vitamin supplements.

Steroid drugs are used to treat acute forms of the disease and other drugs are sometimes used with variable success. Surgery is occasionally necessary to relieve bowel obstruction and remove the fistula and abscesses which may form. Sometimes parts of the bowel that are very diseased are removed, but the disease may recur in the remaining parts of the bowel.

CROSS EYES—see Strabismus

CROUP
A violent, paroxysmal cough, that occurs in an acute *inflammation* of the upper respiratory tract—the larynx, trachea and main bronchi. Croup is caused by a *viral* infection, and usually affects babies and very young children. The cough, which is extremely violent and very alarming, is sometimes accompanied by wheezing, and the sufferer may becomes *cyanosed*, or turn blue, due to lack of oxygen.

The immediate treatment is to humidify and warm the air, either by boiling a kettle or taking the child into the bathroom and turning on the hot tap. A doctor should be consulted, however, because *antibiotics* may also be necessary if there is any *bacterial* infection as well.

CRYOSURGERY
The destruction of tissue by freezing. This is achieved by use of an instrument called a cryoprobe, that has a fine tip into which carbon dioxide or nitrous oxide gas is introduced. The gas expands within the tip and cools it to below freezing point.

Cryosurgery has a variety of applications, but is most often used in the treatment of *cervical erosion*. *Tumours* may also be removed by this technique.

CRYPTORCHIDISM
The medical name for undescended testicles. There are a number of reasons for the condition, probably the most common being that the testicles are retractile. This means that they can and do descend into the scrotum, but quickly shoot back into the abdomen on examination. Another reason may be an anatomical malformation of the inguinal canal through which the testicles descend. This usually affects only one testicle.

Retractile testicles usually descend of their own accord eventually. An undescended testicle on one side, however, will probably need surgery to correct the abnormality. In cases of *intersex*—where a baby has the outward physical appearance of a boy, but no testicles—the chromosomal sex of the baby is decided from an examination of an cervical smear—see *Special Tests, p84*.

In the rare cases where normal testicles fail to descend and remain in the abdomen throughout childhood, they should be removed. This is because they may become malignant if left in the abdomen.

CURETTAGE—see Dilatation & curettage

CVA—see Cerebrovascular accident

CYANOSIS
A bluish coloration of the lips and skin due to lack of oxygen, which may have a variety of causes. Cyanosis may be the result of *heart failure*, a *congenital heart defect*—as in 'blue babies'—lung disease, such as *pneumonia*, an obstruction of the blood vessels supplying the lungs, or any condition in which blood is either prevented from acquiring oxygen in the lungs, or, when oxygenated, is unable to reach the tissues of the body. As the tissues need oxygen to live, cyanosis is an extremely dangerous condition. Permanent brain damage may occur if the brain is deprived of oxygen for more than a few minutes.

The bluish tinge may occur locally, as in chilblains, the itchy swellings which form on the hands and feet during cold weather.

CYST
A growth or swelling containing liquid or semi-solid matter. Cysts often form when the outlets of mucous-producing cells become blocked. A sebaceous cyst, for example, may form in a sebaceous gland in the skin. This type of cyst, called a retention cyst, is unsightly, but harmless. It can be removed by a minor surgical operation—see also *dermoid cyst, ovarian cyst*.

CYSTIC FIBROSIS
A disease that increases the activity of the exocrine glands, which secrete

mucus, sweat and digestive juices The condition, also called fibrocystic disease of the pancreas and muscoviscidosis, is *hereditary* and attacks young people at any time between infancy and adolescence.

The increase in exocrine secretions causes obstruction of the intestine, pancreas and bronchi. Respiratory infection often results from the obstruction to the lungs. Obstruction of the pancreas causes a deficiency of pancreatic enzymes, and so hampers digestion, but these can be administered in synthetic form. Chronic infection can be prevented by *antibiotics*, and *physiotherapy* will help to prevent lung obstruction. The condition cannot be cured, however, and becomes progressively more debilitating, until, by the time they reach adulthood, many sufferers have developed a potentially fatal *cirrhosis* of the liver.

CYSTINURIA—see Metabolic disorders

CYSTITIS

An infection of the bladder. Cystitis is often caused by the bacterium *Escherichia coli*, although a number of other organisms may be responsible. The bacteria usually enter the body through the urethra. The habit of incompletely emptying the bladder when urinating may predispose an individual to cystitis, since urine stagnating in the bladder becomes infected easily. It follows that anything that obstructs normal urination, such as an enlarged womb during pregnancy, any

congenital deformity of the bladder, *calculi* in the bladder, or an enlarged prostate gland makes cystitis more likely to occur.

However, cystitis is much more common in women than in men, partly, it is thought, because the urethra is short, so bacteria can reach the bladder more easily, and partly because it is much closer to the anus than in men. Wiping the anus towards the vagina and urethra, instead of from front to back, after defaecation, is likely to cause such infections—*see Health and Hygiene, p334*.

Cystitis may occur suddenly. It causes frequent and usually painful urination. In mild forms a noticeable increase in the frequency of urination may be accompanied by a burning sensation and cloudy urine; but acute cystitis may cause *fever*, blood in the urine and, if the infection spreads to the kidneys, backache. The pain during urination may be severe.

The cause of cystitis can be established by means of a urine test—*see Special Tests, p84*. If the analysis reveals the presence of the cystitis-causing bacteria, a course of *antibiotics* will be prescribed. Meanwhile, the symptoms can be relieved by drinking quantities of water. If the infection recurs, tests will be made to be sure that *calculi* are not blocking the flow of urine.

'Honeymoon cystitis' is not, in fact, a form of cystitis, but of *urethritis*.

CYTOMEGALIC INCLUSION DISEASE—see Cytomegalovirus

CYTOMEGALOVIRUS

A virus of the *herpes* family which may cause either of two diseases.

The first is cytomegalic inclusion disease, a viral illness similar to *glandular fever*, in which the lymph glands in the region of the infection become enlarged. The second disease is *hepatitis*, of which cytomegalovirus is, occasionally, a cause.

Congenital cytomegalovirus infection, also caused by cytomegalovirus, occurs in infants up to about four months after birth. The unborn baby contracts the disease from the mother through the placenta while still in the womb. There are usually no symptoms, making diagnosis almost impossible other than by a blood antibody test—*see Special Tests, p84*—but the virus may cause severe brain damage, or even death.

There is no specific treatment for cytomegalic disease, other than that designed to relieve the symptoms.

CYTOTOXIC DRUGS

A cytotoxin is an antibody or toxin which attacks specific types of cells. Cytotoxic drugs destroy cells or prevent their multiplication, and are therefore used in treating *cancer*. Cytotoxins are poisons and have unpleasant side-effects, causing feelings of nausea, dizziness, and temporary loss of hair. Medical researchers are looking for the ideal cytotoxic drug: one which would cure fast-growing cancer cells without injuring normal body cells or interfering with normal bodily processes.

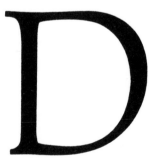

D & C—see Dilatation and Curettage

DANDRUFF

An excessive production of small flakes of dead skin on the scalp. Dandruff occurs when the fine cells of the epidermis or outer layer of skin, are shed at a faster rate than normal. The condition, which is also called *pityriasis capitis* and scurf, is not serious, but, since the cells make the scalp look scaly and stick to the

hair when it is brushed or combed, considerable efforts have been made to find effective ways of treating it.

Dandruff is usually the result of a disorder of the sebaceous glands, affecting the amount of sebum they produce—*see seborrhoea*. If too little sebum is secreted, the hair becomes brittle and dandruff appears as white flakes in the hair; an overproduction of sebum results in greasy hair and yellow flakes. As the scalp is one of the areas of greatest

sebum production, the latter problem is the most common one—dandruff is usually associated with greasy skin and with *acne*.

Dandruff will usually disappear if the hair is washed two or three times a week with an appropriate medicated detergent shampoo. Such shampoos often contain zinc pyrithione or coal tar; soap-based shampoos should be avoided, since they seem to exacerbate the condition.

A form of dandruff is also sometimes caused by certain types of seborrhoeic *dermatitis*. In this case it is often accompanied by *inflammation* and itching. Such conditions need medical treatment with salicylic acid or *corticosteroid* drugs to reduce the inflammation.

DEAFNESS

A partial or total loss of hearing in one or both ears—*see The Nervous System, p32*. Deafness is a common condition affecting over one per cent of the populations of the UK and the USA.

The condition has a wide range of causes. It may be due to a *congenital*, or inborn, malformation of the ear; congenital disease; *inflammation* or some other obstruction within the ear; injury; or *benign* or *malignant* growths. Disorders such as *myxoedema, diabetes mellitus, Ménière's disease* and *hypoglycaemia* may also cause a loss of hearing.

An obstruction to the passage of sound vibrations through the outer and middle ear causes what is known as conductive deafness. *Cerumen*, the waxy substance that lines the external auditory canal, may accumulate and obstruct the passage of sound waves to the ear drum. It can be softened with warm oil and the ear syringed to remove it.

Conductive deafness may also be caused by an infection. In *otitis externa*, an infection of the outer ear, and *otitis media*, an infection of the middle ear, inflammation and the accumulation of pus can lead to a blockage of the ear canal or the chamber behind the ear drum, and so to deafness. This build-up of pus, known as 'glue ear', may be avoided through treatment of the acute attack of otitis media with *antibiotics*, but if this is unsuccessful, or too late, a minor operation may be necessary. An incision, known as a myringotomy, is made in the ear drum and a grommet, a type of valve, is inserted, so that the fluid can drain out. Hearing returns as the membrane of the ear drum heals, after the removal of the grommet.

Such infections are common in childhood. They may occur as *complications* of respiratory diseases, but are more commonly caused by water entering the ear while swimming, or by pushing foreign objects into the external ear canal. Children often push peanuts and other small objects into their ears, while adults try to clean their ears with hairpins, cotton buds, and even paper clips. The outer ear should be cleaned only with a piece of sterile lint dipped in hot water—nothing should ever be pushed down the ear canal.

The eustachian or audito-meatory tube, leading from each middle ear to the throat, can also become blocked by mucus or pus as a result of a cold or infection. This will cause temporary deafness, because the ear drum will only vibrate correctly in response to sound waves striking it if the pressures on either side of it are equal. The blockage in the tube alters these pressures. Air travellers suffer from the same sensation during aircraft take-off and landing, as do deep-sea divers when submerging and surfacing. In these cases, swallowing causes the pressure between the outside air and the eustachian tube to be equalized, thus restoring hearing.

Deafness can also be due to a failure of the stapes bone, the innermost of the three bones called the ossicles bridging the middle ear to transmit sound vibrations from the ear drum to the inner ear. In *otosclerosis*, the stapes, whose function is to vibrate against the oval window leading into the inner ear, becomes immobile. The only effective treatment is to replace the bone with an artificial plastic substitute, or prosthesis. This may not restore hearing completely, however; a hearing aid may also be needed.

A patient with conductive deafness is still able to detect sound through the bones of the skull, and this ability is used by doctors to make an accurate diagnosis of the level of disability. An otologist or audiologist can test hearing to distinguish between the different types of hearing loss. An audiometer—an instrument that measures hearing at different sound frequencies—determines the degree of deafness.

Disorders of the nervous system can also lead to deafness. In such cases, the condition is known as perceptive nerve, or sensorineural, deafness. It is caused by the failure of the nerve impulses to travel along the nerve pathways from the inner ear to the brain. A baby born to a mother who suffered from German *measles, syphilis*, or other *viral* disease, or who took quinine during early pregnancy may suffer from perceptive deafness at birth.

Excessive dosing with certain drugs, including *aspirin*, or injuries to the ear and head, may cause perceptive deafness by damaging the auditory nerve, or the hearing centre in the cerebral cortex of the brain, as may a wide variety of diseases, including *atherosclerosis, meningitis* and *Ménières disease*.

Exposure to excessive noise is a common cause of hearing loss. If the noise entering the ear becomes too loud, the body normally reacts in self-defence by rotating the ossicles to tighten the ear drum so that less sound is transmitted to the inner ear. As this process takes time, a sudden noise of more than about l50 decibels, such as an explosion, can damage the sound receptors in the organ of Corti in the cochlea.

Noise that can damage the ear may be continuous, intermittent or impulsive. If they do not protect their ears, soldiers exposed to the sound of gunfire, and people who work in noisy environments, may suffer permanent damage to their hearing. However, the amount of noise to which the ears can be subjected without damage varies from person to person. Individuals who are particularly sensitive to noise may suffer permanent damage from constant exposure to noise levels of 80 decibels—the level of traffic noise—although others can stand exposure to levels as high as l40 decibels—the noise level produced by a jet aircraft on take-off—without harm.

Gradual hearing loss, known as presbyacusis, also occurs naturally as a result of ageing. Not everyone becomes deaf as they age, however; the onset of hearing loss, its progression and its severity depend upon heredity, physical stress, and environmental factors, such as climate and diet.

Unless the deafness is total, a hearing aid can be used to amplify the sound waves entering the ear. This usually restores the hearing to some extent. Modern hearing aids are extremely efficient in function and unobtrusive in design. Tiny electronic microphones, which pick up sound waves from all directions and not just from the direction in which they are pointing, are now small enough to be fitted behind or into the ear, or in the frame of a pair of spectacles. The amplification such aids provide is considerable, while the volume is easily controlled.

Scientists are now experimenting to improve aids still further to suit people with different kinds of deafness; to make hearing-aid components such as earmoulds and couplings play a part in their performance; and to make them more resistant to shock and wear.

However, although modern hearing aids can improve and restore sound reception to a degree that seems almost miraculous, they still have disadvantages. Patients can find them uncomfortable to wear. They run on batteries, which need to be replaced, and they break down. Moreover, depending upon the type of deafness involved, their wearers may find they are unable to

Deafness is an affliction that can affect us all to a greater or lesser degree as we grow older. There are two types — conductive deafness and perceptive deafness — the first affecting the middle ear and the second the outer ear. Both types produce their own characteristic effects, which can be detected, measured and, in some cases, treated. Conductive deafness is caused by physical damage or blockage; perceptive deafness results from nerve damage and is usually incurable.

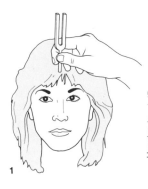

1

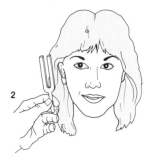

2

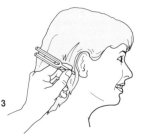

3

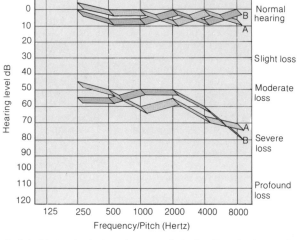

Audiologists test for deafness by measuring the frequency and pitch of the sounds heard by a patient with an instrument called an audiometer and grade the results accordingly on a chart

called a Pure Tone Audiogram. On the chart *(above)*, the results for a patient with normal hearing are shown *(top)* and one with impaired hearing *(bottom)*. A indicates right ear, B left.

By using a tuning fork *(above)*, a doctor can differentiate between the two types of deafness — conductive deafness in the middle ear and perceptive deafness in the inner ear. In the Weber test, the fork is struck and held against the forehead **1**. Normally, it is heard in the middle of the head; if it is heard predominantly in one ear, this indicates deafness. In the Rinne test, the fork is held beside each ear, **2**, and then against the mastoid bone, **3**. The patient tells the doctor in which way he or she hears the note and how long or loud it is. If the note is heard for longer when the fork is held beside the ear, there is perceptive deafness. If the opposite applies, there is conductive deafness.

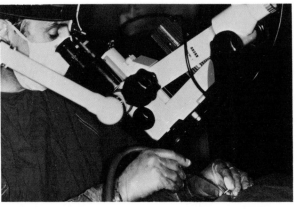

The ear, nose and throat (ENT) specialist uses the technique of microsurgery to perform operations on the delicate structures inside the middle and inner ears. The surgeon employs a binocular microscope *(left)* and specially-adapted surgical instruments to operate upon such disorders as otosclerosis.

Earmould

Volume control

Battery

Microphone

On/off switch

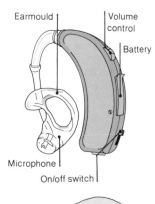

The commonest hearing aids contain a microphone, amplifier and a battery in a plastic case. The amplified sound is transmitted to the eardrum via an earmould, which fits the shape of the ear canal. In a behind-the-ear hearing aid *(left and below)*, the case is worn inconspicuously behind he ear. In a body-worn hearing aid *(right and below)*, the case is clipped to a pocket or article of clothing, usually near the chest. A flexible cord transmits the sound to an earphone, which is attached to an earmould.

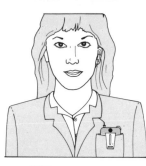

The function of an earmould is to channel sound down the ear canal and into the ear. Because all ears are shaped slightly differently, any earmould has to be individually made. A technician in the audiology department takes an impression of the ear and the acrylic earmould is then processed accordingly, to be fitted when complete. The mould can be used with various types and makes of aid.

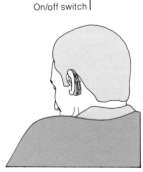

Volume control with on/off switch

Microphone

Battery compartment

Clip

Cord

Earmould

Earphone

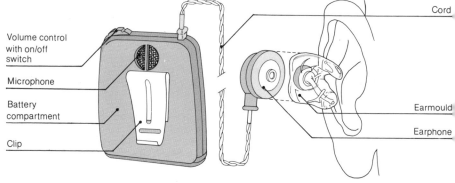

hear very low tones, or that high sounds are always accompanied by an irritating sibilance. Even the newer designs are subject to harmonic distortion.

Victims of deafness are therefore encouraged to use additional methods to help them deal with their hearing loss. Chief among these are lipreading and auditory training. The latter involves learning to search for visual and auditory clues to enhance communication, and to recognize and ignore distracting sounds in the environment. In addition, such facilities as subtitles for the deaf on television help to improve the quality of life for the deaf and people with impaired hearing.

DECOMPRESSION SICKNESS—see Bends

DECONGESTANT
A drug that reduces congestion of the nasal passages. Most decongestants are *anti histamine* preparations, which do not require a doctor's prescription. It is important, however, that a doctor is consulted if congestion persists, since it may be a symptom of a number of conditions, such as *sinusitis*, *hay fever* or a *cold*.

Prolonged use of decongestants can also cause problems, since they have a number of side-effects. They may damage the delicate epithelial tissue that lines the nose and aggravate the symptoms of chronic nasal congestion. This is an *iatrogenic* disorder, which is called *rhinitis medicamentosa*.

DEEP VEIN THROMBOSIS—see Thrombosis

DEFECTIVE COLOUR VISION
The inability to correctly distinguish certain colours. This problem was once called colour blindness, but this term is no longer used—it is considered misleading because it implies that sufferers are unable to see any colours, apart from black and white.

The most common type of defective colour vision is that in which sufferers are unable to dinguish between grey and purple, especially when the two colours are represented only by pale shades. Other types of defective colour vision consist of an inability to distinguish orange and red shades from yellow and green; some people are unable to distinguish green from blue and grey.

Defective colour vision is usually an inherited defect, although a variety of disorders may, on occasions, be responsible. These include chemical poisoning, excess

alcohol or nicotine, and certain disorders of the metabolism, such as *diabetes mellitus*. Since the gene responsible for defective colour vision is carried on the X-chromosome—*see chromosomes*—women are generally carriers of the condition, and men are sufferers.

The condition is thought to be directly due to a defect in one of three types of light-sensitive cone cells in the retina *(p32)* which, respectively, are sensitive to blue, green and yellow. The precise nature of defective colour vision varies according to which type of cone cell is deficient.

Colour vision is tested by showing the patient specially designed colour plates—*see Eye tests, Special Tests, p84*. Unfortunately, however, there is no treatment for the problem. Most sufferers, however, have little difficulty in adjusting to their inability to distinguish between certain colours. Defective colour vision only becomes a serious problem when sufferers have to work with colour-coded machinery, and, in the case of confusion between orange/red shades and yellow/green shades, when they drive.

DEFIBRILLATION
A procedure used to end *fibrillation*. In this state, the heart muscle contracts spasmodically and inefficiently, reducing the supply of oxygen to the body. The jerky, writhing contractions of the muscles of a heart in fibrillation are sometimes said to resemble those of a paper bag filled with worms.

When fibrillation affects the atria alone, there is little disturbance to the pumping action of the heart, although the ECG (electrocardiogram)—*see Special Tests, p84*—is altered considerably and the pulse is irregular. Atrial fibrillation is usually treated with the drug digoxin. This does not end the irregular rhythm, but slows it down to a manageable rate. If, however, the patient is suffering ill effects from rapid uncontrolled atrial fibrillation, attempts may be made to convert it back to sinus rhythm with the use of an electric current—*see cardioversion*. The fibrillation often recurs after a while.

Ventricular fibrillation, on the other hand, is a life-threatening condition and is often the cause of so-called cardiac arrests—*see myocardial infarction*. If the ventricles contract ineffectually, no blood is pumped around the body, and death ensues unless emergency treatment is given.

Ventricular fibrillation is halted by the application of a controlled

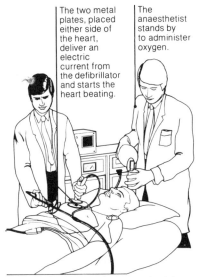

The two metal plates, placed either side of the heart, deliver an electric current from the defibrillator and starts the heart beating.

The anaesthetist stands by to administer oxygen.

Defibrillation The ventricular muscle of the heart normally contracts rhythmically and is coordinated by the heart's natural pacemaker. When the fibres start to contract randomly and independently, the ventricular muscles twitch and fibrillate, causing the heart to stop. A defibrillator *(above)* delivers a shock, so synchronizing the ventricular muscles and restarting the heart.

amount of direct electric current via two paddles, or electrodes, placed on the chest wall, or directly on the heart if the chest is already open for cardiac surgery. The shock causes a *systole*—standstill of the muscle—after which a normal heart beat often returns, either spontaneously or following external cardiac massage.

DEGENERATION
The general deterioration and loss of function of the cells of a tissue or organ. Degeneration can be brought about by *infection*, disease, a defect in circulation, or the natural processes of ageing, but there are many different types. For instance, the fatty degeneration that occurs in the liver in *cirrhosis* is the deposition of abnormal amounts of fat in the liver cells or in the tissue surrounding them.

Diseases in which degeneration is a normal part of the ageing process, such as osteoarthritis—*see arthritis*—and *arteriosclerosis*, are collectively known as the degenerative diseases.

DEHYDRATION
A condition in which there is insufficient water in the body. Dehydration may occur when the amount of water absorbed through food and drink is inadequate. It may also occur when the loss of water from the body, through sweating, *vomiting*, urination or *defaecation* is greater than the intake, as in a serious fever—*see pyrexia*—or when the chemical balance of the body fluids is altered, as in *hypoglycaemia*.

Symptoms of dehydration include excessive thirst, nausea, dizziness and exhaustion. In mild cases, the only treatment necessary is to drink water, but a seriously dehydrated person may need an intravenous infusion, or *drip*, of a *saline* solution to replace lost salts to restore the body's chemical balance, as well as fluids. Dehydration may be prevented during diarrhoea and vomiting by drinking a very weak saline solution at frequent intervals immediately the worst of the attacks seem to be over. The solution should taste no saltier than tears, or further vomiting may result.

People living in hot climates are usually careful not to overexert themselves during the hottest parts of the day, and to include plenty of salt in their diet to replace that lost by heavy perspiration. Through ignorance of such precautions, people unused to such conditions may become dehydrated when on holiday in a hot country, or during an exceptionally hot spell at home. By drinking more water than usual, and taking salt tablets, available from most chemists, every day this type of dehydration can be prevented.

DELIRIUM
A serious disorder of the mental processes that generally develops suddenly, but can, unlike *dementia*, usually be reversed. When delirious, people are normally disoriented in time and place, and restless and excited, with clouded consciousness and *hallucinations*. Their speech is often slurred, and they may also experience double vision and great agitation.

The most common cause of delirium is serious drunkenness. It is also a feature of many conditions that cause a severe fever—*see pyrexia*—as in *cholera*, *typhoid* and *pneumonia*. The disorder may also be caused by *metabolic disturbances*, such as *hyperglycaemia* and *uraemia*, and by problems that result in a lack of oxygen in the body, such as respiratory failure.

Tranquillizers, such as chlorpromazine, are used to treat the symptoms of delirium, but the disorder will persist until the cause is removed. In cases where delirium is symptomatic of *psychosis* and other mental disorders, long-term *psychotherapy* may be the only way to cure it.

DELIRIUM TREMENS
A form of *delirium* that affects alcoholics and opium and barbiturate addicts. Delirium tremens is a *psychosis* characterized by *delusions* and *hallucinations*, which are sometimes pleasant, but more often terrifying. The condition is usually caused by withdrawal from drug or alcohol *addiction*.

An attack of delirium tremens— usually called 'DTs'—may be preceded by *insomnia*, over-excitement, antipathy towards food and *nausea*. The sufferer may become absent-minded or confused, then violently agitated. He or she may experience hallucinations— hearing and seeing huge, vividly coloured insects, or, classically, pink elephants. Behaviour is likely to be abnormal, and may be violent. Occasionally, *convulsions*, similar to epileptic fits, may occur in cases of alcohol or *antabuse* withdrawal.

The condition can be controlled by the administration of a sedative, and by persuading the patient to drink quantities of fluids containing glucose. However, since DTs are potentially dangerous psychologically as well as physically because many sufferers become suicidal, those affected are usually admitted to special detoxication units in a hospital for a spell of rest, sedation, psychiatric help and a specially formulated diet.

DELUSION
A firm conviction that is demonstrably false but that cannot be shaken by rational argument. A person suffering from a delusion may, for example, believe that someone is trying to poison him or her, and may therefore refuse to eat; a person with a hypochondriacal delusion—*see hypochondria*—may be convinced that he or she has *cancer* or some other major illness. Delusion is usually a symptom of *schizophrenia* or another *psychosis*, but milder delusions, perhaps taking the form of vague feelings of persecution by other people may be symptoms of *depression*.

DEMENTIA
Irreversible mental deterioration as a result of physical changes in the brain. *Infection*, chronic poisoning— from lead in the atmosphere, for instance or from drug or alcohol *addiction*, injury, and a cerebrovascular *atheroma*, can all cause the onset of dementia. It also occurs as a final stage in diseases such as *syphilis*, and sometimes after a stroke—*see cerebrovascular accident*—or during mental illness.

Senile dementia is caused by *atrophy* of the brain in old age; the same condition may occur in middle age, when it is known as presenile dementia. *Huntington's chorea* is a typical example. The cause of such diseases is unknown, but some of them may be hereditary.

In the early stages of senile dementia, *insomnia*, restlessness and a slight forgetfulness, especially of recent events, may be the only symptoms. An upheaval in life, such as retirement or the death of a spouse, may precipitate a character change; a formerly cheerful person may become depressed and moody, while a kind person may turn selfish. As the disease progresses, a process which may take many years, memory gradually deteriorates until eventually only events long past can be remembered. Mood swings may become more and more frequent as intellect and personality gradually deteriorate. Eventually the sufferer becomes unable to look after himself or herself, is incontinent and lapses into apathy.

Where poisoning or drug abuse is the trigger for dementia, deterioration may be arrested by removing the cause. Otherwise dementia is incurable and in most cases progresses until death—*see Looking After Old People, p362.*

DEMENTIA PRAECOX—see Schizophrenia

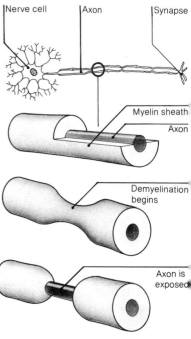

Demyelinating Disease Electric impulses travel along the axon of a nerve fibre from a nerve cell to a synapse *(top)*. Surrounding the axon, a fatty myelin sheath surrounds the axon and insulates it, allowing the impulses to travel at high speeds. When the myelin sheath is worn away, the axon is exposed *(bottom)*. The impulses are no longer transmitted properly and a neurological disorder develops.

DEMYELINATING DISEASES
A number of disorders affecting the central and peripheral nervous

systems—*see The Nervous System, p32*—that result from degeneration of the myelin sheaths which surround the axons of certain nerves, and play an important part in conducting electrical nerve impulses. Among the demyelinating diseases are disseminated or *multiple sclerosis* and acute demyelinating *encephalomyelitis*

DEPENDENCE
The physical and mental state of being unable to achieve a feeling of normality and well-being without taking a specific drug—*see addiction*.

DEPRESSION
A protracted feeling of sadness and despondency. Psychiatric disorders are divided into two main groups: the major disorders or psychoses—*see affective disorders*—and the minor disorders or *neuroses*. Depression may occur in either of these groups, and there is a large degree of overlap between them. It is therefore difficult to differentiate between major or psychotic depression and minor or neurotic depression. Neurotic depression is, however, one of the most common of the emotional disorders, affecting at least one person in seven.

Broadly speaking, a neurotically depressed patient's symptoms are relieved by cheerful surroundings and company. Although the patient usually complains of chronic tiredness, and may brood over minor physical ailments, the depression is not accompanied by physical symptoms, such as slowness of speech, *constipation* or diarrhoea, and *amenorrhoea* in women.

A neurotically depressed patient is usually fully aware that he or she is depressed, and may be anxious to discuss symptoms and feelings, usually attributing them to outside events or other people. The *delusions* that are a common symptom of major depressive reaction are not usually a feature of neurotic depression, but patients tend to feel hopeless and dejected and find it difficult to make decisions. They may feel inadequate and worthless and have crying spells. They may also contemplate or even attempt suicide.

Everyone feels depressed at times, but depression is said to be neurotic when it seems to be disproportionate in intensity or duration. Neurotic depression is often linked to a personal setback or tragedy, such as a bereavement, and is therefore sometimes said to be reactive, or *exogenous*. It may also be accompanied by other problems, such as *phobias*.

Psychotic depression is characterized by more severe symptoms, especially physical ones. Typically, sleep is disturbed and the sufferer wakes early in the morning. There may also be loss of appetite, leading, in extreme cases, to *anorexia*, and a decreased sex drive, or libido. The victim may complain of various imaginary pains—*see hypochondria*—commonly headache, dizziness, and chest or abdominal pains.

Several psychoanalytical theories attempt to explain the causes of neurotic depression. One theory holds that neurotic depression is the result of a conviction that a stressful situation cannot be altered or controlled. Anxiety is believed to be the first response to stress; if this cannot be resolved, the anxiety is replaced by depression. Anxiety and depression are often mixed in a state of mind known as *anxiety neurosis*.

Depression in a person very dependent upon the approval of others may be explained as a way of reliving the loss of a mother's affection. Another theory, that of learned helplessness, explains depression as the result of having learned negative ways of thinking in early life. These and other psychological theories interpret the tendency to depression in terms of defective personality development. However, there are also biochemical views of depression, which link the condition to a relative decrease in the quantity or activity of neurotransmitters—*see The Nervous System, p32*—in the brain.

Treatment for depression depends on the severity of the symptoms. A doctor may refer a person to a psychiatrist if the symptoms are severe and there are marked suicidal tendencies. In addition, *antidepressant* drugs may be prescribed. *ECT* therapy may be used to treat severe, resistant depression. In *manic depressive psychosis*, lithium is thought to reduce the severity and frequency of attacks. However, its dosage must be carefully monitored.

Psychotherapy, behaviour therapy, aimed at replacing negative ways of thinking with positive ones, and *group therapy*, to help people explore their problems with others who have similar problems, have all proved their effectiveness as forms of treatment for neurotic depression. Initially, however, the patient is often too depressed to benefit from any of them. Moreover, long-term psychotherapy is usually prohibitively expensive and may not be available in private insurance schemes or in public medicine.

See also post natal depression.

DERMATITIS
A term used to describe a number of skin disorders, many of which are *allergies*. Dermatitis and eczema are roughly synonymous terms, but certain forms of dermatitis, such as dermatitis herpetiformis, a severe blistering of the skin whose cause is unknown, are not eczemas.

The different forms of dermatitis are divided into two types. *Exogenous*, or externally caused, forms can occur around infected wounds or *ulcers*. However, they are usually the result of skin hypersensitivity to irritants and substances that cause allergies. *Endogenous* forms are due to internal causes, including *metabolic disorders* and hereditary factors.

The commonest single cause of exogenous dermatitis is contact with irritants. Everyday materials, such as wool or nylon, perfume, household cleansing agents, metal, cement or lubricating oil may produce dermatitis in anyone who is especially sensitive to the allergen—the substance that produces the allergic reaction—it contains. The ammonia in urine produces *nappy rash*, or ammoniacal dermatitis, in babies, for example. The nature of the reaction varies from person to person, but symptoms typically include *inflammation*, swelling, raised spots and itching. Any part of the body may be affected.

Scratching aggravates dermatitis and may cause infection, so the application of a soothing, lanolin-based cream may be necessary as a form of first aid to reduce the irritation. Dermatitis artefacta is a skin reaction caused by unnecessary scratching and may require prolonged psychiatric treatment.

The reaction may occur some time after the initial contact—in industry, for example, many workers develop dermatitis when they have been handling a particular substance for years. Similarly, a deodorant, after-shave lotion or particular brand of make-up that is used habitually may suddenly begin to produce an allergic reaction. This may continue for some time after the cause has been removed.

Atopic dermatitis, also called flexual eczema, is a common form of endogenous dermatitis. It takes the form of a chronic itchy *rash*, often complicated by other allergic reactions, such as *hay fever*, *asthma* or *urticaria*. Babies with a form of atopic dermatitis known as *infantile eczema* may react violently to certain old-fashioned *vaccines*, with serious and sometimes fatal consequences. This is why babies with eczema used not to be vaccinated. However, these vaccines, which were made from egg yolks, are now rarely used.

Seborrheic dermatitis is a serious, sometimes *acute* skin disease in which itchy, weeping blisters form on the scalp, face and other areas of high sebum production. They eventually become encrusted and scaly. Like *acne*, it is caused by a disorder of sebum production and may respond to frequent washing of the affected areas with specially formulated shampoos—*see dandruff*.

Generally, these skin disorders are treated with soothing preparations made of coal tar, and steroid cream to reduce the inflammation. Infected eczema may need an *antibiotic* cream, as well as a steroid preparation. Treatment is rarely effective, however, until the cause of the dermatitis has been established and removed. A patch test—*see Special Tests, p84*— may be carried out to discover the cause. In some cases its removal may entail a complete change of life style, such as changing jobs.

DERMATITIS ARTEFACTA—see Dermatitis

DERMATOMYOSITIS—see Myositis

DERMATOPHYTE
Microscopic fungi that grow on or near the surface of the skin, hair or nails. They are responsible for infections such as ringworm and athlete's foot—*see tinea*.

DERMOID CYST
A *cyst* that may contain a variety of different tissues, such as hair, glands and even teeth. Dermoid cysts form as a result of the pinching off of small amounts of tissue during the fusion of different layers in the embryo—*see Embryology, p12*. They are harmless, and can be removed by surgery.

DESENSITIZATION
A term with two different medical meanings. To a psychiatrist, desensitization is a treatment for fears and *phobias*, in which the patient is gradually forced to face up to and come to terms with the cause of the fear. For example, a therapist treating a person with a fear of spiders would first encourage the patient to look at pictures of them, then lead him or her gradually to the point where he or she could look at a live spider, and finally touch one— *see also behaviour therapy*.

To a doctor, the term is more likely to refer to a form of treatment for *hay fever* and other *allergies*. Small dosages of an extract made from the type of pollen to which a patient is sensitive are injected beneath the

patient's skin at regular intervals well before the start of the hay fever season. At first, the quantities injected are tiny, but they are gradually increased over a long period. The theory is that the patient will cease to be allergic to the pollen. Success is not certain, however, and the treatment can also be dangerous—on occasions there is a risk of *anaphylactic* shock.

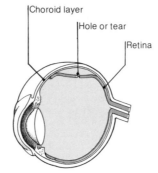

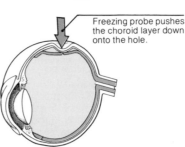

Freezing probe pushes the choroid layer down onto the hole.

Detached Retina When a hole or a tear appears in the retina, fluid from the vitreous humour seeps through and detaches the retina from the choroid layer behind *(top)*. The retina can be reattached and the fluid drained away by using a freezing probe to push the choroid layer downwards on to the hole *(bottom)*.

DETACHED RETINA
A condition in which the retina, the layer of light-sensitive cells that lines the interior of the eyeball, becomes separated from the choroid layer beneath it—*see The Nervous System, p32*. This is usually the result of a hole in the retina caused by *degeneration* of the tissues; or of the vitreous humour, the gelatinous substance that fills the posterior chamber of the eye, shrinking away from the retina and tearing it. Both eyes may be affected, but rarely at the same time. The retina may also become detached as a result of repeated blows to the eye; the condition is a particular hazard for boxers.

The first sign of a detached retina may be flashing lights and black shapes floating in front of the eye. As the retina becomes more and more separated from the choroid layer, the outer field of vision—the border of the image received by the eye—may be lost in the affected eye.

A doctor diagnoses the condition by looking into the interior of the eye with an ophthalmoscope. If a hole in the retina is discovered before the retina becomes detached, it may be sealed by *cryosurgery*, under local *anaesthesia*, or by *laser* surgery, under general anaesthesia.

If the detachment is not too advanced before the operation is carried out, vision usually returns to normal afterwards. However, if detachment is advanced, only blurred vision may be restored and there is a risk of *blindness* in the affected eye.

DETOXIFICATION
The removal, or neutralization, by the liver of poisonous substances, such as alcohol and bacterial toxins—*see Metabolism, p44; The Endocrine System, p48*. The liver makes many of the body's waste products harmless by combining them with other substances.

The term is also used to describe the process by which an alcoholic or drug addict is 'dried out', usually in a special hospital or clinic—*see addiction*.

DIABETES INSIPIDUS
A rare disorder of *metabolism* in which the sufferer produces large quantities of urine and is constantly thirsty. It is caused by a deficiency of the pituitary hormone ADH, which regulates the amount of water absorbed by the kidneys—*see The Endocrine System, p48*.

The most common cause of diabetes insipidus is damage to the pituitary gland after a severe head injury, surgery, or *radiotherapy*. It may also be caused by pressure on the gland from a *tumour*, and occasionally occurs after *encephalitis* or *meningitis*. There is also a rare form of diabetes insipidus called nephrogenic diabetes insipidus, in which the kidneys are unresponsive to the action of ADH.

Special tests are needed to confirm the diagnosis and to distinguish the disorder from *diabetes mellitis* and *personality disorders*, which also cause excessive thirst or *polydipsia*. Diabetes insipidus is treated by replacing ADH. When the condition is caused by a head injury, the defective gland usually rights itself within a year or so and the problem clears up, but if a cure does not occur spontaneously, treatment will be necessary for life.

DIABETES MELLITUS
A condition caused by the underproduction or non-production of insulin by the pancreas. As a result, the body is unable to process glucose, the sugar to which most

Diabetes The graph *(right)* shows how the incidence of diabetes mellitus increases with age in Europe and North America. Among 60-year-old people, 28 in every 1,000 suffer from this form of diabetes. Over-eating is important, for 80% of diabetics over the age of 40 are, or have been, particularly obese.

Do-it-yourself kits *(below)* enable diabetics to test their urine for glucose, **1**. Put five drops of urine, five drops of water and a special pill in a test-tube, **2**. Shake the tube until the pill dissolves, compare the change of colour of the urine in the test tube with the ones given on the accompanying test chart. **3**. Another version of the test involves dipping a test tape or stick in the urine. The colour change can be compared in the same way. Each colour on the chart corresponds to a specific glucose level.

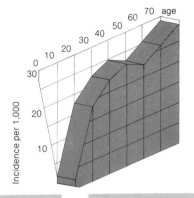

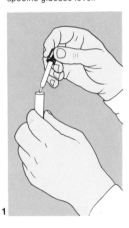
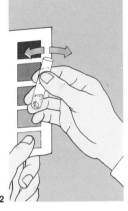
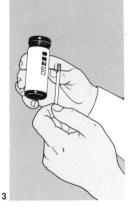

1　　　　　　**2**　　　　　　**3**

carbohydrate in the diet is reduced. The results are a high level of glucose in the blood, and a low absorption of the vital energy-producing glucose by the tissues—*see Metabolism, p44.*

There are two main types of diabetes mellitus. The first, insulin-independent diabetes, usually occurs in adults, and so is sometimes called maturity-onset diabetes. In this condition, the pancreas does not make enough insulin for the body's needs, and what little is produced seems to be ineffective. Sufferers are usually overweight, and nearly one in three has a family history of the disease.

Symptoms include a constant need to urinate, constant thirst, extreme tiredness, weakness and apathy. There may also be tingling in the hands and feet, leg cramps and a reduced resistance to infection. These symptoms often fail to appear until many years after the onset of the disease.

Insulin-independent diabetes is presently incurable, though much research is devoted to finding a cure. However, it can often be controlled if calorie and carbohydrate intake is carefully monitored. The amount of carbohydrate allowed depends upon age and occupation; in the case of a middle-aged woman with a sedentary occupation, for example, it would be very little. However, the diet must contain enough to prevent

acidosis, the minimum being around 100g (3.53oz) a day—*see Diet, p322.* Regular blood samples are taken to gauge progress.

A special diet is not always sufficient, however. Doctors may prescribe *hypoglycaemic* drugs to lower the level of sugar in the blood, but in some cases this may fail to control the blood sugar level. Then, insulin injections may be substituted.

Insulin-dependent diabetes, the second type of diabetes mellitus, tends to occur mainly in young people, and is therefore sometimes called juvenile-onset diabetes. It is thought to be due to an *autoimmune* disorder that destroys the insulin-producing cells of the pancreas. Recent research has centred on viral infection as a possible cause of insulin-dependent diabetes, as some viruses can induce the condition in animals.

Since the pancreas produces little or no insulin in this condition, sufferers depend on insulin injections to utilize the glucose in their diet. Without these, all their energy would be derived from fat, and the result would be *ketosis*, *acidosis* and eventually hyperglycaemic *coma*. These symptoms, along with a loss in weight as fat is burned up, tend to appear rapidly at the onset of the condition.

Treatment involves a

carbohydrate and calorie-controlled diet and daily or twice daily insulin injections. Most people learn how to inject themselves efficiently within a few days, and to check their blood or urine for glucose. A miniature computerized device is now available that constantly monitors the amount of insulin in the body, and the quantity that should be injected.

In both insulin-dependent and insulin-independent diabetes, but less commonly in the latter, the level of sugar in the blood may lead to *coma*. If the level is too high, because of a lack of insulin, *hyperglycaemic* coma may result. If too much insulin has been taken, if the diabetic has not eaten enough, or if he or she has exercised too much, the blood sugar level may drop, and a *hypoglycaemic* coma can develop. The condition is fatal, unless treated, and its onset can be extremely rapid.

Both forms of diabetes may give rise to a number of *complications*. Eye problems are particularly common among diabetics—there is a higher incidence of *cataracts*, for instance. Disorders of the circulation, such as severe *atherosclerosis*, are the most common problem, however. Diabetics are also prone to disorders of the urinary tract, such as *candidiasis*, and to skin disorders. Diabetes may also be a complication of *steroid* drug therapies.

DIAGNOSIS—see The Doctor, The Patient and Disease, p70

DIALYSIS
A technique by which the natural functions of the kidney are performed artificially. To some extent, the technique imitates the action of the kidneys: blood is enclosed within a semi-permeable membrane, which is immersed in a medium of constantly circulating or changing solvent or purified liquid. The impurities filter through the membrane into the solution, leaving the cleansed blood behind.

There are two methods of dialysis. The most common is haemodialysis. A hollow needle attached to a tube is inserted into an artery in an arm or leg and blood is fed through the tube to a machine that acts as a kidney. The blood passes through a filter and back along another tube into an adjacent vein. The machine is usually used for two or three days a week for six to eight hours at a time. Many patients have their own machine and learn to operate it at home, inserting the needle themselves.

This form of dialysis has several disadvantages, however. Kidney machines are extremely expensive

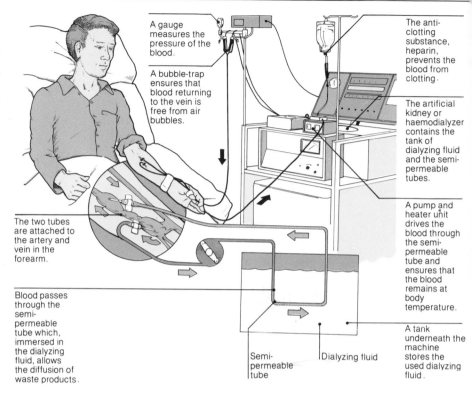

Dialysis Haemodialysis is the technique used to filter waste products from the blood of patients whose kidneys no longer function. Blood from a large artery in the forearm flows through a disposable plastic tube to a kidney machine and is then returned, clean to a vein in the arm. When the machine is not being used, the tube in the artery is connected up to the tube in the vein so that normal blood flow is resumed. Inside the machine, the blood flows through a semi-permeable tube which is bathed in the dialyzing fluid. Waste products diffuse across the semi-permeable membrane of the tube from the blood into the fluid. The blood is cleaned and the fluid is repeatedly replaced.

A gauge measures the pressure of the blood.

A bubble-trap ensures that blood returning to the vein is free from air bubbles.

The anti-clotting substance, heparin, prevents the blood from clotting.

The artificial kidney or haemodialyzer contains the tank of dialyzing fluid and the semi-permeable tubes.

A pump and heater unit drives the blood through the semi-permeable tube and ensures that the blood remains at body temperature.

The two tubes are attached to the artery and vein in the forearm.

A tank underneath the machine stores the used dialyzing fluid.

Semi-permeable tube | Dialyzing fluid

Blood passes through the semi-permeable tube which, immersed in the dialyzing fluid, allows the diffusion of waste products.

and there are not enough of them. The procedure is also time-consuming, and, depending on circumstances, may be physically unpleasant.

Another form of dialysis will, it is thought, provide a viable alternative to the use of a kidney machine. This technique is called CAPD (Continuous Ambulatory Peritoneal Dialysis). CAPD is based on a long-established form of treatment, known as peritoneal dialysis, in which the peritoneum, the membrane surrounding the intestines, is used as the semi-permeable factor. Dialyzing fluid is run into the abdomen through a *catheter* and waste products pass out of the circulation, using the peritoneum as the membrane. After a while, the fluid is drained out, and the process repeated.

In CAPD, the catheter is left permanently in position. About four times a day, the user attaches a new bag, containing dialyzing fluid, to the catheter, and releases the fluid a few hours later. This technique allows the patient on dialysis to walk around during dialysis and, in general, to continue leading a relatively normal life. The main drawback, to date, is the problem of infection entering the peritoneal cavity via the catheter.

DIAPHRAGM
A word with two medical meanings. In anatomy, the diaphragm is the thin muscle separating the chest and stomach cavities, which plays an important part in breathing—*see The Respiratory System, p28*. Every time a breath is taken in, it contracts, pushing downwards to increase the volume of space in the thoracic cavity, and relaxes again on each contraction. The diaphragm is also a contraceptive device, consisting of a rubber cap, fitted over the neck of the womb and used together with a chemical spermicide—*see Sex and Contraception, p338*.

DIARRHOEA
Frequent loose or liquid bowel movements that may be urgent or impossible to control. They often may be accompanied by some abdominal pain. Diarrhoea may be brought on by stress or fear; by eating large quantities of foods with laxative properties, such as prunes or beans; or by taking certain drugs such as *antibiotics*.

'Holiday tummy', one of the commonest forms of diarrhoea, is caused by exposure to bacteria against which the affected person has no natural tolerance or immunity; infective *gastroenteritis*, or gastric 'flu, perhaps the commonest cause of diarrhoea, is a viral *infection* in which diarrhoea is often accompanied by *vomiting*. It may last for no more than 24 or 36 hours, but, in severe attacks, the loss of fluid may cause *dehydration*. A victim should try to take in some liquid, even during the attack.

A baby with persistent severe diarrhoea may lose a dangerous amount of body fluid, especially if there is vomiting as well. The baby should be given plenty of boiled and cooled water and a doctor should be consulted.

Persistent diarrhoea, especially when the stools are accompanied by blood and mucus, may be a sign of other diseases involving the intestines—in particular *irritable bowel syndrome* and *ulcerative colitis*. When diarrhoea is persistent, or when bouts of diarrhoea alternate with *constipation*, a doctor should always be consulted, since this is occasionally a symptom of a serious disease.

DIASTOLE
The period in which the heart muscles contract between contractions—*see The Blood and Lymph Systems, p21*. Diastole usually lasts for about 0.5 seconds in normal circumstances, though it lessens as the heart rate increases. There are, in fact, two diastoles—atrial diastole and ventricular diastole—though the term is usually used to mean ventricular diastole. In atrial diastole, the muscles of the atria relax, allowing the two atria to fill with blood from the veins; this happens towards the end of ventricular *systole*, in which the main pumping muscles of the ventricles are contracting. The atria then contract—atrial systole—and, at the same time, the ventricles relax to receive the atrial blood.

DIATHERMY

A form of treatment is which heat is applied to the skin by means of two electrically-charged electrodes. The heat increases the flow of blood in the area to which it is applied, so helping in the treatment of deep pain, as in *arthritis*. The same principle is used in various surgical instruments; a diathermy knife, for instance, can be used to coagulate blood and tissue. In this case, the knife acts as one electrode, the other being a damp pad applied to the patient's body.

See also cautery.

DIGITALIS

A drug once extracted from foxglove leaves, but now synthesized. It is commonly used in the treatment of atrial *fibrillation* and *heart failure*. Digitalis acts by increasing the strength of contraction of the heart muscles; it also decreases the rate at which the ventricles contract by slowing down the transmission of nerve impulses to them from the atria—*see The Blood and Lymph Systems, p21.*

Although digitalis is extremely effective, it is difficult to prescribe accurately. This is because there is a fine division between how much is necessary for effectiveness and the toxic dosage. The problem is worse in the case of old people, whose kidneys may not be able to cope with the quantities of the drug that must be excreted. In such patients the level of the drug in the body may build up slowly to cause a potentially serious condition known as digitalis toxicity.

The symptoms of digitalis toxicity are the same as those of overdose. Tiredness may be accompanied by visual disturbances, such as blurring and indistinct colour vision. The muscles become weak, making movement an effort. There may be *nausea*, loss of appetite and abdominal pains and, at night, restlessness and vivid dreaming. These symptoms, if ignored, may lead to *bradycardia* or *tachycardia*, and *fibrillation*.

If symptoms of digitalis intoxication are present, ceasing to take the drug for a day or two may be all the treatment necessary. Old people are often advised to take the drug six days a week, but miss out one.

DILATATION & CURETTAGE (D & C)

A minor operation in which the cervix, or neck of the womb, is dilated, so that the endometrium, the lining of the uterus, can be curetted, or scraped. The contents of the uterus are expelled. The operation is often carried out to obtain samples of endometrial tissue for pathological examination in order to discover the cause of a number of gynaecological problems. A D & C, for instance, is often performed as part of the diagnosis and treatment of *menorrhagia*, a heavy loss of blood at menstrual periods; of bleeding between periods; of *endometriosis*; and of bleeding from the uterus after the *menopause*.

In such cases, the endometrial tissue is examined to make sure that the bleeding is not caused by polyps—small, usually *benign* growths—a *uterine cancer*, or, in pre-menopausal women, by an incomplete *abortion*. The action of female hormones in the patient may also be investigated. This is because the appearance of the endometrium alters in response to the hormonal changes of the menstrual cycle—*see Sex and Reproduction, p54.* As a result, a limited D & C, in which only a small piece of tissue is removed, can be useful in an investigation of *infertility*.

Dilatation and curettage is also

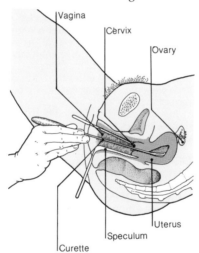

Dilatation and Curettage
A D and C operation involves dilating the cervix with a surgical instrument, so that the gynaecologist can reach into the uterus with a curette *(above)*. The endometrium, or lining of the womb, is scraped away and examined by a histopathologist in the laboratory.

used for abortion in early pregnancy. Occasionally, small fragments of tissue are left in the womb after a spontaneous miscarriage or an abortion. Since they may cause vaginal bleeding, an offensive *vaginal discharge*, pelvic tenderness and *fever*, a D & C is performed to remove them—the procedure being known as an ERPC (Evacuation of Retained Products of Conception).

The operation is carried out under general *anaesthetic* and lasts about 30 minutes. The patient will usually spend the night in hospital, although she is sometimes allowed home the same day. Any pain resulting from the operation is unlikely to be more severe than a mild period pain.

Although a D & C is often primarily performed only to investigate a gynaecological problem, the operation often has the effect of relieving a patient's symptoms and improving her condition. This is especially true in cases of *menorrhagia*. Some doctors, however, recommend that a patient has a D & C for no good reason at all, though most doctors frown on this practice. There is no evidence that an efficiently performed D & C has any effect on future fertility.

DIPHTHERIA

A dangerous, highly infective disease of the upper respiratory tract, most often affecting the nose, larynx or tonsils. It is caused by *bacteria* that produce a powerful toxin, or poison. Diphtheria is spread by droplets expelled when an infected person, or a *carrier*, coughs or sneezes. The incubation period is four to six days, after which the symptoms appear.

Depending upon the patient's degree of immunity to the disease, the first symptoms may include a raised temperature, rapid pulse and enlarged neck glands. A characteristic greyish membrane adheres firmly to the site of infection; if the nose is affected there may be an infected blood-stained discharge from it. If the tonsils are involved, the throat becomes sore. When the larynx is the site of infection, the voice becomes hoarse and there is a cough; there is also a danger that the membrane will obstruct the airway, causing suffocation.

In some cases, there are no further symptoms and the infected person may recover completely, or become a *carrier*—a potential source of infection. Most frequently, however, the sufferer becomes seriously ill.

To prevent the spread of the disease, patients with diptheria are treated in special isolation wards. They are given injections of powerful *antibiotics* and antitoxins. These normally bring about a cure, if the diagnosis has been made in good time. When the airway is obstructed, a *tracheotomy* may be performed. In this, a tube through which the patient can breathe is passed into the trachea below the site of the blockage.

Less than half a century ago diphtheria was *endemic* in the Western world and a common cause

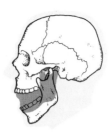

The jaw dislocates easily once it has been weakened by a previous injury. The jaw can only be dislocated in the forward direction and only when the mouth is open.

The thumb joint dislocates when its middle bone moves back and down in relation to its bottom bone *(right)*.

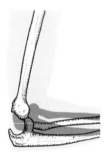

Dislocation of the elbow's pivot joint *(left)* is a common injury which results from falling on the outstretched hand while the elbow is slightly flexed.

Dislocation The bones forming a joint are dislocated *(below)* when they are displaced or separated from one another by the force of an injury. Dislocation is painful when ligaments and tendons are torn and particularly painful when a nerve or artery is compressed or damaged. The brown areas show the bones' normal position, the white the dislocation.

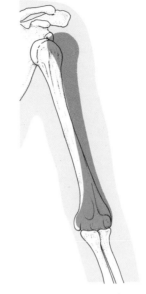

X-rays are usually taken to determine whether or not a joint is dislocated. In the X-ray of the dislocated left shoulder *(above)*, the humerus of the upper arm has clearly been dislocated from the scapula. The shoulder is particularly vulnerable, since its ball-and-socket joint is extremely manoeuvrable and is therefore susceptible to dislocation. The ball of the humerus bone no longer fits into the socket of the scapula and is displaced to the side *(left)*.

of death, especially in children. In recent years, however, new drugs have been introduced that make the disease less likely to be fatal. National *immunization* campaigns combined with compulsory isolation of infected patients have reduced its incidence considerably. However, diphtheria has not been entirely wiped out and it is essential that all babies are immunized against it—*see Health and Your Child, p348.*

When an outbreak occurs, every possible effort is made to trace and test people with whom the infected person may have been in contact during the incubation period. This enables *carriers* to be identified and treated, so that an *epidemic* can be prevented.

DIPLOPIA
The medical term for double vision—seeing two images of a single object. Normally the images from the two eyes appear side by side, but in vertical diplopia one image appears above the other.

Diplopia may be caused by a defect in the optical system of the eye, or by a disorder of the nervous system, such as *multiple sclerosis* or a *lesion* of the cranial nerve supplying the muscles of the eyeball. The most common cause, however, is a squint—*see strabismus.* In this case, the two eyes look along different axes and the image is focused incorrectly. An incipient *cataract*, a displaced contact lens or *astigmatism* may also cause double vision by

distorting the optics of the affected eye. Very rarely, the condition is associated with psychological problems, while excessive amounts of alcohol, drugs, such as *atropine*, and the toxins that enter the body in *food-poisoning*, may all cause diplopia.

Anyone who is suffering from double vision, therefore, should consult a doctor.

DISCHARGE—see Vaginal discharge; Penile discharge

DISLOCATION
The displacement of the bones of a joint from their normal position. If the bones have moved so far that their ends no longer meet, the dislocation is said to be a luxation; if there is still contact between the bones, it is known as a subluxation.

A joint may become dislocated as the result of an injury or accident—as in the case of a dislocated shoulder—or occur repeatedly without apparent cause. This can happen if the fibrous capsule surrounding a joint is unnaturally loose, or, in the case of the hip, when there are *congenital* abnormalities in the structure of the joint.

When a dislocation occurs, the joint becomes immovable, painful and swollen. The area around it may become inflamed and discoloured. A dislocation of the shoulder joint is obvious from its appearance, but dislocations of other joints, such as

the hip, will require an X-ray to confirm diagnosis.

A doctor or surgeon will reduce the dislocation by manipulating the bones back into place, normally under general *anaesthesia*, and then support the joint with bandages, or sometimes a splint. So long as the original injury did not cause any permanent physical damage, the limb will be back to normal after two or three weeks.

See also First Aid, p369.

DISORIENTATION
The loss of awareness of personal identity, location and situation. The condition can be caused by drugs, poisoning and alcohol, and may be a symptom of *delirium, dementia* and *psychosis*.

DISSEMINATING SCLEROSIS— see Multiple Sclerosis

DIURETIC
A drug that increases the amount of urine produced by the kidneys, and so rids the body of excess fluid. Diuretics are used in the treatment of pulmonary *oedema*, the saturation of the lungs by fluid caused by *heart failure*; to treat the generalized *oedema* of kidney disease; and to treat the *ascites* of liver disorders. They are also used to reduce the volume of the blood in mild cases of *hypertension*, or raised blood pressure, and to reduce the pressure of fluid in the eye in *glaucoma*.

Diuretics were once used as a

slimming aid, but, since they sometimes have side-effects, such as rashes, nausea, dizziness, weakness and numbness and tingling in the hands and feet, this practice has largely been abandoned.

DIVERTICULAR DISEASE
The presence of small pouches, called diverticula, in the wall of the digestive tract, most commonly in the large intestine. The condition is also known as diverticulosis.

Diverticular disease is a common problem in the western world. It is thought to be caused by the increased pressure needed to move the hard stools typical of a low-fibre diet through the intestines. The disease often fails to develop until middle age—presumably because the effects of a low-fibre diet and increased intestinal pressures take many years to manifest themselves.

Diverticula often produce no symptoms, though there is occasionally slight tenderness in the lower left side of the abdomen. Their presence may only be detected accidentally, as a result of an unrelated investigation, and no treatment is given other than the advice to adopt a high-fibre diet and to avoid the use of laxatives.

If the diverticula become inflamed due to a *bacterial* infection, the condition is known as diverticulitis. This may cause a severe pain on the left of the abdomen, which feels like that of *appendicitis*, together with nausea and *fever*. If one of the diverticula burst, *abscesses* may form and *peritonitis* can result. *Constipation* may alternate with *diarrhoea*, and there may also be bleeding from the rectum.

Acute diverticulitis is treated with *antibiotics* and, in serious cases, by intravenous feeding through a *drip*, so that the diverticula are given time to recover without being disturbed by food passing through the intestines. The symptoms usually clear up after a few days and patients are put on a high-fibre diet—*see Diet, p320*—to prevent any recurrence of the problem. If colonic diverticulitis does frequently recur, however, an operation may be necessary to remove the diverticula or part of the intestine affected—*see resection*.

DIVERTICULITIS—see Diverticular disease

DIVERTICULOSIS—see Diverticular disease

DIZZINESS—see Vertigo

DOUBLE VISION—see Diplopia

DOUCHE
A stream of water used to clean the vagina. Some women douche the vagina with a rubber bulb fitted with a rigid neck that can be inserted into the vagina. The bulb is filled with dilute antiseptic or soapy water for cleanliness, or with a spermicidal fluid for contraceptive purposes. This is not only an ineffective and unreliable method of contraception, it also may force harmful *bacteria* up into the uterus, causing *infection*, while powerful antiseptics or even disinfectants disturb the normal chemical and biological balance of the vagina, leaving it open to attack. For this reason, douching is not recommended by doctors.

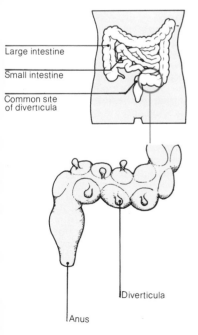

Large intestine

Small intestine

Common site of diverticula

Diverticula

Anus

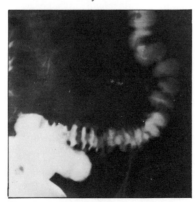

Diverticular Disease Chronic constipation or a low fibre diet can both lead to the development of small pouches called diverticula on the final segments of the large intestine *(left)*. The mucous membrane lining the intestine gives way to internal pressure and bulges out through the muscular coating of the gut wall. The shadowy outlines of the diverticula can be seen in the X-ray *(above)*, taken after a barium enema was swallowed. The barium enables any abnormalities of the small intestine or large bowel to show up on X-ray.

DOWN'S SYNDROME
A *congenital*, or inborn, physical and mental defect caused by a *chromosomal* abnormality.

A child with Down's syndrome is short and squat with a round face, flat nose, slant eyes and straight hair. This characteristic appearance gives rise to the old-fashioned name for the condition—'mongolism'—though this is no longer used. The hands are also squat and have characteristic creases on the palms. These distinguishing features are usually obvious at birth.

The mental development of children with Down's syndrome is abnormally slow, and they are usually retarded, with a mental age of around five or six. Most have a low *IQ*, or intelligence quotient, of around 60. They have friendly and endearing personalities, however, and can usually be taught to care for themselves and to work at simple tasks. Down's syndrome children rarely live longer than the third decade, though this picture is changing. Some sufferers are now living longer, while some women with Down's syndrome have had babies.

The condition is also called trisomy 21 because affected children have three, instead of two, of the 21st chromosome—making 47 chromosomes in all rather than the normal 46. This abnormality usually arises when, on the formation of an ovum, one of the chromosome pairs fails to split, so that the unfertilized egg has two chromosomes instead of one —*see Sex and Reproduction, p54*. Alternatively, it can be the result of an abnormal arrangement of the chromosomes of either parent.

The cause of the defect is unknown, but its incidence increases with the age of the mother—more than 50% of children with Down's syndrome are born to mothers over 40. It can be detected before birth by a special investigation called an amniocentesis—*see Special Tests, p84*. This is a routine procedure for all mothers thought to be at risk in countries where *abortion* is legal; if the results indicate abnormality, they are given the option of terminating the pregnancy.

In some Down's syndrome children, the effect of the extra chromosome is lessened when it is not found in every cell of the body. This form of the condition is known as mosaicism. Such children may achieve an IQ higher than 60.

Specialists who work with Down's syndrome children believe that, because of prejudice and indifference, the children have not been encouraged to develop to their full potential. Professional care in specialized institutions has recently proved that, when well cared for and mentally stimulated, Down's syndrome children are capable of greater emotional maturity and intellectual progress than had previously been thought possible.

A number of associations and charitable organizations exist to provide advice and support for parents of Down's syndrome children. These include MENCAP and Down's Children Organization.

DRIP
A device through which fluid can be passed directly into a vein in a patient's body at a controlled rate.

Intravenous drips are used to give a controlled *transfusion* of blood, *saline* or nutrients. A drip may also be placed in the nose to pass milk, liquefied food or water directly to the stomach when there is difficulty in swallowing, after an operation, or in cases of *dehydration* in babies.

DRUG INTERACTION
The physical effects produced by the reaction of two drugs with each other. Drug interactions may enhance, reduce or alter the effect of either drug, sometimes with fatal results. A huge number of drug interactions have been recorded, so doctors should ensure that there is no risk of unwanted side-effects before prescribing more than one drug at a time.

Many doctors feel that insufficient attention is paid to this problem, and that the use of interacting drugs may often cause *iatrogenic*, or medically induced, disease. One study of hospital patients showed that 40% of those receiving medication were taking six or more drugs at a time, and that these patients experienced side-effects seven times more often than those taking fewer than six drugs.

Some common medications obtainable without a prescription can interact with a drug prescribed by a doctor. Certain drugs, among them some *anticoagulants* and *sulphonamides*, are most efficiently absorbed by the body at a specific stomach acidity. If this acidity is altered by *antacids*, taken to relieve an attack of *dyspepsia*, the rate of absorption, and therefore effectiveness, of the other drug is reduced.

The action of the *antibiotic* tetracycline can also be affected by antacids. The mineral calcium, found in milk, may have the same effect, so it is important that tetracycline is taken on an empty stomach, and never with a glass of milk.

Many drugs are transported or stored in the body as chemical compounds linked with proteins in the blood—*see The Blood and Lymph Systems, p21*. Such drugs are only active in their free, uncombined state. When several drugs are taken at once, one may displace another from its protein link. As a result, there will be a greater concentration of the displaced drug in an active state. This can have serious effects.

Aspirin and indomethacin, an *anti-inflammatory* drug often used to treat *arthritis*, tends to displace anticoagulants, such as *warfarin*, from their protein links, for example. The raised concentration of active warfarin in the blood may cause fatal bleeding in the brain, or from the digestive tract. For this reason, it is vital that other drugs are not taken with anticoagulants, unless they are known not to cause an interaction.

Alcohol should also be avoided during drug therapy, especially if the patient is normally a heavy drinker. In such people, the level of enzymes that break down alcohol in the liver is always high. The same enzymes, however, also break down drugs, often before they have had a chance to work effectively. As a result, alcoholics need larger dosages of many drugs than other people—they have a particularly high tolerance for *barbiturates* and *tranquillizers*.

Not all drug interactions are harmful, however. Some can even be manipulated by doctors to the patient's advantage. One example is the use of drugs to alter the acid-alkali balance of the urine—sodium bicarbonate makes the urine more alkaline, while *vitamin C* makes it more acid.

Doctors often make the urine more alkaline in cases of *barbiturate* or aspirin overdose, because this speeds up the rate of excretion of these two drugs—this technique is known as forced alkaline diuresis. Ascorbic acid (vitamin C), on the other hand, may be given with a drug called mandelamine in cases of urinary infection, because the drug works most efficiently in an acid environment.

Drug interactions have a wide range of side-effects. In some cases, such as those involving the monoamine oxidase *antidepressant* drugs, they may be fatal. In other cases they may be minor and scarcely noticeable.

However, the problem can be avoided to a large extent if the instructions and the 'contra-indications' listed on drug packets are read carefully and followed to the letter; if the course of drugs is

taken exactly as prescribed by the doctor; and if all proprietary medicines are avoided during a course of treatment.

To make absolutely certain, remind the doctor of any drugs that are already being taken before others are prescribed—especially if the contraceptive pill has been prescribed at a Family Planning Clinic, and not by the family doctor—and never, under any circumstances, swap drugs and remedies with friends or relatives.

DUCTUS ARTERIOSUS—see Congenital heart defects

DUMPING SYNDROME—see Gastrectomy

DUCHENNE DYSTROPHY—see Muscular dystrophy

DUODENAL ULCER—see Ulcer

DWARFISM
Stunted growth and short stature, which may be due to an intrinsic inability to grow normally, as in hypopituitary dwarfism, or caused by a number of diseases and conditions. These include *malnutrition*; *congenital heart defects*; *liver* or *kidney* diseases and *coeliac disease* in childhood; *familial* factors; *achondroplasia*, a hereditary disorder in which the skeletal bones fail to develop; and *Turner's syndrome*, which causes short stature in women. Underproduction of the thyroid hormone, a disorder which causes *cretinism*, may result in stunted growth, if the condition is not treated early in life—*see myxoedema*.

True dwarfism, however, is caused by disorders of the pituitary gland, and is known as hypopituitary dwarfism. The anterior lobe of the pituitary produces several hormones —*see The Endocrine System, p48*. One of these, the growth hormone (GH), stimulates the development of the skeleton and the production of substances, such as the proteins which make up the tissues. If, however, these secretions are either deficient or absent, dwarfism will result, but intelligence is not affected.

Since children grow at vastly different rates, it is difficult to distinguish dwarfism from natural smallness of stature or slow growth. The condition can be diagnosed only by comparing X-rays of the left hand and wrist taken at yearly intervals with X-rays showing normal development. Special tests must then be carried out to assess the quantities of growth hormone being secreted into the bloodstream, and to determine whether the secretions are being affected by a *tumour* of the pituitary.

If dwarfism is diagnosed in routine tests at an early age, treatment with GH obtained from human pituitary glands may correct the defect. Intramuscular injections are given twice a week, often for several years, until the patient's growth appears to be completed.

DYSARTHRIA

Difficulty in speaking and enunciating words. Since articulation of speech depends upon perfect co-ordination of lips, tongue and palate, the disorder may have a simple physical cause, such as a swollen tongue, or badly fitting false teeth. However, it may also be due to a *cleft palate*, or defective or damaged muscles and nerves in the lips, tongue or teeth.

Dysarthria also occurs as a result of *paralysis* of the muscles of the larynx in *diphtheria*. It is also a feature of *Wilson's* and *Parkinson's* diseases, *myaesthenia gravis*, and facial palsy. It may also follow a stroke—*see cerebrovascular accident*—affecting the brain stem.

The condition is treated according to its cause; sometimes a cure is impossible. In such cases, dysarthria may be improved by *speech therapy*.

DYSENTERY

A term used to describe an *acute* infection of the intestine whose symptoms include severe and painful *diarrhoea*, and the expulsion of blood and *mucous* in the *faeces*. The infection may be caused by *bacteria* or by *parasites*—*see amoebiasis*.

Bacterial dysentery is usually due to *infection* by *bacteria* of the genus Shigella. Symptoms tend to arise within a week of the infection and range from mild diarrhoea in the form known as Sonne dysentery, which occurs in temperate climates, to severe diarrhoea with cramps, bleeding from the gut and spasmodic contractions of the bowel, nausea, *vomiting* and fever. These symptoms, which occur in the virulent Far Eastern form known as Shiga dysentery, may last for hours or even days, causing exhaustion and *dehydration*.

Bacterial dysentery is transmitted by contact with a patient or a *carrier* of the infection, or through utensils, food or water contaminated with their *faeces*. Mild forms usually clear up without treatment. More severe cases usually respond to treatment with *antibiotics* such as ampicillin, and with *sulphonamide* drugs. If fluid loss can be replaced rapidly, recovery will usually occur in less

than a week.

Although most adults recover from bacterial dysentery, it can be fatal if it occurs in people who are weak from *malnutrition*, or suffering from some other debilitating illness, such as *malaria*. The *dehydration* caused by dysentery may be fatal to children, who cannot tolerate the loss of fluid, nutrients and essential salts as well as adults. Since it is impossible for anyone who is vomiting to take in liquids, children may need an intravenous infusion of fluids, through a *drip*, or, if necessary, by an injection. Although outbreaks of dysentery are fairly common in institutions in the developed countries, the infection is unlikely to spread if standards of hygiene are high, especially in the handling of food. However, in many tropical countries dysentery is rife and a common cause of death, especially among children.

DYSFUNCTIONAL UTERINE BLEEDING

A term used to describe abnormal uterine bleeding, which is usually caused by hormonal variations affecting the menstrual cycle—*see Sex and Reproduction, p54*. A woman who bleeds a little between periods because of *cervical erosion* does not have dysfunctional uterine bleeding, for instance; if, however, physical examination fails to discover any reason for irregular periods, then the bleeding is called dysfunctional.

This pattern of bleeding is often the result of emotional problems, which affect the hypothalamus in the brain (*p32*). The hypothalamus affects the release of the gonadotrophic hormones, which, in turn, influences the production of the female hormones oestrogen and progesterone, which control the menstrual cycle.

Treatment is usually unnecessary, unless the bleeding is causing distress, or problems with contraception, as in the case of the rhythm method—*see Sex and Contraception, p338*. The doctor's main task is to exclude any other possible causes of irregular bleeding and to reassure the patient that there is nothing seriously wrong with her and that her future fertility will not be affected. If the main problem is effective contraception, then the combined oral contraceptive pill can be prescribed. This causes a regular monthly bleed.

DYSLEXIA

A difficulty in recognizing written words. Dyslexia is thought to affect between 5% and 10% of all children to some degree. Four times as many boys as girls are dyslexic, probably

because there are thought to be language centres in both sides of girls' brains, but only one in boys'. The condition defies precise definition, and its cause is not known.

The symptoms of dyslexia vary enormously. Some dyslexic children may confuse certain letters, such as 'b' and 'd', or 'q' and 'p', while others can read well, but find great difficulty in writing. Some may be bad at games, and confuse left with right, but be able to memorize poetry and read music. Vision and intelligence are not normally affected, but, if the condition is not detected, the social and educational effects of the problem may have repercussions in later life.

Dyslexics can be helped considerably by special remedial treatment. In America, a drug called methylphendidate is used to treat the condition, but there are varying reports as to its success—this drug is rarely used in Britain because of the risk of side-effects. The success of remedial teaching depends greatly on the sense of motivation imparted to the child by parents and teachers.

The Dyslexia Institute exists to give advice and support to parents of dyslexic children.

DYSMENORRHOEA

Painful menstrual periods—*see Sex and Reproduction, p54*. Most women feel some pain as a period begins, often because of mild contractions of the womb or of the muscles of the cervix. They may also feel less energetic than usual and perhaps a little tired and irritable. Dysmenorrhoea, however, is a condition in which severe pelvic and *back pain* may occur at the beginning of a period. These often go hand-in-hand with headache, *nausea, vomiting, diarrhoea* and *palpitations*, as well as severe tiredness and irritability.

Primary dysmenorrhoea starts at the *menarche*, the time of the first period, and is common. No physical cause for this has so far been discovered and it is suspected that this type of dysmenorrhoea has a *psychosomatic* origin. Primary dysmenorrhoea often disappears if the contraceptive pill is taken regularly, or after the sufferer has had a baby.

Simple measures, such as resting and getting plenty of sleep during the days immediately before each period, may help deal with the tiredness and tension associated with primary dysmenorrhoea. Pain can be alleviated by painkillers, such as *aspirin, paracetamol* or codeine. Many psychosexual *counsellors* advocate sex and masturbation as remedies for the discomfort of painful periods. Sometimes, however, primary dysmenorrhoea is caused by a hormonal imbalance, in which case it may be necessary to give synthetic hormones to relieve the symptoms.

When periods that are usually normal become painful, the condition is known as secondary dysmenorrhoea. This may have physical causes. It may be due to growths, such as *fibroids*, *endometriosis*, polyps, or even *tumours*; *inflammation* of the lining of the womb, the formation of scar tissue at the neck of the womb, or, rarely, deformities or underdevelopment of the uterus. Surgery may be necessary to remove growths and scars and correct abnormalities; *antibiotics* can be prescribed to reduce inflammation.

Emotional shocks, such as bereavement, the break-up of a relationship, an unsatisfied desire to have children, or fear of sex or of pregnancy can all disturb natural body rhythms, with dysmenorrhoea as the result. *Counselling* and medical help may relieve both the emotional problem and the dysmenorrhoea. *See also pre-menstrual tension.*

DYSPAREUNIA
Painful sexual intercourse, a condition that can affect both men and women and have mental or physical causes.

Primary dyspareunia, also called *vaginismus*, is experienced only by women, and occurs when the muscles around the vagina contract involuntarily. This normally makes penetration by the penis impossible, and attempts to penetrate extremely painful. Primary dyspareunia is usually caused by unconscious fear or dislike of sex and may be the result of a previous frightening, painful, or unpleasant sexual experience. Psychosexual *counselling* and therapy is usually advised if the problem seems to be deeply rooted.

Dyspareunia may also have physical causes. In men it may be due to *balanitis*, an inflammation of the foreskin, or *phimosis*; in women, to inflammation of the vulva, vagina or bladder. Inflammation of the genitals may be due to bacterial or fungal *infection*, such as *chlamydia* or *trichomonas vaginalis*, or be caused by friction or *venereal disease*. The condition requires treatment with *antibiotics* or *fungicides*.

Where dyspareunia in women is caused by an unusually thick hymen, which is difficult or impossible to penetrate, a simple surgical operation will break it. In older women, dyspareunia may be caused by shrinkage of the skin lining the vagina. This condition, which tends to occur after the *menopause*, is called senile *vaginitis*. It can usually be relieved by applying a hormone cream.
See also Sex and Contraception, p338.

DYSPEPSIA
A general medical term, used to describe a group of symptoms that are more commonly known as indigestion.

These symptoms vary widely. They usually include a feeling of pain or discomfort in the abdomen, which may occur at a specific time each day, or after meals. There may also be belching—also called eructation—nausea, *oesophagitis*, flatulence and heartburn—also called pyrosis—in which a severe burning pain is felt behind the breast bone. Sometimes, dyspepsia is associated with waterbrash, in which the mouth suddenly fills with dilute, watery saliva.

Dyspepsia can have a number of causes. Most commonly, it is the result of *gastritis*, an inflammation and irritation of the stomach lining. This may be due to eating or drinking to excess, and is exacerbated by smoking. Generally, dyspepsia from this cause is temporary. However, if excessive drinking, eating and smoking continue, it may become a permanent condition, resulting in the formation of *ulcers*. Ulcers also cause dyspepsia, as do a number of other conditions, including *hiatus hernia* and *gallstones*. Temporary dyspepsia can often be relieved by drinking milk or taking *antacid* preparations. Treatment of chronic dyspepsia is aimed at dealing with the underlying cause. It may involve a change in eating, drinking and smoking habits—*see Diet, p322; Abuses of the Body, p328*—and, if ulcers, a hiatus hernia or gallstones are responsible, drug treatment or surgery.

DYSPHAGIA
Difficulty in swallowing, which can occur for a number of reasons. When the throat is inflamed or sore, as in *tonsillitis*, for example, eating anything is painful and difficult. Fungal infections of the mouth and oesophagus may also cause dysphagia.

More seriously, the swallowing mechanism may be affected by a stroke—*see cerebrovascular accident*—sometimes with the result that liquids become harder to swallow than solids. In *diphtheria* and one type of *poliomyelitis*, the muscles of the palate and pharynx become paralyzed. This makes swallowing very difficult indeed, with fluid sometimes regurgitating through the nose. *Cancer* of the oesophagus, too, makes swallowing a problem.

Treatment of dysphagia involves identifying the underlying disease and treating it. After a stroke, patients can be encouraged to swallow by sucking a piece of ice, which relaxes some of the muscles and so makes swallowing easier. Cancer of the oesophagus is removed surgically whenever possible, while fungal infections are treated with the appropriate drugs.

DYSPNOEA
Breathlessness or laboured breathing. Dyspnoea is often persistent, as in diseases such as *pneumoconiosis*, chronic *bronchitis*, *emphysema*, *tuberculosis* and *lung cancer*. It is also a symptom of severe *anaemia*. It may, however, occur in spasms, as in *acute bronchitis*, *asthma* and the pulmonary *oedema* caused by *heart failure*. People unaccustomed to high altitudes may also suffer from the condition until acclimatized.

The laboured breathing is audible and often loud; there may be wheezing, gasping and *cyanosis*. Rest may be sufficient treatment for high-altitude dyspnoea; asthmatics and people with heart diseases usually carry drugs that will bring them instant relief. In other cases, however, emergency treatment with oxygen and drugs may be necessary.

DYSTROPHY—see Muscular dystrophy

DYSURIA
Discomfort felt while passing urine. Dysuria may be due to an infection of the lower part of the urinary tract such as *cystitis* or *urethritis*, that causes inflammation of the bladder and urethra. The result may be considerable pain on trying to pass urine. Sufferers may have to urinate more frequently than normal and may find that they pass only a small quantity at each attempt. Afterwards, the feeling of needing to pass urine remains.

The inflammation is treated by taking an appropriate *antibiotic* and by drinking large quantities of fluid. This increases the flow of urine and so prevents infected urine from stagnating in the bladder.

Dysuria may also be experienced during attacks of thrush—*see candidiasis*. This is a fungal infection which causes the labia, the lips of the vagina, to become red, swollen and sore. Small skinless areas may appear on the vulva and pain is felt when urine passes over these sores. Treatment is with antifungal creams and pessaries.

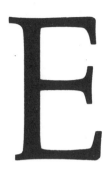

EARACHE

An ache in the ears, which is a common complaint, especially among young children. Infections of the ear, whether of the outer ear—*otitis* externa—or middle ear—otitis media—frequently cause pain. Otitis media is usually the more severe of the two, and is accompanied by loss of appetite, fever and a general feeling of malaise.

Eustachian tube dysfunction, in which the eustachian tube leading from the pharynx to the middle ear becomes inflamed and blocked off, often causes severe earache. This may be associated with infection of the middle ear, as germs may pass along the tube from the throat. Thus, it is common for children with *pharyngitis* to complain of pain and throbbing in one, or both, ears.

Earache may also occasionally be a symptom of dental decay, teething in a young child, or even of a boil in the ear canal. *Sinusitis*, particularly infections of the mastoid sinuses just behind the ear, may similarly cause pain.

Initially, earache can be treated by placing a warm hot-water bottle, wrapped in a pillow case, under the affected ear while in bed. *Analgesics* may also give relief. It is important not to stick cotton buds down the ear canal, as the delicate, inflamed ear drum may be accidentally shattered. If, however, there is severe, uninterrupted pain, a fever, or general malaise, a doctor should be consulted, as *antibiotic* treatment may be necessary. In sinusitis, antibiotics can be combined with steam inhalations, which may help relieve the discomfort.

ECCHYMOSIS

A bruise, or bluish-black mark on the skin that appears when blood is released into the tissues. As the blood is broken down, absorbed by the tissues and carried away, the bruise changes colour to purple, red and yellow before fading away. Such bruising is caused by injury to the dermis or tissues beneath the skin surface. However, in certain diseases, such as *thrombocytopaenia*, blood may leak spontaneously from

the capillary vessels, so that ecchymosis occurs without injury.

ECG (ELECTROCARDIOGRAM)—see Special Tests, p84

ECLAMPSIA

An uncommon complication of pregnancy, in which the pregnant woman suffers fits or *convulsions* during the last three months, during labour or, rarely, after delivery. The convulsions may culminate in *coma* and can result in the death of both mother and baby.

Eclampsia is preceded by a set of symptoms known as pre-eclampsia,of which the earliest is usually *oedema*—swelling—of the legs and feet and sometimes also of the hands and face, which persists even after rest. Weekly weight gain is excessive, blood pressure rises—*see hypertension*—and protein is excreted in the urine. Other symptoms may include headache, dizziness and vomiting, stomach pain and visual disturbances such as spots and flashes of light before the eyes. These latter symptoms usually appear as warning signs of imminent convulsions.

The causes of eclampsia are not entirely understood. It is defined as one of the two *toxaemias of pregnancy*, though this is misleading, as no toxic substances have ever been isolated to account for the pathological changes. However, *lesions* have been discovered on organs such as the kidneys, liver, uterus and placenta of women who have died from eclampsia. It is believed that constriction of blood vessels reduces the blood flow to these organs, causing the blood pressure to rise. Some of the affected organs react by releasing into the bloodstream chemicals that act to restore normal blood flow, but these reduce the blood supply to other parts of the body. As a result, the kidneys fail to eliminate salt, causing water retention and oedema, and *nephritis* develops. This causes the release of proteins into the urine. The placenta begins to deteriorate, with resulting damage to the foetus, while a

reduction in the supply of blood to the mother's brain may cause convulsions in her.

If the symptoms of pre-eclampsia become serious, the mother-to-be may be admitted to hospital and put on a low-salt, fat-free diet. With this treatment the pregnancy usually runs its normal course. If necessary, drugs may be prescribed to lower the blood pressure and promote the excretion of salt. If convulsions occur, both mother and baby are in danger of *hypoxia*, a deficiency of oxygen in the tissues. Sedation and prolonged rest may control the convulsions, but, if they persist, delivery of the baby by *caesarian section* may be the only way of saving both mother and child. However, modern ante-natal care ensures that the first signs of pre-eclampsia are detected and treated as early as possible. Preventive measures have been so successful that the infant mortality rate from eclampsia, formerly as high as 50 per cent, has been reduced to as low as four per cent.

ECT (ELECTROCONVULSIVE THERAPY)

A treatment sometimes used in severe cases of *depression*, also called electroplexy. The patient is injected with a muscle relaxant and a light *anaesthetic*; then an electric shock lasting from 0.1 to 0.5 of a second is administered via one or two saline-soaked electrodes placed on the temples. The shock, in the range of 70 to 150 volts at a very low amperage, causes the patient to lose consciousness and experience a convulsion.

ECT may be administered daily for a few days, or two or three times a week for two or three weeks in succession, depending upon each patient's requirements. It seems to have the effect of relieving severe depression, agitation or restlessness in some patients. However, the reasons for its effects are not precisely understood, and the improvement is not necessarily permanent.

ECT was first used in the treatment of psychiatric disorders

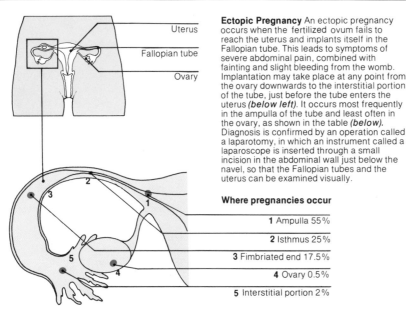

Uterus

Fallopian tube

Ovary

Ectopic Pregnancy An ectopic pregnancy occurs when the fertilized ovum fails to reach the uterus and implants itself in the Fallopian tube. This leads to symptoms of severe abdominal pain, combined with fainting and slight bleeding from the womb. Implantation may take place at any point from the ovary downwards to the interstitial portion of the tube, just before the tube enters the uterus *(below left)*. It occurs most frequently in the ampulla of the tube and least often in the ovary, as shown in the table *(below)*. Diagnosis is confirmed by an operation called a laparotomy, in which an instrument called a laparoscope is inserted through a small incision in the abdominal wall just below the navel, so that the Fallopian tubes and the uterus can be examined visually.

Where pregnancies occur

1 Ampulla	55%
2 Isthmus	25%
3 Fimbriated end	17.5%
4 Ovary	0.5%
5 Interstitial portion	2%

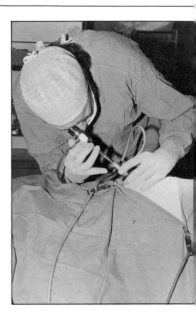

during the 1940s. Although it is reasonably safe, its success rate has proved fairly low. At first it was administered without muscle relaxants or anaesthesia, and the convulsions sometimes resulted in *fractures*. It frightens many patients; it has resulted in loss of memory and confusion, especially in older patients; and consequently it has been much criticized by psychiatrists and psychologists. However, it is still used as a last resort on patients suffering from severe depression or occasionally in the treatment of certain types of *schizophrenia*, and sometimes produces improvement.

ECTOPIC BEAT
Ectopic is a medical term meaning 'out of place'. An ectopic beat, or extrasystole, therefore, is a premature heartbeat, a form of *arrhythmia*.

The electrical impulse for the ectopic beat begins at an abnormal site, rather than at the sinoatrial node, as in normal heartbeats. Healthy people experience this as 'missing' a beat; the effect can be produced by excessive absorption of nicotine from smoking, or caffeine from coffee or tea. If multiple ectopic beats occur regularly, however, this may be a symptom of heart disease.

ECTOPIC PREGNANCY
An abnormal pregnancy in which the fertilized egg becomes implanted outside the womb, and begins to develop there. An ectopic pregnancy most commonly occurs at some point along the Fallopian tube. Very rarely, however, the ovum may implant in the abdominal cavity, or in the ovary.

The first symptom is usually a steadily worsening pain low in the

abdomen. A period may have been missed, but this does not always happen. A doctor will carry out a vaginal examination, and may be able to feel the developing embryo as an abnormal mass in the Fallopian tube or ovary, and the patient usually feels some pain when the doctor moves the cervix from side to side.

Usually the misplaced embryo is absorbed or aborted harmlessly. In more than 30 per cent of ectopic pregnancies, however, the problem is not diagnosed until the foetus has grown large enough to rupture the Fallopian tube. This may happen gradually, with symptoms of pain and bleeding, but it may occur suddenly, with the collapse of the patient due to massive *haemorrhage* into the abdomen. This is an emergency and requires urgent blood *transfusion*. In either type of tube rupture surgery is necessary and, usually, the removal of the affected ovarian tube and its contents—*see salpingectomy*.

ECZEMA—see Dermatitis

EEG (ELECTROENCEPHALOGRAM)— see Special Tests, p84

EFFUSION
The leaking of a fluid, such as pus, *serum*, blood or lymph, into a body cavity. Effusion occurs when an organ or tissue is inflamed or when it is congested with excess blood or tissue fluid.

In pleural effusion, for example, fluid escapes into the pleural cavity between the pleural membranes which surround the lungs. It often occurs in diseases such as *pleurisy*, *pneumonia*, *tuberculosis*, advanced

cirrhosis of the liver and *tumours of the lung*, while it can be a symptom of *heart failure*, and disorders of the kidney, such as *nephrotic syndrome*. Symptoms can include fever, sweating, coughing, laboured breathing, and loss of weight and appetite, but sometimes there are no symptoms at all. The condition is diagnosed by chest X-ray, and the fluid is sucked out and removed from the enlarged pleural space surrounding the lung with a hollow needle.

Pericardial effusion, the leakage of fluid from the pericardium, the membranous sac surrounding the heart, is a symptom of *pericarditis*.

Once effusion has been diagnosed, the doctor will investigate further to determine its cause. A sample of fluid is sent to a laboratory for culture and microscopy; endoscopy and biopsy may also be carried out—*see Special Tests, p84*.

EGO
The part of the personality that deals with the outside world, according to the theory of personality put forward by Sigmund Freud, the Austrian psychoanalyst. Freud claimed that, as a child grows, he or she learns to regulate the demands of the *id*, the basic part of the personality. The ego tries to satisfy the id's demands, but in such a way that they are socially acceptable.

Freud developed his theory as a model, through which he believed both normal and abnormal behaviour could be explained and understood. Many psychiatrists believe that delinquent teenagers may have been deprived of a suitable environment in which to make the all-important transition from id- to ego-controlled behaviour, and that they are therefore unable to recognize socially unacceptable behaviour.

ELECTROCARDIOGRAM—see Special Tests, p84

ELECTROCONVULSIVE THERAPY—see ECT

ELECTROENCEPHALOGRAM— see Special tests, p84

ELECTROLYTES

A number of important substances contained in solution in the fluids of the body—blood, lymph and tissue fluid. The major electrolytes are sodium, potassium, chlorine, calcium, magnesium, bicarbonate, phosphate and protein.

Each electrolyte circulates in the body in the form of electrically charged particles known as ions. Some ions—sodium, potassium, calcium and magnesium ions, for example—are charged positively. Others—the chlorine, bicarbonate, phosphate and sulphate ions—have a negative charge. The health of the body depends on the balance between the two charges, because they provide the necessary electrical environment for chemical reactions to take place. Sodium and potassium are particularly important, because nerve impulses are unable to move along nerve fibres without them.

When the balance between positive and negative ions is altered, or there is too much or too little of a particular electrolyte, the body's essential chemical reactions may be disrupted. This may happen as a result of *dehydration*, which itself may be caused by vomiting, diarrhoea or serious bleeding. The balance of electrolytes may also be disturbed by conditions that affect the body's chemistry, such as *acidosis*, or by a malfunction of a vital organ, such as the liver or one of the kidneys. The balance of electrolytes in the body can be determined by a blood test, in which the different ions are separated out and quantified—*see Special Tests, p84*.

ELEPHANTIASIS—see Worms

EMBOLISM

The sudden blocking of an artery by an embolus. This may be a clot of material such as air, fat, amniotic fluid, a foreign body, or a blood clot which has become detached from a thrombus—*see thrombosis*—and has travelled to another site, often to the brain or the lungs.

The most common form of embolism occurs in the pulmonary artery of the lung—*see pulmonary embolism*. This reduces the circulation of blood through the lungs, which in turn impairs the transfer of oxygen to the blood—*see The Respiratory System, p28*. As a result, the lung may collapse, the blood pressure fall rapidly and the rate of the heartbeat increase. The right side of the heart becomes overloaded and dilated and *necrosis*, or death of the tissues, may occur in the parts of the lung whose blood supply has been blocked. Emergency surgery may be required, but this is often either too late or unsuccessful in the case of large emboli, or usually unnecessary when the emboli are small and scattered.

Embolisms may lodge in other arteries of the body, causing *ischaemia*, or an inadequate supply of blood, and *gangrene* in the areas served by the artery whose blood

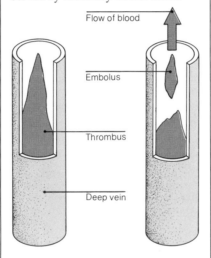

Embolism An embolus is a solid piece of material which circulates in the bloodstream until it becomes wedged in a blood vessel and blocks the flow of blood. It may be a globule of fat, a fragment of a tumour or an air bubble, but usually it is a small clot of blood which has broken away from a large thrombus, lodged in a deep vein.

supply has been blocked. Initial symptoms of this condition, called systemic embolism, are cramp-like pains in the affected area, while the limb becomes very painful, cold and white. If the condition is not treated and gangrene develops, amputation of the limb or part of the body affected will be the only possible form of treatment. Systemic embolism is often the result of a blood clot developing in the heart from disease of the mitral valve or after a heart attack, where a large clot has formed inside the left ventricle—*see myocardial infarction*.

Emboli may obstruct the renal arteries, which supply blood to the kidneys. This causes the affected kidney to release substances which result in a rise in blood pressure; eventually, the kidney will become completely ischaemic and cease to function. An embolism lodging in an artery in the brain may cause a stroke—*see cerebrovascular accident*.

Emboli are treated with *anticoagulants* or sometimes by an enzyme called streptokinase, which liquifies blood clots by destroying their cells. In the most serious cases, however, the embolism will be removed surgically, by an operation called an embolectomy. If the embolism is peripheral, in the femoral artery of the leg, for example, it may be removed with a balloon *catheter*. A thin tube is slipped past the embolism in the artery, a small balloon is blown up, and the tube and the balloon are carefully pulled from the artery, drawing the obstruction with them.

EMPHYSEMA

A condition in which air enters the tissues and distends them.

Pulmonary emphysema is a chronic and incurable disease of the lungs, in which the alveoli, or air sacs, are distended and their walls damaged, so that the surface area available for the exchange of oxygen and carbon dioxide is reduced. The condition is common among people who have smoked heavily over a period of many years, and people with chronic *bronchitis*, *asthma* and other lung disorders.

The main signs of emphysema are *dyspnoea*, or breathlessness, especially on exertion; a cough; and the production of sputum due to the associated bronchitis—emphysema is often seen at an advanced stage of chronic *bronchitis*. As the disease progresses, the chest becomes barrel-shaped due to the pressure of the over-inflated lungs, and respiratory failure may follow eventually. The right side of the heart may become strained—*see cor pulmonale*.

A doctor will usually auscultate, or listen to, the chest, and may have it X-rayed to check that no other condition is present. The patient may also be asked to blow into a peak flow meter to test lung function, or undergo lung function tests to assess lung capacity—*see Special Tests, p84*.

While pulmonary emphysema cannot be cured, the symptoms can be relieved and the progress of the disease delayed, especially by giving up smoking. *Antibiotics* may help to clear up any lung infection. Many patients keep oxygen cylinders permanently on hand at home in case of *dyspnoea*; *bronchodilators* may help to relieve spasm in the bronchi.

Subcutaneous, or surgical

emphysema, is a condition that often arises after a chest operation or a deep chest injury. Air penetrates the spaces in the tissues, making the flesh of the face, arms and chest and, in severe cases, the whole body, swell and crackle to the touch. The air is eventually absorbed and the condition clears up without treatment.

ENCEPHALIN
A group of chemicals made up of amino acids manufactured by the brain. They belong to the same group of natural chemicals as *endorphins*, all of which relieve pain in the same manner as opiate drugs such as morphine—*see opiates, narcotics*.

ENCEPHALITIS
An inflammation of the brain tissue that may be caused by *bacteria*, a *virus*, or *rickettsiae*.

A number of viruses can cause encephalitis, including the ones responsible for *rabies, yellow fever*, and *poliomyelitis*. The viral form of the condition is rare, but occasional outbreaks may be caused by *influenza* viruses, or by *herpes* viruses, either simplex or zoster (shingles). A type of encephalitis affecting mainly children and adolescents seems to be connected with the *measles* or *mumps* viruses. Encephalitis may also occur with *glandular fever*, but this is extremely rare.

Inflammation of the brain may also rarely occur after *chicken pox*, and *vaccination* for *smallpox*. Bacterial encephalitis may be combined with some degree of *meningitis* in the condition called meningo-encephalitis; in encephalomyelitis, the spinal cord is also affected. Brain abscesses may form when bacterial infection spreads from other sites, such as the middle ear. Encephalitis caused by the rickettsia organism is associated with *typhus fever*.

In encephalitis lethargica, or sleeping sickness, a tropical disease, the area of the brain that controls sleep is affected, causing drowsiness, fits and sometimes *coma*.

Encephalitis is a very rare complication of vaccination for *whooping cough*. It can cause permanent brain damage and disability in the very small number of children involved, and enormous anxiety and guilt for the parents. Children with a family history of fits or convulsions in close relations should not be vaccinated for whooping cough.

The symptoms of mild encephalitis are similar to those of other viral infections, and include *fever*, headache, loss of appetite and energy. Irritability, restlessness and drowsiness are symptoms of more severe cases in which there may also be general weakness, *diplopia*, or double vision, *dysphasia* and, eventually, coma.

Diagnosis is by means of blood tests, lumbar puncture, and sometimes an electroencephalogram (EEG) and brain scan—*see Special tests, p84*. The cerebrospinal fluid obtained by means of a lumbar puncture is examined for white cells and protein, and its pressure measured.

Encephalitis is often fatal in small children and old people, but young adults and the middle aged often recover completely, even from serious attacks.

Treatment is mainly to relieve symptoms, to enable the body's defences to overcome the infection. *Steroid* drugs may be given to help relieve inflammation of the brain. Special *cytotoxic drugs* may be used in the treatment of herpes simplex encephalitis. Bacterial encephalitis may respond to *antibiotic* treatment, while brain abscesses are drained surgically.

ENCEPHALOMYELITIS—see Encephalitis

ENDEMIC
A term used to describe a particular disease which occurs frequently in a specific area and has therefore been experienced by the majority of the area's population at some time or other. *Malaria* is a prime example of an endemic disease.

ENDOCARDITIS
Inflammation of the endocardium, the inner lining of the heart and valves. There are two forms of endocarditis—rheumatic endocarditis, caused by *rheumatic fever*; and infective endocarditis, caused by infection by *bacteria* or a *fungus*. Both forms damage the valves of the heart, so, though the disease itself can be treated successfully, a victim may need a surgical valve replacement later in life.

Rheumatic fever is the commonest cause of heart disease in people under the age of 30; it may attack the three layers of heart tissue, and commonly affects the mitral and aortic valves, causing them to become slightly deformed. This may prevent them from closing properly—*see valvular heart disease*.

As living standards have improved, the incidence of rheumatic fever (which is associated with poverty) and therefore of rheumatic endocarditis, has fallen.

Improved heart surgery has also helped to reduce the mortality rate from rheumatic endocarditis.

Infective endocarditis is caused by bacteria or, less commonly, fungi or other organisms. It often occurs in damaged heart valves; in about half these cases the valve damage has been caused by rheumatic endocarditis, while in a smaller proportion the defect is due to a congenital deformity, such as a ventricular septal defect—*see congenital heart defects*. Nowadays infective endocarditis tends to occur in people over 50 who suffered from rheumatic fever when they were young. Other people at risk include drug addicts, whose heart valves, though undamaged, are prone to the disease because of lowered resistance to infection—*see Abuses of the Body, p328*.

The infecting organisms are usually Streptococcal bacteria, which establish themselves in colonies on a heart valve, usually when there is infection elsewhere in the body. Small outgrowths, consisting of thousands of bacteria, fibrin and the minute platelet thrombi that form the bases of blood clots, are formed along the valve cusps. They may cause the valve to rupture.

The condition is always suspected in cases of fever or unusual tiredness in people with congenital heart defects or valvular heart disease. If the heart disease has not been diagnosed, however, the diagnosis of infective endocarditis can also be dangerously delayed, since its symptoms are common to many other illnesses. Other features of the disease are *anaemia* and an enlarged spleen—*see splenomegaly*. Small clumps of outgrowths may break off from the infected heart valves to form *emboli*; these may obstruct the arteries of the circulatory system, leading to *ischaemia* of the organ supplied by the blocked vessel.

Endocarditis is diagnosed largely by blood tests and cultures—*see Special Tests, p84*—to detect the presence of bacteria. Once the diagnosis is confirmed, the disease is treated with *antibiotics*. Sufferers who require dental treatment should tell their dentists about their condition. He or she will then prescribe a course of antibiotics as a preventive measure.

ENDOMETRIOSIS
A condition in which the endometrium, the tissue that lines the womb, somehow escapes from the womb to grow in other parts of the body, such as the ovaries, the Fallopian tubes, the vagina or the intestine. Each month these fragments of endometrial tissue

bleed, just as the lining of the uterus bleeds in menstruation; pelvic *adhesions* occur and large fibrous *cysts* may form. When the endometriosis occurs in the uterine muscle, the blood cannot escape as in menstruation, so it stagnates, and may form fibrous cysts in the uterine wall. This condition is called adenomyosis, and its cause is unknown.

Back pain, lasting throughout the menstrual period and worsening towards the end, is one of the few symptoms of endometriosis. Sometimes periods are irregular or very heavy and may be painful. Sexual intercourse can also cause pain. A few women with endometriosis are infertile. However, in 25 per cent of patients with endometriosis these symptoms are so mild as to be hardly noticeable, and may not appear at all.

If endometriosis is suspected, a doctor may recommend a D & C, or *dilatation and curettage*, for diagnostic purposes. Alternatively, the inside of the abdomen may be examined by means of laparoscopy; this is an exploratory endoscopic operation for which a general anaesthetic is necessary—*see Special Tests, p84*.

In mild cases of endometriosis the symptoms may be relieved with oestrogen or progesterone hormone preparations. In more severe cases, large dosages of hormones or other drugs may be given to stop periods altogether for several months in order to give the body time to disperse the abnormal tissue.

It may be necessary to operate to remove any cysts that have developed. In cases that do not respond to treatment, a *hysterectomy*, an operation to remove the womb, may have to be carried out.

ENDORPHINS

A group of chemicals manufactured in the brain. Endorphins are part of a group of neurotransmitters, chemicals that transmit impulses from one nerve to another across a synapse—*see The Nervous System, p32*. These chemicals were recently discovered in the search for a cure for *addiction* to *narcotics*, and belong to the same group of chemical compounds as the *encephalins*.

Chemicals in this group influence response to pain, and, through their action on the endocrine glands—*see The Endocrine System, p48*—are also believed to affect mood. They are derived from an amino acid found both in the brain and in the pituitary gland, and appear to have a role in regulating body heat, eating, learning, sexual behaviour, and the control of the heart and blood

vessels and respiration. Endorphins, with their pain-relieving properties, are thought to be released when acupuncture—*see Alternative Medicine, p305*—is used as an alternative to chemical *anaesthesia*.

ENEMA

A liquid introduced into the rectum through a tube or nozzle. Enemas are used to loosen faeces in the treatment of *constipation*, and as a means of administering drugs locally, as in the treatment of ulcerative *proctitis*. They are also a diagnostic tool: a barium enema, which contains barium sulphate, enables defects and disorders of the colon to show up on an X-ray—*see Special Tests, p84*.

An enema is also administered to patients in hospital to clear the bowel before intestinal surgery or endoscopy—*see Special Tests, p84*—and sometimes to women before, or in the early stages of, labour.

ENTERIC FEVERS—see Typhoid fevers

ENTERITIS

An inflammation of the small intestine that causes *diarrhoea*. There are two forms—infective enteritis and radiation enteritis.

Infective enteritis is caused by bacteria or by a virus. For example, clostridial enteritis, produced by clostridia bacteria, is a kind of *food poisoning* caused by eating contaminated food. An acute colicky pain and diarrhoea occur a few hours after eating the food. Many viruses live harmlessly in the human intestine, but viral enteritis is the result of infection by the more virulent strains.

Radiation enteritis is a less common form of the disease. It is caused by overexposure to X-rays, or exposure to radioactive substances. It occasionally occurs in patients undergoing *radiotherapy* for the treatment of *cancer*—*See also gastroenteritis*.

ENTERITIS, REGIONAL—see Crohn's disease

EPIDEMIC

A term used to describe a disease which spreads quickly to affect a large proportion of people. Certain types of *influenza*, for instance, occur in epidemics, while the Black Death in the Middle Ages—*see pasteurella pestis*—is also an example.

EPIDIDYMITIS

An inflammation of the epididymis, a tube connecting the testis, the organ in which sperm are manufactured, to the vas deferens,

the duct that carries them to the urethra for ejaculation. The inflammation is caused by bacterial infection that has spread into the sperm ducts from the bladder, or elsewhere in the urinary tract. *Escherichia coli, Streptococci,* Staphylococci, and Neisseria gonorrhoea are the bacteria most often responsible for epididymitis. Most cases of chronic, long-standing epididymitis are *tubercular* in origin.

The first signs of epididymitis are an ache in the groin and a swelling in one of the testicles. They are followed by swelling of the scrotum. Occasionally, it may be difficult to differentiate between epididymitis and *torsion* of the testicle, so it may be necessary to carry out an exploratory operation to confirm the diagnosis.

Treatment is with *antibiotics*.

EPIDURAL

Epidural anaesthesia is a common form of pain relief used during labour—*see Pregnancy and Birth, p60*—though it is opposed by the supporters of natural childbirth. It is administered by means of a catheter, or tube, which allows the anaesthetic to be placed in the epidural space around the spinal column.

An epidural is a very effective method of pain relief during prolonged labour. Nevertheless it has certain drawbacks. For instance, it occasionally takes effect only down one side of the body, and is sometimes completely ineffective. This is probably due to the faulty positioning of the catheter in the epidural space. Moreover, the use of an epidural tends to prolong labour because it relaxes the muscles of the pelvic floor; in normal circumstances, these form a gutter which helps the baby's head to rotate into the correct position for delivery. The lack of sensation in the pelvis also makes it more difficult for the mother to know when to push, as she cannot feel the contractions. The incidence of forceps deliveries is also higher in women who have babies under epidural anaesthesia for these reasons.

One distinct advantage of an epidural is that in cases of emergency the catheter, which remains in place throughout the birth, can be toppped up with more anaesthetic, and an immediate *caesarian section* carried out, rather than face the delay imposed by the administration of a general anaesthetic. With an epidural, the mother is conscious throughout this procedure and although she can feel some sensations of pulling, she cannot feel any pain and is able to hear the baby cry and hold it as soon as it is born.

EPILEPSY

An abnormality of brain function, in which electrical discharges of unusually high voltage occur periodically in the brain tissue, giving rise to one of several kinds of seizure or 'fit'. These recur at intervals varying from a few years to a few minutes; an isolated seizure is not diagnostic of epilepsy.

Epileptic seizures may arise from congenital brain damage, or they may be caused by *oedema*, a *tumour*, an *embolism*, or an injury to the brain. They may be brought about by a disease that affects the blood supply to the brain, such as *atherosclerosis*, by *syphilis* or *fever*, or may result from heavy drinking, excessive dosages of *narcotic*, and a sudden withdrawal from anticonvulsant drugs. Forms of epilepsy due to one of the above causes are known as symptomatic epilepsy. However, the majority of epileptics experience seizures with no apparent cause; this is described as idiopathic epilepsy.

There are as many different kinds of epilepsy as there are areas of the brain to be affected—*see The Nervous System, p32*—but they fall into two major categories. In partial or focal seizures, abnormal electrical discharges occur in a small area of the brain, which may be the site of a *lesion*. In generalized seizures, abnormal electrical activity spreads outward from a localized area to involve other parts of the brain.

The type of major seizure known as grand mal may begin with a cry or a shout, caused by the abrupt contraction of the muscles involved in respiration forcing air through the larynx. There may, however, be a prodromal phase, which lasts a variable length of time and warns the epileptic that an attack is imminent. Respiration ceases briefly, causing *cyanosis*, and since all the muscles in the body contract simultaneously, the patient falls to the ground unconscious. A person in an epileptic seizure may bite his or her tongue, foam at the mouth and urinate or defaecate involuntarily. This spasm, known as the tonic phase of the seizure, lasts for around 15 to 20 seconds. It gives way to a clonic phase, which lasts for 30 to 60 seconds, during which the muscles of the entire body contract rhythmically. The contractions die away gradually, and the patient may either recover consciousness rapidly or subside into a deep sleep. This type of seizure is also sometimes called a tonic-clonic fit.

After a grand mal seizure, a patient may pass through a stage of repetitive behaviour known as automatism. If this state of confusion and *disorientation* lasts for more than a few hours, it is known as epileptic twilight.

Any form of focal epilepsy may progress to a generalized seizure. Petit mal is a relatively mild form of generalized seizure, in which the patient passes through episodes in which consciousness is lost for a few seconds at a time. Petit mal may not be apparent since the sufferer rarely falls, but may suddenly stop what he or she is doing and stare vacantly for a few seconds, then recover consciousness and resume normal activity, perhaps with no awareness of the epileptic episode. This may happen many times a day, or only occasionally.

Epileptics do not always lose consciousness during a seizure. In temporal lobe epilepsy, so called because the abnormal electrical discharge is focused in the temporal lobe of the cerebral cortex *(p32)*, the seizure is characterized by a sense of disassociation, fear, *anxiety*, *déjà vu* *hallucinations*, or even disagreeable thoughts that seem to occur involuntarily. A temporal lobe seizure may not be apparent to an observer unless the patient begins to mutter, appears highly confused, or makes characteristic movements, such as smacking the lips, chewing or swallowing. Rarely, people with temporal lobe epilepsy exhibit wild and violent behaviour, known as epileptic furore, or a disturbance of consciousness known as epileptic fugue.

In a form of focal seizure known as Jacksonian epilepsy, in which the motor cortex of the brain is affected, a group of muscles in one part of the body—one side of the face, perhaps, or a hand—twitch involuntarily. This may subside after a minute or two, but it may spread to involve the whole side of the body.

Epilepsy is a disturbance of brain function, not a disease, and is dangerous only if the affected person falls and injures himself or herself in a grand mal attack, or experiences a series of grand mal seizures in rapid succession without regaining consciousness. This is known as status epilepticus, and, as a result of the continuing dysfunction of the respiratory muscles, can be fatal.

Many epileptics live normal lives, but epilepsy may be a serious social or physical handicap, not least because of ignorance of the disease on the part of others.

A patient who experiences fits several times a day may need strong medication, which may have unpleasant side-effects, such as drowsiness or lack of co-ordination, and may be unable to venture outdoors unaccompanied. Epileptics are forbidden by law to hold driving licences, unless they have not had a fit for at least three years, whether

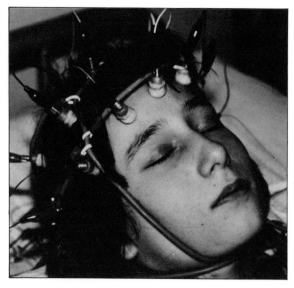

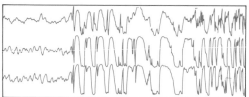

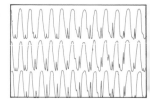

Epilepsy involves disturbances to the normal electrical activity of the brain. These can be detected by means of electroencephalography *(left)*, also known as EEG. A number of electrodes taped to the head monitor the fluctutations of electrical activity, and the EEG records them as a trace on a moving sheet of paper. In the trace *(below left)*, the normal brain waves on the left deteriorate, showing the disruption of electrical activity in a grand mal epileptic fit. The trace *(below right)* shows the characteristic peaks and spikes of a petit mal epileptic fit.

on or off medication.

An electroencephalograph (EEG) test—*see Special Tests, p84*—is used to diagnose epilepsy. The test reveals the presence of abnormal brain waves during a seizure, and perhaps during sleep or between seizures. Once the disorder is diagnosed, the brain may be X-rayed to detect the presence of a tumour or embolism, or other cause of the seizures. A person of normal intelligence with fits that occur only sporadically may need no medication at all, but may be advised to avoid potentially dangerous situations and sports, such as swimming in deep water or hang-gliding. Most patients, however, are treated with anti-convulsant drugs such as phenytoin, which is effective in preventing the spread of an electrical discharge; phenobarbitone, which suppresses focal activity; or sodium valproate, which is reliable in petit mal. Considerable experimentation may be necessary before the correct formula is found.

As our understanding of the brain and its biochemistry progresses, new drugs may become available for the treatment of epilepsy. Nevertheless, some of the more serious cases of epilepsy are untreatable. Once medication is begun, it may be continued for many years, even for life. Withdrawal has to be gradual, since sudden withdrawal from these drugs may precipitate further convulsions.

Some epileptics can learn how to control their attacks by recognizing the 'aura' or symptoms of an oncoming seizure, which may take the form of a sensation in some part of the body, or even a smell, and taking evasive action. This may be as simple as changing position or blinking. Simple measures are also helpful, such as avoiding alcohol and narcotic drugs, eating regularly and plentifully, avoiding stress and ensuring that sleep is adequate and regular.

Outsiders rarely know how to manage an epileptic experiencing a seizure, which can be violent, sudden and startling. It is best to leave well alone during the tonic and clonic phases of a grand mal seizure, unless the person is in a dangerous place, such as in the middle of a road, and has to be moved. Never try to open the mouth or force anything between the teeth, but as soon as the rhythmic muscular contractions appear to be over, turn the person on his or her side so that the tongue cannot block the air passages at the back of the throat—*see First Aid, p369*. If possible, leave the person to 'sleep off' the fit and to

awaken naturally. Remember, however, that on recovering consciousness an epileptic may be confused and disoriented, and may not be able to speak immediately. He or she is likely to have urinated and may need to wash and to change clothing. A grand mal seizure is more embarrassing than painful or debilitating and most epileptics recover completely after a few minutes. If, however, an epileptic seems confused or disoriented after a fit, it is better not to leave him or her unaccompanied.

EPISIOTOMY

A cut made at an angle to the line between the vagina and the anus during the second stage of childbirth—*see Pregnancy and Birth, p60*. The purpose of the cut is to enlarge the vaginal opening, to make delivery of the baby easier. It prevents severe tearing of the tissues when the baby's head is delivered, and preserves the tone of the muscles that make up the pelvic floor, helping to prevent subsequent *prolapse*, or downward displacement of the womb. However, in some countries, notably the United States and to a lesser extent in Britain, an episiotomy is performed almost routinely, whether it is actually needed or not.

Usually the incision is made as soon as the baby's head appears, and after a local anaesthetic has been given. However, in an emergency there may be no time for this; episiotomy may then be performed at the height of a contraction late in the second stage of labour when the perineum, the tissue between the anus and the urethra, is so stretched as to be paper thin. Immediately after delivery, the cut is sewn up. Healing is usually straightforward.

In recent years there has been some controversy about the advisability of performing episiotomies, because they are occasionally the cause of subsequent *dyspareunia*, or painful intercourse. It is claimed that a natural tear may heal better. Currently, various trials are in progress to assess the value of the procedure.

EPISTAXIS

Bleeding from the nose, from whatever cause. Nosebleeds commonly occur in feverish illnesses, blood-clotting disorders such as *haemophilia*, high blood pressure, or *hypertension*, and many other conditions. Among the many possible local causes are skull *fractures, sinusitis*, a foreign body in the nose, a blow and nose-picking.

If the blood is flowing from a blood vessel just inside the nose,

pinching the nostrils together may stop it by allowing a clot to form. When the nose has stopped bleeding, it is advisable not to blow it for a few hours.

If the bleeding is severe, hospital treatment may be necessary. One or both nostrils will be packed with a thin gauze bandage soaked in dilute adrenaline solution, and the gauze will be left in place for a day or more to give the vessel time to heal. If bleeding is recurrent, *cauterization* may be necessary—*see also First Aid, p369*.

ERB'S PALSY

Partial paralysis of the arm caused by excessive stretching of a baby's neck at birth. Erb's palsy is a common complication of *breech presentation*, in which the stretching causes injury to the brachial plexus, the network of nerves supplying the arm. The new-born baby's arm hangs loosely at its side, slightly rotated at the shoulder.

The injury is treated by bandaging the baby's wrist and pinning it to the mattress above the head. Later it is splinted in the correct position. Complete recovery usually takes several months.

ERYSIPELAS

A serious skin infection caused by Streptococcal bacteria. Erysipelas, a *notifiable disease*, usually affects the elderly. The disease begins suddenly, with inflammation and swelling of the skin, usually of the face and scalp, or the legs. Raised patches develop and spread rapidly. The swelling is caused by *oedema* of the *subcutaneous* tissue. The skin is initially red, and spots or vesicles may appear. Patients may also have a high temperature and feel generally ill.

Before the discovery of *antibiotics*, erysipelas was a very serious disease, since there was a danger that the bacteria might enter the bloodstream and cause blood poisoning. Today, penicillin is an effective treatment for the condition.

ERYTHEMA

A reddish discoloration of the skin, caused by dilation of superficial blood vessels, as in conditions ranging from blushing to sunburn.

Erythema marginatum or E. annulare, however, is a specific symptom of *rheumatic fever*, in which short-lived crescent-shaped eruptions, often with slightly raised edges, appear mainly on the trunk and around the junctions between trunk and limbs.

Erythema nodosum often occurs in patients with *sarcoidosis, tuberculosis, ulcerative colitis, streptococcal infections* and sometimes as a side-effect of *sulphonamide* drug therapy. It is a condition in which tender, raised red patches appear on the front of the shins and sometimes on the forearms and thighs. The patches are between two and three centimetres (about one inch) in diameter, and, after a few weeks, usually clear up, leaving no scars.

ERYTHROBLASTOSIS FOETALIS—See Haemolytic Disease of the Newborn

ESCHERICHIA COLI

Bacteria, found in soil and water and in human and animal intestines. Many strains of Escherichia coli live harmlessly in the intestine and play a part in the production of folic acid, an essential vitamin.

Some strains of these bacteria can cause infection, especially when they invade areas of the body outside the bowel. Escherichia coli play an important role in several diseases, including *appendicitis*, *cholecystitis*, *diverticulitis* and *peritonitis*, as well as *cystitis* and other infections of the urinary tract. Invasion by foreign strains of E. coli is thought to be the cause of 'holiday tummy'. In children it can cause infection of the urogenital tract, and *gastroenteritis*, which can be serious in infancy.

Escherichia coli also has an important role in biochemistry. Geneticists can manipulate the *genes* of certain strains to produce other substances, such as *interferon*.

EUPHORIA

An exaggerated feeling of happiness and optimism. A degree of euphoria is a natural reaction to an event of great emotional importance, such as the birth of a baby, or to hard-earned success, such as winning a marathon or passing a difficult examination. However, if the feeling is unfounded, euphoria may be a sign of a mental disorder, such as *mania*. Euphoria alternating with depression is a feature of *manic depressive psychosis*.

A temporary state of euphoria may be induced artificially by alcohol or drugs. It may also be a consequence of steroid therapy.

EUTHANASIA

The active ending of life prematurely, usually to relieve the suffering of a person who is terminally or incurably ill. In voluntary euthanasia, a person asks for his or her life to be taken. Euthanasia is not legal in any country in the world, although, in many countries, pressure groups are lobbying for its introduction. The

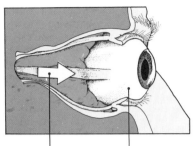

Accumulation of tissue pushes the eyeball forwards.

Eyeball protrudes from its socket.

decision to legalize euthanasia would involve enacting laws to define strictly the circumstances under which it could be carried out; this would be extremely difficult.

However illegal, euthanasia has probably always been practised to some degree by some members of the medical professions: on occasions, for example, they may fail to treat a respiratory infection in a badly deformed infant, and so bring about its early death. Similarly, larger and larger dosages of pain-killing opiates, such as morphine or heroin, may be prescribed to relieve the pain of terminal cancer, but may themselves cause death.

Some doctors and laypeople argue that, in individual cases, such practices are desirable. Others believe they place medical practitioners in an invidious moral and legal position. Many strongly oppose euthanasia, especially since, these days, the terminally ill should not experience agonizing pain. Advances in the control of pain by drugs and improvements in the care of the terminally ill mean that many such patients remain free from pain, conscious and cheerful until their deaths. Hospices, whose function is to care for the dying, place great emphasis on the proper relief of pain and other distressing symptoms— *see Coming to Terms with Death, p366.*

If *brain death* has been established, switching off a ventilator or life-support machine is not considered a form of euthanasia. In some countries, such as the United States, brain death must be certified and permission to disconnect the life-support system must be legally obtained before this can be done.

EXCHANGE TRANSFUSION

A form of blood transfusion used to provide infants suffering from severe *haemolytic disease of the newborn*

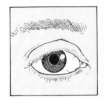

Normal eye

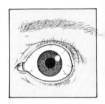

Exophthalmic eye

Exophtalmos is an eye condition which can be caused by a swelling of the eyeball socket as a result of disease, injury, or over-activity of the thyroid gland. Exopthalmic eyes protrude from their sockets, revealing an unusual amount of white eyeball around the iris *(right)*. The eyelids are drawn back and the bulging eyes look as though they are staring. The exopthalmic eyeball is pushed forwards by the accumulation of tissue behind it. Though disfiguring, the condition does not affect sight.

with new blood. It is necessary because the baby's red blood cells are destroyed by the disease, resulting in a high level of circulating bilirubin—a pigment contained in the bile secreted by the liver. This, in turn, may lead to a form of brain damage known as *kernicterus*.

An exchange transfusion is usually carried out in the first two days of life, but it can be carried out on the foetus in the uterus.

Blood is withdrawn from the infant's umbilical vein, using a syringe. The blood is ejected, without removing the syringe, and is replaced by the same amount of compatible blood. This process is repeated many times during the first week of life. An exchange transfusion ensures that damaged red blood cells and their breakdown products in the bloodstream are removed, while the volume of blood in the baby, and the number of red cells in circulation, remains constant.

EXOPHTHALMOS

The protrusion of one or both eyeballs so that the white of the eye can be seen all round the iris. As a result of disease or injury, swelling of the eyeball or socket may cause exophthalmos, but the usual cause is an overactivity of the thyroid gland known as *thyrotoxicosis*.

EXTROVERSION

A tendency to turn one's interests outward and to find pleasure in external things, rather than to be preoccupied with the self. The concept was formulated by the Swiss psychologist C.J. Jung, who divided extroverts into two types: those whose extroversion is brought about by their will, known as active extroverts; and those whose interests are attracted by outside things, independently of the will. These Jung called passive extroverts.

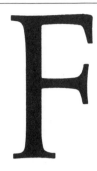

FAINTING—see Syncope

FEBRILE
A term meaning 'feverish'. Febrile *convulsions*, for example, are fits that occur during high fever.

FEVER
An abnormally high body temperature, the medical term for which is pyrexia. The normal body temperature recorded by a thermometer placed in the mouth is 37°C (98.6°F). However, a temperature of 1° or 2° above or below these figures may also be regarded as normal because body temperature fluctuates within a 24-hour period, and there are variations between individuals. The rectal temperature is 0.5° to 1° higher than the oral one, while the underarm temperature is approximately 1° lower—*see Home Nursing, p352.*

In adults, fever is usually a symptom of *bacterial* or *viral infection*. It may be caused by the effect of toxins, the poisonous chemicals released by bacterial activity, on the heat-regulating centres of the body. There are a number of other possible causes in adults, however. These include unusually hot weather, prolonged strenuous activity, injuries, or diseases affecting the body's heat-regulating mechanism, *dehydration*, and the breakdown of dead tissue within the body. Children may also become feverish for these reasons, but on occasions they may experience brief bouts of fever for no apparent cause. These latter episodes are rarely medically dangerous.

A fever may take a variety of courses. Its onset may be gradual or sudden, and the sufferer may be flushed, with a hot, dry skin, and suffer from *nausea, constipation* or *diarrhoea*. He or she may complain of headache and pains all over the body, and have no appetite. The temperature may remain at a constant high, fluctuate considerably, or remain normal throughout the day and rise in the evening. If it rises higher than 40.5°C (105°F), *delirium* may occur, and *convulsions* and *coma* may follow. If it is not treated, the fever may build in intensity to a crisis. At this point the organisms responsible for the illness begin to be destroyed by their own toxins, and the fever starts gradually to subside.

Fevers usually respond to treatment with *aspirin*, which reduces the temperature, and *antibiotics*. A feverish person often feels more comfortable if the skin is washed with tepid water—*see Home Nursing, p352.*

Many diseases in which a high temperature and delirium are major symptoms are called fevers. These include scarlet fever, or *scarlatina*; glandular fever, or *infectious mononucleosis*; *rheumatic fever* and *yellow fever*.

FIBRILLATION
An abnormal quivering of the heart muscle, due to the uncoordinated contraction of thousands of individual muscle fibres. When the heart muscle is fibrillating, or 'in fibrillation', it is not maintaining a steady, rhythmic contraction, and the circulation of the blood is affected as a result.

There are two main types of fibrillation, depending on the areas of heart muscle involved. These are atrial and ventricular fibrillation. In atrial fibrillation, rapid tremors in the muscle of the atria, or upper chambers of the heart, produce an irregular, uncoordinated beat. This may be caused by *rheumatic heart disease, thyrotoxicosis*, and myocardial *ischaemia* or *myocardial infarction*. It may also occur after major surgery to the chest.

Atrial fibrillation is not normally serious unless it is associated with heart failure. It is usually treated with drugs such as *digitalis*, but in serious cases the pattern of muscle contractions can be restored to normal by a process called *defibrillation*.

Ventricular fibrillation, in which the muscles of the ventricles are affected, is a more serious problem. It produces irregular, ineffective movements of the ventricles, which means that the ability of the heart to pump blood is impeded. Respiration ceases and the patient loses consciousness. It is usually caused by a heart attack, or *myocardial infarction*, when it is preceded by a series of abnormal or *ectopic* beats in a condition known as ventricular *tachycardia*. It can also be the result of an accident, such as an electric shock or drowning. If the patient is not to die within five minutes, emergency treatment is essential—*see defibrillation*. After recovery, special anti-arrhythmic drugs are given.

FIBROADENOMA
A *benign tumour* or *neoplasm* that arises in glandular tissue and contains both glandular and fibrous tissue. It is a type of *adenoma*, and is a common, but harmless, cause of *breast lumps*. Although the tumour may compress and push aside the surrounding tissues and structures as it grows, it does not damage them, and can be removed by surgery.

FIBROID
The lay term for a fibromyoma, or *benign tumour* of the muscular tissue of the uterus. Fibroids are so-called because they are composed mainly of fibrous tissue—'fibroid' means containing or resembling fibres. It is thought that they affect around five per cent of all women, and 20 per cent of women over the age of 40. Childless women, and those who have only had one child, appear to be particularly at risk. However, the reason why fibroids grow is not fully understood.

Fibroids usually form in the muscular wall of the womb, either singly or in multiples. They may grow inwards, when they are known as submucus myomata, or outwards into the uterine cavity, when they are called subserous pedunculated myomata. They grow very slowly over a period of years, but may become large enough to fill and eventually widen the uterus. As they grow, fibroids often degenerate into large fibrous *cysts*, harden into *calculi* or, very rarely, become *malignant*. Occasionally a pedunculated myoma may twist, cutting off its blood supply and becoming *gangrenous*.

Although fibroids cause no discomfort to many patients,

depending on their location in the uterus, they may cause vaginal *discharge* and menstrual disturbances, such as *dysmenorrhoea* or *menorrhagia*—heavy periods. Fibroids may also press on the bladder, causing discomfort and a frequent desire to urinate, or on the rectum, causing *back pain* and *constipation*. If a submucus myoma becomes infected, it may cause a continuous bloody discharge. This may lead to *anaemia*. Fibroids may also be responsible for *infertility*, since they often cause the uterus to become distorted. This inhibits the implantation of the fertilized ovum in the uterine wall.

Patients complaining of vaginal discharge, dysmenorrhoea, menorrhagia or an enlarged uterus, together with frequency of urination and back pain, are routinely examined for fibroids. On medical examination, a doctor may be able to feel a large fibroid, but a diagnostic *D & C* may be necessary to detect small and submucus varieties.

Fibroids that cause no discomfort are often left untreated, but, if their growth accelerates, or if they begin to cause symptoms, an operation called a *myomectomy* may be carried out to remove them. Occasionally fibroids may be so large or so numerous that a *hysterectomy* may be necessary.

FIBROSING ALVEOLITIS—see Alveolitis

FIBROSIS

A reaction which takes place in damaged tissues, and usually involves some degree of scarring and consequent loss of normal function. Though fibrosis can be part of the process of healing, it can also be caused by disease, as in the *pneumoconioses*.

FIBROSITIS

A painful *inflammation* in the body's connective tissue—*see Bone and Muscle, p16*. Fibrositis, also called muscular rheumatism, usually affects the muscles of the back and trunk, causing a pain that comes and goes. It may be a symptom of a recognized disease or condition, such as *sciatica*, but in most cases its origin is not known. The pains may be soothed by the use of proprietary linaments.

Many doctors believe that, in the majority of cases in which intermittent pains are attributed to fibrositis, the pains are, in fact, caused by a series of muscular spasms. An alternative theory is that they are the result of minor displacements of the vertebrae, the bones of the spine, which pinch the

nerves that branch from the spinal cord. These may be caused by muscular tension or poor posture.

FILIARIASIS—see Worms

FISSURE

A split in the skin or the mucous membrane lining one of the openings of the body. The most common sites for a fissure are the corner of the mouth and the anus. A mouth fissure, which may be caused by exposure to cold air, is aggravated by constant contact with saliva, which carries *bacteria* into the split. It is treated with antiseptic ointments.

An anal fissure occurs between the skin and the mucous membrane and is usually caused by the passage of hard *faeces*, as in *constipation*. However, sometimes anal fissures are associated with *Crohn's disease*. This tears the membrane, allowing *bacteria* to enter into the wound. As a result, bowel movements are painful and are accompanied by a little bleeding.

The fissure should be kept as clean as possible, and a mild laxative used. This will soften the faeces and prevent the wound from reopening. Anal fissures usually heal in a few days without further treatment, but if they are serious, or persistent, stretching the anal canal under general anaesthetic may be necessary.

FISTULA

An abnormal channel connecting two body cavities, or linking a cavity with the surface of the body. A fistula may result from infection, *abscess* formation, or from an injury—a knife wound, for instance. Sometimes a surgeon may create a temporary, artificial fistula deliberately—between the bladder and the skin, for example, or between the colon and the skin— *see colostomy*.

Most fistulae heal quickly of their own accord, as long as they are kept clean and free from contamination by bacteria. In the case of an anal fistula, however, this is impossible, and minor surgery is required to close off the channel.

Occasionally, fistulae are congenital, that is, they are present at birth. The two most common types are a tracheo-oesophageal-fistula, in which the windpipe and the oesophagus are connected, and a recto-vaginal fistula, in which the rectum and vagina are linked. Such fistulae are closed surgically shortly after birth, and usually heal quickly.

FIT—see Convulsion

FLATULENCE

The distension of the stomach and intestines by gas. The gas may come from two sources—inhaled air and *bacterial* activity.

Small amounts of air are taken into the body while swallowing food, drink or saliva. Some of this is expelled by belching, but the rest passes into the intestine, where it is joined by gas produced by the action of bacteria on food residues. Part of the gas is absorbed, but the remainder is expelled through the rectum.

Flatulence is an embarrassing problem, but it is usually harmless. If flatulence is excessive, the doctor may advise that the sufferer avoids foods that tend to give rise to the condition, such as onions and beans. He or she may also prescribe a charcoal-based drug. This is sometimes effective, though it is not known how it works.

On occasions, however, flatulence is a symptom of a more serious disorder, especially when it is associated with abdominal pain and indigestion. Such disorders include: *hiatus hernia*, *dyspepsia*, a peptic *ulcer*, *irritable bowel syndrome* and *Crohn's disease*. Flatulence may also be a sign of anxiety or *depression*, because many people who suffer from these problems tend to swallow air frequently.

FOETAL DISTRESS SYNDROME

The collective term used to describe a number of conditions, such as foetal *hypoxia*, *tachycardia*, and *bradycardia*, that can affect the foetus while still in the womb. The prime cause for them is an insufficient supply of oxygen from the mother; the foetus depends on this for its energy requirements, since, without it, the conversion of glycogen cannot take place—*see Metabolism, p44*. The oxygen shortfall can be caused by illnesses, such as *anaemia*, in the mother, and also by foetal problems within the womb, such as an entanglement of the umbilical cord.

Symptoms of foetal distress can be detected by electronic monitoring before or during birth. The usual treatment is to deliver the baby as rapidly as possible by *caesarian section* or forceps.

FOLIC ACID DEFICIENCY—see Anaemia

FLUKES—see Worms

FOOD ALLERGY

A term often used loosely to describe a wide range of reactions to food, not all of which are true allergies. Most doctors remain sceptical about the problem, which is unfortunate, since there are indeed some patients who react severely to food, and it can be difficult for them to find doctors prepared to help them.

Some people have an immediate reaction to food, which is usually easy to spot. Their lips swell, their mouth and tongue tingle, and blister-like swellings develop inside the cheeks; there may also be asthma and nettle rash. All these symptoms develop within ten minutes of eating the offending food. More difficult to assess are the claims that have been made for delayed reactions of various kinds. Undoubtedly much of this is due to suggestion: in a recent survey, in which over 18,000 people took part, over 4,000 claimed to experience adverse reactions of one kind or another to foods, food additives, or aspirin. Reactions to food additives were reported by 7.4 per cent of the responders, but when they were tested objectively, only three people were found to be affected.

It is difficult to exclude psychological factors in cases of alleged food allergies. To do so, the patient must be unaware of what he or she is eating or drinking; in other words, the test must be single-blind or, in difficult cases, double-blind. Many of the symptoms attributed by patients to food allergy (tingling, muscle weakness, faintness, palpitations, and chest pain) are typical of the hyperventilation syndrome. There are no fool-proof tests for food allergy; those commonly used are skin tests and the radioallergosorbent test (RAST), but neither is entirely satisfactory.

Some researchers, mainly in the USA, have claimed that food and food additives—especially tartrazine, but also sugar and yeast—cause hyperactivity in children. However, double-blind studies have usually produced largely or wholly negative results. This is important, because some parents have mistakenly believed that their children were responding adversely to various foods and have consequently restricted their diet to such an extent that they have developed severe deficiencies of vitamins and other essential substances.

The foods that most often cause symptoms include milk, eggs, wheat, fish and shellfish, nuts chocolate, and coffee. Pork is often cited, but it is not so much the meat that causes the problem as the substances like papain, a tenderizer, that are added to it.

Most so-called food allergies that are not caused psychologically are really due to direct pharmacological or similar effects. Symptoms affecting the stomach and intestines are not usually due to food allergy. However, some patients have enzyme deficiencies that interfere with digestion and can cause intolerance to certain foods; for example, 80 per cent of Africans and Asians lack the enzyme needed to digest milk sugar. If they drink milk, they experience bloating and diarrhoea. Some patients with *irritable bowel syndrome* react adversely to certain foods, especially those listed above, but this is not a true allergy; the bloating and discomfort experienced by such people is probably due to the action of bacteria in the intestine, which ferment the food and produce gas and acid.

Symptoms can occur outside the intestine. Some patients with migraine react to chocolate and cheese. Asthmatics can be made worse by wine or foods containing sulphur dioxide, added as a preservative. 40 per cent of members of some Asian communities are intolerant of alcohol. Some children with eczema are made worse by eggs, citrus fruit, wheat, and milk. In rare cases, certain kidney problems are caused by food allergy, and a few patients find that their joints hurt and are painful after eating certain foods; however, in spite of the claims made by some, it is rare for arthritis to be made worse by food.

Treatment clearly depends on eliminating the offending food from the diet, but this is sometimes difficult if it is one that is widely used. If the diet has to be severely restricted, supplements of calcium and vitamins may be needed. Anti-allergy drugs seldom help much. Fortunately food allergies are not always permanent; sometimes it becomes possible to eat the offending food again, if it is avoided for a few months.

FOOD POISONING

A disorder of the digestive system, which may have one of a number of causes. In general, the symptoms of food poisoning are abdominal pain, *fever, diarrhoea* and *vomiting.* Depending on the cause, these symptoms may be mild or extremely serious, and sometimes fatal. It is essential, therefore, that anyone suffering from any serious form of food poisoning receives immediate medical attention—*see First Aid, p369.* If possible, a specimen of the food that has been eaten should be saved for analysis, so that doctors can identify the causative agent.

Food poisoning is most commonly caused by eating food contaminated with *bacteria,* in which case it is known as infective *gastroenteritis.* The most common bacterium is Salmonella, although there are others, such as Campylobacter coli which mainly affects children. Salmonella bacteria are found in a wide range of foods—from frozen poultry that has been incorrectly thawed and cooked, or handled by people who have not washed their hands after defaecation, to shellfish caught in sewage-polluted waters. Symptoms such as pain, *fever, diarrhoea* and *vomiting* appear within 48 hours of eating the infected food and may last for several days. The doctor will probably advise a sufferer to rest and drink plenty of fluids, and may prescribe drugs to control the diarrhoea and vomiting.

Similar symptoms are caused by the toxins, or poisonous chemicals, which are produced by certain bacteria. Two varieties of bacteria in particular, called Staphylococcus aureus and Clostridium welchii, grow in uncooked food and excrete toxins into it. While cooking kills the bacteria, it does not necessarily destroy the toxins. Poorly cooked food, or food left warm for a few hours and then partially reheated, is particularly likely to contain such toxins—*see Health and Hygiene, p334.* The symptoms and treatment of this type of food poisoning are the same as those for bacterial food poisoning.

Poisoning from bacterial toxins is rarely serious. An exception to this, however, is the extremely dangerous condition called botulism, caused by the toxin from Clostridium botulinum. This bacterium contaminates badly preserved food and multiplies in the absence of air, so tins, cans or products that have been vacuum sealed can all be affected. Cooking can destroy the toxin, but tinned foods that have been pre-cooked, such as corned beef, are not usually heated before they are eaten. Even tiny amounts of the toxin can paralyze the nervous system and cause death.

Food may also be contaminated by chemicals. These may vary from pesticides, insecticides and preservatives to impurities introduced by accident during food-processing. Certain fungi, roots, berries and leaves may also cause food-poisoning. Examples include the mushrooms Amanita muscaria and Amanita phalloides, the seeds of the laburnum tree, the berries of deadly nightshade and the foxglove leaves. Several hours may elapse before the onset of symptoms, which may include stomach pains, bloody diarrhoea and vomiting. Depending on the precise nature of the chemical or plant, the condition

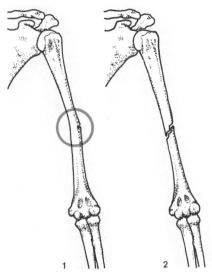
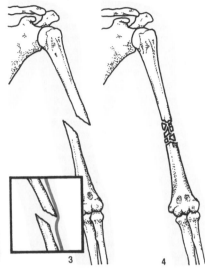
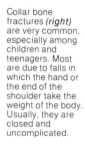
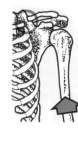

Collar bone fractures *(right)* are very common, especially among children and teenagers. Most are due to falls in which the hand or the end of the shoulder take the weight of the body. Usually, they are closed and uncomplicated.

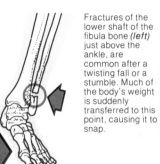

Fractures of the lower shaft of the fibula bone *(left)* just above the ankle, are common after a twisting fall or a stumble. Much of the body's weight is suddenly transferred to this point, causing it to snap.

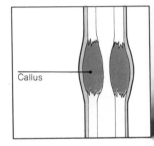

Fracture Bones may be fractured in a variety of ways. In a greenstick fracture, **1**, the bone is partially fractured on only one side. Flexible and soft bones are prone to this type of fracture, which is particularly common in children. In a closed fracture, **2**, the bone is completely broken but the skin is not punctured. In a compound fracture, **3**, the skin is punctured and the wound exposed to infection. When adjacent organs and blood vessels are damaged by the bone, it is called a complicated fracture *(inset)*. In a comminuted fracture, **4**, the bone is shattered or broken in several places.

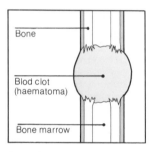
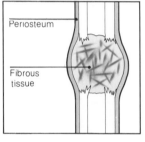
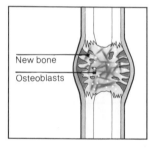

Bone
Blod clot (haematoma)
Bone marrow

Periosteum
Fibrous tissue

New bone
Osteoblasts

Callus

Bone Healing 1. When a bone breaks there is bleeding from the broken ends, giving rise to a collection of blood known as a haematoma.

2. This blood clots, and gradually fibrous tissue grows across it. The blood is gradually absorbed. Periosteum from around the outside of the bone grows round the haematoma to bridge the gap between the broken ends of bone.

3. Osteoblast cells, which form bone, grow out from the periosteum to lay down new bone around the fracture. This new bone is called callus.

4. When healing is complete the bone is joined as strongly as it was before. The callus gradually becomes smaller, and may disappear completely.

may be fatal. Treatment is therefore required immediately.

In all cases of food-poisoning that cause vomiting and diarrhoea, there is a danger of *dehydration*. This condition can be extremely dangerous for children and babies. It is essential, therefore, that sufferers from food poisoning drink plenty of liquid. They should also abstain from food for 24 hours, taking only drugs that have been prescribed by a doctor.

FORCEPS
Pincers of various shapes and sizes designed to perform specific tasks during surgical operations. Delivery forceps are used when complications arise during childbirth. They consist

of two wide blunt blades designed to fit safely but firmly around the infant's head—see *Pregnancy and Birth, p60.*

FRACTURE
A break in a bone that results in pain, bruising, swelling and, occasionally, deformity. In healthy young people, fractures are normally the result of an injury, the most common sites being the clavicle, or collar bone, the wrist and the ankle—see *Bone and Muscle, p16.* However, the bones of elderly people are often weak and brittle as a result of *osteoporosis*—a condition in which bone substance is lost. As a result, they tend to fracture easily, in a light fall, or even without apparent

cause. In old people, the neck of the femur, or thigh bone, at the hip is especially vulnerable.

There are a number of different types of fracture. In a simple, or closed, fracture the break is clean and the ends of the bone do not penetrate the overlying skin. If the skin is punctured, the fracture is said to be compound, or open. This type of fracture may become infected, unless *antibiotics* are given as a preventive measure.

If the bone splinters, the fracture is said to be comminuted, while in an impacted fracture one piece of bone is driven into another. When a broken bone damages neighbouring arteries, nerves or organs, the fracture is said to be complicated.

The bones of young children are

more flexible than those of adults, and instead of snapping completely they may bend or split on one side only, in the same way as a green twig. These types of breaks are known as greenstick fractures.

In a compound or open fracture, bone is often clearly visible, but in other types of fracture the only sign may be an area of discoloration and swelling in the skin over the break. Normally, the area is extremely painful and tender to the touch. It is advisable for anyone who has had a bad fall or blow to consult a doctor, who will arrange for an X-ray examination of the area. This will show whether the bone is fractured.

If a fracture is detected on the X-ray, a doctor will place the broken ends of the bone together, returning the bone to its original shape. This process is known as reduction, and may be done under local or general anaesthetic, depending on the site and severity of the break. To assist healing, the broken pieces are held firmly in place by a plaster cast, or a splint. In serious comminuted fractures the pieces of bone may also be held together by metal pins.

If the fracture is in an area of powerful muscular development, such as the thigh, traction may be necessary. This is because the muscles tend to pull at the ends of bone, pulling them together. If this problem is ignored, the ends of bone may eventually overlap, shortening the limb. In traction, a system of weights and pulleys is used to counteract the pull of the muscles.

The rate at which the fracture heals, and the length of time that the broken bone is immobilized in a plaster, depends on the site of the fracture and also on age: the older the victim the longer the fracture takes to heal. In most fractures, once the plaster has been removed, the site of the break is undetectable. However, the muscles often waste while they are confined within the cast, and a course of *physiotherapy* may be necessary to restore them to their former size and strength.

FRIGIDITY
A loss of sexual desire and an inability to enjoy sexual stimulation. The term is usually applied to women, and tends to mean a general lack of sexual appetite; in men, frigidity is generally referred to as *impotence*. The reasons for frigidity may be one or more of the following: boredom, loss of desire for a partner, lack of orgasm, fear of rejection or of pregnancy, or feelings of shame and guilt. In addition, alcohol and sleeping pills both depress the central nervous system and hence reduce desire.

The psychological problems may stem from *traumas*, such as the painful loss of virginity, childbirth, rape and gynaecological surgery. Stress and tiredness also play an important role in upsetting mental and physical well-being, as does chronic and painful illness.

Frigidity can be, and frequently is, treated successfully. The problem often becomes worse if sufferers worry about it; this vicious circle can often be broken by the advice of a doctor or a course of psychosexual therapy—*see Sex and Contraception, p338.*

FROSTBITE
Damage to the skin and underlying tissues due to prolonged exposure to temperatures below freezing point. In response to the cold, blood vessels near the skin contract, cutting off the supply of blood to the surface tissues. Ice crystals may also form in the cells, damaging the cell membrane and causing cell death.

Prompt action is necessary to prevent this. The first sign of frostbite is an intense pain in the affected area—most commonly the hands, feet, ears and nose—followed by numbness, with the skin turning hard and pale.

As soon as these signs are noticed, the frostbitten parts should be immersed in warm water and gently covered with a clean dressing. *Antibiotics* may be necessary to prevent infection, for a frostbitten area has no supply of blood and thus no defence against bacteria.

If frostbite is treated quickly, there are usually no permanent effects. However, if infection is allowed to set in, *gangrene* may develop, and it may become necessary to amputate the affected part.

FROZEN SHOULDER
A disorder in which the shoulder becomes painful and stiff. There can be many causes of shoulder pain, some of which are completely outside the shoulder, but frozen shoulder denotes a disease affecting the shoulder itself. It is common; about one per cent of referrals to orthopaedic surgeons are for this condition. This is without taking account of the many patients who are seen by their general practioner and never come to hospital.

The majority of patients are women, and most are in the 50 to 70 age group. The condition may begin suddenly, or there may be a preliminary phase of slight shoulder ache. At the onset of the condition proper, the pain can be very severe, requiring the use of strong analgesics to control it. There is loss of movement at the shoulder joint, which may be complete – hence the term frozen shoulder, though the joint is not cold, but hot. Certain movements are particularly affected; thus, the patient may be unable to move the arm away from the body, while putting the hand behind the back is also difficult. However, even when all movement between the humerus and the scapula is lost, there is still movement between the scapula and the chest wall, so the disability is less than it would be otherwise.

After some time, usually several months, the pain gradually diminishes, but the stiffness persists for longer. Eventually that, too, may disappear to give full recovery; the whole process takes from one to two years. However, recovery of movement is sometimes incomplete, though the patient may not be aware of this, while in some cases the pain lasts much longer.

There is no single satisfactory treatment for frozen shoulder. At least 14 different kinds of treatment have been tried, ranging from massage to radiotherapy, but few of them have been properly evaluated by scientific trials. Probably the commonest methods in use at present are local injection of corticosteroids into the joint and manipulation under anaesthesia. Both of these work well on occasion, and so does acupuncture, but in most of the trials that have been done heat plus physiotherapy were as good, or almost as good, as any of the other treatments. It seems that not enough is known about the condition to say which patients are suited to which treatment.

FRUCTOSURIA—see Metabolic disorders

FUNNEL CHEST
A congenital deformity, also called pectus excavatum, in which the sternum, or breast bone, is depressed backwards towards the spine and the ribs are curved inwards. As a result, the heart is pushed to the left and may be compressed between the sternum and the spine. This may reduce the capacity of the lungs, but rarely causes any reduction in efficiency of the heart.

The condition does not require treatment unless it is extremely serious, when the deformity may be repaired by surgery. The operation is occasionally performed for cosmetic reasons.

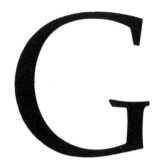

GALACTORRHOEA
The persistent abnormal secretion of milk from the breast. The term is used to describe continuation of secretion after breast feeding has finished, an excessive flow of milk during breast feeding, or secretion of milk in women who are not pregnant. The cause is usually over-production of prolactin—the hormone that stimulates milk production—by the pituitary gland (p48). In this case, drugs may be prescribed to correct the hormonal imbalance. It is often accompanied by an absence of menstruation. Very rarely galactorrhoea occurs in men, when it may also be associated with impotence and infertility.

GALACTOSAEMIA
A very rare inherited disorder in which a baby is unable to convert galactose, a sugar which is made in the body from lactose—the sugar found in both breast and cow's milk—to glucose, the sugar the body uses as fuel. The reason for this failure is the lack of the appropriate enzyme in the baby's liver. The galactose builds up in the body; the baby becomes lethargic and jaundiced and suffers from persistent vomiting which may itself be fatal. If the condition is not treated, a surviving baby's growth will be stunted and it will become mentally retarded.

Treatment consists of giving special galactose-free milk, and later avoiding milk products altogether.

GALLSTONES
Hard, insoluble stones—see calculi—that may collect in the gall bladder. Composed of bile pigments, cholesterol and calcium salts, they may be large and smooth, small and sharp, single or multiple. Gallstones occur most frequently in middle-aged women and older people of both sexes who have a high level of cholesterol in their blood, but why they develop is not fully understood.

Sometimes gallstones travel along the bile duct, carried by the bile that is stored in the gall bladder. If they get stuck in the duct, intense pain builds up in the upper right abdomen and sometimes between the shoulder blades. This is often followed by nausea and vomiting, probably due to the tube contracting in an effort to get rid of the stone. The problem is known as biliary colic. Infection or inflammation of the gall bladder and jaundice are possible complications, and the organ's removal may be necessary by cholecystectomy.

GAMMA GLOBULIN
A protein found in the blood which plays an important role in the body's natural defence system—see Natural Defences Against Disease, p52. Because it can confer immunity from disease, it is also known as immunoglobulin. Unlike many blood proteins, which are formed in the liver, gamma globulin is made by the lymphatic system.

Gamma globulin is particularly useful in helping to deal with some diseases because it can be taken from a person who is immune to a disease and used to confer temporary immunity on another. Although they are not infallible, gamma globulin injections have been used to combat infectious hepatitis, measles, poliomyelitis and tetanus.

Special injections of gamma globulin are usually administered to Rhesus negative mothers who have just given birth to a child with a rhesus positive blood group—see haemolytic disease of the newborn—to prevent a reaction in the mother's blood to the incompatible blood cells passed to her from the baby through the placenta during birth. This can affect subsequent babies.

GANGRENE
Decay and eventual death of part of the body's tissue, due to prolonged loss of blood supply. It may be triggered by a number of causes. These include a crushing injury, frostbite, burns, a blood clot, or circulatory problems, which in turn

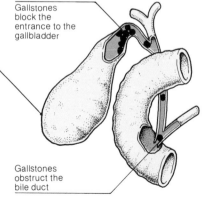

Gallstones The gallbladder *(left)* is the storehouse of bile, a liquid rich in fatty substances, such as cholesterol, and bilirubin which is a breakdown product of haemoglobin. A gallstone is a hard crystal that starts as a tiny solid particle and grows as the substances in the bile crystallize around it. Gallstones are harmless if they remain in the gallbladder or pass unhindered into the duodenum.

Gallstones block the entrance to the gallbladder

Gallstones obstruct the bile duct

Gallstones may grow large and smooth, as shown in the X-ray *(left)*. When they block the entrance to the gall-bladder or obstruct the bile duct leading to the duodenum, they cause severe pain and nausea. If the obstruction persists, the gall-bladder may have to be removed and the bile duct cleared.

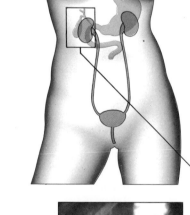

Spine

Gallstones

Gallbladder

can be caused by *diabetes mellitus, atherosclerosis,* or excessive smoking.

Gangrene is either dry or moist. Dry gangrene is simply the drying out or dehydration of tissue, which may take months to develop, and affects elderly people in particular. Moist gangrene typically develops after a crushing injury, when bacteria have infected tissue which cannot be reached by the body's defence mechanisms.

Gas gangrene develops after infection by one of the Clostridia family of soil bacteria, which then manufactures gas in the infected part. This was responsible for many deaths during World War I.

Gangrene can sometimes be prevented from spreading by means of *antibiotics,* but it usually requires the amputation of the affected limb.

GARDNERELLA VAGINALIS

An organism commonly present in the vagina of women of child-bearing age. It sometimes causes a whitish, slightly offensive discharge, and some degree of *vaginitis,* or inflammation of the vagina. Apart from the discomfort it causes, it is not a serious infection. If the discharge or soreness becomes excessive, it can be treated with metronidazole, an antimicrobial drug taken in tablet form. It is not thought to cause symptoms in men.

GARGOYLISM—see Lipid storage disease

GASTRECTOMY

The surgical removal of the stomach. In a total gastrectomy, the entire stomach may be removed; this may be necessary in cases of *stomach cancer,* for instance. A loop of intestine, usually the duodenum, is then joined to the end of the oesophagus to preserve the continuity of the gastrointestinal tract. Part of the stomach may be removed in an operation called a partial gastrectomy. This is normally done as a treatment for a serious gastric *ulcer.*

After a total gastrectomy, patients should eat small quantities of food fairly frequently, and will need frequent vitamin B12 injections, as they will have lost their capacity to absorb this vitamin. They may also have to face a collection of symptoms known collectively as dumping syndrome after the operation. Following a meal, the sufferer feels weak, faint, and may become pale and sweat. The symptoms are caused by the rapid emptying of the stomach and a consequential fall in the blood sugar level and the drawing of fluid into the intestine from the blood. They

are brought on by excessive carbohydrate intake and can last for a minimum of half an hour. Reducing the carbohydrate intake may relieve the symptoms.

GASTRIC ULCER—see ulcer

GASTRITIS

An inflammation of the mucous membrane that lines the stomach. Gastritis is often the result of drinking, smoking or eating to excess. It may also be due to taking drugs such as aspirin. In these cases, the symptoms resemble those of *indigestion.* A period of moderation or abstinence should clear up any symptoms. However, if symptoms such as pain or vomiting continue after 24 hours, a doctor should be consulted. Habitually heavy drinkers and smokers run the risk of serious erosion of the stomach lining and of developing an *ulcer.*

GASTROENTERITIS

An inflammation of the stomach and intestines which leads to *vomiting* and *diarrhoea.* Gastroenteritis is caused by a virus. An attack usually lasts for a few days, with or without treatment, during which it is best not to eat anything—in any case, vomiting and loss of appetite make it difficult to do so.

An effort should be made to drink plenty of water to prevent *dehydration.* In severe cases, anti-emetic and anti-diarrhoea drugs can be prescribed.

Gastroenteritis can also be caused by *food poisoning,* where the organisms responsible may be bacteria or protozoa such as those that cause *amoebiasis* or *giardiasis.* See also *enteritis* and *Crohn's disease.*

GAUCHER'S DISEASE—see Lipid storage disease

GENDER IDENTITY—see Transsexualism

GENES

The fundamental units of inheritance, a complete set of which are found in the *chromosomes* of every cell in the body. Each gene is made of DNA (deoxyribonucleic acid) and is located in the same place on each chromosome.

Although each cell in the body has a complete set of genes, which regulate the workings of the cells and the body as a whole, each cell is programmed to play a specific role, and only those genes that contribute to this role are used in that cell.

No two human beings are identical, except for identical twins, who have developed from the same

fertilized egg, and therefore have exactly the same chromosomes and the same genes.

Every characteristic of an individual, such as hair colour, eye colour or blood group, is governed by at least one pair of genes. These genes, located opposite each other on a pair of chromosomes, are inherited, one from each parent. The characteristic to be inherited often depends upon one of these two genes being dominant and the other recessive. The gene for brown eyes, for example, is dominant, while the gene for blue eyes is recessive; this means that a person with one gene for brown eyes and one for blue eyes will be brown-eyed. Only when both chromosomes carry the genes for blue eyes will blue eyes be the result. Two brown-eyed parents can give birth to a blue-eyed child only if both carry the gene for blue eyes, and if these genes happen to combine in the right way at the moment of conception of the child.

Other characteristics carried by recessive genes include *albinism, cystic fibrosis* and *galactosaemia.* In a few diseases, such as *Huntington's chorea,* the gene responsible for the disease is dominant. In this case anyone who inherits the gene will contract the disease. Some recessive genes are carried on the sex chromosomes. For example, *haemophilia,* colour blindness, and *Christmas disease* are carried on the X chromosome. Men are far more likely to suffer from these conditions, because they have only one X chromosome. Since women have two X chromosomes, a gene for such a disease would be dominated by a healthy gene. The chances of a woman having the gene on both her X chromosomes are very small; however, women in a family where the disease appears are often carriers. (Queen Victoria was such a carrier; see *haemophilia.*) A man cannot pass such a gene on to his son, but only to his daughter, who then becomes a carrier.

Over the generations, any group of people that continually interbreeds will reduce the size of its 'gene pool', increasing the chances of inherited diseases appearing in future generations. The people who live in the Appalachian Mountains in the eastern United States have remained a small and relatively exclusive gene pool since their one-time ancestors came to the area from 16th-century England; the result is that *albinism* is common among them.

These sex-linked characteristics are nearly always carried on the X chromosome. The only gene known to be linked to the male Y

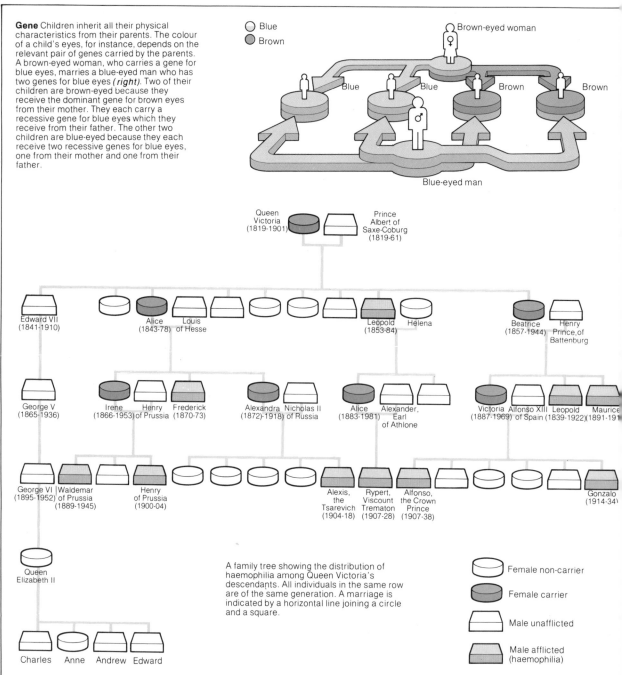

Gene Children inherit all their physical characteristics from their parents. The colour of a child's eyes, for instance, depends on the relevant pair of genes carried by the parents. A brown-eyed woman, who carries a gene for blue eyes, marries a blue-eyed man who has two genes for blue eyes *(right)*. Two of their children are brown-eyed because they receive the dominant gene for brown eyes from their mother. They each carry a recessive gene for blue eyes which they receive from their father. The other two children are blue-eyed because they each receive two recessive genes for blue eyes, one from their mother and one from their father.

Blue
Brown

Brown-eyed woman
Blue
Blue
Brown
Brown
Blue-eyed man

Queen Victoria (1819-1901)
Prince Albert of Saxe-Coburg (1819-61)

Edward VII (1841-1910)
Alice (1843-78)
Louis of Hesse
Leopold (1853-84)
Helena
Beatrice (1857-1944)
Henry Prince, of Battenburg

George V (1865-1936)
Irene (1866-1953)
Henry of Prussia
Frederick (1870-73)
Alexandra (1872)-1918) of Russia
Nicholas II
Alice (1883-1981)
Alexander, Earl of Athlone
Victoria (1887-1969)
Alfonso XIII of Spain (1839-1922)
Leopold (1891-19..)
Maurice

George VI (1895-1952)
Waldemar of Prussia (1889-1945)
Henry of Prussia (1900-04)
Alexis, the Tsarevich (1904-18)
Rypert, Viscount Trematon (1907-28)
Alfonso, the Crown Prince (1907-38)
Gonzalo (1914-34)

Queen Elizabeth II

A family tree showing the distribution of haemophilia among Queen Victoria's descendants. All individuals in the same row are of the same generation. A marriage is indicated by a horizontal line joining a circle and a square.

Charles   Anne   Andrew   Edward

Female non-carrier
Female carrier
Male unafflicted
Male afflicted (haemophilia)

chromosome is the rare gene for hairy ears. It is transmitted by a man to all of his sons, but not to his daughters, who can never be carriers either, as they do not have a Y chromosome.

Most gene pairs, however, do not follow this dominant-recessive pattern. Most characteristics are determined by several genes acting together rather than by a single pair of genes.

The message in a gene is a chemical one, and is coded by the DNA. When it is needed, the message in a gene is transcribed by a messenger molecule called RNA (ribonucleic acid). The RNA

communicates with the rest of the cell by interpreting the genetic code and issuing chemical orders. Whenever a protein, such as an enzyme or a hormone, is needed, the gene issues the appropriate instructions and the RNA sees that they are carried out.

Some illnesses and diseases are caused by a malfunction in this system. People may be born with errors in their metabolism, for example, because a gene does not work properly; either it issues the wrong instructions or none at all. So a key protein is either lacking in one or more of its components, or it is absent altogether.

Genetic research has now made it possible to scrutinize genes in great detail. Genetic counselling services are now available in many hospitals. Couples who come from families with a history of inherited disorders, or who have already given birth to an abnormal child, can seek advice. Tests can show whether couples are carriers of certain diseases. If one or both parents-to-be are carriers, the chances of their child having the disease can be calculated.

Screening unborn babies for potentially fatal genetic diseases is becoming standard medical practice. A test called amniocentesis—*see Special Tests, p84*—can detect some chromosomal abnormalities in an embryo which may be due to an inherited disorder. The test is carried out early in pregnancy; the foetal cells from a fluid sample are cultured and their chromosomal patterns studied. If the test shows that the unborn baby is likely to be affected by the disease, the parents are offered an *abortion*.

Duchenne's disease, the most common form of *muscular dystrophy*, is the first disease to have been linked to specific genes. A technique is now available to test whether these genes are defective or not. In the future this technique will be used in pre-natal screening for most of the 200 or so genetically transmitted diseases.

GERMAN MEASLES—see Rubella.

GESTALT THERAPY
'Gestalt' is a German word meaning form or shape, and is used in the gestalt method of *psychotherapy* to refer to the patient's total environment. The focus is on the present (rather than on the past, as in *psychoanalysis*), taking the attitude that the present is of the greatest importance, since only the present can be changed. The patient's environment includes physical, social and psychological elements which cannot be separated. The patient is encouraged in a variety of ways to express his or her feelings, and to overcome psychological blocks which limit awareness of the possibilities of the present.

GIARDIASIS
An intestinal disease caused by a parasitic protozoan which interferes with the absorption of fat. Two weeks after eating contaminated food, the symptoms—diarrhoea, cramps, nausea, flatulence and *steatorrhoea*—begin. Encountered all over the world, particularly in children, the disease is successfully treated with the drug metronidazole.

GIGANTISM—see Acromegaly

GINGIVITIS
Inflammation of the gums, which leads to swelling and bleeding. It is one of the commonest of dental problems; surveys show that nine out of ten people suffer from the disease to some extent. Its main cause is poor dental hygiene or ill-fitting dentures, but it can also occur during pregnancy, in women taking the contraceptive pill, or as a side-effect of phenytoin therapy— phenytoin is an anticonvulsant drug used to control epileptic seizures.

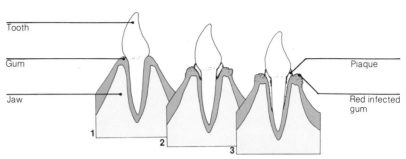

Gingivitis This condition is one of the commonest dental problems, since few people have healthy gums, pale pink flesh that fits firmly around the tooth but does not bleed easily, **1**. Most people have some degree of plaque which slowly accumulates between the teeth and gums, causing slight inflammation, **2**. When toxins from the tiny ulcers in the gums spread, gingivitis develops and the gums become red, infected and swollen, **3**.

Treatment involves the use of an antibacterial mouthwash, the removal of plaque and calculus from the base of the teeth and careful, regular brushing in the future—*see Routine Health Checks, p346*.

If ignored, gingivitis can develop into periodontitis, an inflammation of the structures supporting the teeth. This is another common dental problem. In it, pockets of pus may accumulate around the teeth and resulting bacterial infection may lead to Vincent's angina, or trench mouth. The result of this is serious ulceration of the inside of the mouth.

Minor cases of periodontitis can be treated by taking the same kind of hygienic precautions described above; major ones, however, may require a minor operation called a gingivectomy. In this, the gums are trimmed. This reduces the depth of the pockets, while the teeth themselves are given a protective coating of oil of cloves, zinc oxide and cotton wool. This stays in position until the gums heal. A full follow-up programme of careful dental hygiene is essential.

GLANDULAR FEVER—see Infectious mononucleosis.

GLAUCOMA
A painful eye condition in which the pressure of the aqueous humour, the fluid inside the eye, is raised.

Normally the fluid flows easily between the two compartments separated by the iris: the anterior chamber, in front of the lens of the eye, and the posterior chamber, behind the lens. In glaucoma, however, part of the iris blocks the narrow channel so that there is a build-up of fluid in the anterior portion of the eye, or sometimes the aqueous humour is produced faster than it can be absorbed into the veins of the eye. It results in a hard, red, painful eyeball, with visual disturbances, such as haloes around

lights, and tunnel vision (loss of peripheral vision). If the condition is not treated it will lead to blindness.

Glaucoma can be *acute* or *chronic*; if it is chronic it can slowly develop for years without detection until vision has deteriorated. Since peripheral vision is affected first, the binocular or overlapping vision of the two eyes can mask the problem for a time. Glaucoma seems to run in families, but why it develops is not known. People with a family history of glaucoma should have frequent eye checks from middle age onwards.

Treatment is with eyedrops that constrict the pupil, allowing more drainage; drugs that reduce the production of aqueous humour; or surgery. Part of the iris can be removed, by an operation called *iridectomy*, so that it no longer obstructs drainage, or a tiny hole can be made to assist it.

GLOMERULONEPHRITIS
Inflammation of the glomeruli of the kidney, the networks of capillaries in each of the kidneys where filtration of wastes from the blood begins. As a result, proteins are lost into the urine, blood may pass into the urine, and fluid retention—*see oedema*—may cause local swelling. This is seen in the face as swelling around the eyes and also affects the ankles.

The disorder is usually a complication of an upper respiratory tract infection, such as *scarlet fever* or *tonsillitis*. The damage to the glomeruli is due to deposition of chemical compounds made up of antibodies and antigens—*see Natural Defences Against Disease, p52*—which circulate in the blood because of the infection.

The patient is admitted to hospital for various tests, possibly including a renal biopsy—*see Special Tests, p84*. Treatment consists of bed rest, restriction of salt and fluids to rest the glomeruli during the acute phase of the disease, and usually penicillin to combat infection.

Glomerulonephritis usually occurs in children and young adults, and complete recovery is the rule. In older people the condition may become *chronic*, contributing eventually to *hypertension* and possible kidney failure—*see kidney disorders; nephrotic syndrome*.

GLOSSITIS
Inflammation of the tongue which becomes smooth and dark red. The tongue often feels sore, particularly if spicy foods are eaten. Glossitis can be a symptom of either iron-deficiency *anaemia* or *pernicious anaemia*. If there is no such underlying disorder, glossitis normally heals quickly. Hot, spicy foods should be temporarily avoided.

GLUTEN-FREE DIET
A diet that does not contain gluten, a protein found in wheat, rye and other grains. Gluten is often the aggravating factor in *coeliac disease*, a digestive disorder. Any cakes, bread or biscuits must be made from specially prepared gluten-free flour. Vegetables such as beans, cabbage, turnips, dried peas and cucumbers should also be avoided. The diet has also been suggested for sufferers from multiple sclerosis, though there is no evidence to show that it is more effective than other treatment.

GLYCERYL TRINITRATE
A drug which dilates blood vessels and rapidly relieves the pain of *angina pectoris*. Known also as nitroglycerin, it is traditionally administered as tablets which are either chewed or allowed to dissolve under the tongue. More recently, it has been manufactured as a metered aerosol to spray under the tongue, and as a slow release preparation, which can be applied to the skin either as a paste or as a plaster.

GLYCOGEN STORAGE DISEASES—see Metabolic disorders

GLYCOSURIA
The presence of glucose in the urine. While traces of this sugar may be found in normal urine, for example during pregnancy, the presence of larger amounts is an indication of *diabetes mellitus*. Diagnosis is made using the glucose tolerance test—*see Special Tests, p84*—in which glucose levels in the blood and urine are monitored after a measured dosage of glucose is eaten.

Disorders of the kidney and of the pituitary and adrenal glands can also be reponsible for glycosuria. In women, glycosuria can predispose to *candidiasis*.

GOITRE
A swelling in the front of the neck due to an enlarged thyroid gland—*see The Endocrine System, p48*. The thyroid needs iodine to produce its hormone; when iodine is missing from the diet, the gland swells as it tries to make more of the hormone in the absence of this key ingredient. Goitre is endemic in areas where iodine has been leached from the soil and is absent from drinking water. The addition of iodine to the water supply in these areas, or to salt, is the usual way of preventing the condition. If the swelling is very large and presses on other parts of the neck, it may require surgical removal.

A goitre may also develop of its own accord, either when the cells of the gland multiply excessively, or because of a tumour—*see also thyrotoxicosis*.

GONORRHOEA
An infection by the bacterium gonococcus of the mucous membranes lining the genitals, which may affect people of either sex. The disease is transmitted sexually.

Colloquially known as the 'clap', gonorrhoea affects the urethra in both sexes; in women the cervix may also be infected. In addition, the rectum can become infected after anal sex, or the throat after oral sex.

Male symptoms appear about ten days after infection; urination becomes painful, and a yellowish-white discharge seeps from the tip of the penis. A woman may not have any symptoms at all, or there may be a vaginal discharge or occasional pain when urinating. The only certain way of identifying gonorrhoea in a woman is to examine smears.

Special clinics, where confidentially is guaranteed, exist for the treatment of sexually transmitted diseases. These clinics estimate that the people who are treated for gonorrhoea are predominantly those who have more than one sexual partner, and that two-thirds of the patients are men. The disease is treated with a course of antibiotic tablets, during which it is best to stop drinking alcohol.

If the disease is ignored and allowed to progress, the gonococcus can spread to deeper tissues. Severe inflammation of the urethra may lead to a *stricture*. If infection spreads throughout the reproductive system, *sterility* may result. Further complications may include *arthritis*, or *conjunctivitis*.

GOUT
A painful disease of the joints that usually begins in the foot, especially the joint of the big toe. Gout most commonly affects middle-aged or elderly men, and women after the menopause. It occurs when one of the body's waste products, uric acid, accumulates in the blood and cannot be excreted properly by the kidneys. The uric acid crystals then collect in the joints, restricting their movement and inflaming their tissue.

Apparently, some people are predisposed to gout, and there is a family history of gout in most cases. Sometimes, however, gout is a secondary effect of a disease such as *leukaemia* or *polycythaemia*, in which there is a high level of uric acid in the blood.

The first pain comes without warning, affects the big toe, and is excruciating. It lasts only a few days and may not reappear for a long time. Subsequent attacks last longer, recur more often and affect more joints.

Gout is easily treated with drugs which either increase the excretion of uric acid salts or slow down their formation; these are known as uricosuric drugs. Eating plain food and cutting down on alcohol is also advisable. If left untreated, gout can cause high blood pressure, or *hypertension*, destruction of the joints and kidney failure.

GRAFT
The replacement of damaged tissues with healthy ones. In the case of serious burns, for example, a healthy piece of skin is taken from elsewhere on the body and grafted on to the burnt area. In *keratoplasty*, a replacement cornea is grafted on to an eye to repair a damaged cornea. Arteries and bones can be grafted, while *transplantation* of a kidney or a heart is also a kind of graft.

Artificial tissues, such as heart valves, artery walls and tendons, can be grafted to replace or repair faulty tissues. Since they are made of inert materials, such as dacron fibre or silicone, they are not rejected by the body's defence mechanisms—*see Natural Defences Against Disease, p52*.

All human graft tissue must be of the same type as the tissue it is replacing; skin, bone and nerve should come from elsewhere on the same body. Otherwise the graft operation must be accompanied by *immunosuppressive* drugs. These subdue the body's defences while the graft heals, though in some cases —notably in a kidney transplant— they must be taken for life. Only the cornea, which has no blood or nerve supply, can be grafted from one body to another without these drugs.

GRAND MAL—see Epilepsy

GRAND PARALYSIS OF THE INSANE—see Syphilis

GRAVES'S DISEASE—see Thyrotoxicosis

GROUP THERAPY

A way of treating psychiatric illness which has gained popularity since World War II. Small groups of patients gather together at regular intervals under the guidance of a psychotherapist. Patients are usually those suffering from *neurosis*, borderline *psychosis* or *personality disorders*. Sufferers from *depression* seldom benefit from group therapy.

Participants become 'intimate strangers'—that is, they talk freely about their own and each others lives and problems, and each learns that others suffer from the same anxieties, doubts and fears. The establishment of a group cohesiveness—a sense of solidarity —is seen as an important curative factor, because a patient coming to grips with a problem is a source of encouragement to the others.

The role of the psychotherapist is essentially a passive one. Once the group has been set up, the therapist takes a back seat, stepping in only when it is important to draw attention to a particular point.

GUILLAIN-BARRÉ SYNDROME—see Neuropathy

GYNAECOMASTIA

The enlargement and tenderness of the mammary tissue in the male breasts. It may affect one or both breasts. Adolescent boys often suffer from a temporary gynaecomastia, which lasts from one to three years and causes social embarrassment. In this case, growth hormones are thought to be responsible, since the condition disappears as growth stops.

Gynaecomastia is a common symptom of *Klinefelter's syndrome*. It may also be seen in cases of tumours of the adrenal glands or testis, and it is a frequent side-effect of the oestrogen treatment given to sufferers of prostate cancer.

Male transsexuals cause gynaecomastia deliberately by taking oestrogens. People who use oestrogen-containing hair creams to prevent baldness may also develop the condition after many years.

Several other diseases, including *cirrhosis* of the liver, may precipitate gynaecomastia, and so may a number of drugs. Treatment depends on the cause: a tumour may be removed by surgery, a particular drug withdrawn, or, as in the case of Klinefelter's syndrome, the breasts may be removed by surgery.

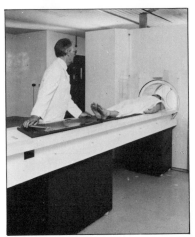

H

HAEMANGIOMA

A congenital malformation of the blood vessels, often seen in newborn babies as a birthmark. It is a benign tumour of the blood vessels which usually disappears within a few years—*see naevus*.

HAEMATINIC

An iron compound, such as ferrous sulphate, that stimulates the production of red blood cells and increases the level of haemoglobin in the blood. Haematinics are used to prevent or treat iron-deficiency *anaemia*, which can be a particular problem during pregnancy. Occasionally, however, they may upset the digestion and cause constipation.

HAEMATOMA

A solid swelling full of clotted blood, caused by bleeding from a broken blood vessel. Some haematomas are minor—a bad bruise or a blood-blister, for example—and will disappear on their own. In some circumstances, however, a haematoma can be extremely serious.

A fractured skull and damage to the middle meningeal blood vessels

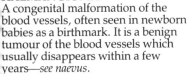

Haematoma A haematoma is an accumulation of clotted blood, which, if it develops in the brain, can be dangerous. Haematomas can occur in various areas. Until the brainscanner *(left)* was developed, such haematomas were difficult to detect. The scanner produces a horizontal image of

may cause a haematoma to develop between the skull and the brain. There are three meninges, or protective membranes, in this region, the outermost layer being the dura mater. A haematoma between the skull and the dura may

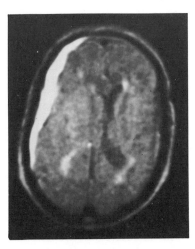

the brain, locating and showing the exact nature and extent of disorders such as haematomas and tumours. The scan *(right)* shows a subdural haematoma — the white area in the picture — where a blood clot has developed beneath the dura mater, one of the meninges of the brain.

put pressure on the brain tissues and cause permanent brain damage, or even death. Immediate surgery is needed to remove the clotted blood and so relieve the pressure.

A haematoma that develops between the brain and the dura is

called a subdural haematoma. It is often the result of a seemingly trivial injury, and may cause serious damage. It can take several days before symptoms appear, however. These include drowsiness, confusion, headaches, and numbness on one side of the body. The condition often occurs in elderly people who have fallen over, or had a bump on the head. Surgery is necessary to remove the clot and relieve the pressure.

Haematomas may also occur in the middle of the brain, sometimes as a result of a violent injury but more often because of high blood pressure—see hypertension.

Straining to pass faeces sometimes ruptures a small vein in the anus. A perianal haematoma may then develop, but this usually clears up of its own accord—see also haemorrhoid.

HAEMATURIA

The passing of blood in the urine. This may be a symptom of a number of potentially serious medical problems. If blood is noticed in the urine, a doctor should always be consulted. The blood may come from a kidney that has been ruptured or bruised by an injury, or damaged by a stone in the renal pelvis. Alternatively, the blood may come from the bladder, the prostate gland, the ureters or the urethra as a result of infection or injury.

HAEMOCHROMATOSIS

An uncommon disease in which excessive amounts of iron are absorbed and stored in the body, particularly in the liver, pancreas, endocrine glands and heart. The disease is inherited, and usually affects men over the age of 45. Women are ten times less likely to suffer from haemochromatosis, probably because menstruation and pregnancy naturally deplete the stores of iron.

Haemochromatosis is also called bronze diabetes, because the accumulation of iron turns the skin a bronze colour and *diabetes* develops. The liver may fail from a form of *cirrhosis*, and the heart is weakened. Men may also become impotent, as the testes stop producing male hormones.

If the condition is diagnosed and treated promptly, recovery from the symptoms is normally complete. The usual treatment for haemochromatosis is *venesection*: half a litre (0.87pt) of blood is removed from a vein every week for about two years, or until such time as the level of iron in the blood returns to normal. Subsequently, the level of iron in the patient's blood is tested at intervals in case it begins to rise again.

Similar symptoms are caused by a separate rare condition called haemosiderosis. In this, the iron excess is the result of an excessive number of blood transfusions, or an excessive consumption of iron.

HAEMOLYTIC DISEASE OF THE NEWBORN

A disease of newborn babies caused by an interaction between the blood of a mother and that of her foetus—see Pregnancy and Birth, p60. The disease is also known as erythroblastosis foetalis, icterus neonatorum and hydrops foetalis, according to its consequences and severity.

The name of the disease refers to the newborn baby, because, at one time, the disease was not apparent until the baby was born, although a *stillbirth* or a premature birth was often the result. Nowadays routine blood tests—see Special Tests, p84—during pregnancy reveal the danger, and in some cases the foetus is treated while still in the womb.

Depending on the nature of the problem, the foetus can suffer from *anaemia*, as a result of the haemolysis—destruction of blood cells—and *jaundice* in varying degrees of severity. In mild cases, the jaundice is not a problem and the anaemia is mild and treatable.

In more severe cases, the foetus develops jaundice so seriously that an *exchange transfusion* is necessary to prevent *kernicterus*, or brain damage. At its most severe, the anaemia is so

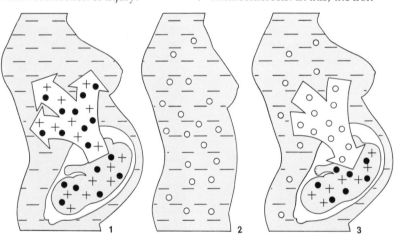

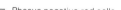

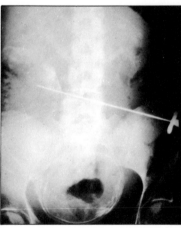

Haemolytic Disease of the Newborn On the surface of red blood cells there are a number of proteins called antigens which enable haematologists to group a person's blood. In addition to the A, B and O antigens, there is also a Rhesus antigen — so-called because of a similar antigen in Rhesus monkeys. 84% of the population inherit this Rhesus antigen, also called the Rhesus factor, and their blood is typed Rhesus positive. The remaining 16% do not inherit this factor and their blood is therefore Rhesus negative.

When a Rhesus negative woman conceives a Rhesus-positive child, the foetal Rhesus antigen may enter the woman's bloodstream via the placenta, **1**. This usually happens during labour. The woman produces antibodies which circulate in her serum and attack the 'foreign' Rhesus antigens.

While her first baby is unaffected, the woman still retains the antibodies in her body, **2**. When she conceives another Rhesus positive child, her anti-Rhesus antibodies enter the foetal circulation via the placenta, **3**. They attack the Rhesus antigen and, in doing this, destroy or haemolyze the foetal red cells. This causes haemolytic disease of the newborn, in which the foetus is anaemic, due to lack of red cells, and jaundiced, due to the yellow bilirubin released from the breakdown of haemoglobin from the damaged cells.

— Rhesus negative red cells

+ Rhesus positive red cells

● Rhesus antigen (factor)

○ Anti-Rhesus antibodies

To prevent this, an exchange transfusion is performed, either while the foetus is still in the womb **(above)**, or the moment it is born. An intrauterine transfusion can be performed from the twentieth week of pregnancy onwards. It involves the repeated removal of blood from the umbilical vein and the injection of Rhesus negative blood into the peritoneal cavity of the foetus.

acute that it causes gross heart failure and the premature birth of the child, who usually dies. In this case, the condition is known as hydrops foetalis.

In each case, the red blood cells of the foetus have been destroyed by antibodies (52) from the mother's blood which have passed through the placenta. These antibodies are produced because of an incompatibility between the mother's blood group system and that of her foetus. This is bound up with the presence or absence of a blood factor known as the Rhesus factor on the surface of the mother's red blood cells.

Occasionally, a rhesus negative mother conceives a rhesus positive child. The first time that this happens the child is rarely affected, because the foetal blood cells are normally too large to cross the placenta. Some foetal cells may enter the mother's circulation during labour, however. In response, the mother's body manufactures antibodies against the rhesus positive blood.

If the mother conceives another rhesus positive child, these antibodies cross the placenta and attack the blood cells of the foetus, destroying them and causing serious anaemia and jaundice.

Whether a mother has rhesus positive or negative blood is determined by routine blood tests taken during pregnancy. If the mother has rhesus negative blood, and the father's blood is rhesus positive, there is a possibility that the baby will also have rhesus positive blood. The mother's blood is tested throughout pregnancy to make sure that the level of antibodies against Rh+ blood is not building up. Normally, pregnancy proceeds without incident—on very rare occasions, however, it is found during a first pregnancy that a mother has been sensitized to Rh+ blood by a previous rhesus incompatible blood transfusion.

After the birth, the mother will be given an injection of *gamma globulin* within 48 hours. These kill the foetal blood cells before the mother's body has time to manufacture antibodies against them, so desensitizing the mother against a Rh+ foetus in a future pregnancy.

When the mother is found to have Rh+ antibodies in her blood before the birth, action can be taken to prevent damage to the foetus. Before 34 weeks, it can be given intrauterine transfusions of blood which is compatible with that of the mother. After 36 weeks, labour can be induced, since the risks of premature birth are considered to be less than those of the disease.

ABO haemolytic disease is a rarer and less serious condition than the form of haemolytic disease caused by rhesus incompatibility. In it, a mother with an O blood group gives birth to an A, B or an AB child. This is treated, if necessary, with a intrauterine transfusion of type O blood.

HAEMOPHILIA

An incurable inherited disease in which the blood either fails to clot properly or takes a long time to do so. Its degree of severity ranges from being mild and inconvenient to being fatal.

Haemophilia is caused by the absence of a crucial blood-clotting substance, a protein known as Factor VIII—*see The Blood and Lymph Systems, p21.* Haemophiliacs inherit the inability to make this factor from their parents. It is a sex-linked characteristic carried on the X *chromosome*, which means that almost all sufferers are male, and female offspring are carriers; the only way a female can be a sufferer is if her mother is a carrier and her father is a sufferer. Queen Victoria was a carrier, and passed haemophilia on to many males in European royal families.

In a haemophiliac, the smallest injury, such as a scratch or a bruise, can trigger off prolonged bleeding, though sufferers are affected in varying degrees. Some have the problem only after dental extractions, but in others bleeding may occur spontaneously without any apparent cause. As a result, the joints may swell up painfully and can even become deformed. In the past, many haemophiliacs died in childhood, but nowadays many survive to adulthood, though some are chronic invalids.

A number of treatments can prevent bleeding from becoming excessive and fatal. Haemophiliacs usually carry some identification and sometimes a supply of Factor VIII, which they can inject themselves to stop the bleeding. More serious cases of bleeding are treated in hospital, either with Factor VIII, or a *transfusion* of a concentrated plasma called cryoprecipitate, which is rich in the factor. *See also Christmas disease.*

HAEMOPHILUS

A group of bacteria, of which two types can cause disease in humans.

Haemophilus influenzae is a contributory factor in a variety of infections of the upper respiratory tract, among them *otitis media*, *pneumonia*, and *meningitis*. It is especially dangerous to children, because when their resistance is lowered by another infection, such as influenza, the bacterium may multiply and cause serious complications, such as *pneumonia* and, occasionally, *meningitis*. However, H. influenzae is often found in the throats of healthy adults where it is harmless. This is because most adults have acquired immunity to the bacterium during childhood.

Another haemophilus bacterium. called H. ducreyi, causes *chancroid*, a sexually transmitted disease.

Both forms of haemophilus bacteria are treated with *sulphonamide* drugs or other *antibiotics*.

HAEMOPTYSIS

The coughing up of blood. Although this is not necessarily a symptom of serious disease, haemoptysis may be an indication of *tuberculosis* or *lung cancer*. It can also be a symptom of an infection of the respiratory tract, such as *pneumonia*, or a heart disease, such as mitral stenosis—*see valvular heart disease*—in which the blood pressure in the lungs is higher than normal. Because of this, the coughing up of blood should always be reported to a doctor, no matter how small the quantity of blood produced. He or she will probably investigate the problem by means of a chest X-ray.

HAEMORRHAGE

Loss of blood, which may be external and obvious, or internal and more difficult to diagnose.

Haemorrhage from superficial skin wounds is usually minor, and can be stopped with firm pressure—*see First Aid, p369.* Where there is a deep, penetrating injury, however, the amount of damage and blood loss is substantial and often fatal.

Blood vessels and organs may also bleed internally. The only immediately detectable signs of this are the lowering of the blood pressure and the increase in pulse rate this causes. A perforated peptic *ulcer* may haemorrhage into the stomach, and the blood will then either be vomited up, or passed out via the rectum as black, tarry stools. A ruptured spleen will bleed, stretching its capsule and causing abdominal pain, pallor, low blood pressure, and *tachycardia*. A ruptured aortic *aneurysm* will cause a massive internal haemorrhage, which is often fatal.

An injury to the head may cause the vessels inside the skull to rupture and bleed, leading to a subdural or extradural *haematoma*. Bleeding may also take place into the subarachnoid space surrounding the brain—*see subarachnoid haemorrhage*.

Blood loss from haemorrhage must be replaced to restore the blood pressure, and ensure an adequate supply of blood to the body's vital organs, such as the kidneys. This loss may be replaced by *transfusion* of what is termed whole blood, of a compatible blood group—*see The Blood and Lymph Systems, p21*—plasma, or synthetic fluids called plasma expanders.

HAEMORRHOIDS

Swollen, or *varicose*, veins in the wall of the anus, also called piles. Haemorrhoids are usually caused by the increase in the abdominal pressure needed to pass a hard stool in *constipation*. Abdominal pressure also rises in pregnancy, *obesity* and in those who have a chronic cough, making the formation of piles more likely in all these cases. A sedentary life, *diarrhoea*, *cirrhosis* of the liver or an excessive use of laxatives are all contributory factors.

Haemorrhoids vary in severity and extent, but are typically accompanied by bleeding, usually after defaecation, and some degree of pain or itching. They may form either internally or externally. Internal haemorrhoids are varicosities of the superior rectal veins, and may prolapse—that is, they fall downwards and protrude out of the anus, appearing as small brown swellings of skin. External haemorrhoids are small *haematoma* around the anus, formed from the rupture of an inferior rectal vein.

Sufferers from piles should consult a doctor, since prolonged bleeding caused by haemorrhoids can lead to iron-deficiency *anaemia*. In rare cases moreover, bleeding from the anus may be caused not by piles, but by *cancer* of the bowel. Piles can be treated successfully. If they are not serious, a soothing ointment or suppositories may be prescribed, for use after defaecation, and the patient will be advised to keep the anal area clean with a sponge and hot water. At the same time, the doctor will probably recommend that the patient adopt a high-fibre diet—*see Diet, p322*—in order to relieve constipation and ensure that the stools are soft.

If the condition is more severe, the affected veins are injected with a sclerosing fluid, which hardens them and stops the bleeding. In serious cases, however, surgery may be required. The operation, called a haemorrhoidectomy, involves removing the piles, often by freezing, or *cryosurgery*, and widening, or dilating, the anus. The operation is usually completely successful, but the patient may experience severe discomfort and some pain for several weeks after it.

HALITOSIS

Bad breath. Halitosis is often the temporary result of eating aromatic foods, such as garlic or onions, but it can also be a symptom of poor oral hygiene, *constipation*, chronic *sinusitis*, or *bronchiectasis*. In the latter two conditions, infection causes the build·up of foul-smelling pus in the airways. Halitosis is treated according to its cause, but the condition can often be improved by following the simple rules of oral hygiene—*see Health and Hygiene, p334*.

HALLUCINATION

Seeing or hearing things that do not exist in physical terms. The other senses—touch, taste and smell—may also be involved. Hallucinations are false perceptions and may be triggered by *schizophrenia, hysteria, epilepsy* or *psychotropic* drugs such as LSD or mescaline. They are not *illusions*, because these are usually seen to be false, while hallucinations are often very real to the sufferer.

Hallucinations are usually indicative of a *psychosis*, as, for example, in the case of a chronic alcoholic who experiences *delirium tremens*. Smells are usually foul or chemical, often being associated with decay. Tactile hallucinations usually centre around the genital regions, and are experienced by schizophrenics who are convinced that someone has made a sexual approach to them.

Sometimes, psychiatric patients think that they have heard voices, but questioning reveals that they were hearing their own thoughts. Fleeting hallucinations can be experienced by people in a state of exhaustion, or in the transition period between wakefulness and sleep. Hallucinations may also occur during moments of emotional or religious ecstasy.

HALLUX VULGUS—see Bunion

HANSEN'S DISEASE—see Leprosy

HAY FEVER

A disorder with symptoms similar to those of the common *cold* that tends to occur seasonally. It is caused by antibodies found in the blood as an *allergic* reaction to pollens from weeds, flowers, trees or grasses. The reaction causes *inflammation* of the mucous membranes of the nose, which leads to stinging and watering of the eyes, nasal obstruction, sneezing and a runny nose. Attacks usually occur in early summer, and normally last for several hours.

Hay fever is a form of rhinitis. An all-year form of the latter complaint is caused by a reaction to *antigens* in house dust, fungus spores or dander, the dust from the fur of domestic animals such as cats. This form of rhinitis may also occur in some people after exposure to chemical fumes and strong odours or extremely cold or dry atmospheres. It is not an allergy, but its symptoms are similar to those of hay fever, though they are less severe.

In mild cases of hay fever, the symptoms may be relieved by taking a mild *antihistamine*, but, because these drugs cause drowsiness, they are unpopular with many patients. If symptoms occur for only a few days a year, a *decongestant* nasal spray used up to six times a day may keep them at bay. However, decongestants tend to damage the delicate mucous membranes of the nose if they are taken regularly. When hay fever is severe enough to interfere seriously with work, it is sometimes treated with injections of *steroids*; however, these drugs often have serious side effects, so their prescription for such minor complaints is discouraged.

The reaction that causes seasonal hay fever may be prevented by a process of *desensitization* to the particular variety of pollen responsible for it. Patch tests—*see allergy*—are carried out to discover which pollen is causing the reaction and a preparation containing minute amounts of the extract is injected into the patient's blood. Injections are repeated at regular intervals for three months or more until the patient becomes desensitized and the reaction no longer occurs. The treatment gives some patients lifelong immunity against certain pollens, but with some the immunity may last for no longer than a year.

As far as perennial rhinitis is concerned, such measures are rarely effective. Sufferers from this condition can only try to avoid exposure to the agent that causes it as much as possible.

HEADACHES

Headaches, with their characteristic pain or throbbing sensation in the head, are an extremely common complaint, experienced by almost everyone at some time or other. Occasionally, they are a symptom of an underlying disorder, but, if they occur on their own, developing gradually and clearing up with no side-effects, the probability is that they are totally harmless, apart from the discomfort they cause.

Probably the commonest form of headache is caused by tension, from the contraction of the muscles of the neck, shoulders and scalp. The second commonest is the result of the swelling of local blood vessels. There can be many contributing factors. These range from stress, sleeplessness and drinking and eating too much, to noise and stuffy rooms, but, insofar as tension headaches are concerned, one of the commonest causes is poor posture. The muscles of the neck become tense and sore because they have to support the considerable weight of the head in an awkward position. Another common cause is eye strain. This can be due to the simple need for glasses. If headaches persist, it is as well to go to an optician for a check-up, and to work in a good light.

The treatment for all these forms of headache is similar. Rest, relaxation—either by, say, massaging the muscles, having a bath, applying a warm or cold compress, or using relaxation techniques—see Stress, p332—and mild pain-killers will normally do the trick. If, however, the headaches last for more than a day or frequently recur, a doctor should be consulted, particularly if the headaches develop into migraine. By discovering, among other things, how long each headache lasts, how frequently it occurs, which area of the head it chiefly affects and whether it goes hand-in-hand with other symptoms, such as feeling sick, the doctor can establish if there is an underlying cause. Examples of these include hypertension, or high blood pressure, probably because it dilates the blood vessels inside the skull, and meningitis. This causes a severe headache, which worsens if the neck or back is bent. Headaches are also a symptom of a brain tumour, but this condition is rare. Dental disease and sinusitis may cause headaches, although the primary infection is in the mouth and face. Treatment involves good dental care, antibiotics and, in the case of sinusitis, decongestants.

Anxiety and depression often manifest themselves as psychosomatic symptoms, of which headache is a very frequent feature. The headache disappears when the underlying problem is treated.

HEART ATTACK—see Myocardial infarction

HEART BLOCK

The interruption of the regular flow of electrical impulses which keep the heart beating normally. These impulses originate in the heart's natural pacemaker, the sinoatrial node, which is under the control of the vagus nerve. They travel to the atrioventricular node and from there spread out through the ventricles, stimulating the heart muscle to contract.

Heart block can occur anywhere along this path and can be detected by an ECG or electrocardiogram—see Special Tests, p84. If the impulses are delayed, or if some of them are not conducted at all, then an incomplete block results. The beating of the heart, and hence the pulse, is slower than normal. As long as there are no fainting episodes, there is little cause for concern.

In a complete heart block, no impulses reach the ventricles and so they beat with their own intrinsic rhythm of 30-40 beats per minute. The condition may be left untreated if there are no concurrent symptoms. If the heart rate drops too far, however, there will be dizziness and faints, due to an inadequate supply of blood to the brain. In a Stoke Adams attack, the heart may stop beating altogether.

Some heart block cases are due to a congenital defect of the electrical impulse system. The remainder are due to heart diseases, such as cardiomyopathy, myocardial infarction and myocarditis. Heart block may also be caused by the drugs used to treat cardiac arrhythmias. In serious cases, either the drug is withdrawn or an artificial pacemaker is implanted.

HEARTBURN—see Dyspepsia

HEART DISEASE

An imprecise term, used to describe a variety of cardiac problems, including coronary artery disease, cardiomyopathy, valvular heart disease, and heart failure. It may also be used to describe the condition of a patient suffering from angina, or a recent heart attack or myocardial infarction. The term can similarly serve as a broad description of a congenital heart defect, such as a hole in the heart, or other physical abnormalities.

In ischaemic heart disease, the heart muscle is short of blood, or ischaemic. The consequences of this are likely to be angina and, possibly later, a heart attack.

HEART FAILURE

An imprecise term, which, though commonly used by both doctors and patients, can lead to considerable confusion. It generally describes what happens when the heart is unable to work efficiently, for whatever reason.

Usually, with every heart beat, the right ventricle pumps a certain amount of blood into the lungs through the pulmonary artery—see The Blood and Lymph Systems, p21. At the same time, the same amount of blood flows from the lungs into the left ventricle and then around the body via the aorta. If either ventricle pumps less blood than normal, this careful balance will be upset and the result will be heart failure.

There are several reasons why the heart's pumping action becomes less efficient. Either the heart muscle can be weakened by ischaemic heart disease, in which the muscle receives an inadequate supply of oxygen over a long period, or cardiomyopathy, a disorder of the heart muscle, may also cause heart failure. When a piece of heart muscle dies, in a heart attack, or myocardial infarction, the working of the heart may be affected and heart failure result.

Another cause of reduced cardiac pumping efficiency is a mechanical fault in one of the heart valves, affecting the control of the blood flow—see valvular heart disease. If a valve opening is narrowed, for instance, the heart has to pump harder to force the same volume of blood through it. Similarly, if a valve is unable to close properly and is therefore incompetent or regurgitant—see valvular heart disease—blood rushes back through it every time the heart pumps. Again, the heart has to pump harder to eject sufficient blood.

Heart failure can affect the whole heart, in which case it is described as congestive heart failure, or one ventricle only, when it is said to be right- or left-sided, depending on which is affected. The symptoms of right- and left-sided heart failure differ, primarily because the function of each ventricle is different. In the former, where the right ventricle cannot pump its load of blood into the lungs efficiently, the chief initial symptom is extreme tiredness. This is accompanied by swelling of various parts of the body, particularly the ankles. The problem is that blood stagnates in the major veins of the body, because back pressure discourages its return to the heart. The blood pressure therefore increases in the veins, forcing fluid to seep out of them into the surrounding tissues. This process is known as oedema.

In left-sided heart failure, the primary symptom is breathlessness. In this, blood accumulates in the pulmonary circulation—see The Blood and Lymph Systems, p21—and, as in right-sided heart failure, fluid leaks out to cause pulmonary oedema, or fluid on the lungs, and chest pain.

Treatment is generally along the same lines for both right- and left-sided heart failure. This involves

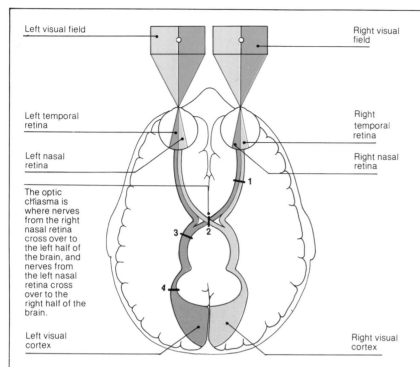

Left visual field

Right visual field

Left temporal retina

Right temporal retina

Left nasal retina

Right nasal retina

The optic chiasma is where nerves from the right nasal retina cross over to the left half of the brain, and nerves from the left nasal retina cross over to the right half of the brain.

Left visual cortex

Right visual cortex

Left visual fie d

Right visual field

Hemianopia Optic nerve fibres carry information about what both eyes see in the visual field to the visual cortex at the back of the brain *(left)*. Damage by lesions, **1-4**, to the optic nerves causes hemianopia, in which half the visual field cannot be seen *(right)* and partial blindness results. The lesion, **1**, causes total blindness in the right eye. The lesion, **2**, causes loss of the outer half of the visual field on each side. The lesions, **3** and **4**, cause hemianopia in the corresponding halves of both eyes.

removing the cause wherever possible—for instance, an operation to replace a heart valve—and the use of *diuretic* drugs to encourage urination and so reduce the quantity of fluid. Rest is important, and *digitalis* may be prescribed to stimulate the heart beat. The disease need not be incapacitating provided it is effectively treated; even in acute heart failure—a medical emergency which may follow a serious heart attack and requires immediate hospital treatment with oxygen and drugs—the outlook for the future is frequently good.

HEART-LUNG MACHINE—see Cardiopulmonary bypass

HEMIANOPIA
A condition in which only half the field of vision can be seen. This may occur after a stroke—*see cerebrovascular accident*—in which part of the visual pathway of the eye has been affected, or may be a sign of a tumour of the pituitary gland that is impinging on the pathway.

HEMIPLEGIA
The paralysis of one side of the body due to a *lesion* in the opposite side of the brain. The face and the arm are particularly affected, and there may be a loss of sensation as well as the power of movement. The lesion may be caused by a *cerebrovascular accident*, or stroke, a *tumour* or by an injury to the brain. Many hemiplegics can be helped to regain a certain amount of sensation and movement in the affected areas through *physiotherapy* and

occupational therapy—*see cerebrovascular accident*.

HENOCH-SCHONLEIN PURPURA
A disorder of the body's immune system, which mainly affects children aged between five and 11. The cause is unknown, but the onset of the disease is often preceded by an infection of the upper respiratory tract, such as a sore throat. Typically, the disorder occurs in the spring and begins with a skin rash which looks like purple bruising. This normally appears on those areas of the body that are subject to pressure, such as the buttocks. A form of *arthritis* makes the joints swell. The bowels may also be involved, leading to abdominal pain, blood in the stools and *intussusception*.

In the majority of cases, the kidneys are eventually affected. Blood may appear in the urine and *immunoglobulins* may be deposited in the glomeruli, the capillaries inside the kidneys that filter blood.

There is no specific treatment for the disorder itself, though, in more than 75 per cent of cases; treatment of the symptoms brings about a complete recovery. However, a small but significant proportion of cases are left with serious kidney damage—*see kidney disorders*.

HEPATITIS
An acute inflammation of the liver. There are two forms of hepatitis, each caused by a different virus. These are type A, which is also called infectious, epidemic or short

incubation hepatitis; and type B, which is also called serum or long incubation hepatitis.

Infectious hepatitis is usually transmitted from one person to another through food and water that has been contaminated by faeces. Sea-food taken from waters polluted by sewage is a major source of infection. The incubation period is about one month, after which the early symptoms appear. These include headaches, fever, chills, vomiting, loss of appetite, distaste for tobacco and general malaise. A week or so after this *jaundice* begins: first the whites of the eyes, and then the skin, turn yellow. The urine darkens and the stools turn pale. The liver enlarges to stretch its capsule, causing continuous abdominal pain.

There is no specific treatment for infectious hepatitis, though sufferers should rest and drink plenty of fluids. Recovery takes only a few weeks, but depression and tiredness may last for much longer. Alcohol should not be drunk for at least six months to give the liver time to recover fully. The patient may excrete viruses in his or her faeces for about three weeks before the jaundice appears and for about two weeks afterwards, so it is important that the rules of hygiene are observed scrupulously at all times—*see Health and Hygiene, p334*.

The virus that causes type B, or serum, hepatitis is transmitted in the blood, saliva, urine, vaginal secretions and semen. It is therefore commonly seen in drug addicts, who tend to re-use needles without sterilizing them adequately, and is sometimes a hazard for those visiting a tattooist or acupuncturist who fails to observe strict standards of hygiene. Close physical contact, both oral and sexual, is also a common means of transmission and serum hepatitis is currently endemic among male homosexuals.

Very occasionally, the virus is transmitted by a blood transfusion. Sometimes, however, if hepatitis is contracted after a blood transfusion it cannot be attributed positively to either a type A or type B virus. This condition, known as non-A, non-B hepatitis, is rare in Britain, but more common in North America.

Unlike the infectious type A variety, it is possible to carry serum hepatitis without actually suffering from it, sometimes for many years. Diagnosis can quite frequently come about accidentally, as part of a routine blood test. If an expectant mother has, or is a carrier of, serum hepatitis, she may easily pass it on to her child. In addition, doctors and dentists have to take special precautions when treating such carriers, in order to avoid contaminating any open cuts with blood or saliva from the carrier.

The symptoms of serum hepatitis are similar to those of the infectious variety, but more severe, and there is also pain and *arthritis* in the joints. The incubation period is much longer—from two to six months. Which virus, type A or B, is responsible for the symptoms can be determined by an Australia antigen test—*see Special Tests, p84.*

The virulence of the type B virus and the chances of dying from it are far greater than with type A. As with infectious hepatitis, however, there is no specific treatment for the condition, other than rest and stopping drinking. It is important that the sexual partners of sufferers from serum hepatitis are traced and their blood tested, to rule out the possibility that they are carrying the disease.

Sometimes the inflammation of the liver caused by hepatitis persists, in which case the condition is called chronic hepatitis. This may also be caused by alcohol abuse—*see Abuses of the Body, p328*—by drugs, such as carbon tetrachloride, or dry-cleaning fluid, and sometimes develops into *cirrhosis.* About 50 per cent of patients who develop cirrhosis die within five years of diagnosis.

An injection of *gamma globulin* can provide some protection from hepatitis for three months. It is not an infallible method, but is usually recommended to people about to visit the tropics, where the disease is common.

HEPATOMA

A *malignant tumour* of the liver, which is associated with *cirrhosis* in about 80 per cent of cases. A hepatoma may also develop after treatment with testosterone, a male hormone, over a long period. The condition is rare in those of European race, but more common among Africans and Orientals.

The first symptom is a loss of appetite, and this is followed by a rapid loss of weight and strength. The hepatoma will normally show up on a liver scan—*see Special Tests, p84*—and the diagnosis can be confirmed by a needle biopsy—*see Special Tests, p84*—of the area. Surgical removal of the tumour is the only effective treatment, though it is not often successful. However, this operation can only be contemplated if the tumour is confined to a single lobe of the liver and cirrhosis is not present.

HERMAPHRODITISM—see Intersex

HERNIA

An abnormal protrusion of the abdominal contents, usually through some part of the abdominal wall. The condition is commonly known as a 'rupture', and there are three common types.

Inguinal hernia may occur in both men and women, but is more common in men. It occurs in the groin, and can be either direct or indirect. In the indirect type, a part of the peritoneum protrudes down through the inguinal canal, sometimes as far as the scrotum in men. This causes a swelling that bulges when the patient coughs, or strains while defaecating. In the direct type, the abdominal organs push their way through the weakened muscles of the wall of the groin.

The danger of inguinal hernia is that a loop of bowel may slip down inside the peritoneal sac, and become twisted or strangulated. This, in turn, cuts off the blood supply to that part of the gut, resulting in *ischaemia* and eventually in infection or *peritonitis.*

Treatment depends on the size of the hernia, and whether or not it can easily be pushed back through the opening in the inguinal region. If this is possible, the hernia is said to be easily reducible, and may be controlled by wearing a truss. In more complicated cases, or if wearing a truss is unacceptable, surgery may be necessary.

Femoral hernia is more common in women than in men. It is a protrusion of the abdominal contents through the femoral canal.

The condition shows up as a swelling at the top of the leg, which may disappear on lying down. This type of hernia cannot be treated by wearing a truss, and requires an operation to replace the contents of the abdomen, and to strengthen the weakness through which it protrudes.

Diaphragmatic or hiatus hernia may affect either men or women. It is caused by a weakness or hole in the diaphragm, through which a portion of the stomach protrudes. It may stick out so far that it is in the thoracic or chest cavity rather than the abdomen.

Hiatus hernias tend to cause *flatulence* and *dyspepsia*, because the stomach contents regurgitate into the oesophagus—*see oesophagitis.* These symptoms are worse on bending down or lying flat. Treatment may consist of taking drugs that form an artificial seal at the top of the stomach to cut down the amount of regurgitation. Alternatively, surgery may be carried out to correct the problem.

Other, rarer, types of hernia are incisional hernias, which can occur at the site of a surgical scar, and umbilical hernia, a soft bulge of protruding tissue around the navel of a newborn baby. if either is serious, surgery is the usual form of treatment, *see over page.*

HERPES

The family name of a very large group of viruses, of which two species—herpes simplex and herpes zoster—are of medical significance. Both are responsible for skin infections.

There are two types of herpes simplex, designated HSV1 and HSV2. Most people carry the HSV1 type, experiencing no symptoms of infection until their body's defences are weakened in some way. The cold sore is the most common manifestation of this virus, which may be activated by exposure to sunlight or cold, or by an infection of the upper respiratory tract. The *lesions*, which appear as an inflamed, blister-like sore, occur most commonly on the face or lips and may last for a week or more.

Genital herpes may also be caused by HSV1 (which may be transmitted by oral sex with a person who has a cold sore), but is more often due to HSV2. This is a sexually transmitted disease, the incidence of which is increasing at an alarming rate. In the USA its incidence is now second only to *gonorrhoea.*

The incubation period of genital herpes is about two to four days. There are usually some warning signs, including pain or burning on

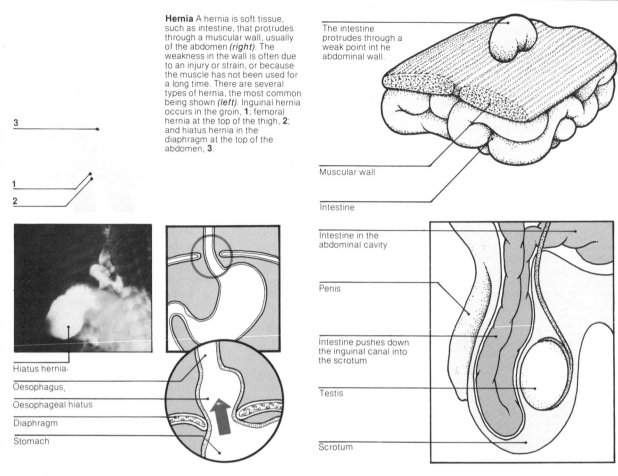

Hernia A hernia is soft tissue, such as intestine, that protrudes through a muscular wall, usually of the abdomen *(right)*. The weakness in the wall is often due to an injury or strain, or because the muscle has not been used for a long time. There are several types of hernia, the most common being shown *(left)*. Inguinal hernia occurs in the groin, **1**; femoral hernia at the top of the thigh, **2**; and hiatus hernia in the diaphragm at the top of the abdomen, **3**.

3

1
2

The intestine protrudes through a weak point int he abdominal wall.

Muscular wall

Intestine

Intestine in the abdominal cavity

Penis

Intestine pushes down the inguinal canal into the scrotum

Testis

Scrotum

Hiatus hernia

Oesophagus

Oesophageal hiatus

Diaphragm

Stomach

The oesophagus leads into the stomach just after it has passed through a hole in the diaphragm called the oesophageal hiatus *(top right)*. When part of the stomach rises up and protrudes through this opening, a hiatus hernia results *(above right)*, as shown in the X-ray, taken after a barium meal has been swallowed *(above left)*.

Inguinal hernias are more common in men than in women. The male testes pass down the inguinal canal from the abdominal cavity to the scrotum during foetal development. Although the canal usually closes after the testes have passed through it, there is still a weak point in the abdominal wall where the thigh and the abdominal muscles meet. Injury or strain may rupture this weak point, allowing

part of the intestine to push through and cause an inguinal hernia *(above right)*. The intestine may not be able to move back into the abdominal cavity and so may cause pain and distress. The danger of this is that the trapped intestine may become strangulated and lose its blood supply, in which case surgery is essential.

the areas of the penis or vulva where the blisters are about to appear, pain on passing urine, vaginal discharge, numbness of the genitalia. Often, however, there are no initial symptoms.

Once the infection begins to make itself apparent, initial patches of sore, red skin erupt into one or several groups of spots. These develop into shallow ulcers that crust over and may join. They are extremely painful and may be itchy. In women they are often accompanied by swelling of the lymph glands in the groin.

In men, the glans, foreskin and shaft of the penis and the scrotum are usually affected. In women the usual site is the vulva, but cervical herpes is not uncommon and has been associated with subsequent *carcinoma* of the cervix. It is possible, but not yet certain, that some women may be carriers of cervical herpes and some men carriers of

anal herpes.

An attack of genital herpes lasts from two to three weeks. Besides the spots and blisters, there may be a feeling of general malaise, and also fever. New lesions may continue to develop for up to ten days, but the patient continues to be infectious for two weeks, even after the lesions have ceased to be painful. This is the time when infection is most likely to be passed on, since with the disappearance of the lesions, the infected person assumes himself or herself to be cured. Once the crusts have disappeared, the red marks fade and leave no scars.

After the first infection, which tends to be severe in terms of duration and discomfort, the complaint may recur, but in milder form. In recurrent attacks the infectious period may last only four or five days, or may fail to occur at all. However, recurrence is more common with an HSV2 infection

than with HSV1. The mechanism for recurrence is unknown, but while attacks recur for no apparent reason, certain factors, such as stress, tiredness, other infections, sexual activity and even menstruation, may be linked with recurrences.

The risk for women is potentially greater than for men. Not only are attacks more severe and cervical complications possible, but a pregnant woman may pass on the infection to her unborn child. It is possible for the foetus to be infected via the placenta or, more commonly, during delivery when the baby passes through the infected birth canal.

Babies affected by the herpes simplex virus are at high risk. If infected while in the womb, they may be born with congenital abnormalities of the eyes and central nervous system, and suffer brain damage. The chances of survival for a baby with an infected central nervous system are poor. It is difficult to treat new-born babies since the drugs that have any effect on the disease are highly toxic; administered intravenously, they are probably as dangerous as the virus. If a baby is infected during birth, the lesions usually appear from two to ten days afterwards, when it is possible that they may be mistaken for nappy rash.

In adults there is a slight risk of the infection being disseminated to other parts of the body, such as the eyes or central nervous system. This may lead to aseptic *meningitis*, herpetic *encephalitis* or infection of the heart, lungs or other internal organs.

Vaccines that have been developed have not, so far, been very effective. A number of drugs may be applied to the infected area, or administered orally or intravenously, but, again, they do not always work and have a fairly high level of toxicity. These are common problems encountered in trying to treat virus infections. Treatment available is therefore most effective in relieving pain and irritation. Since no cure has been discovered, it is essential that infected people should take great care not to transmit the disease, abstaining from intercourse for at least a week after an attack.

Shingles is an attack of herpes zoster that commonly occurs on the chest. It can occur in people who have had *chickenpox* in childhood, when it is thought that the virus lies dormant in the nervous system until it reappears. After two or three days of a feverish illness, a rash breaks out, following the distribution of the intercostal nerves which run under the ribs. It can be extremely painful, especially in the elderly. The pain may precede the appearance of red spots, which then blister; the rash encircles only half the chest. Special anti-viral 'paint' can be applied. This cuts short the attack, but as the paint should be used before the spots appear, when diagnosis is still uncertain, this is not a very useful form of treatment. The pain may

continue after the rash has disappeared; this is called post-herpetic syndrome. It is very debilitating and depressing, usually worse than the shingles itself, again particularly in the elderly. Treatment is with strong *analgesics*, and *antidepressants* if necessary.

Ramsay Hunt syndrome, or geniculate herpes, is an infection of the seventh cranial, or facial, nerve, by herpes zoster. Infected blisters appear on the roof of the mouth, behind the back teeth and in the exposed part of the ear, causing *deafness* and *dizziness*. The fifth, or trigeminal, nerve is affected in facial shingles, a more common infection caused by herpes zoster. This is an extremely painful condition, for which there is no treatment other than *analgesia*. The lesions tend to affect a quarter of the face, and may damage the cornea of the eye on the affected side.

HICCUP, HICCOUGH
Involuntary and abrupt inhalation of air, due to an irritation of the nerves of the diaphragm.

Traditional remedies include drinking plenty of cold water, a tablespoon of peppermint or cinnamon water, or a few drops of spirit of chloroform. Increasing the amount of carbon dioxide in the lungs, by holding the breath or breathing into a paper bag, may also do the trick. If hiccups are prolonged, medical advice should be sought.

HIP REPLACEMENT
The insertion of an artificial joint, or prosthesis, to replace a damaged hip. This form of orthopaedic surgery is a very common procedure.

Probably the most frequent reason for a hip replacement is a fracture in the neck of the thigh bone or femur in the elderly. Unless the fracture is rectified, the head of the bone will eventually die, because its blood supply has been interrupted. Thus, the bone is either mended with a metal plate and screws, or the whole

head of the bone is replaced with a prosthetic one. These replacements are made of various materials, including stainless steel, titanium, and various plastics, which do not react with the surrounding tissues.

The operation is relatively quick, and may be carried out either under general anaesthetic, or under spinal block if the patient is frail. Patients are encouraged to be up and about within days of the operation.

Joints damaged by both osteoarthritis and rheumatoid *arthritis* can also be replaced by artificial ones.

HIRSCHSPRUNG'S DISEASE
An inherited disorder of the newborn, also called congenital megacolon. In this, the lower parts of the large intestine—particularly the rectum—have no nerve cells to control the contractions of the bowel, which normally push the contents of the intestine through to the rectum. As a result, the bowel dilates, its contents accumulate and the newborn baby experiences severe abdominal pain, swelling, constipation and, in some cases, vomiting.

Diagnosis is by rectal biopsy, to confirm the absence of the parasympathetic nerve supply, and barium enema—*see Special Tests, p84.* Surgery is necessary to remove the affected area and to join up the remaining healthy intestine to the anus.

HIRSUTISM
The abnormal growth of body hair. It is the coarseness of the hair, rather than the number of hair follicles, that is increased.

Much of what patients describe as abnormal hair growth is really due to individual, familial, or racial predisposition, and is not a strictly medical problem. Hair of this type can be removed by shaving, plucking, or depilatory creams; electrolysis is another method, though it is expensive, time-consuming, and only suitable for small areas. It should only be carried out by properly trained operators.

Some tumours and other diseases of the endocrine glands can cause hirsutism, while it can also result from the use of hormones, such as testosterone and corticosteroids. Even if a cause for hirsutism is found, removing it will not necessarily cure the condition, since once the hair follicles have become sensitized they may continue to be over-active for a long time.

HISTAMINE
A substance found in almost all the tissues in the body. When a tissue is damaged, histamine widens the

Herpes Zoster Commonly called shingles, herpes zoster is an infection caused by the same virus that causes chicken pox. It usually develops in a long thin band, following the line of the intercostal nerves under the ribs and running under the armpit to the back; it can also spread from the face, infecting the shoulders. The rash consists of small blisters, which gradually dry to form scabs. The condition can be extremely painful, the pain sometimes continuing after the rash has disappeared.

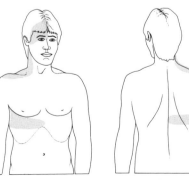

blood vessels, so increasing the supply of blood. This helps the delivery of the factors necessary for tissue repair. The chemical is often released after a bee or nettle sting, or a snake or insect bite.

Histamine has some side-effects. As well as dilating the blood vessels, it contracts the body's smooth muscle, particularly in the lungs. Thus, excessive amounts can sometimes make breathing difficult. Its release during *anaphylaxis* and in response to *allergies* may cause a characteristic rash and, in some cases, can trigger an attack of *asthma*.

Hayfever, too, causes the excessive release of histamine. Its effects can therefore be reduced by *antihistamine* drugs, though these must be taken before an attack.

HODGKIN'S DISEASE

A form of cancer in which the lymphatic nodes gradually enlarge. The disease is one of a number of *lymphomas* and is also called lymphadenoma. Its cause is unknown and theories that it may be infectious have not been proven. It is a rare disease, yet it is the most common cancer among teenagers and young adults; it is more likely to affect men than women. Superficial lymph nodes *(p21)* enlarge painlessly—often a gland in the neck is the first to be noticed and reported to a doctor. The malignant nodes are rubbery, mobile and insensitive; they usually appear in the left side of the neck, although sometimes also in the armpits, the groin, the thymus, and the abdomen.

Sufferers experience weight loss, fever, tiredness, anaemia, backaches, sweating at night and itching. There may also be local pain at the site of a node, which occurs a few minutes after drinking alcohol. If the disease is detected while still localized, it can be treated and often cured with radiotherapy. After it has become widespread, chemotherapy is used, often involving a combination of *cytotoxic* drugs. These have unpleasant side-effects and do not provide a cure, although life may be prolonged for some years.

HORMONE REPLACEMENT THERAPY (HRT)

The use of natural or artificial hormones to replace those which are not being secreted in adequate amounts in the body. Replacement therapy is used, for example, to treat *myxoedema*, *Addison's disease*, and pituitary dwarfism; the use of insulin in *diabetes mellitus* is also an example of HRT, although it is not usually described as such.

As a rule, however, the term refers to the use of female sex hormones as a treatment for menopausal symptoms, such as hot flushes, dizziness, palpitations, and headaches. The hormones used for this are the same as those that are given for oral contraception, but the dosages are smaller. They may be given by mouth, by implantation under the skin, or in a medicated sticking plaster; the last two methods are more convenient and have theoretical advantages over the first one.

It may seem surprising that middle-aged women should be prescribed these substances, considering that not very long ago the contraceptive pill was not advised for women older than 35. However, increasing experience of the use of the pill has led many doctors, though not all, to believe that the benefits outweigh the possible dangers. The benefits, in addition to relief of menopausal symptoms, include a considerable degree of protection against the loss of bone mass (osteoporosis) that can follow the menopause. Theoretically, at least, it might also protect against coronary artery disease, since premenopausal women have a reduced incidence of this, presumably owing to their oestrogen levels. However, two recent US studies produced diametrically opposite results: one showed a decrease in coronary problems in women receiving HRT, the other an increase. This illustrates the uncertainty that currently attends the whole question of the safety of HRT.

Theoretically, again, there may be an increased risk of cancer of the womb, breasts, and ovaries in women prescribed HRT. Unfortunately the evidence about this, too, is conflicting, although some studies have actually shown a decrease in the incidence of breast cancer. The risk of cancer is probably decreased if oestrogen and progestogen are both given, rather than oestrogen alone, and this is now standard practice.

Doctors advise against the use of HRT for women with a history of cancer, venous thrombosis, coronary heart disease, and high blood pressure. But, if these are absent, does a menopausal woman need HRT?

Much depends on the severity of her symptoms. HRT itself may cause symptoms, such as breast tenderness and slight vaginal bleeding, so unless the menopausal symptoms are really troublesome or there is a serious risk of osteoporosis, it is probably better to avoid it. (Factors that increase the chance of osteoporosis include an early menopause, a family history of osteoporosis, and a thin small build. It can, to an extent, be prevented by a healthy diet, vitamin D supplements and regular exercise).

HOUSEMAID'S KNEE—see Bursitis

HUNTINGTON'S CHOREA

A rare inherited disease of the central nervous system, which occurs in middle age. In it, speaking, walking and movements of the hands become seriously impaired. Spasmodic and jerky movements, characteristic of *chorea*, gradually become worse and more frequent. *Dementia* and mental deterioration eventually alter the personality so seriously that sufferers usually require institutional care. The disease is commonly fatal within about 15 years of the onset of the symptoms. There is no known treatment, although *tranquillizers* are used to calm the nervous system.

The disease is inherited as a dominant *gene*, which means that the children of an affected parent have a 50-50 chance of suffering from it. Specialist genetic counsellors recommend that anyone suffering from this form of *chorea* should not have children, since it is impossible to tell if such a child will develop the disease later in life.

HYDATIDIFORM MOLE

A rare and usually benign tumour, which develops in early pregnancy. It affects the chorion, the membrane surrounding the embryo *(p12)*, and is a collection of tiny fluid-filled sacs resulting from the degeneration of the chorion. The tumour looks like a bunch of grapes and prevents the development of the embryo, which dies. Symptoms include irregular vaginal bleeding and very bad morning sickness, and should be reported to a doctor immediately they occur. The tumour may be expelled spontaneously, although, once the diagnosis has been established, oxytocin is often injected to initiate uterine contraction, causing a therapeutic abortion.

Occasionally there is a malignant change, giving rise to a *cancer*. This is treated by cytotoxic drugs and a total *hysterectomy*.

HYDATID DISEASE—see Worms

HYDRAMNIOS

An excessive amount of amniotic fluid surrounding a foetus during pregnancy. It is caused by a defect in the circulation of the amniotic fluid. If the condition develops, it usually does so after the fifth month. The womb may swell, causing breathlessness, indigestion and aching.

Hydramnios occurs in around five per cent of twin pregnancies, and may also develop in women with *diabetes* or *pre-eclampsia*. The condition is usually harmless, but if the symptoms appear suddenly, there is a risk of premature labour. In mild cases, an obstetrician will simply advise more rest, but this may be combined with drug treatment to relax the uterus and lessen the chance of premature labour.

Hydramnios is also sometimes associated with foetal abnormalities of the digestive tract or of the spinal cord, such as *anencephaly* or *spina*

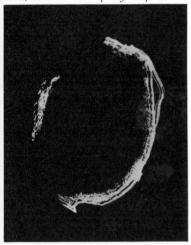

Hydrocephalus The brain and spinal cord are bathed in the cerebrospinal fluid, which is constantly absorbed and replaced. When the absorption of this fluid is prevented, either by a defective membrane or a blockage, the fluid accumulates and hydrocephalus develops. The condition is usually a disease of babyhood and is frequently associated with spina bifida. Ultrasound, the technique of using high frequency sound waves to see inside the body, can detect the condition when it is well advanced in pregnancy *(above)*. The outline of the skull shows a swelling on the right, where fluid has pushed the soft skull outwards.

bifida. This is because an affected foetus may be unable to swallow the fluid and excrete it in the urine, as happens normally. Treatment in such a case is to remove the excess amniotic fluid by amniocentesis—*see Special Tests, p84*—but the outlook for the baby is poor.

HYDROCEPHALUS

An increase in the volume of cerebrospinal fluid in the brain. Hydrocephalus is popularly referred to as 'water on the brain' and usually occurs in babies. About one in 500 babies is born with a degree of hydrocephalus, which is frequently associated with *spina bifida*. The

condition can also arise in late childhood as a consequence of brain damage caused by a *tumour* or an infection.

A blockage preventing the normal circulation of spinal fluid prevents it from draining away into the bloodstream and causes the skull to swell. The fontanelles and sutures of the infant's skull widen, and the skull enlarges. This may cause difficulties with delivery through the vagina at birth.

If hydrocephalus is not detected, serious brain damage and an early death from infection are likely. Ultrasound—*see Special Tests, p84*—and X-ray can detect the condition during pregnancy, if it is well-established. However, treatment is possible only after birth, and its success depends on the severity of the condition. In advanced cases, there is little chance of success, which is why such babies are often delivered by *caesarian section* to protect the mother. If the circumference of the baby's head at birth is greater than 350mm (13.5in), the disease may be in its first stages. To check this, the head's rate of growth is monitored to see if further growth is excessive. In such cases, further investigations are carried out to establish a definitive diagnosis.

Treatment involves surgery as soon as possible after birth. In this, a small hole is drilled in the skull and a fine tube or shunt with a one-way valve is inserted. The other end of the tube is inserted into a major blood vessel or the left atrium of the heart. The tube allows the excess fluid to drain directly into the bloodstream, and the swollen head becomes reduced in size. There is always a danger, however, that the shunt will become blocked or infected, so that regular check-ups are needed. If necessary, the shunt can be replaced, but it must be worn for the rest of the patient's life.

HYDRONEPHROSIS

A swollen kidney, resulting from an obstruction in the ureter which blocks the flow of urine. As a result the urine builds up in the kidney, and the increased pressure causes damage to kidney tissue. An occasional ache in the lower back may be the only symptom until the kidney fails completely. When this happens, the level of waste products in the blood becomes excessively high, and uraemia develops.

Hydronephrosis can be diagnosed by X-ray, while the associated uraemia is detected in blood tests— *see Special Tests, p84*. Any infection must be treated at once, and the obstruction removed. If grossly

enlarged the damaged kidney may be removed—*see nephrectomy*.

HYDROPS FOETALIS—see Haemolytic disease of the newborn

HYPERACTIVE CHILDREN

Children who are restless, prone to tantrums and who find it hard to concentrate. They have lots of energy and sleep very little.

There are various theories as to the cause of this problem. Some doctors see it as a medical problem, caused by a minor disorder in the brain's functioning, which itself cannot be detected but may have been brought on by trauma in birth, an allergy to food additives or a marginal vitamin deficiency. In this case treatment is with *amphetamines* to control the condition and a special diet. Others see it as a behavioural problem, caused by stresses within the family and advise the appropriate *counselling*.

HYPERCALCAEMIA

An excess of calcium in the blood. There are a number of possible causes; the most common are an excess of parathyroid hormone, and too much vitamin D in the diet.

One of the main functions of parathyroid hormone is to release calcium from the bones in order to maintain the level of calcium in the blood. Too much of the hormone therefore releases too much calcium, as in *hyperparathyroidism*. Excessive dosages of vitamin D have the same effect by increasing the absorption of calcium from the intestine.

The symptoms of hypercalcaemia include nausea, vomiting, diarrhoea and possibly *anorexia*; mental disturbances such as *depression*, fatigue and even *dementia*; and extreme thirst, requiring large amounts of liquid with, as a consequence, copious urination.

If the hypercalcaemia is caused by an excess of vitamin D, then this must be excluded from the diet. If it is due to *hyperparathyroidism*, this must be treated. Other possible causes of hypercalcaemia include excess milk and alkali consumed by *ulcer* patients; and *cancer*, which may or may not have spread, or metastasized.

Idiopathic hypercalcaemia is a condition of unknown cause which occurs in infancy and may cause mental retardation and *hypertension*. It is thought to be caused by a sensitivity to vitamin D. Sometimes the condition is fatal, but often it can be treated with a special diet.

HYPEREMESIS GRAVIDARUM

Excessive vomiting, which may occur in *gastroenteritis*, intestinal obstruction, and pregnancy. Hyperemesis gravidarum is a severe form of the morning sickness from which many pregnant women suffer to some degree. Usually this is just *nausea* and occasional vomiting; if the vomiting is severe, however, it may lead to weakness and dehydration. The mother may develop *acidosis* and the foetus may suffer as a result. Treatment involves rest in hospital, sedation, replacement of the lost fluid by means of an intravenous *drip*, and sometimes anti-nausea drugs.

HYPERGLYCAEMIA

Excess glucose in the blood, which occurs in *diabetes mellitus*. Hyperglycaemia may be due to insufficient dosages of insulin and may progress to serious diabetic *coma—see diabetes*.

HYPERMETROPIA

Long-sightedness, or the inability to focus on close objects. The most common reason for this is that the eyeball is too short from front to back. Hypermetropia can also be due to a weakness in the focusing ability of the lens.

In hypermetropia, nearly all objects, except for distant ones, appear to be blurred. This is because the light rays reflected from these objects are not quite focused on the retina. The nearer the object, the more blurred it appears to be. Reading a book, for example, is out of the question unless special contact lenses or spectacles with corrective converging lenses are used.

Hypermetropia can be inherited or acquired, usually after the age of 40, when the lens of the eye hardens and becomes less elastic.

HYPERNEPHROMA

A malignant *tumour* of the kidney, the most common form of kidney cancer. The tumour is caused by the uncontrolled division of the cells of the kidney's tubules, and grows on the surface of the kidney.

Hypernephroma is twice as common in men as it is in women, and usually occurs over the age of 40. *Haematuria*, or blood in the urine, is the usual symptom, the urine being red or smoky. Sometimes there is abdominal pain accompanied by a long continued fever.

Hospital tests, including X-rays, arteriograms, and ultrasonic scanning—*see Special Tests, p84*—will reveal the presence of a tumour. The whole of the affected kidney must be removed and tests made regularly to ensure that the problem does not recur. If diagnosis is late, the tumour may have broken up, or *metastasized*,

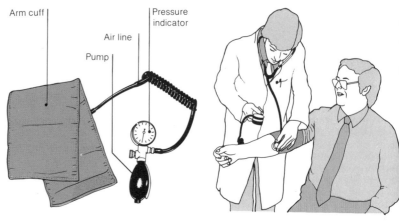

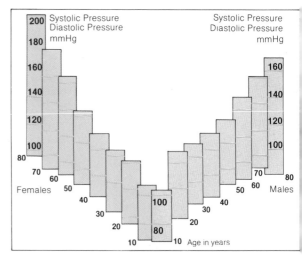

Hypertension or high blood pressure is an extremely common complaint. Its consequences can be serious, which is why blood pressure is checked routinely in a doctor's examination *(above right)*. A soft cuff *(above left)* is inflated around the upper arm until it stops the blood flow and then deflated until the doctor can hear the flow starting again. This gives the systolic pressure. The cuff is deflated further until the blood flows freely, when the diastolic pressure is taken. The chart *(right)* shows how average blood pressure varies

with cancerous cells becoming lodged in other tissues, particularly the lungs and bone.

HYPERPARATHYROIDISM

An overactivity of the parathyroid gland, leading to overproduction of the parathyroid hormone, The result is an increase in the level of calcium in the blood, which comes largely from the bones. A benign *tumour*, an *adenoma*, in one or more of the four glands is usually reponsible, although the condition can also be an indirect result of failure of the *kidneys*.

Symptoms are similar to those of *hypercalcaemia*, while stones can form in the kidneys, since they cannot cope with a normal load of calcium. The surgical removal of the tumour cures the condition; thereafter calcium supplements have to be taken, normally in the form of vitamin D tablets. If kidney stones have formed, they too will have to be removed.

HYPERSPLENISM—see Splenomegaly

HYPERTENSION

Consistently high blood pressure, in

the West the chief cause of premature deaths. Sometimes hypertension is a disease in itself, and has no apparent cause, when it is known as essential hypertension; at other times it is a symptom of a number of different diseases.

As blood circulates around the body, it presses against the walls of the arteries. The force with which it does this is called blood pressure, and is a measure of the work done by the heart in pumping the blood. In a person with hypertension, this force is greater than normal, and slowly causes the arterial walls to thicken and become narrow; it also wears out the heart, which has to perform more work than normal.

The blood pressure is not the same every second. When the left ventricle of the heart pumps out blood, the pressure rises to a maximum; this is the systolic blood pressure. As the heart fills up with blood, the pressure falls to a minimum; this is the diastolic blood pressure.

A doctor or nurse measuring blood pressure takes two readings and produces two figures. These are expressed as a fraction, the higher figure coming first. This refers to the systolic blood pressure, while the lower one refers to the diastolic blood pressure.

There is no normal blood pressure, only an average one. Most adults have a systolic blood pressure between 100 and 140, and a diastolic pressure between 60 and 90. However, even this can be misleading. Thin people and young women, for example, often have a blood pressure reading of 90/60.

Hypertension is diagnosed if both measurements, but more particularly the diastolic, are consistently elevated above the range considered normal for the particular age group.

Hardening of the arteries, or *arteriosclerosis*, is probably the most common cause of hypertension. The arterial walls lose some of their usual elasticity. This causes the peripheral resistance to rise, and so the heart has to work harder to pump blood. The systolic pressure rises, but the diastolic pressure remains about the same. If the systolic pressure rises to 200 or more, arteriosclerosis can cause problems, but otherwise it is rarely serious.

Another cause of hypertension is *atherosclerosis*, in which cholesterol and other fats are deposited on the inner lining of the arteries. This means that the arteries become narrower; therefore the heart has to work harder to pump the usual volume of blood through them. Once again only the systolic pressure rises. However, atherosclerosis is more serious than arteriosclerosis, especially in the coronary arteries. Here it is the major cause of *angina pectoris* and *coronary thrombosis*.

The real dangers of hypertension begin when both the diastolic and the systolic pressures remain high. The left side of the heart, which does the pumping, thickens as the muscles have to work ever harder. The heart becomes enlarged and may eventually weaken so much that some degree of heart failure results. Arteries also have to take the strain, and sometimes one ruptures. This usually happens in the small arteries of the brain and results in a stroke, or *cerebrovascular accident*.

High blood pressure which has no apparent cause is given the ambiguous name of essential hypertension. It may be an inherited characteristic, suddenly appearing of its own accord.

However, some disorders are known to contribute to or directly cause hypertension. Many of them are involved with the kidney, the adrenal glands and the blood vessels. These include kidney diseases, *Cushing's syndrome*,

phaeochromocytoma, coarctation of the aorta, and *aldosteronism*.

Hypertension may also be associated with pregnancy, *gout, obesity, thyrotoxicosis*, certain oral contraceptives, a high salt diet, smoking, and the natural process of ageing.

Though there is much still to learn about the nature and causes of hypertension, there have been some important discoveries. Firstly, part of the body's nervous system, the so-called sympathetic nerves—*see The Nervous System, p32*—is involved in some cases of hypertension. Stimulation of these nerves causes a rise in blood pressure; adrenaline from the adrenal glands is noted for doing this. The nicotine in tobacco also stimulates the sympathetic nervous system. Cutting these nerves—a form of treatment used in the past—results in a dramatic fall in blood pressure. However, the benefits of this kind of surgery are no longer considered worthwhile.

Secondly, it is known that the kidney is one of the most important organs involved in hypertension. Whenever the kidney's blood supply is reduced, the blood pressure rises, because the kidney tissue releases a substance called renin whenever it receives an inadequate supply of blood or it is stimulated by the sympathetic nerves. Once in the bloodstream, renin reacts with a protein to produce another substance called angiotensin. Angiotensin causes the blood pressure to rise temporarily, by constricting the blood vessels in certain muscles. It also indirectly increases the blood pressure in the long-term by stimulating the adrenal glands to produce the hormone aldosterone, which prevents the kidney from removing salt and water from the blood. A high level of salt and an excess of water in the circulation always causes hypertension. The renin-angiotensin system of raising blood pressure is associated with various kidney diseases, but it has not been established whether kidney disease causes hypertension, or vice versa.

The third important discovery is that the endocrine system—*see The Endocrine System, p48*—is involved in hypertension, particularly the adrenal glands. Sometimes a *tumour* called a *phaeochromocytoma* grows there, causing increased production of adrenaline. The blood pressure may suddenly rise to 220/140, and only the removal of the tumour will reduce it. Another type of tumour produces large amounts of aldosterone which, as already stated, raises blood pressure by preventing the kidney from

removing salt and water from the blood. This is known as Conn's syndrome, and it is one of the treatable causes of hypertension.

The dangers of untreated hypertension are often deadly. Apart from the potentially fatal consequences of a stroke, a heart attack or a burst *aneurysm, uraemia* can develop from kidney disease, or the kidney itself may fail. Uncontrolled hypertension in pregnancy can lead to *haemorrhage*, eclampsia, and retarded growth or even death of the foetus.

Diagnosis of hypertension starts with several blood pressure readings. If these are consistently high, the doctor will then examine the retina at the back of the eye with an ophthalmoscope. Here the blood vessels are visible, and their condition may reveal signs of hypertension. An electrocardiogram, or ECG, may also be performed to see if there are any signs of hypertrophy of the left ventricle.

There is no cure for hypertension at present, and it is generally agreed that patients with moderate or severe hypertension must continue to undergo treatment indefinitely to reduce the risk of complications. There is controversy, however, about the need to treat mild or borderline hypertension, since although in such cases drugs may possibly reduce the chances of a heart attack or stroke slightly, most patients would not have suffered these even without treatment. The consequence of such treatment, therefore, can be unnecessary prescription and the consequent risk of side effects.

There has therefore been much interest in methods of treating mild and borderline hypertension that do not involve the use of drugs. Salt reduction helps some patients; it should not be severe, and should consist in not adding salt during cooking or at the table. Relaxation has a modest, but possibly useful, effect. Exercise reduces blood pressure both immediately after the session and for some hours afterward. Obesity, if present should be treated. Excessive alcohol intake is another cause of hypertension. Tackling all, or some, of these may enable people to avoid taking drugs for mild hypertension. The need for treatment in any individual case will depend, not just on the actual degree of hypertension, but on age, sex, race, family history of strokes and heart attacks, serum cholesterol level, whether or not the patient smokes, and so on.

For patients requiring medication,

two main classes of drugs are usually prescribed. The first line of treatment is often a *diuretic*, which reduces the quantity of water and sodium in the body and also relaxes the blood vessels, which lowers the blood pressure. Alternatively a *beta blocker* may be used; the way in which these drugs lower blood pressure is not fully understood. If necessary, a diuretic and a beta blocker may be given together.

For patients who find these drugs ineffective, or for whom they are unsuitable, some new kinds of treatment have been introduced in the last few years. Angiotensin-covering inhibitors (ACE inhibitors) block the pathway by which angiotensin raises the blood pressure; they are effective and produce few side effects, but, because they are fairly new, they are still regarded as a second choice. Calcium-channel blockers (also used to treat angina) act by interfering with the passage of calcium into cells. Again, they are given only when the usual drugs are unsuitable or ineffective.

Other drugs for hypertension exist, but are used comparatively infrequently. Methyldopa, though effective, has numerous side effects and is now seldom used.

Screening for hypertension is one of the most valuable public health measures, since it is easy, cheap, and effective. Hypertension, unless severe, produces few or no symptoms, but it can nevertheless lead to serious illness, so it is important to detect it sooner than later.

HYPERTHYROIDISM—see Thyrotoxicosis

HYPERTROPHY

The enlargement of an organ or a tissue due to the increase in number or size of its cells. *Hypertension* may cause hypertrophy of the heart, for example; removal of one kidney may result in the hypertrophy of the remaining one—*see kidney disorders*. Hypertrophy of the prostate gland is a common problem in older men— *see prostate disorders*.

HYPERVENTILATION

The act or process of breathing more deeply and faster than normal. It can be due to a metabolic *acidosis*, as in diabetic coma or aspirin overdose, but it can also occur as part of an *anxiety* state. Nowadays many doctors believe that hyperventilation as a result of anxiety is an important cause of many symptoms. The patient acquires the habit of breathing a little too much; perhaps this is only temporary at first, but after a time it becomes habitual.

Patients who habitually overbreathe in this way may experience palpitations, chest pain, sweating, tingling, faintness, giddiness, and other symptoms; possibly in some cases it can actually precipitate *angina pectoris,* or even a heart attack. Hence a vicious circle is established. The patient overbreathes and produces symptoms, which alarm him or her; he or she then starts to breathe even faster, which makes the symptoms worse.

Ideally, diagnosis of the hyperventilation syndrome requires the taking of a sample of arterial blood for measurement of the carbon dioxide level. Because this is not always practical, the patient may be asked to take rapid deep breaths for two minutes. Normal people are able to do this, though they may feel dizzy, but hyperventilators stop quickly and may find that the over-breathing produces the symptoms of which they complain.

If hyperventilation is confirmed as the cause of the patient's symptoms, she should carry a paper bag at all times to use in an emergency. The bag is placed over the nose and mouth and the patient breathes in and out inside the bag, so that she is re-breathing her own air. This quickly brings the acid-alkali balance of the blood back to normal and relieves the symptoms. Long-term treatment involves re-educating the patient's breathing pattern.

HYPOCHONDRIA

A psychological condition in which a person has an exaggerated preoccupation with the workings of his or her body. Nearly everyone is occasionally worried that something is going wrong, but hypochondriacs constantly imagine they are ill. Serious hypochondria is a type of *neurosis*.

Hypochondria is often a complication of *anxiety*, each condition making the other worse. The hypochondriac imagines the symptoms of the anxiety as symptoms of a serious illness— which only aggravates the original anxiety. *Depression* may also lead to hypochondria, when the sufferer is convinced that his or her body is irreversibly decaying. This delusion dominates the hypochondriac's perception of reality to the exclusion of everything else.

Hypochondria is difficult to treat. Simple reassurances from a doctor will not work, because the patient wants to believe that he or she is ill. In some cases *antidepressant* drugs or *psychotherapy* may be helpful.

HYPOGONADISM

The total or partial malfunction of the gonads or sex glands. This means that at puberty normal sexual development does not take place.

Treatment depends upon the cause of the disorder, but in general involves *hormone replacement therapy*. A patient is given whichever hormones he or she is lacking. Women are given oestrogen and/or progesterone therapy, and men are given testosterone. The degree of success of the treatment depends upon the cause; in many cases, for example, the infertility cannot be treated successfully.

HYPOPITUITARISM

A disorder of the pituitary gland, in which it fails to manufacture one or more of its hormones. The pituitary gland is of such importance to the endocrine system—*see The Endocrine System, p48*—that hypopituitarism can have wide-ranging repercussions throughout the body.

Among the hormones secreted by the anterior pituitary gland are growth hormone, thyroid stimulating hormone, adreno-corticotrophic hormone, prolactin, and the follicle-stimulating hormone. Hypopituitarism can therefore affect the functions of the body's general metabolism, the thyroid gland, the adrenal glands and the ovaries.

The most common cause of hypopituitarism is a tumour in the cells which secrete the hormones. Other possible causes include serious head injuries, and more rarely, severe haemorrhaging and shock during childbirth. Rarely, the disease may follow conditions such as tubercular *meningitis*, or *sarcoidosis*.

People with hypopituitarism are pale, weak, in constant ill-health, infertile and prematurely aged. They show a set of symptoms that are similar to those of *anorexia nervosa*, a well as a combination of several hormonal disorders. *Dwarfism* occurs in children, women suffer from *amenorrhoea*, and all those affected will show some of the symptoms of *Addison's disease* and underactivity of the thyroid gland. Alternatively, there may be isolated deficiencies of certain of the hormones, which only affect the target organs.

Hypopituitarism is an incurable long-term disorder. It can be controlled if treated soon enough, otherwise it can quickly become fatal. The usual therapy is the substitution of the hormones which are lacking. Patients often respond well to *corticosteroids*, which may be given in conjunction with thyroid hormone. Sometimes an oestrogen is given to female sufferers and an androgen to men.

HYPOTENSION
Low blood pressure. The most familiar example of hypotension occurs when a person stands up suddenly from a sitting or lying down position. The blood pressure falls abruptly and may result in a faint, or *syncope*. Normally, a nervous reflex constricts the blood vessels and prevents this postural hypotension. Older people and those who take drugs to combat high blood pressure, are particularly prone to such fainting episodes. They go pale, their pulses are weak and their pupils dilate.

Hypotension also occurs after a considerable amount of body fluid is lost, as in *diarrhoea, vomiting,* or *haemorrhage. Myocardial infarction,* the allergic shock following an insect sting or a snake bite, and heart *arrhythmias* are other causes of low blood pressure.

One serious consequence of hypotension is the risk of *kidney failure.* After a massive haemorrhage or a heart attack, the blood pressure is lowered so dramatically that the kidneys do not receive an adequate blood supply, and the tissue dies—*see ischaemia.*

HYPOTHERMIA
The lowering of the body's temperature below 35°C (95°F). Hypothermia may be induced deliberately by an anaesthetist during surgery to reduce the patient's need for oxygen; more commonly it results from prolonged exposure to low temperatures, or immersion in cold water.

The body normally responds to coldness by shivering, which produces heat. Hypothermia sets in when this shivering response breaks down or cannot cope with the prolonged cold of the environment. Old people, babies and people suffering from illness or disease are all particularly prone to hypothermia. Diabetics, paraplegics, and sufferers of *hypothyroidism, hypopituitarism* and peripheral blood vessel diseases also have a reduced response to cold. However, even fit people, such as mountaineers and hill climbers, are subject to hypothermia when exposed to conditions of extreme cold.

The skin turns a pale blue colour, and the body is very cold to the touch. Shivering continues until body temperature falls below 30°C (86°F), below which the muscles become spastic. Mental processes gradually slow down, confusion sets in and the victim becomes unconscious before dying. The cause

of death is a heart attack, or *myocardial infarction,* which occurs when the body temperature falls to about 26°C (78.8°F).

If the body temperature, which is taken with a special low-reading thermometer, is above 32°C (89.6°F), nursing in a warm room is all that is necessary for an otherwise healthy patient. Below this temperature the body has to be actively rewarmed, usually by immersion in a bath at 40°C (89.6°F), and hydrocortisone injections are given to fight the effect of physical *trauma—see also frostbite, First Aid, p369.*

HYPOTHYROIDISM—see Myxoedema

HYPOXIA
A deficiency of oxygen in the body's tissues. Hypoxia is also called anoxia, and the term is usually used to describe high-altitude sickness which results from breathing rarefied air. While there is still the same percentage of oxygen in the air as there is at sea level, the atmospheric pressure is reduced. This means that insufficient oxygen can enter the blood from the lungs.

Above 3,000 metres (about 10,000ft) most people will experience the effects of hypoxia, unless the air has been artificially pressurized, as in an aircraft. The symptoms include breathlessness, headaches, palpitations, nausea, tiredness and impairment of vision. After a few days, however, the body begins to compensate and people acclimatize themselves. They breathe in more quickly and deeply, the heart increases its output, more red blood cells are produced and the haemoglobin in the blood gives up its oxygen more readily.

Hypoxia may also result from certain chemicals and diseases. Morphine, *barbiturates,* alcohol and nearly all *anaesthetics* depress the respiratory system and initiate some degree of hypoxia. Cyanide creates immediate and fatal hypoxia in the cells of the tissues themselves.

However, when hypoxia is a symptom of a disease, it is rarely as debilitating as the disease itself. For example, an abnormality in the respiratory system, as occurs in *poliomyelitis* and *pneumonia,* will reduce the amount of oxygen that enters the blood. A disorder of the red blood cells, such as *anaemia,* means that not enough oxygen can be carried to the cells. Carbon monoxide poisoning, in which haemoglobin combines with carbon monoxide instead of oxygen, will also reduce the carrying-capacity of oxygen in the blood. A reduction in the volume or the flow of blood to

the tissues, which occurs in all cardiovascular diseases, also means that there will be a reduction in the amount of oxygen reaching the tissues.

HYSTERECTOMY
An operation to remove the uterus, or womb. The cervix, or neck of the womb, may be removed as well. It is usually performed for treatment of *fibroids* or cancer. Hysterectomy is a major operation, requiring a general *anaesthetic;* the tissue is sometimes removed through the vagina and sometimes through an incision in the abdominal wall.

Total hysterectomy means removal of the ovaries and Fallopian tubes, as well as the womb. While hysterectomy means sterilization and the end of menstrual periods, the ovaries are not nowadays removed before the menopause unless there is good medical reason for the procedure. If total hysterectomy is necessary in a pre-menopausal woman, *hormone replacement therapy* may be used to treat the loss of oestrogen, the hormone produced by the ovaries.

After a hysterectomy, normal procedure is to keep the patient in hospital for approximately 10 days. The period of convalescence varies from individual to individual, but the minimum is two weeks. One of the common consequences of the operation is a psychological one—many patients believe that a hysterectomy makes intercourse impossible, stops the sex drive, or *libido,* and leads to *obesity.* None of this is true. A normal sex life can usually be resumed about six weeks after the operation. The only permanent legacy of the operation is its scar, which becomes less noticeable in time.

HYSTERIA
A type of *neurosis* which may manifest itself in an apparent physical illness, accompanied by an assortment of psychological symptoms. Hysteria is one of the most ill-defined of psychological disturbances, because its manifestations are so varied, and often subtle.

The word 'hysteria' is derived from the Greek word for uterus. However, despite the fact that women are associated with hysteria, men suffer from the problem as well.

The personalities of hysterics are usually childish. Such behaviour has led psychiatrists to attribute hysteria to a childhood trauma, or to insensitive parental treatment during adolescence. However, normal people under prolonged stress can also become hysterical.

In general, hysterical people are overtly selfish and are obsessional about attracting attention and admiration. Their manner, speech and dress is often extrovert and their habit of forgetting their mistakes and behaviour leads them to frequently change friends. Their hysteria usually manifests itself in specific circumstances. They appear to conjure up physical symptoms in order to avoid situations they consider unpleasant. For no apparent reason they suddenly go blind, deaf or mute, or they may suffer from paralysis. Pain may occur anywhere in the body, and headaches, backaches and lumps in the throat are common. Once the situation that the patient has found threatening or unpleasant disappears, the symptoms may subside.

Such behaviour may be taken to extremes, as in *Munchhausen's syndrome*. Hysterics with this condition exhibit so convincing a set of symptoms that doctors may assume that organic causes are present, and even surgery may be undertaken. True hysterics, however, are not pretending; the symptoms are quite real to them. Sometimes an emotionally threatening situation will result in terrifying screams and convulsions resembling *epilepsy*; however, such a patient never loses consciousness.

Only hypnotism—*see Alternative Medicine, p305*—or long-term psychotherapy seem to benefit the true hysteric, while tranquillizers may provide temporary relief from a hysterical fit. One symptom of the hysterical personality is its denial that it is hysterical; patients therefore do not see any reason why they should need treatment. However, there is a danger that, on rare occasions, a doctor may mistakenly diagnose hysteria in a patient who is, in fact, suffering from a disease whose symptoms are hard to define and can be confused with those of hysteria. Multiple sclerosis is an example of this.

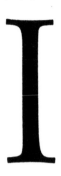

IATROGENIC
A Greek term meaning 'caused by doctors', used to describe a condition that arises as a result of medical treatment. Iatrogenic disorders may be the result of *drug interactions* or be side-effects of drugs; they may follow surgery—as, for example, when *adhesions* form, or bowel habits are altered after surgery on the digestive tract—or be caused by an infection by resistant *bacteria* or other organisms, following the use of *antibiotics*.

Since one disease may closely resemble another, iatrogenic disease is occasionally caused by inappropriate treatment based on incorrect diagnosis.

ICTERUS—see Jaundice

ICTERUS GRAVIS NEONATORUM—see Haemolytic disease of the newborn

ID
A term coined by the Austrian psychologist Sigmund Freud to describe the aspect of the personality that is concerned with the satisfaction of basic needs. The id is the most obvious aspect of the personality in babies; their need for food and demonstrations of love is expected to be gratified instantly, regardless of the needs or desires of the parents.

As children grow, this part of the personality becomes tempered by the judgements of the developing *ego*, the aspect of the mind that, according to psychological theories, mediates with the outside world, or interacts with it. Children learn to control the expression of these physical and psychological needs until times when they seem most likely to be satisified.

IDIOPATHIC DISEASE
A disease with no discernible cause. For example, when a case of *epilepsy* is not caused by an injury or a *lesion* of the brain, or by some other discoverable cause, it is called idiopathic epilepsy.

ILEOSTOMY
An operation in which the ileum, the lowest portion of the small intestine *(p40)*, is diverted from its usual position in the intestinal tract to a stoma, or artificial opening, on the abdominal wall. The contents of the small bowel then empty into a detachable bag that is fixed to the abdominal wall around the stoma and worn under the clothes, instead of passing into the colon, the large bowel.

An ileostomy may be performed as part of the surgical treatment of severe, advanced ulcerative colitis, for example. In the procedure the diseased colon and rectum are removed and an ileostomy fashioned so that the faeces pass into a bag. The operation is usually permanent, and the patient uses the bag for the rest of his or her life.

Although an ileostomy may be distressing initially, most people adjust quickly, and live a normal life—*see colostomy*. The Ileostomy Association can give advice on the special problems experienced by those who have an ileostomy.

ILEUS PARALYTICUS
A condition, also called adynamic obstruction or paralytic ileus, in which the normal passage of food through the digestive tract *(p40)* is halted by a breakdown of peristalsis, the rhythmic contractions of the intestinal muscles. The condition may be caused by *peritonitis*, a bacterial infection in the cavity of the abdomen, by an obstruction to the intestines—for example, by *adhesions*—or may follow major surgery to the bowel. It is sometimes a complication of a serious disorder elsewhere in the body, such as a perforated peptic *ulcer*. Symptoms include nausea and vomiting, abdominal distension and severe constipation.

When paralytic ileus has been caused by bowel surgery, the problem usually clears up by itself within a few days. Otherwise, the condition is treated according to its cause. A peritoneal infection, for example will be treated with *antibiotics*, and an intestinal obstruction caused by adhesions will normally be removed by surgery. In all cases, the discomfort can be relieved if a tube is passed into the stomach through the nose to remove any stomach contents and to relieve pressure, and food and liquid are given directly into a vein by means of a *drip*. Impacted faeces, the result of serious constipation, are removed from the rectum by hand, or by means of an enema.

ILLUSION

A mistaken impression, which can involve any of the senses, but is most commonly visual. Illusions arise when the senses are unable to interpret the information that they receive. For instance, a mirage is an optical illusion, created when heat rising from a desert distorts the light reflected from the crystalline particles of sand, giving the impression of a shining expanse of water.

Illusions are more pronounced during the altered states of consciousness caused by *fever*, excessive alcohol in the bloodstream, or by drugs—*see Abuses of the Body, p328*. People whose brain tissue has been damaged by the abuse of alcohol or drugs, or patients with mental abnormalities, may experience persistent illusions which eventually become *delusions*—illusions or false impressions that cannot be corrected by rational argument or by a demonstration of the truth.

IMMUNIZATION

A method of protecting the body against a disease by artificially sensitizing it to that disease. This is achieved by introducing antigens, the *viruses* or *bacteria* that cause the disease, into the body. The antigens have been rendered harmless, and are contained in a vaccine; this is introduced into the body by a procedure known as *vaccination*, or inoculation. The vaccine stimulates the body's immune system to produce *antibodies*, proteins capable of rendering the specific antigens harmless—*see Natural Defences Against Disease, p52*. The body is then primed to recognize any future invasion by this type of antigen, and has the means to repel it.

The technique was first used successfully against *smallpox* in the 18th century—*see vaccination*—but for more than a hundred years no further advances were made, because it was not understood how vaccination worked. In the 20th century, however, a greater understanding of immunology has made it possible to protect people against a wide range of diseases that

might otherwise be common. These include: *diphtheria, tetanus, whooping cough, poliomyelitis, measles, rubella, tuberculosis, cholera, typhoid* and paratyphoid, and tropical diseases such as *yellow fever*. In many countries, protection against some of these diseases is provided free of charge, especially for children, while protection against others is offered only in special circumstances, for example during an epidemic.

There are several different types of protection against a disease, depending on the type of vaccine used. 'Active' protection is provided by the use of a vaccine that contains a similar, but less potent antigen to that which causes the disease. This is normally a specially modified, or attenuated, strain of live virus. It provokes a mild reaction that stimulates antibody production, creating an immunity against the more serious disease. This is the type of protection given by smallpox vaccination and by the vaccination programme against *poliomyelitis* that began in the 1950s. However, attempts to provide a 'live' vaccine against other diseases, such as *leprosy* and *syphilis*, have failed.

Some vaccines, for example those that give protection against cholera and typhoid, contain dead viruses or bacteria. Unfortunately, this type of vaccine does not give permanent immunity. It is mainly used by people who intend to visit those countries in which typhus and cholera are common, and the vaccination has to be repeated at intervals of one to three years.

In the case of diseases such as tetanus and diphtheria, where the danger is from the toxins—the poisons manufactured by the bacteria—rather than from the bacteria themselves, a different method is used. Vaccines for these diseases contain modified toxins, called toxoids. The protection given by this method is not permanent, but usually lasts longer than that given by dead antigens.

There is a time lapse between vaccination and protection, during which the body's immune system is stimulated to produce the necessary antibodies. This is why people travelling to certain countries are required to have their 'shots' a number of days before departure. If immediate protection is required, when, for example, a patient is suspected of already having contracted a disease, an injection of immune serum can be given. This consists of plasma, from which the platelets and clotting factors have been removed—*see The Blood and Lymph Systems, p21*—taken from a patient who has recently been

infected with the disease but has recovered. This serum will contain the necessary antibodies in the form of *gammaglobulins*. Immune serum is also given in the treatment of diseases such as *Lassa fever*, for which there is no effective vaccine.

IMMUNODEFICIENCY DISEASES

A group of rare diseases that arise when the body's immune response fails, leaving the affected person open to infection—*see Natural Defences Against Disease, p52*. There are three main causes for the breakdown. In some sufferers from immunodeficiency diseases, there is a failure to manufacture immunoglobulins, the proteins that act as antibodies; in others the number of lymphocytes and white blood cells, which fight infection, is reduced. The third category of patients suffer from both these problems.

The most serious form of immunodeficiency disease, in which no immunoglobulin is produced at all, is inherited; it is called congenital agammaglobulinaemia. The *gene* responsible is sex-linked, and the disease affects around one in 100,000 male babies. This condition is usually fatal, but other, less serious, forms can be treated by a transplant of bone marrow from a donor who has similar marrow. However, this type of transplant is not always successful, and affected children are at risk of dying from minor conditions, such as *influenza*, from which, under normal conditions and with full immunity, they would recover. Such infections are kept at bay by means of immune serums—*see immunization*—and *transfusions* of blood that is rich in white blood cells.

Immunodeficiency diseases can also be acquired, that is, they develop during adult life. Until recently, this problem was uncommon. Those affected suffered from a succession of minor infections, and had a tendency to develop *auto-immune disorders*, in which the immune system turned on the normal tissues of the body. However, during 1981 and 1982, acquired immunodeficiency disease became much more common, and much more serious. The problem is now classified as a separate, identifiable disorder—*see AIDS (acquired immunodeficiency syndrome)*.

IMMUNOSUPPRESSIVE

A drug that reduces the immune response, the body's reaction to invasion by foreign matter. Immunosuppressive drugs enable surgeons to transplant organs, such

Modern medicine has developed many vaccines to protect you against the risk of infection from disease. The way these work is easy to understand; antigens — the viruses or bacteria that cause the disease — are made safe and incorporated into a vaccine, which stimulates the body's own natural defences to produce the appropriate antibodies. These counter-attack and defeat any subsequent infection.

The technique itself is not new; it was first used successfully as long ago as the 18th century, when the British doctor Edward Jenner developed the first smallpox vaccine. It is only in the present century, however, that greater knowledge of the processes of immunology has made it possible to protect people against what, in the past, were often killer diseases.

Some of the commonest infectious diseases are shown here (right), together with basic information about them. Always remember the following points. First, some infectious diseases have no vaccine against them. Second, just because vaccines exist, this is no reason to relax the proper rules of hygiene and health, especially when travelling in areas where certain diseases are endemic. Third, if you do have to deal with a case of infection, always make sure the quarantine period is observed.

TRAVELLING ABROAD

When planning to travel abroad, always check with your doctor, who will be able to advise you whether there are any special precautions you should take, such as specific vaccinations, and what you should do about any other potential medical problems endemic to the area you will be visiting. There is no anti-malarial vaccine, for instance. Tablets must be taken before, during, and for a month after a visit to a malarial area. Always observe the following precautions. Wash your hands thoroughly before eating and drinking. Make sure the drinking water is safe; otherwise drink bottled water and avoid ice in drinks. Be cautious about eating raw vegetables, unpeeled fruit, ice-cream, raw shellfish, underdone meat and fish, and reheated food.

Disease	Incubation period	Contagious period	Rash, if any
Chickenpox	12 to 19 days (usually 13th or 14th day)	From one day before appearance of rash to six days after appearance of rash.	Small pink spots develop into pinhead-size pimples. Blister forms on top of pimple which turns to scab in about 4 days.
Diphtheria	Usually two to six days	Varies — usually 2 weeks or less. Considered completed when three successive nose and throat cultures are negative at daily intervals.	None.
German measles (Rubella)	14 to 25 days (usually 17th or 18th day)	From start of symptoms to at least four days after disease subsides. Contagion considered over three days after start of rash.	Pink and mottled rash, which usually appears first on face and neck and spreads down, covering whole body.
Infective hepatitis	10 to 50 days (average 25 days)	Unknown. Virus may be in faeces two to three weeks before onset of disease.	None.
Influenza	Usually one to three days.	Shortly before and up to one week after onset of symptoms.	None.
Measles	Seven to 14 days (usually 10 days)	From four days before until five days after rash appears.	Mottled pink rash on face and neck extending down over whole body within three days before starting to fade from the head down.
Meningitis	One to 10 days (usually three to seven days)	As long as the bacteria remain in the nose and throat of infected person.	Tiny dark red spots appearing mainly on trunk, and buttocks in about 40% of cases of meningococcal meningitis.
Mumps	14 to 21 days (average 17 days)	Until swelling of affected glands has completely subsided.	None.
Poliomyelitis	Usually seven to 14 days but may be less.	Not known. At least 5 days from nose and throat secretions. Virus may be present in faeces for several weeks.	None.
Smallpox	Eight to 16 days (usually 12 days)	From first symptoms until all scabs have been shed.	Small dark red spots which form pimples appear over body. Dimpled blisters form, each about the size of a pea. Scabs form.
Typhoid	Seven to 21 days (average 14 days)	As long as patient or carrier harbours the typhoid organisms in faeces or urine.	Usually scanty pink spots on trunk a few days after onset of symptoms.
Tetanus	Three to 21 days (average 10 days)	None.	None.
Tuberculosis	Approximately three to eight weeks from time of infection to tuberculin allergy as indicated by skin tests.	First infection generally not contagious. Tuberculosis lung cavities or draining tuberculous sinuses are contagious as long as tubercule bacilli are present.	None.
Whooping cough	Five to 21 days (usually under 10 days)	Greatest in early stages before cough becomes repetitive. Contagion is believed to last 6 weeks from onset.	None.

Symptoms	Treatment	Care	Immunization
Usually fever and headache, followed by rash within 24 hours. Rash develops fully in two to three days, followed by drop in temperature. Itching usually subsides by fourth day.	No specific treatment. Cut fingernails, apply calamine lotion. Oral antihistamine may help.	Quarantine for one week after the rash appears.	None.
Headache, fever, and sore throat with white spots over tonsils, throat, and throat, and soft palate. There may be difficulty swallowing, a croupy cough, and bloody discharge from nose.	Diphtheria antitoxin. Penicillin. Erythromycin.	Penicillin by injection and by mouth for five to seven days.	Diphtheria toxoid with booster inoculations given at periodic intervals.
Low fever and occasional headache. Usually swollen glands behind neck and on back of head appearing either before or during rash. Eyes may be slightly inflamed.	No specific treatment.	Quarantine from diagnosis for five days. Pregnant women may suffer complications.	Live German measles vaccine should be given to all girls approaching puberty.
Malaise, weakness, headache, and loss of appetite are initial symptoms. These are followed by discomfort in the upper stomach. Pain, nausea, and vomiting usually occur. Urine is dark, faeces light-coloured. Soon afterwards jaundice appears.	No specific treatment. In severe cases corticosteroids may be prescribed.	Injections of gamma globulin usually give immunity for five weeks or longer.	Temporary immunization for five weeks or longer may be obtained with injections of gamma globulin.
Sudden headache, malaise, chills, and aches and pains in arms, legs and back. Nose congested. Hard, dry cough common. Symptoms last for approximately three days.	No specific treatment.	None.	Polyvalent vaccine against known viruses. Yearly booster injection to maintain immunity.
Fever, followed by hard dry cough, red eyes, and running nose. Tiny white spots then appear on inner cheeks, gums, and palate. A rash appears, fever rises and continues for several days until rash has covered body. Then fever drops, cough subsides, and eyes clear as rash subsides.	No specific treatment. Antibiotics often used to prevent complications.	Quarantine for one wek. Can be prevented by injections of gamma globulin during incubation period, but this is of no use once symptoms show.	Live measles virus vaccine will immunize for long period, possibly for life.
Fever, headache, vomiting. Later, delirium and loss of consciousness. A stiff neck is a common symptom, the child being unable to rest the chin on the chest.	Intensive antibiotic treatment directed at the organism causing the infection is required in meningitis.	Penicillin, sulphonamides, or erythromycin by mouth in cases of meningococcal meningitis.	None.
Occasionally fever and vomiting, but often no signs or symptoms before tender swelling appears in front of and below ear, usually on one side of the face. The swelling on the other side appears in two or three days.	No specific treatment.	Rest. Quarantine until the swelling has subsided.	Live mumps vaccine but vaccination usually unnecessary as the disease is mild.
Usually starts with fever, vomiting, and irritability, which may subside after several days. A flare-up then occurs, with severe headache, fever and neck and back stiffness. Pain in affected muscles follows. Paralysis occurs in 10 to 15 per cent of cases.	No specific treatment.	None of proved value, though Gamma globulin has been used.	Oral live polio vaccine usually protects for life.
Headache, backache, fever, and characteristic rash.	No specific treatment. Antibiotics may be given to lessen scarring from secondary bacterial infection.	Immediate vaccination.	Smallpox vaccine repeated every 3 years. Disease now almost eradicated.
Fever, headache, malaise, loss of appetite, backache, and bronchitis. Diarrhoea is usually but not always present. Mild abdominal tenderness and distension also are common symptoms. Condition usually lasts one to three weeks.	Antibiotics.	Rest. Family contacts are not allowed to handle food until three successive negative tests of faeces and urine.	Three doses of typhoid vaccine given by injection at weekly intervals. Booster every two years.
Increasing stiffness of jaw, making it difficult to open mouth. Later, stiffness of back and abdominal muscles with neck thrown back and back curved in. Muscle spasms are extremely painful.	Tetanus antitoxin, sedatives, sometimes tracheostomy, and artificial respiration.	Rest.	Tetanus toxoid, two injections at monthly intervals. Booster every few years. For immediate immunization, tetanus antitoxin is given.
Usually few specific symptoms in children. The signs and symptoms may be only those of a mild infection with low fever and a dry cough. Complications such as an infection through the bloodstream will produce more severe symptoms.	Isoniazid for at least a year or rifampicin. In severe cases, one of these drugs may be combined with streptomycin and para amino-salycic acid.	Repeated tuberculin tests and X-rays if tests are found positive.	Heaf test and BCG vaccination.
A dry cough gradually gets more severe at night. At about the third week cough becomes very severe, spasmodic, and paroxysmal. The child may become breathless and blue. At end of the paroxysm there is a long crowning whoop. Vomiting may occur.	Ampicillin or amoxycyillin may be helpful. Severe cases require hospital treatment. Improvement occurs after three weeks.	When a child develops whooping cough, it is probably too late to immunize brothers and sisters if they have not already received vaccine.	Three doses of pertussis vaccine injected at intervals of at least one month.

as the heart or kidneys, from a donor to a patient, since without them the body would quickly reject the transplanted tissue.

However, immunosuppressive drugs are double-edged. They do not merely suppress the body's reaction to transplanted tissue; they also lessen the natural reaction to invasion by harmful micro-organisms, leaving the body open to infection. This is one of the reasons why sterile conditions are so important in hospital units in which transplant surgery is performed. In addition, they may have other side-effects; *steroids*, for example, an important group of immunosuppressive drugs, cause the deposition of a layer of fatty tissue around the face, neck and trunk.

IMPETIGO

An infectious skin disease that is usually caused by Staphylococcal and sometimes by *Streptococcal* bacteria. In impetigo, inflamed, puffy patches appear on the skin—usually of the face, scalp and neck; pus, seeping from infected blisters or pustules, forms a crust over this. The disease is common in children, and is spread by scratching the infected areas and then touching a part of the skin that is not affected, or the skin of another person. Impetigo responds rapidly to treatment with *antibiotics*.

IMPOTENCE

The inability to have sexual intercourse. Impotence, meaning 'loss of power', is used to describe this problem in men.

In order to have sexual intercourse, a man must have an erection of the penis; he must sustain the erection for long enough to penetrate his partner, and he must ejaculate—*see Sex and Reproduction, p54*. Impotence may be due to any of these three events failing to occur. The problem may have either a physical or psychological cause, and be temporary or long-standing.

The most common form of impotence is temporary, and is caused by anxiety. It is sometimes experienced by adolescent boys at the time of their first sexual experience, and by middle-aged men who are going through an emotional crisis. Impotence may also be a sign of general malaise: most men experience a temporary loss of *libido*, or sexual drive, if they are not feeling well. In these cases, no treatment is necessary. However, long-standing impotence, without physical cause, is usually due to deep-rooted psychosexual problems and *psychotherapy* may be necessary to cure them—*see Sex and Contraception, p338*.

The most common of all physical causes of impotence is over-indulgence in alcohol. However, the problem may also be a side-effect of treatment with *barbiturates*, or with methyl dopa—a drug that is be used to treat *hypertension* in some patients. In these cases potency is restored once the drugs are withdrawn. Men are often temporarily impotent after they have had their prostate gland removed—*see prostate disorders*—but potency usually returns within a few months.

Since penile erection and ejaculation are controlled by the nerves that link the genitals with the spinal cord, any damage to the nerves of the lower spine may result in impotence. The damage may be caused by injury, or by *neuropathy*—a disease of the peripheral nerves—a *tumour* of the brain or spinal cord, and *syringomyelia*. It may sometimes be irreversible, making impotence permanent. The condition may also be a result of longstanding *diabetes mellitus* in which there is involvement of the autonomic nervous system (*p32*). It may also occur in some disorders of the endocrine glands (*p48*), such as *hypogonadism, Cushing's syndrome* and *myxoedema*. In these cases potency is restored when the condition has been treated successfully.

INCOMPETENT VALVES—see Valvular heart disease

INCONTINENCE

The partial or complete loss of control over urination, defaecation or both. Urinary incontinence is much more common than faecal incontinence, which is known as encopresis.

Continence, or full control of the bladder, is usually learned during the first few years of life. However, children who suffer from *mental handicap* or a disorder of the nervous system (*p32*), such as *spina bifida*, may take much longer to become continent, and in severe cases, never achieve control over the bladder at all. Some children who are otherwise normal learn bladder control much later than others, and may become incontinent at times of emotional stress, wetting the bed at night—*see nocturnal enuresis*. The reason for this is not known, though the problem tends to run in families.

Once bladder control has been learned, there are rarely any problems with continence until old age. However, there are several exceptions to this. People whose nervous system has been damaged by an injury—*see paraplegia*—or by a disease, such as *multiple sclerosis*, may suffer from urinary incontinence, and the condition is also a problem for women who have a *prolapsed* womb. In this case, a specially shaped pessary may be placed in the vagina to support the womb and relieve the pressure on the bladder, until the prolapse can be repaired surgically. Some women find it difficult to control their bladders for a few months after the birth of a child, because the muscles of the floor of the pelvis have been weakened by the delivery; this condition is sometimes known as stress incontinence. A course of post-natal exercises, designed to strengthen the muscles, usually clears up the problem—*see Exercise, p316*.

However, incontinence is a common problem among elderly people. Many elderly men suffer from *prostatic hypertrophy*, a condition in which the prostate gland (*p54*) becomes enlarged and constricts the urethra that passes through it. As a result, urine builds up in the bladder, a condition called *retention of urine*. As the pressure builds up, urine may be forced past the constriction, causing a problem known as overflow incontinence. Men with prostatic enlargement may have to get out of bed as many as five or six times during the night to pass water—a condition known as nocturia. If the sufferer has *arthritis*, with stiffness and immobility of the joints, or is taking sleeping pills, this may not be possible, and so there is nocturnal enuresis, or bed-wetting.

Another cause of urinary incontinence in the elderly is *senile dementia*, a condition in which standards of personal hygiene often deteriorate drastically. In serious cases, there may be faecal incontinence as well. However, a more common cause of incontinence of faeces, which is sometimes, but not necessarily, associated with a degree of dementia, is long-standing *constipation*. This results in the faeces becoming impacted, forming a solid mass in the rectum. The mass does not form a complete blockage, and liquid faeces often overflows around it. This problem is treated by curing the constipation with drugs in the short-term and preventing its recurrence by mean of a high-fibre diet—*see Diet, p322*. The impacted faeces are removed by hand.

Many elderly people who are otherwise healthy are admitted to geriatric hospitals because they suffer from incontinence. This is often unnecessary, because a number of welfare agencies provide services that can greatly improve the quality of life for sufferers from incontinence and their relatives. Among these services are the supply of commodes that can be placed by the bed, incontinence pads to be used in bed and access to an incontinence laundry—*see Looking After Old People, p362*.

INCUBATION PERIOD

The time that elapses between the invasion of the body by infecting organisms such as *bacteria, viruses* and *protozoa*, and the onset of symptoms of disease. For example, the *common cold* and *cholera* may have an incubation period of 24 hours, while *syphilis* or *leprosy* may remain latent in the body for several years before symptoms appear. On average, however, bacterial diseases, of which *gonorrhoea, scarlet fever* and *whooping cough* are examples, have an incubation period of less than a fortnight, while viral diseases, such as *mumps, hepatitis* and *poliomyelitis* have incubation periods of two weeks or more.

Within a few hours to a few days of exposure to an infectious disease, an infected person may be capable of transmitting the disease to others, yet unaware that he or she has contracted it. In most countries, cases of serious contagious disease—*see notifiable diseases*—must be reported to the appropriate medical authorities, so that all those who have been in contact with the infected person can be traced, isolated and treated, in order to prevent an *epidemic* of the disease.

INCUBATOR

A life-support system, usually consisting of a transparent container with a clean, warm, controlled atmosphere, used to support prematurely born babies until they have grown strong enough to survive in normal conditions. Hospital incubators are specially designed with inlets in the side through which hands can reach the child. The inlets enable a baby to be fed and changed and allow contact with the mother to be maintained. This is crucial to the emotional well-being of both mother and child.

INDIGESTION—see Dyspepsia

INDUSTRIAL DISEASE

A group of diseases that are contracted as a direct result of conditions at places of work. Also called occupational diseases, a number of such conditions have been recognized by health authorities. These include: *pneumoconioses*, the lung disorders, such as *asbestosis* and *silicosis* caused

Incubator Premature babies may need the life-support system provided by an incubator *(right and below right)*, because some of their bodily functions are not yet fully developed. The more premature the baby is, the less developed are its bodily functions and the longer it must remain in the incubator. Low birth weight babies need an incubator to maintain their body temperature. Milk may be given through a tube passed into the stomach or other nutrients may be passed directly into a vein via a drip. The baby's heart rate and respiration are constantly monitored, while he or she can be touched, fed and changed through inlet holes in the side of the incubator.

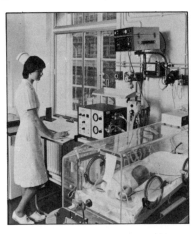

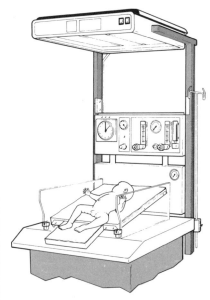

Special baby care units are equipped with neonatal resuscitation units *(above)*. The unit is a mobile system, which provides vital facilities for any baby who is born with respiratory problems. Oxygen cylinders for instant resuscitation and a lung ventilator are on hand to deal with any emergency. Heat from an overhead radiator is designed to keep the baby warm.

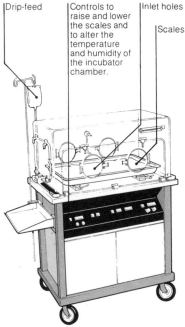

Drip-feed | Controls to raise and lower the scales and to alter the temperature and humidity of the incubator chamber. | Inlet holes | Scales

by an inhalation of particles; *brucellosis*, a hazard for farm workers; and the formation of *cataracts* in the eyes of glassblowers.

Doctors are required to notify the coroner and the national health authorities of all cases of death from industrial disease—*see Coming to Terms With Death, p366*—and living victims are entitled to claim compensation from their employers. In addition, certain disability pensions and other rights may be claimed by anyone who has been disabled by an industrial disease. In the event of the sufferer's death, these benefits pass to the widow or next of kin.

Anyone who believes that their health is being, or has been, affected by their working conditions should consult a doctor. Should the diagnosis be confirmed, general practitioners and specialists will not only treat the disease. With the patient's permission, they will

report their findings to the appropriate official bodies. Citizens' advice bureaux, and municipal and national health authorities can give advice on how to apply for compensation.

INFANTILE ECZEMA

A form of *dermatitis* that affects mainly male children from the age of about three months. It usually begins as a bright red inflammation on the cheeks and forehead on which itchy, weeping blisters rapidly form. This rash may spread all over the body.

Infantile eczema is an *allergy*, and occurs more often in temperate than in tropical climates. It is more common in babies who have been fed on cows' milk than on breast milk or goats' milk; the reasons for this are not fully understood, but it is possible that an allergy to cows' milk is involved. A number of factors appear to make infantile eczema worse, among them contact with woollen or nylon clothing. Parents should watch for any other factors that seem to cause or irritate the condition in order to avoid them.

It is important to keep a child suffering from infantile eczema cool, to keep the fingernails short and to prevent him or her from scratching. This can often be achieved by keeping the child's attention distracted as much as possible. The condition cannot be cured but it can be brought under control, especially if the causative factor can be identified and eliminated. In mild cases the doctor may prescribe a cream containing coal tar and a mild *corticosteroid* preparation to control the rash. However, children suffering from infantile eczema tend to have relapses, in which the condition becomes worse. If the rash is widespread and the blisters are weeping, hospital treatment may be necessary. The child's arms may be restrained, sometimes by splints, and a succession of lotions and pastes used to dry the blisters and soothe the skin.

INFANTILE SPASMS
A rare form of *epilepsy* that affects infants between six months and two years old. It is also called 'lightning fits', since the seizures take the form of a spasm of the entire body that lasts for a second or two. The child's head drops and the arms fly out, and he or she may draw up the legs or straighten them. The seizure is followed by a cry.

Often, infantile spasms occur for no apparent cause, though sometimes the child already has some degree of brain damage from a previous illness—for example, from post-vaccination *encephalitis*, a very rare complication of immunization against *whooping cough*. The spasms cause a retardation of mental development and, occasionally, blindness. Although the attacks usually begin to die out by the age of two, the damage that they cause is permanent.

As the spasms are so short-lived, they are often not noticed by parents. However, when the baby's slow development becomes apparent, the diagnosis of infantile spasms can be confirmed by means of an electroencephalograph test (EEG—*see Special Tests, p84*). After diagnosis, the spasms can be prevented by treatment with *corticosteroid* drugs and the hormone ACTH *(p48)*.

The disease has no connection with the convulsions that are often a feature of *fevers* in childhood. These convulsions are very different in character from infantile spasms, and

they do not cause changes to show up on an EEG test. However, parents should consult a doctor.

INFARCT
The death of tissue due to an interruption in its blood supply. Infarction occurs most commonly in three areas of the body: the brain, the heart and the lungs.

In a cerebral infarction, an area of brain tissue dies after a stroke or *cerebrovascular accident*, when normal blood flow is impeded due to bleeding or a blood clot in a blood vessel. The clot is called a *thrombus* when stationary and an *embolus* when carried from another part of the body. In *myocardial infarction*, an area of heart muscle dies as a result of the formation of a blood clot in the coronary artery that supplies the particular area of muscle. In a pulmonary infarction an area of lung tissue dies when an embolus blocks off the artery that is supplying it.

INFECTION
The invasion of the tissues of the body by harmful micro-organisms, usually *bacteria, viruses, fungi* or *protozoa*. An elaborate system of traps and defences protects the body from infection—*see Natural Defences Against Disease, p52*—but this cannot always prevent microbes from invading the tissues.

Once micro-organisms have found a way into the body, they establish colonies in the bloodstream or on the inner surface of a vessel or organ. After an *incubation period*, during which the colony multiplies, the area becomes inflamed. This is the result of a build-up of toxins, or poisonous chemicals, that are released by bacteria as a by-product of their biological activity, and of the fight between the body's defences—the white cells *(p21)* and antibodies—and the microbes. The battle may also give rise to other symptoms, such as a *fever*.

In most cases, the body's defence systems eventually triumph, and the symptoms of infection die down. Sometimes the microbes assist in their own downfall, because some toxins are poisonous not only to the body but to the microbes that produce them. At other times, the microbes are killed by drugs such as *antibiotics*, which destroy bacteria. The remaining toxins are either broken down by the liver *(p44)* and excreted, or mopped up by antibodies.

INFECTIOUS DISEASES—see Contagious diseases

INFECTIOUS MONONUCLEOSIS
A viral infection, also called

glandular fever, that is commonly known as the 'kissing disease', since it may be spread by mouth-to-mouth contact. It tends to occur in children and young adults. The incubation period is about one week, after which the first symptoms appear. These include tiredness, headache, muscular pain and a sore throat. A week or two after this, the lymph nodes *(p21)* in the groin, neck and armpits may enlarge.

Infectious mononucleosis is difficult to diagnose, because the symptoms are similar to those of several other conditions. The muscular pains may lead a doctor to suspect *influenza*, and the symptoms sometimes also mimic *tonsillitis*: the throat becomes very sore and is covered with a whitish material and the trunk is sometimes covered by a faint red rash. The virus may also be responsible for a mild form of *hepatitis*.

As a result, a special type of blood test called a Paul-Bunnell test—*see Special Tests, p84*—may be necessary to confirm the diagnosis. The test reveals the presence of antibodies that are specific to the virus in the patient's blood, and, characteristically, an increase in the number of monocytic white cells *(p21)* that gives the disease its medical name.

The disease usually lasts for a few weeks, during which time the patient feels generally ill and weak. However, in some cases it may last for several months, clear up and then recur. There is no specific treatment other than rest in bed. Oddly, sufferers from infectious mononucleosis who are given the *antibiotic* ampicillin, as a result of a misdiagnosis, develop a severe red rash all over the body. This is a peculiarity of the disease, and does not mean that the sufferer is allergic to this form of penicillin.

INFERTILITY
The inability to conceive children. There are many possible causes of infertility: scientists estimate that in about one-third of cases infertility is due to the woman's inability to conceive, in one-third the man is infertile, and in the final third both partners have some degree of infertility.

While not a disease as such, infertility can cause a great deal of anguish to the partners and requires a sympathetic approach and careful explanations, both of the often bewildering reasons for its cause, and of the methods of investigating and treating it.

Sometimes the problem is a simple one of technique and timing. Either the sperm do not reach the cervix, or do not do so at the appropriate moment in the menstrual cycle—see *Sex and Reproduction, p54; Sex and Contraception, p338*. In this case, a brief explanation of the mechanisms of sex and reproduction may be all that is necessary to treat the problem.

However, normally infertility is due to a physical defect of one partner or the other. In men, this may be lack of sperm, which may be total—see *azoospermia*—or relative compared with the normal sperm count. The sperm may be abnormal, either in shape or mobility. Both of these factors may adversely affect their chances of fertilizing the ovum, or egg. Occasionally, an illness such as *mumps*, when it affects an adult man, may cause an *orchitis*, or inflammation of the testes. The inflammation can cause permanent damage to the affected testicle, seriously reducing the quantity of sperm produced.

Infertility in women can also have a number of causes. Sometimes it may be because an egg is not produced each month, or that, having been produced, it is unable to travel along the Fallopian tubes to the womb because they have been blocked and distorted by previous infection—see *salpingitis*. The problem may be mechanical, due to an abnormally shaped womb, although women with this congenital abnormality often become pregnant and later miscarry. Sometimes the mucus that covers the cervix, or neck of the womb, is hostile to the sperm and destroys them before the ovum can be fertilized.

The precise cause of infertility is often investigated in a special unit within a hospital. However, there are a number of tests and observations that can be carried out in the doctor's surgery. First, the woman is asked to keep an accurate temperature chart for a few months to see if she is ovulating regularly. Next, a sample of her partner's seminal fluid may be taken for a sperm count. The couple are made aware of the most appropriate time of the month to concentrate their efforts to conceive, and of the positions in which sexual intercourse is most likely to culminate in conception. Certain techniques after sex are also helpful; if the woman lies quietly with her bottom on a pillow and her knees bent for half an hour, she is more likely to conceive than if she gets up immediately to have a bath or to resume other activities.

If the initial results are normal, but infertility persists, the couple is referred to a hospital infertility clinic. There, an internal examination called a laparoscopy and dye is performed on the woman to see if the tubes are functioning normally. A fibre-optic device called a laparoscope—see *Special Tests, endoscopy, p84*—is inserted into the pelvis, and a dye injected into the Fallopian tubes via a catheter or thin tube passed through the cervix into the womb. If the tubes are not blocked the dye can be seen coming out at the other end, near the ovaries. If the tubes are blocked, an operation to attempt to restore their function may be performed. However, if the Fallopian tubes are found to be clear, the problem is usually caused by a defect in the mechanism of ovulation *(p54)*. This can often be corrected by treatment with the hormones oestrogen and progesterone *(p54)*, depending on the precise nature of the defect.

Where either the quantity or quality of the man's sperm is insufficient for fertilization to take place, a procedure known as artificial insemination by husband, can be used—see *AIH*. In this technique, a doctor places large quantities of the man's sperm, collected over a period of several weeks and stored by freezing, high up into the woman's womb. If the man's ejaculate contains no sperm at all, a technique called *AID*, or artificial insemination by donor, may be suggested. In this, a doctor places a quantity of a donor's sperm inside the woman's womb.

Sometimes it proves impossible to unblock the Fallopian tubes by surgery. In this case, a recently developed technique called in vitro fertilization may be used to produce a so-called test-tube baby. The man's sperm is used to fertilize an egg, which has been removed from the mother's ovary by means of a laparoscope, in a test-tube. At an early stage of its development, the embryo *(p12)* is then implanted in the mother's womb. However, this technique is only available in a few special centres, and is not always successful.

If, after investigation and treatment, childless couples are still unable to conceive, and are unwilling to contemplate AID or in vitro fertilization, they may wish to consult their family doctor about adopting a child. Not all couples are considered suitable for this, and there is a long waiting list for young babies. Many months of counselling and discussion are required before a couple is accepted; thereafter, there may be many delays before a child is actually adopted. Eventually, however, the rewards for both the adoptive parents and the child are often considerable.

INFLAMMATION
The response of the tissues of the body to injury or *infection*, that takes the form of redness, local heat, pain and swelling. These are the symptoms of the body's attempt to heal itself: the blood supply to the area of infection increases, so that more white cells *(p21)* are available to fight the microbes responsible. At the same time, the microbes produce toxins, or poisonous chemicals, which irritate the tissues. By-products of the fight against infection, such as dead white blood cells, dead tissue cells and dead bacteria, accumulate at the site as pus. *See also The Blood and Lymph Systems, p21; Natural Defences Against Disease, p52*.

INFLUENZA
One of the most common viral illnesses, that usually occurs in epidemics during the winter. There are three main type of 'flu, caused by three different types of virus; these are designated A, B and C. For example, Asian 'flu, the most serious form, is caused by an A-type virus, while the small outbreaks of milder 'flu that occur in cold and temperate climates are caused by a type B virus. The C-type virus is least common, and causes only a mild illness.

Influenza is highly infectious. It is usually spread by droplets from an infected person's sneezes and coughs. The incubation period is usually little more than a day or two, after which the symptoms appear. These include a headache, aching joints, muscular pain, and often nausea and lack of appetite. Often there are symptoms of upper respiratory tract infection, such as breathlessness, cough, sneezing and general malaise, together with a moderate *fever* with the temperature about 39°C (102°F).

There is no medical treatment for influenza. A sufferer should stay in bed, drink plenty of fluids and take *aspirin*, or paracetamol preparations to reduce the temperature. The illness usually clears up in a few days, but it may lower the body's resistance to a bacterial infection, such as *bronchitis* or *bronchopneumonia*. This is a particular hazard for the elderly and infirm, in whom a bout of 'flu is often the forerunner of a serious and possibly fatal disease. In such cases, doctors try to prevent the onset of bacterial infection by prescribing *antibiotics*.

Vaccines that confer immunity against influenza for up to a year are now available. However, they are usually recommended only for the elderly or for patients with chronic chest complaints such as *bronchitis* or *emphysema*, in whom influenza would be a particular danger. This is because there are hundreds of different strains of the influenza-producing virus, which continually mutate, or change slightly, making it very difficult to prepare an effective vaccine against them. However, if the particular strain of virus can be identified early enough in an epidemic, a specific vaccine can be produced and the spread of the infection halted.

INGUINAL HERNIA—see Hernia

INOCULATION—see Vaccination

INSOMNIA
The inability to sleep. Insomnia is a common disorder that affects almost everyone at some time or other. However, it is difficult to define since people differ greatly in their assessment of the quality and quantity of sleep they need.

Most people feel ill, losing mental and physical co-ordination when deprived of sleep; prolonged sleeplessness may eventually cause complete mental breakdown. But individuals vary considerably in the amount of sleep they need. Some evidence suggests that people who appear ill-adjusted to life, experiencing periods of depression, for example, or psychological difficulties in their relationships with other people, tend to need more sleep than individuals who appear well-adjusted and have no serious personality problems. The young need considerably more sleep than the old, women seem to need more sleep when they are pregnant, and in general, people need more sleep when they are ill. This is probably because, in all these cases, a large proportion of the body's energy is being devoted to the growth of new tissue, or the repair of damaged tissues.

People who find their sleep pattern changing over a period of weeks, or even years, may believe, wrongly, that they have insomnia. Older people in particular often complain of insomnia and ask for sleeping pills to remedy what they see as a disorder, though in fact the relative sleeplessness may be a normal accompaniment of ageing. Since sedatives are habit-forming if taken regularly, and since it may be even more difficult to sleep when sedatives are discontinued, it is important that older people learn to adjust to the change in their sleeping habits, rather than attempting to correct them with sleeping pills.

Anxiety is a constant companion of insomnia. Difficulty in falling asleep, and early morning waking, are usual in states of *anxiety* and *depression*. All too often, however, sufferers try to treat the insomnia rather than the underlying causes of the problem. They become even more anxious about the insomnia, exacerbating the problem and creating a vicious circle.

Although it is frustrating to be unable to sleep when everyone else is sleeping, especially if early rising is essential, worrying is unnecessary. The amount of sleep actually needed is surprisingly small. Relaxing in bed with a warm drink and a book, or a radio or television programme, is better than worrying. In all cases, sleep will come when the body needs it.

If the insomnia is part of a depressive illness, *antidepressants* may be prescribed to be taken at night, since they have a sedative effect and thus treat both complaints.

Cases of chronic insomnia, in which it is impossible to sleep until shortly before it is time to wake up—the result being perpetual overtiredness—are extremely rare. Relaxation therapy is the modern treatment for this type of insomnia. The therapy is based on the principle that the insomnia is caused by physical and mental tension. Patients are taught to relax by carrying out a series of tensing-and-relaxing and breathing exercises before going to bed, not unlike those practised in yoga—see *Stress, p332*. Simple meditation techniques help to control the spiral of anxiety and tension that tends to exacerbate insomnia. These new techniques may eventually replace the traditional drug therapy.

See also REM sleep.

INSTITUTIONALIZATION
A state of mind and form of behaviour that occurs in people who have spent many years in institutions. These may be orphanages, old-fashioned mental hospitals, or even modern long-stay geriatric units. Such people become totally dependent on the routines that operate in the institution in which they are resident, and upon the staff to provide everyday needs, ceasing to choose or think for themselves. Eventually, they may become incapable of looking after themselves at all, and thus unable to exist outside the institution.

Now that the problem of institutionalization is recognized, staff in such institutions try to prevent this state of mind from

developing. They aim to make everyday activities interesting by encouraging the residents to live as full and active a life as possible, and ensuring that they retain and use their powers of decision-making, even in minor matters, such as deciding what to wear or to eat each day.

INTERFERON
A protein produced naturally by a cell that has been infected by a *virus*. Interferon is thought to form part of the body's defences against infection, because it prevents viruses from multiplying. Interferon was discovered as a result of a research programme that took as its starting point the observation that the body does not usually suffer from two viral illnesses simultaneously. This made it likely that a substance produced by one infecting virus somehow interfered with the process of infection by another. Eventually, the substance was isolated, and called interferon.

At the time of this discovery, some scientists believed that *cancer* might be caused by a virus. Interferon, therefore, was tested as a cure for the disease. At first, the results were promising, and attracted considerable publicity. However, after controlled trials it became evident that interferon has little or no effect on cancer, and it is now no longer considered a suitable treatment for the disease. The theory that cancer is caused by a virus remains unproved.

Even though interferon is ineffective against cancer, it may still be possible to use it as a treatment for known viral diseases.

INTERMITTENT CLAUDICATION
Pains in the calf muscles which develop during exercise and disappear when the legs are at rest. Intermittent claudication is caused by a reduction in the supply of blood reaching the muscles of the legs and feet.

This is usually caused by *atherosclerosis*, in which fatty atheroma forms on the inner wall of the arteries, and may develop into a blood clot, or *thrombus*. The atheroma blocks the artery, depriving the tissues it supplies of blood and oxygen. The result is cramp, a coldness of the feet and pain whenever the demands for oxygen increase, as when walking. There is no specific treatment for intermittent claudication although it is improved by regular, moderate exercise. Sometimes, synthetic grafts are used to replace the narrowed vessel.

INTERSEX

A rare condition in which an individual shares some or all of the sexual characteristics of both sexes. It may be due to a *chromosomal* defect or a variation from the normal levels of sex hormones (*p54*).

Intersex can be caused by several different chromosomal abnormalities. The two most common forms are *Turner's syndrome*, which affects women, and *Klinefelter's syndrome*, affecting men. Women who suffer from the former have the sex chromosomes XO, instead of the normal female configuration XX. Such women tend to be very short, and have either underdeveloped ovaries, or no ovaries at all. In Klinefelter's syndrome the chromosomal pattern is XXY, as opposed to the normal male configuration of XY. As young boys, sufferers from this condition often appear normal, but after puberty the testes remain small and soft, and there may be *gynaecomastia*, an abnormal development of the breasts.

There are two further chromosomal abnormalities that cause intersex: hermaphroditism and pseudohermaphroditism. The first condition is extremely rare in humans; hermaphrodites have the chromosomes and sexual organs of both sexes. Psedohermaphroditism is more common. In this condition the sex glands conform to the chromosomal sex—that is, if the chromosomes are XX then the sex glands are ovaries—but the external genitals resemble those of the opposite sex.

Pseudohermaphroditism may be caused by factors other than chromosomal abnormalities. One such factor is congenital *adrenal hyperplasia*, in which a defect of the metabolism (*p44*) stimulates an excessive formation of androgens (*p54*), or male sex hormones, by the adrenal glands (*p48*) of female foetuses. The baby girl has two ovaries at birth, but a large clitoris and a single opening for the vagina and urethra (*p54*). The condition may also rarely be caused by treatment of the mother with androgens during pregnancy—at one time androgens were given to women who had a tendency to *miscarry*—or a *tumour* of one of the mother's ovaries, which secretes androgens as a result.

Male pseudohermaphroditism, in which the testes are present and the chromosomes are XY, but the external genitals resemble those of women, is a rare hereditary disorder, for which the cause is not known. Because the testes often do not descend, affected children are often thought to be girls. However, at puberty breasts develop, but menstrual periods are absent, because the child has no ovaries or uterus. When their condition is recognized, such children are normally encouraged to continue dressing as women, and their undescended testicles are removed by surgery to prevent the possibility of *malignant* changes later in life.

The diagnosis and treatment of the various forms of intersex is extremly difficult. Where there is any question of sexual ambiguity, the chromosomal sex is identified by means of a buccal smear—*see Special Tests, p84*. The levels of the sex hormones in the blood are measured, and, as a last resort, a laparotomy is performed. This is an operation in which the surgeon opens the abdomen to examine the sex glands.

Cosmetic surgery can make the appearance of the external genitals conform to that indicated by the chromosomal sex. However, it is impossible for sufferers from intersex to perform in the normal reproductive role of members of their chromosomal sex. This may cause a number of psychological problems which must be treated by sensitive *counselling* and support.

INTERTRIGO

An inflammation of the skin that usually affects the moist folds of the body, especially in the elderly and overweight. Intertrigo is caused by skin-chafing, followed by maceration, or softening of the skin, due to the production of sweat in the affected areas, from which it cannot evaporate. The softened areas usually become infected with fungi such as thrush—*see candidiasis*. Intertrigo is treated by keeping the areas clean and dry, and by applying a soothing, anti-fungal cream to the affected parts.

IQ

An abbreviation of the term 'intelligence quotient', a standard index by which psychologists attempt to measure intelligence. IQ is classified on a scale that rises from the profoundly retarded (below 20), those who are retarded but can benefit from education (50 to 70), normal or average intelligence (90 to 110), very superior intelligence (120 to 140), to 'genius' (above 140). IQ is estimated by means of one or other of a variety of standardized tests; performance in one of these is measured against the individual's age to give an indication of mental age.

Intelligence testing is no longer as widely used as it was in the first half of this century, because it has become apparent that there are a number of inherent inconsistencies in the tests. For example, children from deprived backgrounds will not do as well on a given test as children from homes where the parents are themselves well-educated, but this does not necessarily mean that the less privileged children are less intelligent in any meaningful sense. Apart from social and educational background, there are other factors which affect intelligence as measured by IQ tests, such as the degree of emotional security and the unimpaired ability to see and hear. *Institutionalization* is also known to have an adverse effect on intellectual development.

In an attempt to offset this bias, modern IQ tests attempt to measure many aspects of mental ability, rather than selected ones such as mathematical skills, for example, or reasoning ability. They are often preceded by routine tests of language comprehension, of sight and hearing, and of personality.

IRIDECTOMY

An eye operation performed on the iris (*p32*), the coloured part of the eye, to relieve ocular pressure in *glaucoma*. Under general *anaesthesia* part of the iris is removed, making the pupil larger and irregular in shape. This relieves the pressure by enlarging the channel through which the transparent substance which fills the eyeball, called vitreous humour, circulates.

IRITIS

An inflammation of the iris (*p32*), the coloured part of the eye. It causes redness and pain, and sometimes also blurred vision. Unlike *conjunctivitis*, which is a superficial inflammation usually due to bacterial infection or an *allergy*, iritis is a serious condition that is often associated with other diseases. It may occur in *rheumatoid arthritis*, *ankylosing spondylitis*, *tuberculosis* and *ulcerative colitis*. Prompt treatment of iritis is important, because the condition may progress until vision is lost. Iritis is usually treated with *steroid* eye drops.

IRRITABLE BOWEL SYNDROME

A common disorder, also called spastic colon and mucous colitis, which is characterized by abdominal pain, disturbance of bowel habit (constipation, diarrhoea, or each alternately), bloating, flatulence, and the passage of small stools, which may be pellet-shaped and covered with mucus. There are often symptom-free intervals, the disorder tending to recur over a long time in episodes lasting for days, weeks, or months. It may begin at any age, but usually first appears in adolescence or early adult life.

Irritable bowel syndrome is generally regarded as being due to disturbance of the autonomic nervous control of the bowel. It seems to be one form of a wider group of disorders affecting smooth muscle – that is, the involuntary muscle that forms the wall of the gut, the blood vessels, and many other structures. There may be an overlap with chronic constipation, especially in women, and with *dysmenorrhoea*. There is a tendency for sufferers to be tense and anxious; the condition is certainly made worse by psychological tension, even if that is not its whole cause.

Mild degrees of irritable bowel syndrome are very common, particularly at times of emotional tension. In mild cases the usual symptom is constipation, with pain in the lower left part of the abdomen that is relieved by defecation. A minority have more severe symptoms, with acute pain, diarrhoea accompanied by the passage of large amounts of mucus, and other more generalized symptoms, such as headaches, fatigue, and shortness of breath on mild exertion.

Diagnosis of the disorder is usually made on medical history alone in the case of a young person. Even so, a full physical examination should be carried out and most patients will have a sigmoidoscopy and barium enema as well as examination of the stools. The purpose of these tests is to rule out other causes for the symptoms; there are no diagnostic findings in irritable bowel syndrome itself, although, if the patient is seen during an attack, the barium enema may show spasm of the large intestine. Middle-aged or older patients certainly require thorough investigation to exclude the possibility of a more serious disease, such as cancer of the colon.

Treatment, unfortunately, is often difficult. Drugs based on peppermint help some people, while medicines that relieve colonic spasm are also used. A high-fibre diet is usually advised, though this does not always help (some people find it makes things worse). Recently, some patients with severe irritable bowel syndrome have been treated by hypnosis; autogenic training can help some patients.

It might seem logical to look for food allergies in this disorder, and some doctors have found this a useful approach. Others, however, have not; and there is a danger that patients may become confused by constantly altering their eating pattern in a vain attempt to identify the food or foods that are causing their symptoms. On the other hand, some patients find that they are made worse by certain foods, particularly during an attack. This is not an allergy, but rather an intolerance of the foods in question. Milk is often a problem, especially whole milk; skimmed milk, buttermilk, and cheese are tolerated better. Vegetables of the cabbage and turnip families should be avoided, as should alcohol, coffee, and tobacco. The only laxatives that should be given are those that work by increasing the bulk of the stools.

ISCHAEMIA
A reduction in the supply of blood and, therefore, oxygen and nutrient to an area of tissue. This can cause permanent damage, including the necrosis, or death, of the tissue, in the affected part. Ischaemic heart disease, therefore, is a long-standing reduction of the blood supply to the heart that is caused by *coronary artery disease*, and may lead to a heart attack, or *myocardial infarction*, or to *heart failure*.

ISLET CELL TUMOURS OF THE PANCREAS
Small, rare *tumours* that form clusters in the pancreas, and are usually benign, but occasionally become malignant. The islets of Langerhans are groups of two types of cell—alpha and beta— in the pancreas. Alpha cells produce a hormone called glucagon *(p44)*; beta cells produce a hormone called insulin *(p44)*, which lowers the blood glucose level. Tumours in the islets may therefore secrete insulin which causes *hypoglycaemia* or much more rarely, glucagon, which causes diabetes and muscular wasting. There is a third substance which is rarely secreted by the islet cells. This is gastrin, a hormone which is usually produced in the stomach and plays a part in digestion. An excess of gastrin causes a high level of acid in the stomach which, in turn, causes peptic *ulcers*. This is known as the *Zollinger Ellison syndrome*.

Islet cell tumours are treated by surgical removal of the pancreas. A patient can live without a pancreas, if the digestive enzymes that it produces *(p40)* are replaced with food additives and the insulin deficiency is made up by means of injections.

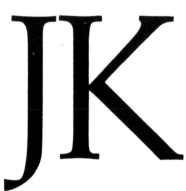

JACKSONIAN EPILEPSY—see Epilepsy

JAUNDICE
A condition, also called icterus, in which the skin and the whites of the eyes take on a yellow tinge, and the colour of the urine deepens. This is the result of an increased level of the yellow bile pigment bilirubin in the blood. Bilirubin is a component of haemoglobin, the dye that gives red blood cells *(p21)* their colour. It is released when red blood cells are broken down. Normally, bilirubin is itself broken down by the liver and excreted into the duodenum with the bile *(p44)*.

Jaundice, therefore, can be a symptom of any disease that interferes with one of these three processes. If there is an excessive breakdown of red blood cells, which overloads the liver, the resulting jaundice is said to be haemolytic. When the blood is healthy, but there is a malfunction of the liver, the

Jaundice The characteristic yellowing of the skin and whites of the eyes in jaundice is due to the large amounts of bilirubin circulating in the blood. This yellow pigment is the main breakdown product of haemoglobin from the red blood cells. Normally, it is filtered from the blood by the liver, transported to the gall-bladder as a constituent of bile and then secreted into the duodenum *(right)*. It is then broken down by bacteria in the intestine and excreted in the faeces. Jaundice usually results from a malfunction of the liver due to infectious hepatitis, cirrhosis, anaesthetics such as halothane or drugs such as chlorpromazine. Jaundice is also caused by gallstones, which block the bile duct, and tumours of the pancreas *(far right)*, which prevent bile from entering the duodenum.

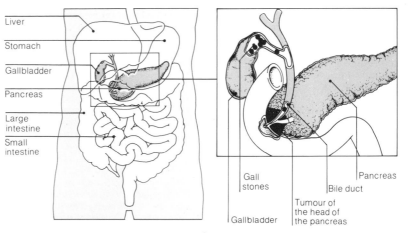

Liver
Stomach
Gallbladder
Pancreas
Large intestine
Small intestine

Gall stones
Pancreas
Bile duct
Tumour of the head of the pancreas
Gallbladder

condition is called infective jaundice; when the bilirubin is processed by the liver but cannot be excreted because of a blockage in the bile duct, the condition is called obstructive jaundice.

Haemolytic jaundice is a complication of conditions in which red blood cells are destroyed in excess. Such conditions include *sickle-cell anaemia, haemolytic disease of the newborn*—when the resultant jaundice is known as icterus neonaturum gravis—and a mismatch of blood groups *(p21)* in a blood *transfusion*. The jaundice clears up once the underlying blood disorder has been treated, and, in adults, does not cause any permanent ill-effects. However, in young children, *kernicterus*, the deposition of bilirubin in immature brain cells, may cause permanent damage.

Infective jaundice occurs when a *viral* infection of the liver interferes with the organ's normal functions *(p44)*. The most common viral infections of the liver are caused by the *hepatitis* A and B viruses. There is no specific cure for either type of hepatitis, but the jaundice normally disappears as the infection clears up.

Obstructive jaundice occurs when the common bile duct *(p44)* becomes blocked, and prevents the normal passage of processed bilirubin to the duodenum. This may be caused by a *gallstone* or a tumour of the pancreas *(p48)*. The condition is treated by surgical removal of the obstruction, or, if this proves impossible, by grafting an additional section of tube to the bile duct to by-pass the obstruction. After the obstruction has been removed or by-passed, the jaundice clears up.

JET LAG
A disturbance in the rhythms of the body caused by rapid transit across a number of time zones. The body has many cycles of activity, which are called *circadian rhythms*. The most

obvious of these is the sleep-wake cycle, but there are numerous others, including the secretion of cortisol, which is lowest between 10pm and 12pm and highest between 6am and 8am. These cycles tend to be upset by changes in time, especially in older people; this results in tiredness, disturbances in bowel function, menstrual irregularities, and a loss of efficiency; the effects last for at least 24 hours and frequently longer. As a rough guide, one day of impaired efficiency should be allowed for each hour that has been lost or gained.

There are certain steps that travellers can take to minimize these effects. Fly by day if possible. Adjust your cycle, if you can, for a day or so before flying. Set your watch to the new time as soon as you get on the plane. Take care not to eat too much, or drink a lot of alcohol, on the day before you fly; avoid alcohol on the plane, but drink plenty of water or fruit juice (flying tends to dehydrate you). Avoid having to take important decisions soon after you arrive.

Recent research has linked jet lag to disturbance in the secretion of melatonin, a hormone produced by the pituitary gland. The function of melatonin is unknown, but in evolutionary terms it appears to have some relation with the way in which our circadian rhythms are tied in with the day-night cycle. Giving melatonin by mouth seems to provide a degree of protection. However, melatonin is not yet generally available.

KERATITIS
An inflammation of the cornea, the circular, transparent layer at the front of the eye *(p32)*, in which the eye becomes watery and painful, and vision may be blurred.

The condition may be caused by *bacteria*, in which case it is treated by *antibiotics*, or by a virus, such as *herpes simplex*. It can also be caused

by foreign objects, such as dust or grit, in the eyes, or by excessive exposure to ultraviolet light. The inflammation usually heals if the eyes are kept covered, and any pain or irritation can be soothed by eyedrops.

A more serious form of the condition, known as interstitial keratitis, is caused by congenital *syphilis*, passed from mother to child at birth. Interstitial keratitis usually develops after the age of five. The eye normally heals, after *steroid* treatment, but sometimes the cornea is permanently scarred.

See also conjunctivitis.

KERATOCONJUNCTIVITIS
An inflammation of both the cornea, the circular, transparent layer at the front of the eye *(p32)*, and the conjunctiva, the delicate mucous membrane that covers the front of the eye.

See keratitis and conjunctivitis.

KERATOPLASTY
An operation, also known as a corneal graft, in which either all or part of the cornea, the circular, transparent lens at the front of the eye, is replaced by a graft of corneal tissue. The replacement tissue is usually taken from a dead human donor.

The operation is performed to restore vision when the cornea has been scarred by chemicals, as in an industrial accident, or by a disease, as in *trachoma* or interstitial *keratitis*. Because the healthy cornea does not contain blood vessels, the body's immune system *(p52)* cannot reject the replacement tissue. As a result, corneal transplants have become almost routine, and have a high success rate.

KERATOSIS
A group of conditions in which the skin is disfigured by the formation of *callosities*, or hard, thick areas of tissue. This is caused by the

excessive production of *keratin*, a horny protein, by the skin cells. Pigmented, scaly spots may also develop, making the skin look harsh and rough. The condition most commonly affects the middle-aged and elderly, and may take a number of forms.

Solar keratosis is one of the more common varieties of the disease. It is caused by overexposure to the sun, and results in the formation of pinkish *warts*. Seborrheic keratosis, also common, results in the appearance of *benign*, or harmless, yellow or brown skin tumours.

Other forms of the condition are less common. Follicular keratosis, also known as 'toad skin', is a rare hereditary disease. In this the hair follicles, usually of the head and trunk, become blocked with horny plugs of keratin. These give the skin a lumpy appearance. In smoker's keratosis, spots with red dots at their centres form in the mouth at the outlets of mucus-producing glands that have been irritated by smoke. This problem is more common among pipe-smokers than cigarette-smokers, and can be cured completely by giving up tobacco—*see Abuses of the Body, p328.*

The causes of most other forms of keratosis are unknown. The callosities that develop are usually treated by *curettage*, in which the affected skin is scraped away under a local *anaesthetic*. New, normal skin cells then grow to replace the ones that have been removed.

KERNICTERUS
A disorder of new-born children in which the basal ganglia of the brain—*see The Nervous System, p32*—become stained with, and damaged by, yellow bile pigments. The pigments are products of the chemical breakdown by the liver of haemoglobin (*p21*), a constituent of red blood cells. Normally, these are excreted from the body in the bile (*p44*).

When large quantities of red blood cells are broken down, as in *haemolytic disease of the newborn*, the liver cannot cope with the increased quantity of bile pigments. As a result, these continue to circulate in the blood, causing serious *jaundice*. Once brain damage has occurred, symptoms of cerebral *palsy*, such as deafness and lack of co-ordination, are inevitable.

The best cure for kernicterus is prevention. The haemolytic disease, which is a result of a rhesus blood group mismatch between mother and foetus, must be treated before or at birth, by means of an exchange *transfusion*.

KETO-ACIDOSIS—see Acidosis

KETOSIS
A condition in which excessive quantities of chemicals known as ketones accumulate in the blood. This may result in *acidosis*.

Ketones are chemical compounds produced during the metabolism of fats (*p44*). Fat is rarely used as a fuel unless carbohydrates are not available, as in starvation, or cannot be utilized because of disease. In *diabetes mellitus*, for example, carbohydrates cannot be properly metabolized because *insulin* is not present, so fat is used as fuel for the cells instead. Pregnant women who suffer from severe *morning sickness* occasionally develop ketosis, since frequent vomiting leads to carbohydrate deficiency.

As a result of the increase in fat metabolism, ketones circulate in the blood until they are excreted in the urine, where their presence can be detected by a urine test—*see Special Tests, p84*. Normally the condition can be diagnosed without difficulty, because the breath of sufferers from ketosis smells distinctly of acetone. This smells like nail-varnish remover.

KIDNEYS
Two organs which lie in the lower back, beneath the diaphragm, one on either side of the spine. Each kidney (*p40*) contains thousands of nephrons that filter wastes, such as urea, from the blood to be excreted in the urine. The kidneys can be affected by a number of serious conditions.

Failure of the kidneys, called renal failure, is a very serious condition which quickly leads to *uraemia*. In this, the waste products, many of which are poisonous, accumulate in the blood. Renal failure may be *chronic*, or long-standing and progressive, or *acute*, starting suddenly. There are many possible causes.

Unless they are treated, chronic complaints may affect the kidney tissue progressively until its function is impaired to such an extent that renal failure results. Among these conditions are kidney infections such as *glomerulonephritis*, chronic *pyelonephritis* and renal *tuberculosis*; *hypertension*; and diseases of the connective tissue (*p16*) such as *polyarteritis nodosa* and *lupus erythematosus*.

Another cause of chronic renal failure is polycystic kidney disease. This is an inherited disorder in which cysts form in the tissue of the kidneys. There are two forms of the disease, of which the rarest and most severe occurs in infancy and is usually fatal before the age of three. The milder and more common form may not become apparent until late middle age, when it may be associated with pain, *haematuria* and *hypertension*. The cysts may cause chronic renal failure because their presence reduces the amount of active renal tissue; as more and more cysts form, they may also cause the kidneys to enlarge to such an extent that they can be felt through the abdomen. There is no specific treatment for the disease.

Acute renal failure may occur when the kidney is *ischaemic*, or deprived of blood. The kidney is one of the first organs to suffer if the blood pressure drops significantly—following a *haemorrhage*, for example. Sudden renal failure may also be caused by a blockage of the flow of urine by a *calculus*, or stone, a *tumour*, or by a *stricture* in the ureter. The blockage causes the kidney to swell up; it is then termed hydronephrotic.

Most stones are formed from calcium, and can occur anywhere in the urinary tract. Any disease causing a high level of calcium in the blood and the urine, such as *hyperparathyroidism* and *Paget's disease*, as well as an overdose of vitamin D, can contribute to the formation of stones.

If the stone is inside the kidney, there may be no symptoms. In this case, treatment is not necessary, and the stone may be passed spontaneously in the urine. However, if the stone is jammed in the ureter or pelvis of the kidney, there may be a sudden, excruciating pain at intervals. To avoid a serious build up of fluid in the kidneys, which may lead to renal failure, it may be necessary to remove the stone. Until recently, this could only be done by an operation called a pyelolithotomy. This treatment may be superceded by a new technique that has proved successful in trials in Germany. In this, the patient lies in a warm bath, and the stone is dissolved by a precisely directed beam of high-frequency sound waves.

Several types of malignant tumour, or *cancer* can cause kidney failure, but all of them are uncommon. A *nephroblastoma*, or Wilm's tumour, occurs in infancy, and is treated by surgery and *radiotherapy*. Renal *adenocarcinoma*, is rare, but occasionally occurs in people between the ages of 40 and 60. If the tumour is diagnosed early and removed by surgery, the chances of a complete recovery are good. The most common type of kidney cancer in adults is called a *hypernephroma*, or Grawitz tumour. It

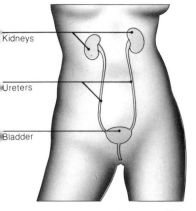

Kidneys

Ureters

Bladder

Kidney Stones Kidney stones form in the middle of the kidney, where the ducts which collect the urine from the nephrons enter the kidney's pelvis. A stone starts as a tiny particle which grows larger as more and more calcium crystallizes around it. Over a period of years, stones as large as 25mm (1 inch) may develop, although this is uncommon. The stones vary in size and shape and they may also be smooth or sharp. Very small smooth stones *(below left)* will pass without hindrance through the urinary system and out of the body. If a stone has a sharp edge, however, it is likely to cause bleeding, so that blood appears in the urine. Large long stones *(below and below left)* may block the ureter. Staghorn stones occupy all the pelvis area of the kidney and take on the charcteristic shape of the cavity *(below and below left)*.

Swollen pelvis of the kidney

Swollen ureter

Stones

Bladder stones

Stone at the exit of the ureter

Stones in the urethra

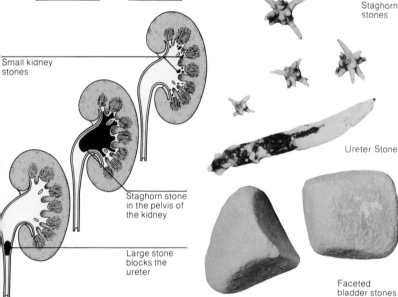

Small kidney stones

Staghorn stones

Staghorn stone in the pelvis of the kidney

Large stone blocks the ureter

Ureter Stone

Faceted bladder stones

Urine from the kidneys passes down both ureters and is temporarily stored in the bladder until it is excreted during urination. Kidney stones can obstruct this flow at any point. A stone takes two or three days to pass down a ureter to the bladder and causes a sharp pain in its wake. Small stones pass out of the body without difficulty, but faceted stones formed inside the bladder *(left)* are usually removed surgically. They are often larger than kidney stones.

usually invades the renal vein, but it is not diagnosable until it has spread to other organs.

Kidney tumours are difficult to diagnose, since they rarely cause obvious symptoms. They may, however, cause abdominal pain and the presence of blood in the urine, and they are very occasionally the cause of prolonged and unexplained bouts of fever. Unfortunately, by this time such tumours are often well advanced. They are diagnosed by contrast X-rays, such as a pyelogram, or by angiography, which may show up the abnormal blood supply to the tumour—*see Special Tests, p84.*

Drugs such as the *sulphonamides*, when taken in abnormally high dosages, and poisonous substances such as mercury, may also cause acute renal failure because of the damage they cause to the kidney's nephrons.

Before *dialysis* and transplant surgery, kidney failure was invariably fatal. Now the filtering function of the kidneys can be taken over by a dialysis machine, or by constant ambulatory peritoneal

dialysis (CAPD)—*see dialysis.* The most effective treatment for kidney failure, however, is a transplant. If the problems of tissue rejection and infection can be surmounted , the patient can lead a near-normal life. The replacement kidney is often taken from a dead donor, but if a near relative can donate a kidney, the risk of rejection is lessened. (The donor can live normally on one healthy kidney).

KLEPTOMANIA—see Personality disorders

KLINEFELTER'S SYNDROME
A genetic disorder in which males have 47, 48 or 49 chromosomes, instead of the normal 46. The majority of the extra chromosomes are X (or female) sex chromosomes, in the formation XXY, XXYY, XXXY or XXXXY—*see chromosomes and genes.* This chromosomal abnormality is believed to occur in two of every 1,000 live male births.

Klinefelter's syndrome is rarely diagnosed in childhood, since there are no outward physical symptoms, with the exception of unusually long

legs in occasional cases. Many sufferers do not realize that there is anything wrong with them until they try to have children. Then they find that they are sterile, because there is a complete absence of sperm in the semen.

In rare cases, however, breasts may start developing at the onset of puberty; the genitals may remain immature and soft; and the fusion of the epiphyses *(p16)*, or growing points of the long bones, may be delayed. The result may be that the child does not experience the normal spurt of growth of adolescence, but may continue to grow steadily throughout his teens, becoming unusually tall.

These symptoms of *hypogonadism*, the failure of the sex glands to function properly, are socially and psychologically distressing for the sufferer. If the condition is diagnosed in early adolescence, the symptoms can be controlled by hormone therapy with androgens, or male hormones *(p54)*. However, this usually boosts sexual desire, so the treatment must be carefully monitored. Abnormally enlarged breasts, or *gynaecomastia*, may be removed by plastic surgery.

KOILONYCHIA
A disorder in which the nails become thin, flat, spoon-shaped and brittle. The condition is associated with iron-deficiency *anaemia*. Koilonychia usually disappears when the *anaemia* has been successfully treated.

KORSAKOFF'S PSYCHOSIS
A disorder of the brain, caused by *alcoholism*, that is also known as alcoholic *dementia*. The damage to the brain tissue is caused by a lack of thiamine, a B-vitamin, which is destroyed by alcohol.

Most sufferers from Korsakoff's psychosis have severe *amnesia*. They are often unable to remember events for a year preceding the onset of the condition, and typically make up stories to cover the memory gap. This tendency is known as *confabulation*. Judgement may also be affected.

The condition of the patient may be slightly improved by giving up alcohol; rest; vitamin B injections and a high vitamin diet. However, the damage to the brain tissue usually cannot be reversed.

KWASHIORKOR
A disease caused by a protein deficiency, or a deficiency of protein and carbohydrate *(p40)*. Both these problems are the result of *malnutrition*.

Kwashiorkor can affect both sexes and all age groups, but children and women who are pregnant or are breast-feeding are particularly at risk. This is because their need for

protein and calories is higher than normal—*see Diet, p322*.

In a child suffering from kwashiorkor, both weight and height are below normal for his or her age, although *oedema* around the hips and legs, the result of a diet high in salt and water, may make up for some of the weight loss. The stomach may be distended, while other parts of the body are emaciated. Such children are listless and depressed, and may also lose their appetites.

In both children and adults, the muscles become wasted if protein and carbohydrate are lacking in the diet. The hair becomes sparse, straight and soft, and the skin may become pigmented or depigmented. Ulcers develop and the liver enlarges. The disease causes vomiting and *diarrhoea*. Usually, people with kwashiorkor also suffer from *anaemia*.

Kwashiorkor is sometimes difficult to diagnose. This is because its symptoms can be easily confused with those of chronic *dysentery*, abdominal *tuberculosis*, *coeliac disease*, *pellagra*, *beriberi*, fibrocystic disease of the pancreas, *hookworm* and *nephritis*. Once it has been identified, however, kwashiorkor can be treated with rest and an adequate diet. Infants may have to be fed six or more times a day with whole milk, or a mixture of skimmed milk powder, butter, flour and water, until appetite and physical condition return to normal. This mixture is often given through a polythene tube passed into the stomach.

KYPHOSCOLIOSIS—See Kyphosis

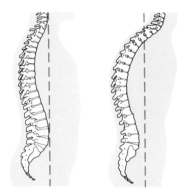

Kyphosis The normal curvature of the spine is a gentle S-shape *(left)*. When the outward curve is exaggerated, the hunch back appearance is known as kyphosis *(right)*.

KYPHOSIS
An exaggeration of the normal outward curve of the spine that gives rise to a hunchbacked appearance known as Pott's curvature. The condition is sometimes congenital, or present at birth, but more often is the result of adopting a bad posture over many years, allied with a weakness of the muscles in the back. Occasionally it is a symptom of another disease

Kyphosis tends to develop most often in the elderly, and more often in women than in men. In women, the condition is sometimes known as 'dowager's hump'. If the spine is curved backwards and sideways, the condition is called kyphoscoliosis—*see also scoliosis*.

Depending on its cause, kyphosis may be treated with varying degrees of success. Treatments include exercise, physiotherapy, an orthopaedic brace, or an operation known as an *osteotomy*.

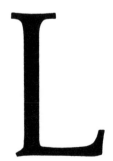

LABYRINTHITIS—see Otitis

LACTIC ACID—see Cramp

LAMINECTOMY
An operation in which some of the laminae—the thin plates of bone that make up the vertebrae *(p16)*—are removed to expose the spinal cord and *meninges*. A laminectomy may be performed to remove a spinal

tumour, to repair or treat a spinal injury or to relieve pressure on a spinal nerve.

LARYNGITIS
An *inflammation* of the larynx, the part of the trachea, or windpipe, in which the voice box is located *(p28)*. It may be caused by either a *bacterial* or a *viral* infection, and usually occurs when resistance has been

lowered by a *cold*, by inhaling noxious fumes, or by infection with a *contagious* disease, such as *measles*.

In *acute* laryngitis the throat is inflamed and coated with mucus, and there is a painful cough in which no phlegm is produced. The voice becomes hoarse and speaking may be painful. The condition is not serious, and usually clears up after a day or two of rest in a warm room and regular treatment with a suitable cough medicine; the voice should be rested and sufferers should not smoke. Regular inhalations of steam from boiling water may also help. To prevent other conditions from developing, such as *tracheitis*, *bronchitis* and *pneumonia*, antibiotics may sometimes be necessary. In children, mucus may block the narrow laryngeal opening, causing *croup*.

If attacks occur repeatedly, laryngitis may become *chronic*. This is common in mouth breathers and people working in dusty atmospheres where the voice is frequently used. In chronic laryngitis the surface of the larynx becomes dry and inflamed, and the vocal cords become swollen, causing permanent hoarseness and difficulty in speaking, with a permanent, irritating cough.

Treated as for acute laryngitis, each attack of chronic laryngitis will clear up. But to achieve a permanent cure, the sufferer may have to change his or her occupation.

LASER
A concentrated beam of light of a single colour or wavelength; the name is formed from the initial letters of the words 'light amplification (by) stimulated emission (of) radar'. Lasers have many uses in medicine. The heat of a precisely focused laser beam will burn *malignant* cells, leaving the healthy cells surrounding a *tumour* untouched. A laser can also be used to make an incision, which bleeds far less than one made with a scalpel, because it is sealed immediately by the laser's own heat. Since a laser beam can penetrate the fluid in the eyeball, it can be used to repair a *detached retina*, or to destroy the abnormal blood vessels that occur on the back of the retina in advanced *diabetes mellitus*. Laser surgery is now also being used in a delicate operation to remove spinal tumours in children.

LASSA FEVER
A serious *viral* disease discovered in 1969 in West Africa, caused initially by eating food contaminated by rats, Mastomys natalensis. It may also be spread by contact with the vomit, urine or *faeces* of an infected person; by droplets of saliva transmitted by coughing and sneezing; and by contact with infected blood or blood products, such as serum.

The *incubation period* is thought to be between three and 21 days. The condition can be diagnosed within a few days of the onset of the first symptoms—general tiredness and a sore throat—by blood tests and tissue cultures—*see Special Tests, p84*.

The first symptoms are followed by a *fever*, lasting from one to just over two weeks, with severe muscular pains, *vomiting, diarrhoea*, and leucopenia, a reduction in the number of white cells (p21) in the blood. The throat becomes inflamed and a sticky yellow secretion makes swallowing difficult. In severe cases a thick membrane covers the pharynx (p28), and may ooze blood. Blood pressure falls, and the heartbeat slows down; renal *anoxia* develops, causing a reduced excretion of urine and *uraemia*. Mild cases have been recorded, from which patients have recovered fairly quickly, but in severe cases extreme *shock* leads to death from kidney and heart damage—*see kidney disease; heart failure*.

Anyone who has been exposed to Lassa fever is isolated as soon as possible, and as soon as symptoms appear is placed in an intensive care unit. Treatment is mainly supportive. Symptoms of shock and *dehydration* are treated as soon as they appear, and patients may also be treated with immune serum—*see immunization*.

Nursing a patient with Lassa fever is particularly difficult since the patient continues to be infectious for several weeks after recovery. Nurses and doctors have to wear masks and special protective clothing.

LEAD-POISONING
A collection of syndromes caused by the ingestion of lead particles. Lead-poisoning may occur in both *chronic* and *acute* forms.

Since the body has no means of eliminating lead, minute amounts absorbed through the lungs or gastrointestinal tract are stored, usually in the bones. If the level of lead becomes sufficiently high, the symptoms of chronic lead-poisoning develop. These include: *anaemia*, colicky abdominal pains, *vomiting* and *diarrhoea*, *paralysis* of certain muscles, such as those of the wrists and fingers or the foot, and a tell-tale blue line around the gums. There may also be pains in the joints and loss of appetite, and on microscopic examination a characteristic stippling can be seen on the blood cells (p21). In severe cases there may be headache, *epilepsy* and sometimes brain damage.

These days lead is ingested mainly by inhaling air polluted with particles of tetra-ethyl lead added to petrol. It may also be found dissolved in drinking-water running through new lead pipes, or in fruit preserved in tins sealed with lead solder. There are now strict controls on the use of lead in paint, but children may still suffer from lead-poisoning after sucking old paintwork or imported toys coloured with lead paint. Lead-poisoning is still an occupational hazard for lead-smelters, plumbers and other people who work with lead.

Acute lead-poisoning is rare, but it occurs occasionally among workers in industry who accidentally inhale lead fumes or dust, or in children who consume lead paint. When this happens, a metallic taste in the mouth is followed by the characteristic pain of 'lead colic', accompanied by vomiting, and diarrhoea with black stools. In some cases the brain and peripheral nervous system (p32) are affected and there may be serious damage to the blood circulation.

Patients with severe chronic or acute lead-poisoning are treated by pumping out the contents of the stomach and administering penicillamine. This is a chelating agent, a drug that promotes the excretion of metals. Alternatively, they may be given intravenous injections of a calcium chelating agent diluted in dextrose, a sugar, followed by injections of *diuretics*. In milder cases, regular dosages of epsom salts and large amounts of calcium in the diet help to remove the lead from the bones. EDTA (ethylenediamine tetra-acetic acid), a chelating agent that forms a compound with lead and is excreted in the urine, may be given by injection. Further treatment may be necessary to prevent brain damage.

Legislation has recently been enacted in many countries to remove common sources of lead-poisoning from the environment. Lead additives in petrol have been banned in many states in the USA, and in most countries the use of lead in paint has also been banned. In addition, most new houses now have lead-free water pipes, and stringent safety measures have considerably reduced the risk of lead-poisoning in industry. However, these measures are not universal and as the consumption of petrol with lead additives rises, the risk of lead-poisoning grows. As a response to studies showing conclusively that even small levels of lead can retard children's intellectual development, pressure to ban lead additives in petrol has increased considerably in the last few years.

LEGIONNAIRES' DISEASE
A disease first identified in 1976 following an outbreak of pneumonia among members of the American Legion who had attended a convention in a Philadelphia hotel. Since then, outbreaks have been

recognized in other parts of the world, including Britain.

The bacterium responsible for Legionnaires' disease probably lives naturally in moist soil. It is often found in water from cooling towers of air-conditioning systems, and fine droplets containing the organism can spread from these to contaminate the neighbourhood. It can also be present in hot water systems and can be spread by showers. The incidence of the disease is highest in August and September in temperate climates; it is not infectious.

The incubation period is usually about a week. Most patients are aged from 40 to 70, with the death rate being higher in those over 55 and in people with disease of the heart, lungs, or kidneys. However, for many people the disease is no more serious than an attack of influenza, and 80 per cent of those infected probably recover without any special treatment. Some, however, develop pneumonia, and in these the kidneys may become involved.

The best antibiotic to treat Legionnaires' disease is erythromycin, which should be taken for three weeks since there is the risk of relapse and death if treatment is stopped too soon.

LEPROSY
A disease of the skin and nerves caused by Mycobacterium leprae. Leprosy is now seen only in tropical and sub-tropical countries, but in ancient times it was common throughout Europe and Asia. It is still a major cause of suffering, however: scientists believe that today the disease affects between fifteen and twenty million people.

Leprosy, also called Hansen's disease—after the doctor who first identified the bacillus in 1873—is thought to be spread by droplets from the nose and mouth of an infected person, although whether the organism enters the body through the skin, the lungs or the digestive tract is not known. The *incubation period* is usually between three and five years, but may be as long as 30 years.

There are two main kinds of leprosy. Tuberculoid leprosy, a benign form, is rarely *infectious* and eventually heals without treatment. Lepromatous leprosy is the virulent form, in which large numbers of organisms attack nerve tissue, muscles and the endothelial tissue that lines blood vessels. In addition, there are a number of types of leprosy that are intermediate between these two main types.

Leprosy usually begins as a *macule*, or thickening of the skin, usually of the face. The macule multiplies, and large and unsightly nodules appear on the sites of the macules. *Oedema* may obstruct the nasal passages and broaden the nose. At times the infected person may experience recurrent attacks of tiredness with *fever* and swelling of the joints or glands. The peripheral nerves may also swell and are eventually destroyed, leading to loss of sensation, usually in the hands, feet, nose and ears. The bones in these parts of the body may be entirely absorbed, so that the affected part—the nose, fingers or toes—completely disappears. Less commonly, *iritis* develops in the eyes, leading to blindness and, if the larynx *(p28)* is affected, the voice disappears.

The wasting away of fingers, hands, feet and other areas of the body was the almost inevitable result of leprosy until the 1940s. Then a range of sulphone drugs was discovered to be an effective method of treatment. These drugs, the most common of which is dapsone, do not cure leprosy, but if they are taken regularly over a long period they do contain the disease, especially if treatment begins in the early stages. *Physiotherapy*, aimed at maintaining mobility in the affected limb, has also proved effective in delaying or preventing gross deformity; and plastic and orthopaedic surgical techniques can be used to repair some deformities once they have occurred.

These medical advances have led to the disappearance of the traditional leper colony, since they enable lepers to live safely among uninfected people while regularly attending day clinics for treatment. Recent research gives hope that leprosy may one day be eradicated, in the same way as *smallpox*, by the use of a vaccine. Such a vaccine has been developed, and has already proved successful in trials in South America.

LEPTOSPIROSIS
A *zoonosis*, a disease that affects both animals and humans, caused by Leptospira, a type of *bacteria* that infects many wild and domestic animals. There are various different varieties of Leptospira: L. canicola, found in dogs and pigs, causes aseptic *meningitis* and *fever* in humans, while L. icterohaemorrhagiae, found in the urine of infected rats, causes a serious condition called Weil's disease. These types of bacteria occur world-wide, while less common species cause leptospirosis in eastern Europe and in the East.

Weil's disease, also called spirochaetal jaundice, swamp fever and Japanese seven-day fever, is an occupational hazard of people who work with animals, but the disease can also be contracted by bathing in stagnant water that has been contaminated by the urine of infected rats. The bacterium enters the human body either through a graze or wound in the skin, or through the mucous membranes in the mouth and nose. After an *incubation period* of between a few days and three weeks, the sufferer develops *fever*, with *rigors*, or cold sweats, a headache, muscular pains, *nausea* and *vomiting*. This feverish stage is followed by enlargement of the liver and *jaundice*.

In areas where Weil's disease is known to be *endemic*, the condition is suspected as soon as the symptoms appear, and the diagnosis is confirmed by blood and urine tests—see *Special Tests, p84*. The sufferer is then treated with *antibiotics*, and the problem usually clears up within two to three weeks. However, in severe cases, and when the diagnosis is delayed, the condition may progress to cause severe *jaundice, liver failure, kidney disease* and sometimes *heart failure*. These symptoms are treated in an intensive care unit, but, nevertheless, around 20 per cent of patients in whom the disease develops to this stage die within a few weeks.

LESION
An area of damaged tissue anywhere in the body, the result of disease or injury. Grazes, cuts, sores, *abscesses, ulcers*, spots, rashes and *tumours* are all said, in medical terms, to be lesions.

LEUKAEMIA
A group of serious diseases in which there is an excess of white cells *(p21)* in the blood and bone marrow. In leukaemia, a proportion of the leucocytes, or white blood cells, manufactured by the bone marrow, spleen and lymph nodes fail to mature. Since once they have matured cells lose the ability to reproduce, these abnormal, immature cells multiply rapidly and eventually outnumber other types of blood cell, in the same manner as cancerous cells.

The causes of leukaemia are not understood. However, *viruses* are known to cause leukaemias in certain animals and birds, and may do so in humans. In addition, since the incidence of leukaemia in Hiroshima and Nagasaki rose significantly after the explosion of atomic bombs over those cities in

1945, irradiation is also known to be a contributory factor.

The leukaemias are classified according to the type of white cell that is overproduced. They may be *acute*, or of sudden onset, or *chronic*—that is, long-standing and progressive.

Acute leukaemia is so called because without treatment most patients die within six months. There are two main forms of this: acute lymphoblastic leukaemia tends to affect children under five; and acute myeloblastic leukaemia, although most common in children and young adults, may affect people of all ages.

The various types of acute leukaemia have similar symptoms. Since the over production of leucocytes interferes with the production of red blood cells, a sufferer from acute leukaemia becomes *anaemic*, pale, tired and highly susceptible to *infection*. *Thrombocytopaenia*, a reduction in the number of platelets *(p21)* in the blood, may interfere with normal blood clotting and so cause bleeding into the skin and from the nose, mouth and digestive tract. The spleen, liver and lymph nodes *(p21)* may become enlarged, affecting their function. In children, in particular, there may be pain in the joints and bones, and *splenomegaly*, an enlarged spleen.

There are also several forms of chronic leukaemia. Of these, the two most common forms are chronic lymphatic leukaemia, which tends to affect men aged between 40 and 60, and chronic myeloid leukaemia, affecting people of both sexes between the ages of 20 and 50. Both forms of leukaemia progress gradually, beginning with excessive tiredness, especially after exercise. The abdomen may become swollen and the glands in the neck, armpit or groin enlarged. Eventually the symptoms of anaemia appear.

Leukaemia is usually diagnosed from blood and bone marrow tests— *see Special Tests, p84*—in which the number of white blood cells is found to be higher than normal. Treatment with drugs has replaced *radiotherapy* as the major form of treatment for both acute and chronic leukaemia; different combinations of drugs are used in each case. Doctors experienced in the complicated procedures involved can effect a cure in some cases, and prolonged remission in others. *Cytotoxic* drugs are used to suppress cell division in conjunction with drugs to reduce haemorrhage and *antibiotics* to fight infection. *Corticosteroid* drugs have been found to cause a sudden, but temporary, remission in many

patients. Blood *transfusions* may be used to arrest the progress of the disease until the drug treatments take effect.

The drug therapy has unpleasant side-effects, but in cases of acute leukaemia they may prolong the life of the patient by more than a year and may lead to remission for six years or more in cases of chronic leukaemia.

LEUKOPLAKIA

White spots or patches that appear most often on the cheek or tongue, and sometimes on the vulva *(p54)*. They are hard, smooth and painless when they first appear, and cannot be removed by scraping; later they crack, giving rise to painful fissures.

Leukoplakia in the mouth may be caused by excessive friction from pipe- and cigarette-smoking, or by the smoke itself, when it is associated with smoker's *keratosis*. Either in the mouth or the vulva, the spots may be caused by the spirochaetes that cause *syphilis*. However, many have no apparent cause, though there is some evidence that they may be the result of an infection by the *Herpes simplex* virus.

There is no treatment for leukoplakia, though a sufferer whose condition is caused by smoking will be advised to give up the habit. However, since the patches occasionally develop into *carcinomas*, a biopsy—*see Special Tests, p84*—is usually performed to check that no cancerous cells are present.

LIBIDO

The sexual drive. Libido is said to be at its peak in men in their teens and early twenties and in women in their late thirties and early forties. Loss of libido may be due to fatigue, illness, stress or psychological factors—*see frigidity; impotence, Sex and Contraception, p338*.

LICE—see Pediculosis

LICHEN PLANUS

A skin disease, which may also produce changes in the mouth (sometimes the latter appear first). The skin lesions are raised violaceous patches (papules), which may be very itchy. In the mouth, there are white areas with a lacy appearance. The genitalia may be affected as well. The cause is uncertain, although the immune system seems to be involved.

Most sufferers are aged between 30 and 60. There is no curative treatment, but most people recover spontaneously in about a year. However, the changes in the mouth

can persist and should be monitored.

LIPID STORAGE DISEASES

A group of rare diseases, sometimes called lipidosis, that occur as a result of *disorders of the metabolism* of lipids by the body. Lipids are fats and fat-like substances in food—*see Metabolism p44*.

Most lipid storage diseases are inherited *congenital* disorders in which lipids accumulate in the liver and spleen. For example, in Gaucher's disease, the spleen enlarges massively, and fats may accumulate in other major organs of the body. When it appears in new-born babies, this disease is fatal, but it may not become apparent until childhood or early adulthood. Symptoms include *anaemia, jaundice*, a yellowish pigmentation of the skin, and a thickening of the conjunctiva, the lining of the eyelid.

Unfortunately, most lipid storage diseases are incurable. A splenectomy, an operation to reduce the size of the spleen, may be performed to relieve some of the symptoms.

LIPOMA

A slow-growing *tumour* made of fat cells that can occur wherever fat is found in the body. Lipomas are among the most common tumours. They are usually small, but often occur in multiples. Most are benign, but occasionally a lipoma develops into a *sarcoma*.

LISTERIOSIS

Infection with one of the group of bacteria known as *Listeria*, which lives in the soil and is carried by animals as well as humans. Usually it causes no disease, but it can do so occasionally, mainly in the very young, the very old and in pregnant women.

In pregnancy, listeriosis usually causes two or more episodes of feverishness. On the first occasion there is headache, fever, backache, a sore throat, and diarrhoea. A second bout of symptoms may occur after delivery of the baby. Babies may be infected before birth, when they are usually premature and have difficulty in breathing; about a third are born dead. They may also be infected after birth, in which case they often suffer from meningitis and encephalitis. Antibiotics, however, are effective.

LITHIUM

A metallic element, compounds of which are used to treat patients with *manic-depressive psychosis*.

LITHOTRIPSY

A relatively new technique for the destruction of kidney stones or gallstones by means of ultrasound. The obvious advantage of this is that it avoids the need for surgery. At first the patient had to be under general anaesthetic and be immersed in a tank of water for the treatment to be given. With improved machines, however, it became possible to break up the stones using only sedation and analgesia, and there was no longer any need for the large water tank; instead, it is enough to have water contact over a much smaller area of the body. Modern machines allow over 95 per cent of renal stones to be broken up, the fragments then passing down the ureter by themselves, or by being washed down if they stick.

Lithotripsy has also been used to deal with gallstones, but there are several difficulties with this. The fragments of stone have to leave the gall bladder via the cystic duct, which is narrow, and if they stick on the way down it, they are more difficult to remove here than in the ureter. In addition, not all of the several kinds of gallstones are suitable for lithotripsy. For these and other reasons there is not such a clear-cut preference for using lithotripsy in this instance. However, gallstone lithotripsy will probably be carried out increasingly often in the future, as equipment improves.

LIVER DISEASE
The liver is one of the body's most important organs. It has a variety of functions—see *Metabolism, p44*—many of which are vital for life. When these are disrupted by damage or disease, the consequences for the victim are widespread and serious.

A number of different conditions can affect the liver and disrupt these functions. It may be damaged by the excessive consumption of alcohol, or by drugs and poisons—see *cirrhosis*—or by a disease, such as *biliary cirrhosis*; it may become infected by a virus, as in *hepatitis*; or be invaded by parasites, such as *flukes*. The liver may be the site of a primary *cancer*, called a *hepatoma*, and is often the first site in which secondary cancers form after *metastasizing* from a tumour in the lungs, breast or abdomen.

If any of these diseases remains untreated, and does not clear up on its own, the result may be a serious condition called liver failure. This may develop gradually after a disease, such as *cirrhosis*, has affected the liver for many years. However, sometimes it occurs suddenly, and is known as fulminant hepatic failure or acute massive liver necrosis. This may rarely follow acute *hepatitis*, or be due to liver-poisoning by a large overdose of drugs such as paracetamol, chemicals such as carbon tetrachloride and yellow phosphorus, or the poisons contained in certain fungi. Very occasionally, a disorder known as acute fatty liver of pregnancy causes massive liver necrosis in pregnant women. The reason for this is not known.

Liver failure initially causes *jaundice*, a yellowish pigmentation of the skin, and mental confusion. There is also *nausea*, loss of appetite and *vomiting*, and sometimes troublesome hiccups. There may be *ascites*, in which the abdomen becomes distended by fluid and *oedema*—this is because the chemical balance of the blood is disturbed by the decrease in the liver's manufacture of plasma proteins *(p21)*. The lack of plasma proteins, from which antibodies *(p52)* are made, means that the body's resistance to infection is greatly reduced.

The patient is generally gravely ill. He or she has sweet-smelling breath and a tremor in the hands if they are held out. There may also be bleeding into the skin and digestive tract *(p40)* because the level of blood-clotting factors *(p21)*, which are made in the liver, is reduced.

Sufferers from liver failure are treated in an intensive care unit, where the disease that has led to the condition is treated, and the symptoms of liver failure are kept in check. This involves correcting the lack of plasma proteins and blood clotting factors by *transfusions* of plasma.

In severe cases this treatment is ineffective, and the patient usually sinks into a profound coma and dies within a week. Patients whose condition is less serious, who are not in coma but only drowsy, have a much better chance of survival. If the disease that has caused liver failure is treated successfully, the liver normally regenerates and its full functions are restored.

In cases where the liver is so severely damaged as to be incapable of normal functioning, a liver *transplant* is now possible. Such operations have been performed both in Britain and America, with varying success. The operation is technically more difficult than a heart transplant, and the same problems of infection, rejection and organ availability apply.

Some liver functions may be taken over by a mechanical filter in much the same way as kidney function can be carried out by dialysis. However, this is practical only in the short term; it is used, therefore, in cases where liver failure has been caused by a drug overdose, to allow the liver time to recover.

LOBECTOMY
An operation to remove a lobe of an organ such as the lungs, a gland or the brain. A lobe is usually separated from the rest of the organ only by connective tissues. Thus it can be removed without seriously affecting the organ's other parts. For example one broncho-pulmonary segment of the lungs *(p28)* can be removed without affecting the function of the other segments.

A lobectomy is usually performed as a treatment for chronic infection or to remove a malignant *tumour*.

LOCHIA
Material, such as blood, mucus and cells from the womb, that is normally discharged through the cervix and vagina for about two weeks after the birth of a child—*see Pregnancy and Birth, p60*. During the first four days after birth more blood is discharged than subsequently, so the lochia gradually diminishes in quantity and changes from a brownish red to a creamy colour, an indication that the womb is returning to normal after the delivery.

LOCKJAW—see Tetanus

LONG SIGHT—see Hypermetropia

LUMBAGO
A lay term for any severe persistent or recurrent ache or pain that occurs low in the back. Sufferers often report the sudden onset of an excruciating pain while bending, standing up from a sitting position, twisting round or lifting a heavy weight, and difficulty in moving from the position in which the spasm occurred. Such an attack does not usually last for long.

Lumbago often responds to heat and massage treatments. However, acute pains in the lumbar region of the back may be due to a slipped disc—*see prolapsed invertebral disc*. In this case, the pain can be relieved only by resting, taking *analgesics* when it is severe.

See also back pain.

LUNG ABSCESS
The formation of an *abscess*, a pocket of pus, in the tissue of the lungs *(p28)*. Lung abscesses are occasionally complications of infections of the lung, such as *pneumonia*, when large quantities of pus are formed as a result of the

body's fight against the invading bacteria—*see Natural Defences Against Disease, p52*. However, nowadays, when most such conditions are treated by *antibiotics*, which prevent pus from forming, this is uncommon.

The commonest cause of a lung abscess is the presence in the lungs of particles of foreign material, such as dust or dirt. These particles carry *bacteria*, the source of infection, into the body. They are sometimes inhaled by an *anaesthetized* patient during an operation on the throat or mouth, even in the scrupulously clean, sterile conditions of an operating theatre. They may also be inhaled during the near-anaesthesia experienced by chronic alcoholics after a drinking bout. Foreign particles may also enter the lungs from the bloodstream. As a result, lung abscesses are a particular hazard for drug addicts who 'mainline', or inject drugs directly into a vein, using dirty syringes, especially when they inject an impure solution made from crushed tablets.

Lung abscesses cause shortness of breath and a *fever*, with chronic cough and the production of pus-laden sputum. Their presence can be confirmed easily, by means of a chest X-ray, but treatment is difficult, because antibiotics do not always penetrate to the centre of the abscess, where the source of the infection is to be found. Sometimes an abscess may rupture spontaneously with the result that the patient coughs up a large amount of foul-smelling pus. However, if this does not happen, and antibiotics prove ineffective, the abscess is drained surgically: a long needle is passed into the lungs and the pus sucked out through a syringe.

After treatment, the abscess cavity grows smaller and finally disappears, the accompanying fever subsides and the patient begins to feel much better.

LUNG CANCER

A serious condition in which a malignant tumour, or *cancer*, develops in the tissue of the lungs. Around 30,000 to 40,000 people in Britain die from lung cancer each year.

A number of different types of tumour may cause lung cancer. The most common, responsible for more than half of all cases, arises in the cells lining the bronchi (p28), the medium-sized air passages. This type is called a bronchial

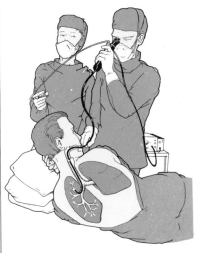

Lung cancer Internal examination of the bronchi inside the lungs is carried out with an instrument called a bronchoscope (*above*) in a procedure called bronchoscopy. It is a standard procedure in cases of suspected bronchial carcinoma, a common lung tumour. A narrow, flexible, fibre-optic tube is introduced through the mouth and guided down the trachea into the lung. A light is shone down the tube, allowing the surgeon to inspect a portion of the bronchus.

carcinoma—a term that is often used as an alternative to lung cancer. A second type, accounting for around ten per cent of all cases, arises in the mucous glands of the air passages,

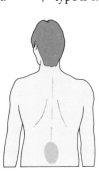

Lumbago is a severe aching pain in the lower back (*right*), which is muscular in origin. It is brought on by exposure to cold, damp conditions or by straining the muscles of the lumbar region. It often begins with an abrupt spasm in the lower back while bending, standing up from a sitting position or while lifting something heavy. To protect the muscles of the lower back, precautions should be taken (*right and below*).

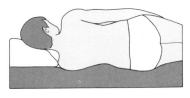

Make sure you sleep on a firm flat mattress, This will support your back and keep your spine straight (*left*). A mattress that curves and bows in the middle (*below*) is likely to distort your spine.

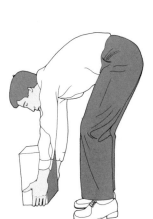

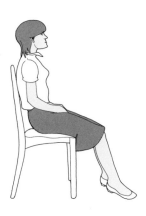

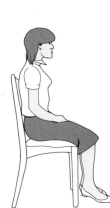

When you sit on a chair, make sure it has a back which is high enough to support you and then sit erect (*right*). Do not sit in a slouched position (*above*) in which your back takes the strain of your body.

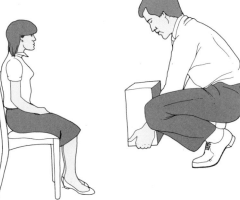

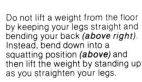

Do not lift a weight from the floor by keeping your legs straight and bending your back (*above right*). Instead, bend down into a squatting position (*above*) and then lift the weight by standing up as you straighten your legs.

and is called an adenocarcinoma. The remainder of tumours are undifferentiated—that is, they belong to no specific type.

The most important cause of bronchial carcinoma is cigarette smoking—see Abuses of the Body, p328—and statistics show that the risk of dying from lung cancer is 30 times higher in smokers than in non-smokers. Adenocarcinomas are not, however, linked statistically to cigarette smoking. Other causes of lung cancer include nuclear radiation, atmospheric pollution, and the pneumoconioses, industrial diseases caused by the inhalation of substances such as asbestos and silica.

Early diagnosis of lung cancer can be difficult, because there are often no lung symptoms until it has reached a late stage. This is true of around five per cent of cases. In a further ten per cent the cancer may only be detected when it has already spread, or metastasized, to cause symptoms in another part of the body. However, in the remainder of cases, there are lung symptoms, normally taking the form of a persistent cough and haemoptysis, or coughing up of blood. Such symptoms should be reported to a doctor immediately.

If the tumour has already grown to such a size that it obstructs a bronchus there may be shortness of breath. If it has invaded the pleura, the membranes surrounding the lungs, there will also be chest pain. As the disease progresses these symptoms worsen, until, in the late stages, there is a serious loss of weight. Secondary tumours may develop, most commonly in the liver—see liver disorders— where they may cause more pain. Occasionally, secondary tumours invade the brain tissue, causing fits similar to those of epilepsy. If it reaches the stage at which secondary tumours develop, lung cancer is almost invariably fatal.

The first step in the diagnosis is a chest X-ray—see Special Tests, p84. Usually this shows up the presence of a tumour, but sometimes the X-ray can appear perfectly normal, even though the cancer is at a late stage. If the X-ray appears normal, but the doctor still suspects cancer, a CAT scan may be performed, or the bronchi examined by means of a fibre-optic bronchoscope—see Special Tests, p84. If a growth is then seen, a biopsy (p84) may be taken, so that the tissue can be examined under a microscope.

The treatment of lung cancer depends on the size, position and type of the tumour. Small tumours that have not yet spread can be removed by surgery; radiotherapy is used to reduce the size of a large tumour and to prevent or treat secondary tumours. Cytoxic drugs, which kill cancerous cells, are used in conjunction with both these techniques. Such treatments often slow down the growth of a tumour, but rarely cure it. Thus, lung cancer is usually fatal unless it is detected and treated at an early stage.

See also cancer.

LUPUS ERYTHEMATOSUS (LE)
A rare inflammatory disease of the connective tissues—the skin, joint linings, ligaments and muscles (p16). Mild forms of the disease may affect only the skin, but generally the whole body is involved. In this case, the disease is sometimes called systemic lupus erythematosus, or SLE. The cause of the disease is unknown, but it appears to run in families and has similar symptoms to those of rheumatoid arthritis. Like this condition, lupus erythematosus is thought to be an auto-immune disorder, in which the body turns against its own tissues.

In common with rheumatoid arthritis, the condition usually affects women in their early twenties to thirties. Pregnancy makes lupus erythematosus worse, whereas rheumatoid arthritis usually improves at this time.

The symptoms—caused by an inflammation of the small blood vessels and connective tissues— include arthritis, or stiffness and immobility of the joints, a red, scaly skin rash, inflammation of the eyes, kidneys, heart and nerves, and the deposition of fibrous tissue in the lungs. The immune response to disease is disrupted, and consequently the body's resistance to infection is lowered.

The diagnosis can be confirmed by an antibody test—see Special Tests, p84. Almost invariably, this shows up the presence of antibodies that attack the sufferer's DNA, a chemical found in the nucleus of every cell in the body—see chromosomes. Treatment is mainly with steroid drugs, to reduce inflammation and limit the damage to the kidneys. This holds the condition at bay for some time, but after about ten years, many sufferers succumb to kidney failure and die.

LYMPHADENOMA—see Lymphoma

LYMPHOEDEMA
A swelling of areas of tissue caused by a build-up of lymph within them—see Blood and Lymph, p21. The condition occurs most often in women and tends to affect the legs. It may be the result of an obstruction to the lymphatic ducts, for example by a tumour, by abnormalities in the lymphatic circulation, or, in the tropics, by parasitic worms. Sufferers from lymphoedema are advised to rest as much as possible, with the legs elevated, and to wear surgical stockings or tights, and are given diuretics to reduce the volume of fluid.

LYMPHOMA
A malignant tumour that forms in a lymph gland—see Blood and Lymph, p21—also called a lymphadenoma. There are three main types of lymphoma. Around a third of all lymphomas are associated with a condition called Hodgkin's disease, and a much smaller proportion with Burkitt's lymphoma. The remainder, sometimes called non-Hodgkin's lymphomas (NHL), are not associated with any specific condition, and are normally fatal in time.

NHL lymphomas usually affect only middle-aged and elderly people, and slightly more men than women suffer from the condition; around one in 20,000 people in Britain die as a result of a such a lymphoma each year.

The first sign is a small swelling, or group of swellings, most commonly in the neck, armpit or groin. Any such swelling should be reported to a doctor immediately. Some lymphomas grow slowly, over a period of years, and there are no initial symptoms, while others spread rapidly over a period of weeks. In the latter group, there are often early symptoms, such as an enlargement of the spleen, a mild fever, loss of appetite and tiredness.

The exact nature of the lymphoma is determined by microscopic examination of a sample of the tumour that has been taken in a biopsy—see Special Tests, p84. Once the diagnosis has been confirmed, the lymphoma will be treated by radiotherapy if it is confined to one site. Otherwise, treatment has to rely on steroid drugs, such as prednisolone, and cytotoxic drugs, such vincristine. These often slow down the growth of slow-growing tumours, and temporarily arrest the growth of fast-growing tumours. The period of remission is variable, however, and decreases after each attack.

The outlook depends on precise nature and structure of the cells of the lymphoma. In some cases, there is a good chance of remission with treatment, and even a total cure. In other cases, however, the condition usually proves fatal within a few years. See also cancer.

M

MACULE
A flat patch of discoloured and sometimes thickened skin. Macules appear for a variety of reasons, and are generally harmless. Sometimes, however, their appearance can be confused with that of a *melanoma*, a mole which may become malignant. For this reason, any sudden growth of a discoloured patch of skin, or bleeding from it, should be reported to a doctor.

MAGNETIC RESONANCE IMAGING (MRI)
MRI, also known as nuclear magnetic resonance (NMR), is a relatively new technique for obtaining pictures of the inside of the body. When certain elements, chiefly hydrogen, that occur naturally within the body are placed within a strong magnetic field and subjected to radio-frequency waves, the nuclei of the atoms resonate, and it is possible to use this phenomenon to obtain a cross-sectional image of the body similar to that obtained by computerized tomography (CT). Because X rays—and, hence, radiation—are not involved, MRI is almost certainly completely safe.

MALABSORPTION SYNDROME
A collection of symptoms caused by the body's inability to absorb essential nutrients from the diet. This, in turn, may be the result of a number of disorders. The symptoms vary according to the root cause of the problem, but may include weight loss, diarrhoea, *steatorrhoea*, *oedema*, *anaemia*, and the problems associated with *vitamin deficiency diseases*.

Malabsorption is a symptom of a number of diseases, such as *cystic fibrosis* and the *coeliac disease*, a condition in which an intolerance to the gluten found in many foods causes changes in the wall of the small intestine—see *The Digestive System, p40*. In addition, major surgery of the stomach and bowel may result in malabsorption. In the first case, it may prove necessary to *resect*, or cut away, the enzyme-producing glands; in the second, the removal of large sections of the colon

or small intestine reduces the body's ability to absorb its essential nutrients, since the length of gut through which food can pass is considerably shortened.

Damage to the mucus lining of the stomach and intestines can also cause malabsorption, because this reduces the surface area available for absorption. Such damage may be caused by a number of diseases, including *chronic* diseases of the digestive tract, such as *ulcerative colitis*, chronic *pancreatitis* and *diabetes mellitus*.

When malabsorption is caused by an enzyme deficiency, the necessary enzymes can usually be supplied in powder or tablet form as a dietary supplement. Special diets help to alleviate the symptoms of malabsorption caused by damage to the lining of the gut, or by major surgery to the digestive tract.

MALAISE
The general feeling of non-specific illness, tiredness and lethargy that often precedes the onset of an *infection* and accompanies a *chronic* illness.

MALARIA
An infectious disease, also called ague, jungle fever, marsh fever, periodic fever and paludism. Malaria is common in the tropics and subtropics, and its incidence is steadily increasing. It occurs when parasitic *protozoa* called Plasmodia invade the red blood cells. There are different forms of the disease, depending on the specific type of protozoan involved, which can be identified in a sample. Plasmodium vivax and, less commonly, P. ovale and P. malariae, cause *benign* tertian malaria, in which attacks recur every three days; P. malariae causes benign quartan malaria, in which attacks recur every two days and P. falciparum causes malignant tertian malaria. (In this context, the term 'malignant' does not mean that the

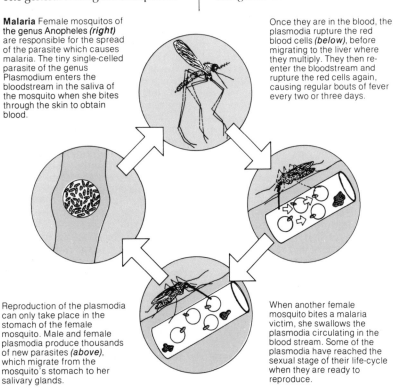

Malaria Female mosquitos of the genus Anopheles *(right)* are responsible for the spread of the parasite which causes malaria. The tiny single-celled parasite of the genus Plasmodium enters the bloodstream in the saliva of the mosquito when she bites through the skin to obtain blood.

Once they are in the blood, the plasmodia rupture the red blood cells *(below)*, before migrating to the liver where they multiply. They then re-enter the bloodstream and rupture the red cells again, causing regular bouts of fever every two or three days.

Reproduction of the plasmodia can only take place in the stomach of the female mosquito. Male and female plasmodia produce thousands of new parasites *(above)*, which migrate from the mosquito's stomach to her salivary glands.

When another female mosquito bites a malaria victim, she swallows the plasmodia circulating in the blood stream. Some of the plasmodia have reached the sexual stage of their life-cycle when they are ready to reproduce.

condition causes cancerous changes).

Malaria is transmitted from person to person by mosquitos belonging to the genus Anopheles, which feed on human blood. The parasites are carried in the mosquito's stomach before being injected into a victim's blood stream in the insect's saliva when the mosquito bites. Once in the human body, the immature protozoa reproduce, first in the liver, then in the red blood cells, which are destroyed in the process. When an infected person is bitten by an Anopheles mosquito the protozoa in the blood are sucked into its stomach, and the cycle begins again.

The first symptoms of malaria appear anything from 10 days to six weeks after the bite, depending on the type of protozoan. They include tiredness, a headache, muscular pains, and a slight temperature. As the parasites multiply, these symptoms intensify, until, at the point where the protozoa move from the liver to the bloodstream, there may be rigors, a feeling of intense cold and shivering combined with a raised temperature. After about an hour, this gives way to hot flushes and a high *fever*, with generalized aches and pains, nausea, dizziness and *delirium*. This is called the hot stage; it slowly subsides into a sweating stage, during which the temperature falls and the patient temporarily recovers.

In quartan and tertian fever these attacks recur every two or three days. However, in the malignant form, also called aestivo-autumnal or subtertian malaria, each attack lasts for longer than a day. As a result, there is little or no recovery period. The victim may also be reinfected by another mosquito bite between attacks, so that the bouts of fever occur successively. This can be extremely serious, because the recurrent daily attacks of malignant malaria, which are sometimes called quotidien fever, may lead to a condition known as cerebral malaria. In this, millions of protozoa block small blood vessels in the brain, causing unconsciousness and death.

The most effective anti-malarial drug is chloraquine, which is used to treat all forms of the disease. However, certain strains of P. falciparum have become resistant to the drug. As a result, malaria is now treated in some areas by other anti-malarial drugs, such as quinine, and by *sulphonamides*. If malaria is not treated adequately, there is a danger that *blackwater fever* will develop. This condition is extremely serious, and sometimes fatal.

Treatment for the benign forms of malaria is usually given between attacks, so that the severity of each attack is gradually reduced. It is essential, however, that treatment is continued until the parasites are entirely destroyed. Any parasites that remain in the body may multiply, and as a result the sufferer may be subject to relapses for several years. This condition, known as chronic malaria, causes *anaemia* and wasting of the tissues.

It is easier to prevent malaria than to cure it. There is no vaccine against the disease, but anyone travelling to an area where the disease is common should take anti-malarial drugs for a few days before setting out, should take them daily during the visit and for four weeks after returning.

Since different species of the parasite are prevalent in different areas, it is essential that the correct drug is prescribed. People travelling to areas in which malaria is common can obtain up-to-date advice on which anti-malarial drug to take by contacting the School of Tropical Medicine in London.

MALIGNANT

A term used to describe certain serious progressive and often fatal conditions. A *cancerous tumour* that invades surrounding tissues is described as malignant, as distinct from a *benign*, self-limiting tumour. In addition, the types of *hypertension*, *smallpox* and other diseases that lead to death if untreated are described as malignant, as is the form of *malaria* that affects the brain.

MALFORMATION—see Congenital abnormalities

MALNUTRITION

The name given to a condition in which the body does not receive an adequate supply of essential nutrients.

There are a number of medical causes of malnutrition—*see malabsorption syndrome*—and the symptoms of the condition may be the result of a number of major diseases. These include: *anorexia nervosa*; certain *cancers*; *cirrhosis*; *diabetes mellitus*; and diseases of the digestive tract, such as *Crohn's disease* and *ulcerative colitis*.

However, by far the most common cause of malnutrition is a diet containing insufficient protein and *calories*. There may be several reasons why the diet is inadequate. The most common of these is poverty and a lack of resources. Estimates vary, but it is likely that more than half the people in the world are inadequately fed for this reason. In Third World countries, where population growth tends to be high, chronic malnutrition is a major problem. This is because the climate, poor soil resources, and primitive agriculture make the production of sufficient food almost impossible, and a lack of financial resources means that it cannot be imported.

Poverty is sometimes the main cause of cases of malnutrition in the developed countries, but ignorance is often also a factor. The diets of low-income families, for example, tend to be high in fats and carbohydrates and low in proteins and essential minerals. The result is often slight malnutrition. People whose jobs involve hard, physical work and women who are pregnant or breast-feeding may also become undernourished because they require more calories and proteins than they realize are necessary—*see Diet, p321.*

Cases of malnutrition in the developed countries are not confined to these groups. People on their own, especially the elderly, may suffer from malnutrition because they become too apathetic to feed themselves properly, even though they are able to afford food. Alcoholics and drug addicts often do not eat regularly because of apathy and mental confusion.

Initially, malnutrition causes a rapid loss of body fat and muscle as the body draws on its reserves to keep up with the demand for energy. Eventually, it adjusts to a regular shortage of proteins and calories and the weight stabilizes at a point below that normal for a person's age, sex and height. The cost is high, however. Sufferers from malnutrition are listless and become tired easily; their bones protrude; the skin becomes pale; and blood pressure, blood sugar levels, body temperature and basic metabolic rate *(p44)* all fall. In addition, there may be symptoms of specific deficiencies—*see kwashiorkor; vitamin deficiency diseases*. Malnutrition stunts growth in children and creates a tendency to *hypothermia* in the elderly; it also reduces the body's resistance to disease, with the result that minor infections may have serious consequences, and may even cause death.

The symptoms of malnutrition begin to disappear once the patient is fed an adequate diet, though he or she will not be fully fit for several months. A patient who has been semi-starved can digest only small quantities of bland foods, such as milk and syrups rich in vitamins, and has to be weaned gradually on to solid foods and a normal diet.

MALPRESENTATION

The presentation of the foetus at the

neck of the womb in a position other than head-first—*see Pregnancy and Birth p60*.

The most common type of malpresentation is a *breech presentation*, in which the foetus lies with its head in the upper part of the uterus and its buttocks in the lower part. There are two other main types of malpresentation. The first is a shoulder presentation, which occurs only at the onset of labour. In this, the foetus lies transversely across the womb, so that the lower shoulder presents. In the second, the foetus lies in the normal position, but with the head forced backwards, so that the face or brow presents. A foetus in the shoulder or brow position can usually be delivered without harm to the baby, but a face presentation may require a *Caesarian section*.

MAMMARY DYSPLASIA—see Breast lumps

MAMMOPLASTY

A surgical operation in which the breast is either enlarged—in which case the operation is known as an augmentation mammoplasty—or reduced in size—when it is known as a reduction mammoplasty.

Mammoplasties are most commonly performed for cosmetic reasons. Most such operations are performed at private clinics, and are extremely expensive; cosmetic mammoplasty is only available on the National Health Service if doctors consider that the size of a woman's breasts is causing her serious psychological problems. Otherwise, an augmentation mammoplasty may be carried out as part of a sex-change operation—*see transsexualism*; a reduction mammoplasty is sometimes necessary when the breasts are so large that their weight presses on the chest and impedes breathing.

A breast augmentation operation is carried out under general *anaesthetic*. A small incision is made underneath the breast and a **prosthesis**, a soft polythene sac filled with silica gel, is inserted under the skin. The patient usually spends one night in hospital and the stitches are removed after about ten days.

There is some bruising and discomfort for two or three weeks after the operation, and strenuous physical activity should be avoided during this period. The sac is inert and does not interfere with the development of the breast during pregnancy, or with breast-feeding. However, a fibrous capsule may occasionally form around the prosthesis and become hard to the

touch. Once this capsule is fully formed, a process that takes about one year, it can be removed under a local anaesthetic. The fibrous capsule is then softened and the prosthesis reinserted.

In a reduction mammoplasty, tissue is removed from the breast and also from the area around the nipple. This is in order that the nipple can be moved to a higher position that looks more natural on the smaller breast. Several stitches are necessary; these are removed within the two weeks after surgery. Since fluid collects within the breast while it is healing, small drainage tubes may be inserted during surgery and the patient kept in hospital for three or four days until these are removed. There is more bruising and general discomfort, such as aching and itching, than in an augmentation operation.

Strenuous exercise must be avoided for about two months after a breast reduction mammoplasty. By then, most of the discomfort will have disappeared, but there may be permanent loss of sensation in the nipple and considerable scarring, especially in people who have a tendency to scar easily. There are rarely any other side effects. It is essential that a mammoplasty is performed by a reputable plastic surgeon. A badly performed operation may result in an implant slipping out of place or, worse still, in a septic infection of the breast. Your family doctor will be able to recommend a reputable plastic surgeon who accepts private patients.

MANIA—see Affective disorders

MANIC DEPRESSIVE PSYCHOSIS—see Affective disorders

MARBURG DISEASE

A disease of green (vervet) monkeys, caused by a virus. **Extremely infectious, it** occasionally breaks out among laboratory technicians who handle infected tissue and cell cultures from this African monkey. Its symptoms include fever, headache, vomiting, diarrhoea, bleeding from internal mucous membranes and a rash. Although an *antiserum* is sometimes helpful, a quarter of all sufferers die within a couple of weeks.

MARFAN'S SYNDROME

An inherited disorder of the bones and connective tissue *(p16)*. The condition may not become obvious until a child reaches puberty. At this time, a person suffering from Marfan's syndrome becomes

exceptionally tall—over two metres (six feet)—and develops a marked stoop and a 'pigeon' or 'funnel chest', long, spindly arms and legs, and abnormally long, thin fingers and toes. The irises of the eyes may be different colours, or the cornea may have a blue tinge, and defects of the eyes, including short-sightedness or *myopia*, *detached retina* and partial dislocation of the lens, are common. Heart defects, including dilatation of the *aorta* and *aortic incompetence* are also characteristic symptoms.

It is not possible to cure Marfan's syndrome. However, the funnel chest may occasionally be surgically repaired, and, if the syndrome is recognized in early childhood, it may be possible to arrest the growth of the bones by hormone therapy, so that the child's height remains within normal limits. In the past many patients with this disorder died in early life from heart disease, but it is now possible to treat dilatation of the aorta and incompetent valves, and so prolong the patient's life.

MASOCHISM

A psychological disorder in which a sufferer derives pleasure from the infliction of mental or physical pain on himself or herself.

There are many different degrees of masochism. Many people who suffer from *neuroses* and *depression* derive an unconscious satisfaction from their problems; similarly, some neurotics take an unconscious pleasure in their physical illnesses and fail to recover as quickly as other patients. Both these cases are symptomatic of a slight degree of masochism. In the higher degrees of masochism, sexual satisfaction can only be obtained through the threat of the infliction of pain, and the sexual act may be accompanied by beating or whipping.

The tendency towards masochism develops in childhood, but usually becomes obvious during adolescence or early adulthood. Many patients do not recognize the need to seek treatment unless urged to do so by others. *Counselling* may help some patients to recognize and overcome their masochistic feelings. However, the deep-rooted psychosexual masochism is more difficult to treat and requires long-term *psychoanalysis* or *psychotherapy*.

MASTECTOMY

A surgical operation to remove part or all of the breast tissue in order to prevent the spread of breast cancer to the rest of the body—*see breast lumps*. Both sexes may be affected by breast cancer—men account for

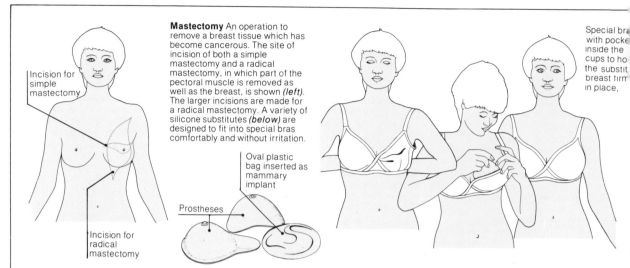

Mastectomy An operation to remove a breast tissue which has become cancerous. The site of incision of both a simple mastectomy and a radical mastectomy, in which part of the pectoral muscle is removed as well as the breast, is shown *(left)*. The larger incisions are made for a radical mastectomy. A variety of silicone substitutes *(below)* are designed to fit into special bras comfortably and without irritation.

Incision for simple mastectomy

Incision for radical mastectomy

Oval plastic bag inserted as mammary implant

Prostheses

Special bra with pocket inside the cups to hold the substitute breast firm in place.

0.6% of all cases—so a mastectomy may be performed on either men or women.

There are three types of operation: a simple mastectomy, in which the whole breast is removed, but the chest muscles and tissues of the armpit are left; a radical mastectomy, in which the majority of the underlying muscles and the fat, connective tissue and lymph nodes of the armpit are removed; and an extended radical mastectomy, in which a string of lymph nodes, called the internal mammary lymphatic chain, is also removed. The lymph tissue is excised because malignant cells can spread to other part of the body through the channels of the lymph system—see *Blood and Lymph, p21*.

The procedure for a mastectomy has changed in recent years. In the past, a woman who had a breast lump would be anaesthetized and taken to the operating theatre for a *biopsy*. A piece of the lump would be removed, a frozen section made—see *Special Tests, p84*—and the malignancy or otherwise of the lump established while the woman was still anaesthetized. If the lump was malignant, a mastectomy would be performed, the type of operation depending on the specific nature and extent of the cancer.

Research has now shown that a mastectomy is unnecessary unless the cancer is already widespread. As a result, a simple 'drill' biopsy is often taken nowadays, under a local anaesthetic. If the lump proves to be *malignant*, it is removed along with the surrounding tissue in an operation called a lumpectomy. The unaffected breast tissue is left in place. A radical mastectomy is only recommended when the surgeon is certain that no simpler operation will be effective.

The patient spends several days in hospital after a mastectomy.

Drainage tubes, inserted so that fluid accumulating beneath the wound may be drawn off, are kept in place during this time, and the patient's arm is supported by a pillow so that the wound can heal. Nevertheless, some movement may be lost in the arm if a large amount of the pectoral muscle *(p16)* has been removed.

Treatment continues after the woman has left hospital, with *chemotherapy*, or drug treatment, and *radiotherapy*, on an out-patient basis. The drug treatment may include the use of synthetic sex hormones, because different types of tumour are either stimulated or suppressed by sex hormones. After the menopause, women do not produce sex hormones in sufficient quantity to stimulate the growth of tumours. However, if older women have had a breast cancer of a type that can be suppressed by sex hormones, they will be given synthetic oestrogens *(p54)*. Similarly, younger women may be given drugs to suppress their production of oestrogen, or, in extreme cases, their ovaries may be removed in an operation called an *oophorectomy*. (In men, the testicles may be removed, for a similar reason, in an *orchidectomy*). In order to control the level of hormones circulating in the body, women are also advised not to take the contraceptive pill, and not to become pregnant for three years after treatment.

After the mastectomy wound has healed, the woman is fitted with a special bra containing a prosthesis, in order to make her appearance entirely natural. However, she has to make a major psychological adjustment, both to the fact of her illness and to the loss of a breast. Ideally, *counselling* should begin before the operation is carried out, and continue for some time afterwards to help the woman deal

with the psychological problems that may arise. It is particularly helpful if her partner is invited to attend counselling sessions, particularly since the loss of a breast often makes a woman feel less attractive. Unfortunately, such counselling is not always routinely given. In cases of difficulty, the Mastectomy Association can advise on where to obtain informed help and support.

The chances of complete recovery after a mastectomy depend on how far the cancer had progressed before the operation. In all cases, the woman will have frequent check-ups for many years after the operation, and in some cases the cancer recurs. The statistics concerning the recovery of patients are compiled according to the stage that the cancer had reached before the operation. In one ten-year study it was found that if the cancer was confined to the breast at the time of operation, around 54% of patients had no recurrence of breast cancer; if the lymph nodes in the armpit were involved, the figure was 24%; and if the cancer had spread to other sites, only 4% survived without a recurrence. This emphasizes the need for routine self-examination of the breasts to detect any cancers as early as possible—see *Routine Checks, p346; breast lumps*.

MASTITIS

An acute inflammation of the breast. This is distinct from a condition called chronic cystic mastitis, in which small cysts develop in the breast—see *breast lumps*. Inflammatory mastitis occurs most commonly in mothers who are breast-feeding, when it is usually caused by bacteria that enter the breast through a cracked nipple; on other occasions bacteria from an infection elsewhere in the body may reach the breast through the bloodstream.

The first symptoms are a slight tenderness in the affected area of the breast. As the condition develops, the tenderness rapidly worsens and a hard swelling is formed, causing a feeling of fullness in the breast. If the condition is not treated at this stage, the breast begins to ache, and breast-feeding is extremely painful. An *abscess* gradually develops in the affected area, causing a high *fever*.

Treatment is by *antibiotics*. These normally prevent the formation of an abscess, if they are prescribed as soon as the first symptoms appear. For this reason, it is important that any pain and swelling in the breasts should be reported to a doctor as soon as they arise. If the abscess has already formed, bathing or dipping the breast in warm water several times a day may help. Often, however, the condition is so painful that a doctor will prescribe painkillers and lance the abscess under a local anaesthetic to release the pus. The wound will be covered with an antiseptic dressing, which must be changed daily until healed.

Some doctors recommend that a nursing mother who suffers from mastitis should stop feeding with the affected breast until the problem has cleared up. The breast should be regularly emptied with a breast pump to prevent engorgement with milk, and the nipple covered with a dressing of sterile cotton wool.

Mastitis can usually be prevented by careful attention to hygiene. A number of special precautions should be taken during pregnancy and breast-feeding. In the later stages of pregnancy, the breast should be washed at least once a day with cotton wool dipped in warm, soapy water. If the nipples start to retract, they should be drawn out every day, and the skin around them stretched to prevent cracks from developing later.

Once breast-feeding starts, the mother should make sure that her breasts are emptied of milk at each feed. This is because stagnant milk is an ideal breeding ground for the bacteria that cause mastitis. The nipples should be kept scrupulously clean, and, if cracks appear in them, they should be treated with antiseptic cream between feeds. A nipple shield can also be worn to guard against further damage. Some doctors advise mothers to rub antiseptic cream over the baby's body on alternate days, in order to **reduce the risk of bacteria being** transferred from baby to breast.

MASTOIDITIS
An inflammation of the mastoid process, a spongy, air-filled bone behind the ear.

Mastoiditis is normally caused by the spread of pus or bacteria from an untreated infection of the middle ear—*see otitis*. The condition is painful and causes *fever* and deafness. It is also potentially serious, because there is a risk that pus will drain into the skull, causing an *abscess* in the brain tissue. An X-ray *(p84)* is sometimes taken to check whether this has happened and to confirm the diagnosis.

Mastoiditis is treated by *antibiotics*. This is normally successful, but when the infection persists an operation may be necessary to drain the pus and remove the infected bone. This is called a mastoidectomy: it is performed under general anaesthetic and may involve staying in hospital for about a week.

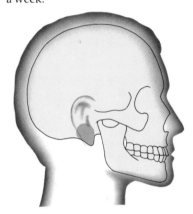

Mastoiditis An inflammation of the mastoid process, the spongy air-filled bone behind the ear *(above)*, is caused by the spread of infection from the middle ear, with fever and deafness as the result.

MASTURBATION
The act of obtaining sexual pleasure or orgasm by manipulating one's own or another person's genitals. During the nineteenth century masturbation was considered wicked and physically and mentally damaging. Today, however, solo masturbation is recognized as a natural expression of the sexual development of children and adolescence, and as a normal sexual activity during adulthood. Mutual **masturbation is considered to be a** normal part of love-making.

Repeated, uninhibited masturbation in public is a symptom of certain mental disorders, such as *schizophrenia*. However, a child who often plays with his or her genitals when surrounded by family or friends is not showing signs of mental disturbance. Instead, he or she is displaying a healthy response to the stresses involved in growing up, and a natural curiosity about, and a pleasure in, his or her body.

See also Sex and Contraception, p338.

MEASLES
A highly infectious disease whose medical name is morbilli or rubeola. It mainly affects children, but is sometimes contracted by adults, and tends to occur in winter *epidemics* every two years.

Measles is caused by a *virus* that is found all over the world. It is spread in droplets of saliva ejected into the air when an infected person coughs or sneezes—*see Health and Hygiene, p334*. After an incubation period of between eight and 12 days, the disease may begin suddenly with a *catarrhal* stage. In this, the symptoms of a cold—coughing, sneezing, a dry cough and watery eyes—are commonly accompanied by a slight *fever* and a feeling of tiredness. In some children these symptoms may be so mild as to be scarcely detectable, while in others they may be severe, and accompanied by *croup, diarrhoea* and sometimes *convulsions*. These symptoms may disappear after two to three days.

The characteristic rash usually appears within a week of infection. It is often preceded by the appearance of clusters of Koplik's spots—whitish spots on the insides of the cheeks. These increase in numbers until the rash appears, and then gradually fade.

The rash consists initially of scattered pink spots that quickly merge to form reddish patches. It usually begins around the hairline and spreads downward over the trunk to the legs. At this stage the temperature rises to between 37.7° and 38.9°C (100°F-102°F) and the child may be thirsty, restless and irritable and complain of a headache. The rash takes around 48 hours to reach its full extent, and then begins to fade from the legs upward. The temperature begins to fall and the child immediately begins to feel better.

If the symptoms are mild, measles may be difficult to diagnose, especially in black-skinned children, since the rash merely gives black skin a granular appearance. Once the disease is diagnosed, however, the patient should be isolated from other children, kept warm in bed and given a light, nourishing diet with plenty of fluids—*see Home Nursing, p352*. There is no specific treatment for measles, though aspirin may help to reduce the temperature and so control the fever. Careful attention should be given to hygiene, especially of the mouth and teeth. Contrary to popular belief, it is not necessary to nurse a child with measles in a darkened room since light will not damage the eyesight.

Measles is rarely serious in

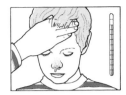

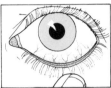

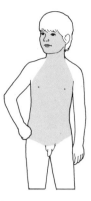

Measles A severe, feverish cold is the first symptom of measles, followed by a dry cough, runny nose and conjunctivitis of the eyes *(left)*. The first sure signs are tiny white spots, surrounded by red inflamed skin, which appear in the mouth, inside the cheeks and around the back teeth. Four days after the cold starts, a rash appears behind the ears and across the forehead *(right)*.

The chart *(below)* shows the daily rise and fall of temperature, together with the rash that accompanies the fever, during an eight-day bout of measles.

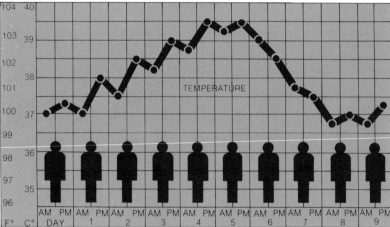

healthy children, and isolation can end as soon as the temperature has returned to normal and the rash has entirely disappeared—usually about ten days after the appearance of the first symptoms.

Very young and delicate children should be nursed carefully during the early stages of the disease since there is a danger that bacterial infections may arise. Such infections include *otitis media, bronchitis, bronchopneumonia, encephalitis* and eye infections such as *conjunctivitis* and *blepharitis*. These conditions are all common complications of measles, and are treated with *antibiotics*.

Poorly nourished children are also susceptible to a rare *malignant* form of measles in which acute *catarrh* and serious weakness leads to collapse and sometimes death. The mortality rate from measles, which is one per l,000 in the UK and the USA, is as high as 20% in some Third World countries.

Vaccines are available for *immunization* against measles. When the disease breaks out on a hospital ward, other patients are usually vaccinated as a preventive measure. Children who have had measles have a degree of immunity, but some children may on rare occasions contract the disease a second time. Babies, however, absorb antibodies

(p52) from the mother's blood through the placenta while in the womb, and are immune to measles for the first three months of life.

MECONIUM
The greenish brown semi-fluid waste matter that collects in the bowel of a foetus during the weeks before birth and is excreted a few days after birth. It is made up of secretions from the liver and the mucous lining of the intestines.

Before birth doctors and nursing staff examine the amniotic fluid for traces of meconium. This may be done by means of an amniocentesis—*see Special Tests, p84*—or by looking at the amniotic fluid produced when the waters break before labour *(p60)*. If any traces are detected by amniocentesis, or the waters appear brown, the foetus may be unwell—*see foetal distress*. Special treatment is required to ensure the safe delivery of the baby.

After the birth, doctors take careful note of the excretion of meconium and, shortly afterwards, of faeces, to ensure that the baby's excretory functions are normal.

MEGACOLON—see Hirschsprung's disease

MEGAVITAMIN THERAPY

The use of very large doses of vitamins to treat various diseases. It derives from the work of the Nobel Prize-winning chemist Linus Pauling and others in the 1950s. Initially, the therapy was used to treat *schizophrenia*—nicotinamide (vitamin B3) being the vitamin involved—but others have tried megavitamin therapy to help treat other conditions, such as learning difficulties in children; while popular books and leaflets have advised its use to treat allergies, colds, cystitis, diabetes, eczema, and many other diseases. Not only is there no scientific foundation for this; giving prolonged large doses of vitamins can be dangerous.

It has been known for a long time that vitamin A can be dangerous in over-dosage. Polar explorers who ate polar bear's liver, which is rich in vitamin A, became ill, while patients who have taken large doses of the vitamin have also done so. However, large doses of certain vitamins are justified in the treatment of certain conditions. Such treatment should only be undertaken on the advice of a specialist.

MEIBOMIAN CYST—see Chalazion

MELANOMA
A *tumour*, which may be *malignant*, arising in the cells of the body that contain melanin, the pigment that gives human skin its colour. Melanomas commonly occur in white-skinned people who live in tropical and sub-tropical areas where they are exposed to strong sunlight.

There are various types of melanoma. A juvenile melanoma, which tends to occur on the face, is a small red spot that grows to about one centimetre (about ½in) in diameter. A different type of melanoma, called lentigo maligna, affects middle-aged and elderly people. This appears as a raised, circular patch anywhere on the skin, normally it is benign and grows slowly, but it may become malignant after a time. As a malignant melanoma grows, it may change colour and start to itch and bleed; the surrounding skin may become depigmented—this is called a halo naevus.

Melanomas arise most commonly in a wart—*see Verruca*—or mole and any change of size or colour, or bleeding in a wart or mole should be reported immediately to a doctor. Since melanomas are fast-growing tumours that metastasize rapidly, particularly to the lymph nodes and liver, they should be removed by surgery at the earliest possible stage of their development.

MENARCHE

The onset of menstruation, an event that occurs during puberty, the time of life in which a girl develops the ability to bear children—*see Sex and Reproduction, p54*.

Female puberty usually begins two or three years before the menarche—usually at around the age of 10, but in some girls at eight or nine and in others as late as 15, and continues for some years afterwards, usually up to the age of 18.

Between the onset of puberty and the menarche the female body undergoes major hormonal changes. The pituitary gland begins to secrete gonadotrophins, hormones that stimulate the ovaries to produce oestrogens. The vagina lengthens and the lining of the womb thickens and becomes richly supplied with blood. The pubic and axillary hair and the breasts develop and the secretion of human pituitary growth hormone causes the rate of growth to increase from an average of five centimetres (two inches) a year before puberty to as much as 10 centimetres (four inches) a year. The menarche occurs at the height of this growth spurt.

In industrialized western countries the average age of the first period has fallen from 18 to 13 during the last century, but there is no evidence that this trend, which may be due to improved standards of living, is continuing. 'Average' means, however, that 95 per cent of girls begin to menstruate between the ages of 11 and 15, so there is considerable variation. Records show that girls whose parents are in the lower income groups begin to menstruate on average a few months later than those with richer parents; that girls living in cities have an earlier menarche than country girls; and that those living at high altitudes begin to menstruate significantly later than those living near sea level. Girls who have several brothers or sisters begin to menstruate slightly later than those who have none and younger sisters earlier than older sisters.

There are significant racial differences in the average age of the menarche. The Chinese, for example, begin to menstruate considerably earlier than Europeans —there are recent records of girls of eight and nine having conceived and borne children—while girls in tribal communities, such as those inhabiting the highlands of New Guinea, begin to menstruate at an average age of 18. The reasons for these differences are not understood.

The menarche often occurs without warning, but it may be preceded by a slight vaginal discharge. The first few periods are usually anovulatory—that is, no ovum is released from the ovaries. Both the blood flow and the timing of the periods may be very irregular; many girls find that the bleeding is extremely scanty at first, or heavy and prolonged for longer than a few days. Others experience oligomenorrhoea—menstruation occurring at intervals of more than 42 days but less than one year—or have periods at intervals of less than 21 days. *Dysmenorrhoea* and *amenorrhoea* are also common in adolescence.

Although hormone therapy may be prescribed to regulate menstruation during the first five years after menarche, it is no longer considered good practice for doctors to prescribe the contraceptive pill for this purpose. There are two reasons for this: first, treatment with the pill carries a risk of side-effects—*see Sex and Contraception, p338*; second, there is no specifically medical reason why a woman should have regular periods unless she is contemplating becoming pregnant.

The changes brought about in the body during puberty are mentally disturbing to all adolescent girls and require a considerable adjustment. This may lead to major swings of mood and unpredictable behaviour, as the teenager adjusts to a maturing body and an adult sexual role. This normally combines with increasing independence from family and perhaps the start of a career. Life becomes rapidly more complex, a phenomenon that is sometimes stimulating, but often exhausting and frightening. Few girls are able to pass through the years of adolescence without withdrawing now and again into a prolonged spell of depression, bad temper, or awkward behaviour, to which parents should respond by showing a high degree of good-humoured understanding.

MÉNIÈRE'S DISEASE

A disorder of unknown cause affecting both hearing and balance, associated with an accumulation of fluid in the inner ear that damages the receptor cells of the cochlea *(p32)*. Ménière's disease affects both men and women, and tends to begin in middle age and to worsen progressively over a number of years.

Initially, sufferers may experience attacks of *vertigo* or become aware that their hearing is failing in one ear. *Tinnitus*, a persistent, usually high-pitched noise, sets in as the deafness worsens. Attacks of vertigo often occur suddenly and wake a sufferer up if he or she is asleep. Otherwise, an attack of vertigo may be preceded by an intensification of the tinnitus, giving the person time to sit or lie down before the attack reaches its climax, or it may occur without warning, causing the sufferer to fall to the floor. It is often accompanied or followed by nausea, vomiting and a feeling of faintness. The skin pales and the patient sweats profusely. A mild attack may last for as little as 15 minutes, passing off as suddenly as it began, but a sufferer may feel giddy and ill for several hours after a severe attack. Some people also experience dizziness and nausea on awakening in the morning.

These symptoms often disappear for several months, but if the disorder progresses they recur at gradually more frequent intervals. The deafness spreads to the other ear, and, eventually, damage to both inner ears causes total loss of hearing, and paralysis of the organs of balance. The result is that the tinnitus and the attacks of vertigo diminish and disappear, and the sense of balance is completely lost.

The cause of Ménière's disease is not yet known, and it is incurable. Its progress may be arrested, however, by restricting the patient's intake of fluid to 1.5 litres (2½pts) a day and by a diet low in salt. *Diuretics* may also be prescribed. The attacks of vertigo are aggravated and often stimulated by sudden movement, and may be reduced in severity if the patient regularly takes drugs to prevent vomiting, and regularly rests in bed. Drugs may also be prescribed to dilate the blood vessels and so increase blood flow.

MENINGISM—see Meningitis

MENINGITIS

A disease caused by an inflammation of the meninges, the three membranes that enclose the brain and spinal cord—*see The Nervous System, p32*.

There are several different types of meningitis: cerebral meningitis affects the meninges of the brain, and spinal meningitis affects the meninges of the spinal cord. In addition, the disease is classified according to the micro-organism that causes it. Meningococcal meningitis, for example, is caused by the *bacteria* of the Neisseria family, of which other members cause *gonorrhoea*; tuberculous meningitis is caused by the bacillus responsible for *tuberculosis*. Viral meningitis, a third type, is caused by a *virus*. While the symptoms of all types of meningitis are similar, the meningococcal form is the most serious; viral meningitis

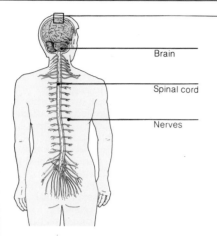

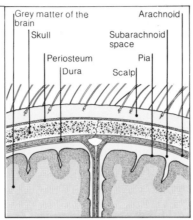

Grey matter of the brain
Skull
Periosteum
Dura
Arachnoid
Subarachnoid space
Pia
Scalp

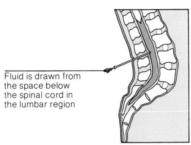

Fluid is drawn from the space below the spinal cord in the lumbar region

Brain

Spinal cord

Nerves

Meningitis is the inflammation of the membranes or meninges which protect the brain and the spinal cord. There are three meninges — the dura, the arachnoid and the pia *(right)*. The inflammation is the result of a bacterial or viral infection which usually begins elsewhere in the body, such as the upper respiratory tract, and spreads to the meninges via the blood. The condition is diagnosed by examining a sample of the cerebrospinal fluid that circulates between the arachnoid and pia meninges in the subarachnoid space, since meningitis changes its composition.

is the most common and the least serious. Tuberculous meningitis is now rarely seen.

Meningococcal meningitis, also called cerebrospinal or spotted fever, is an infectious disease and often occurs in epidemics. As a result, it is *notifiable*. Neisseria meningitis, the bacteria responsible, lives harmlessly in the nose and throat of many people. It tends to cause infection when the natural resistance of the body is lowered, and, for this reason, young children and the elderly are the most commonly affected.

The first symptoms in adults are sometimes a sore throat, cough, headache and slight *fever*. More commonly, however, its onset is sudden and violent, with no warning symptoms. A sufferer can suddenly feel an intense, throbbing pain, centred in the back of the head, then begin to vomit severely and to shiver; he or she may fall to the ground in a *convulsion*. The temperature rises to 38.9°C (102°F) or higher and the sufferer becomes irritable and photophobic—that is, unable to stand light—and often semiconscious and *delirious*. He or she typically lies to one side with the back towards the light. A spotty rash usually develops on the trunk within two or three days and the muscles of the neck stiffen.

In infants, the first symptoms are usually repeated *convulsions* and severe attacks of *vomiting*. Between attacks the child is irritable, cries with a high-pitched sound when

picked up, and refuses to feed. The fontanelle, the opening in an infant's skull, may appear swollen, a symptom of raised pressure within the skull.

A doctor faced with these symptoms will take a sample of the cerebrospinal fluid *(p32)* from the spinal cord by means of a lumbar puncture—*see Special Tests, p84*. The sample is examined to identify the infecting organism and determine the specific form of meningitis, and to ensure that the patient is not suffering from meningism. In this condition the stiffness of the neck, headache and vomiting are relatively innocent. They are due to a mild form of meningeal irritation that often occurs in chest infections and diseases of the *upper respiratory tract*, as well as *enteritis*, *nephritis* and other infections.

Without treatment sufferers from meningococcal meningitis often die, sometimes within a week of the appearance of symptoms. In some patients, however, the symptoms gradually die down and there is a complete recovery; in others the initial symptoms lose their severity, only for the disease to pass into a chronic stage in which the body becomes wasted and *hydrocephalus* develops. Some patients become blind or deaf or mentally handicapped as a result. However, this untreated, persistent form of meningitis is now very rare.

Treatment involves isolation in hospital and the administration of large dosages of *sulphonamide* drugs

or penicillin. Since their discovery, these drugs have reduced the mortality rate from between 70% and 80% to below 10%. *Sedatives* may be prescribed, together with *analgesics* to relieve the headache. As the disease is contagious, people who have been in close proximity to the victim may be given sulphonamides as a preventive treatment.

Tuberculous meningitis is a complication of tuberculosis and may develop during any stage in the disease. Like meningococcal meningitis, it is more common in children than in adults. The main symptoms—headache, vomiting, stomach pains and a rise in temperature to 38.9°C (102°F) — may preceded by a period of increasing irritability, loss of appetite and apathy. The patient becomes feverish and photophobic and, over a period of three weeks, increasingly drowsy. Paralysis of one or more of the cranial nerves *(p32)* may result in *strabismus*—a squint—*diplopia*—double vision—or facial paralysis.

Without treatment the patient sinks into a *coma* and usually dies within three weeks. If the disease is diagnosed at an early stage, however, the *antibiotic* streptomycin is given, together with two other drugs to which the bacillus is known to respond. This treatment usually ensures complete recovery, but drug therapy may be continued for several years. *Corticosteroid* drugs may be administered to patients in coma. Patients who are diagnosed early in the course of the disease usually recover completely as a result of this treatment, but those who have already fallen into a coma before treatment often suffer from permanent brain damage.

Viral meningitis may be caused by a number of viruses, among them those responsible for *mumps*, *poliomyelitis* and *glandular fever*. Meningitis is therefore a complication of these and several other diseases. However, the headache, fever, vomiting and stiffness of the neck symptomatic of bacterial meningitis are usually less severe in viral meningitis. There is no specific treatment for viral meningitis, other than bed-rest, and the affected person usually recovers within a week. Occasionally, patients suffer from convulsions and some mental deterioration, but this only happens in severe cases.

MENOPAUSE
The medical term for the a woman's last menstrual period—*see Sex and Reproduction, p54*—the opposite of *menarche*. In physiological terms, the male menopause does not exist:

there is no sudden change in the production of sex hormones. The term refers to a mid-life crisis of confidence experienced by some men. In women, the menopause is an inevitable and natural part of life.

The menopause takes place during the period of life known as the climacteric, or change of life, during which a woman's ability to bear children gradually diminishes; 75% of women experience the menopause between the ages of 45 and 55, while the remaining 25% may have their final period as early as 38 or as late as 58. The average age at which it occurs has remained constant at 50, apparently since mediaeval times.

Several factors may influence the age at which the menopause occurs. The most important of these is smoking. Though the exact mechanism is not known, recent research in America has shown that women who smoke experience the menopause significantly earlier than those who do not; the more cigarettes smoked, the earlier the last period. An early menopause may also be the result of *radiotherapy* or removal of the ovaries—*see oophorectomy*—as part of the treatment of disease. By contrast, a late menopause may be the result of *fibroids* in the womb. Women who suffer from fibroids sometimes have their last period as much as seven to eight years later than the average.

The climacteric begins some eight to ten years before the menopause, and lasts for up to ten years after it. During the climacteric there is a gradual, but radical change in the balance of hormones (*p48*) circulating in a woman's body. After the age of 30, the secretion of female hormones by the ovaries gradually diminishes and ceases altogether within a decade after the menopause. There is also gradual decline in fertility from the age of 30—when it is around 30%—to around 3% at 40.

In some women menstruation ceases suddenly with little warning, but more commonly the process is gradual, often taking several years, during which menstruation occurs less and less frequently. It is often difficult, therefore, for a woman to know when the menopause finally occurs. Periods during the months before the menopause are often anovulatory—that is, no ovum is released by the ovaries. However, there is a theoretical possibility of pregnancy, so contraceptive measures should be taken to avoid an unwanted pregnancy. If no bleeding occurs for one year in women over 50, or for two years in younger women, the last period can

be safely reckoned to have taken place. A woman on the pill will be advised to use other contraceptive methods for a month, so that hormone tests can be made to determine whether or not the menopause has taken place.

In some women the climacteric passes with few obvious signs other than the cessation of menstruation. Others, however, suffer from one or more of a number of symptoms and disorders, both physical and psychological. Since the study of hormones and their precise role in the human body is still in its infancy the causes of many of these problems are not yet fully understood and treatment is still in the experimental stages. It is particularly difficult, for example, to establish whether symptoms such as depression and insomnia are due to the imbalance of hormones, or reactions to the psychological stresses brought about by the change of life and by problems common at this age, such as bereavement and the behaviour of adolescent children.

The most common physical problem, experienced by about 60% of women, is hot flushes. These take the form of a sudden sensation of heat in the face, often combined with flushing of the skin and profuse sweating, followed by a period of cold shivering. Some women only experience hot flushes occasionally—when they are excited or nervous, for example—but in others they may occur many times each day and even interrupt sleep. In addition, 40% of menopausal women suffer from excessive perspiration, often occurring at night. These disorders are caused by the effect of hormonal changes on the autonomic nervous system (*p32*). The precise mechanism is not fully understood, but both problems are considerably improved by treatment with the hormone oestrogen.

The hot flushes and excessive perspiration often gradually subside after the last period. From this time, any physical problems are caused not by an imbalance of hormones, but by a lack of one of them, oestrogen. The ovaries continue to secrete oestrogen until the menopause takes place, but after this the amount of oestrogen produced falls off quickly. Small quantities, however, continue to be produced by the adrenal glands—*see The Endocrine System, p48*.

The lack of oestrogen may cause a number of changes: the skin gradually thins; the hair on the head and body decreases in density, becoming dry; and the sebaceous

glands, sweat glands and mucous membranes tend to dry up. There are also changes in the reproductive organs (*p54*): the vulva gradually becomes less fleshy, and the vagina becomes shorter, narrower and dryer; the cervix, Fallopian tubes and uterus become smaller; and the breasts become either smaller and flatter or pendulous. However, the vagina and vulva degenerate considerably more slowly in women who continue regular sexual activity than in those who do not.

As a result of these changes women become more susceptible to complaints such as *pruritis, urethritis* and *vaginitis*. These often cause pain on sexual intercourse, or *dyspareunia*, and, as a result, affected women may lose interest in sex—normally, however, they clear up after treatment. There is also an increase in the incidence of *cysts* and *benign* and *malignant tumours* in the reproductive organs.

The lack of oestrogen also affects bone, with the result that women lose, on average, 1% of their skeletal bone each year after the menopause. This condition, known as *osteoporosis*, is exacerbated by smoking and causes the bones to fracture easily.

Many of the physical problems caused by the decline in production of oestrogen can be relieved, or held at bay, by *hormone replacement therapy*, or HRT. Pruritis, urethritis and vaginitis, for example, become much less common, and there is some evidence that HRT prevents thinning of the skin and hair. Shrinkage and wasting of the genitals is prevented, and osteoporosis is avoided.

Until recently, HRT was also thought to give women a degree of protection against *heart disease*. As a result, the therapy was once thought of as a panacea for ageing. Recently, however, the dangers and side-effects of such treatment have become evident. Modern research shows that oestrogens are unlikely to have any beneficial effect on heart disease. In addition, it is now realized that there are links between oestrogen therapy and the excessive growth of the endometrium, the lining of the womb, which may, in some cases, lead to *cancers*. The problem can be avoided if patients are given oestrogens for three weeks in every month, with progesterone supplements for seven to ten days during that time. However, this treatment causes the woman to have a monthly withdrawal bleed.

Several problems caused by the lack of oestrogen after the menopause can be relieved without recourse to hormone therapy.

Oestrogen creams are widely used for the relief of problems such as vaginitis, and pain on intercourse can be avoided by the use of a lubricating jelly, available without a prescription. Osteoporosis can to a large extent be prevented by a healthy diet, regular vitamin D supplements, and regular exercise. This will also have a beneficial effect on the heart and lungs—*see Diet, p322; Exercise, p316.*

Although the climacteric does not cause any psychiatric illness, many women seek medical help during their 40s and 50s for relief of symptoms that can be broadly classified as psychological. These range from headache, *vertigo*, or giddiness, *dyspnoea*, or shortness of breath, and fatigue to apathy, inability to concentrate, depression, tension, anxiety, feelings of inadequacy and sudden fluctuations of mood. Such symptoms may be fairly mild, but disruptive to work or family life, or occasionally so serious as to require treatment in a psychiatric hospital.

There is little doubt that hormone imbalance causes some depression and see-sawing of mood; the argument is made more convincing by the fact that HRT generally gives post-menopausal women a feeling of mental wellbeing. However, the effects of hormone imbalance on mood during the climacteric are, like the mood swings of adolescence, rarely so severe that the individual cannot handle them.

It is inevitable that the approach of the menopause should bring a series of conflicts into many women's minds. Their effects may exacerbate downward swings of mood and cause ailments to become magnified into illnesses. At the menopause many women have to reconcile themselves to their inability to bear children, though some welcome this. In addition, the menopause is a sign of ageing, which some people find hard to accept. The stresses that often occur in women's lives at around the age of 50 may exacerbate these problems. During the climacteric many women lose one or both parents and their children are often on the brink of leaving home or going through adolescence, with all the accompanying family problems. These stressful changes can make the burden of adjustment to the upheaval of the climacteric intolerable.

Psychologists have classified womens' reaction to the menopause in four main ways. Some women passively accept the inevitable; some resist both the menopause and the ageing process, the resistance being expressed as nervousness,

depression, irritability and sometimes as a *psychosomatic* illness; some simply refuse to recognize what is happening, throwing themselves into their careers or into hobbies. The majority, however, adjust well to the climacteric. Such women tend to be those who are satisfied with their occupation and relationships, and who have a frank, open attitude to menstruation and female sexuality. In fact, many women look forward to the prospect of sex without the worry of contraception or pregnancy.

Women who develop minor symptoms of *neurosis* during the climacteric are often treated with drugs such as analgesics, tranquillizers and sleeping tablets. These may be helpful in the short term, but psychologists find that *counselling* or, if the symptoms are particularly severe, *psychotherapy*, are generally extremely effective in helping women to adjust to their new circumstances. Physical symptoms such as palpitations, vertigo, headache and dyspnoea, none of which have any proven relationship with blood hormone levels, often respond to such treatment as well.

Just as the menarche symbolizes the end of childhood and the beginning of adult life, the climacteric and menopause represent not merely the end of reproductive activity, but the start of a new phase of creative life.

MENORRHAGIA
An excessive loss of blood during a menstrual period. The period may be longer than usual and the menstrual blood heavily clotted.

Menorrhagia occurs most commonly in women under 35, when it is usually caused by an imbalance in the ratio of oestrogen to progesterone in the blood—*see Sex and Reproduction, p54.* However, it may also be caused by disorders of the uterus, such as *fibroids.* Women who complain of menorrhagia are usually examined, therefore, for uterine abnormalities. In the first instance, there is a routine examination of the vagina and womb by the family doctor, but the doctor may recommend that a *D & C* is performed.

If the uterus is found to be healthy, the hormone imbalance can be corrected by the prescription of the hormone progesterone, which is taken for a specific number of days during the menstrual cycle. The progesterone-only contraceptive pill is also effective in the treatment of menorrhagia, but carries the risk of certain side-effects—*see Sex and Contraception, p338.*

MENSTRUAL DISORDERS—see Amenorrhoea; Dysmenorrhoea; Menorrhagia

MENTAL SUBNORMALITY
A symptom of a number of conditions, affecting between 2% and 3% of people, in which the intelligence quotient is below the normal range of 90 to 110—*see IQ.*

Mental subnormality may be the result of a number of factors. Sometimes there is no specific cause: just as some people have an IQ higher than the normal range, others have an IQ below it. However, mental subnormality can result from a number of conditions that affect the mother during pregnancy, such as German measles—*see rubella—mumps, alcoholism,* drug addiction, a rhesus blood group mismatch—*see haemolytic disease of the newborn—*infection with *cytomegalovirus* and *syphilis.*

Mental subnormality may also be caused by problems arising during birth or by disorders affecting the baby itself. For example, a difficult or prolonged labour may cause bleeding inside the baby's brain or a reduction in the supply of oxygen to it, resulting in permanent damage. *Encephalitis, meningitis, abscess* in the brain and *Down's syndrome,* or mongolism, can also cause mental subnormality as a result of their effects on a baby's brain.

In such cases, damage to the brain tissues often results in permanent mental subnormality. Other conditions, however, only retard mental development and, as a result, their effects can be reversed if the condition is diagnosed early enough and treated. Examples include *cretinism,* a condition due to defective development of the thyroid gland, and *phenylketonuria,* a disorder of the metabolism.

Some children suffer from retarded mental development because they suffer from a lack of mental stimulation early in life. A child whose partial *deafness* or inability to speak is not diagnosed until he or she has spent some years at school, or a child with a physical illness who has been isolated from other children, may fail to develop normally. Emotionally deprived children often do not realize their full intellectual potential. Such children often recover completely, if these handicaps are diagnosed early enough for special training to be given.

The diagnosis of mental subnormality is often a difficult one to make. Parents may worry that a baby is mentally subnormal when he or she is unresponsive, and fails to take an alert interest in the surroundings, to smile or to recognize them by the expected age—*see Routine Health Checks, p346.* However, this worry is often unnecessary. Many tests are needed to make the diagnosis in children, since visual and auditory defects, emotional disorders, speech disorders, *autism* and clumsiness can all be wrongly interpreted as mental subnormality. Because of this, children suspected of being mentally subnormal are observed for prolonged periods, usually in special diagnosis and assessment centres.

Until shortly after World War II, mental subnormality was considered incurable and people whose IQ was lower than average were often interned in institutions, usually for life. Since the 1950s, however, considerable knowledge has been gained about the causes and treatment of mental subnormality. As a result, patients are now, if possible, treated from home in diagnostic and assessment centres, special schools or training centres.

Only people with an IQ of less than 50, usually classified as severely subnormal, are totally dependent. They may be unable to protect themselves from danger, to care for themselves or to respond to training. They have only a limited ability to form relationships with others, may be unable to express themselves or understand others and may suffer from other handicaps such as fits or deafness. Wherever possible, severely subnormal people are brought up in small residential institutions in which emphasis is placed on stimulation and development.

More than 80% of mentally subnormal people have an IQ above 60 and, with specialized education, they can learn to live almost independent lives. Training is normally given in special centres, on an out-patient basis whenever possible. This is because a mentally subnormal child tends to respond to treatment much better when able to live with his or her family.

Training consists of maximizing personal development and independence. The emphasis is placed on social adjustment, since mentally subnormal people often have behavioural problems and find it difficult to tolerate frustration. With the benefit of such training, most mentally subnormal people are able to undertake simple employment in special centres and to lead nearly normal, semi-independent lives.

MESOTHELIOMA
A rare *malignant tumour* that arises in the pleura, the membrane surrounding the lung *(p28).* Mesotheliomas are particularly common among people who work in the asbestos industry, and in other industries in which blue asbestos is used. Tumours have been found in people as long as 20 to 40 years after they have worked with asbestos for only one year, and also in people who have lived near an asbestos factory.

The first symptom of a mesothelioma is often an ache in the chest. As the tumour invades surrounding organs, fluid escapes into the pleural cavity, causing *dyspnoea*, or breathlessness, and the sputum produced by coughing is blood-stained. Fluid may also leak into the cavity of the abdomen, causing *ascites*, pain and distension. The tumour also causes *clubbing* of the fingers, and *crepitation*, a crackling in the lungs, audible when a doctor listens to the chest with a stethoscope. A mesothelioma is difficult to diagnose, however, since these symptoms are common to a number of conditions. A doctor will normally recommend that an X-ray and biopsy are taken—*see Special Tests, p84*—if the patient's work history leads to the suspicion that a mesothelioma may be present.

There is no effective treatment for a mesothelioma, and death usually occurs within a short time of the diagnosis of the tumour. Preventive measures include wearing respirators and efficient dust-damping and ventilating systems in factories in which asbestos is worked.

See also asbestosis.

METABOLIC DISORDERS
Any disorder in which one or other of the millions of chemical processes necessary for life is deficient—*see Metabolism, p44.* Metabolic disorders can be classified according to the type of chemical process that is deficient: protein, carbohydrate or fat metabolism. The exception is *gout.* This condition results from a disorder in the metabolism of purines, compounds of nitrogens.

The most common of all metabolic disorders is *diabetes mellitus*, which affects the metabolism of carbohydrates. Other, rarer, disorders of carbohydrate metabolism include *galactosaemia*, an abnormality in the metabolism of the sugar, galactose; fructosaemia, in which fructose, the sugar found in fruit, is excreted in the urine; and glycogen storage diseases.

Fructosaemia is a rare hereditary disorder caused by a deficiency in liver enzymes. Affected infants vomit when fructose, in the form of cane sugar, is added to the diet, develop *hypoglycaemia* and an enlarged liver, and fail to gain weight. Treatment is by substituting glucose for any fructose or sucrose in the diet, and by teaching the child to avoid foods that contain fructose for the rest of his or her life.

The glycogen storage diseases are also rare, hereditary illnesses. They are caused by a deficiency in the enzymes responsible for the breakdown of glycogen, the storage form of the sugar, glucose. Most of these diseases result in an abnormal accumulation of glycogens in the body, giving children an obese, stunted appearance, hypoglycaemia and an enlarged liver. Others may have serious consequences, causing the sudden onset of a hypoglycaemic coma.

People with glycogen storage diseases are advised to eat small quantities of food frequently, especially late at night, and may be prescribed carbohydrate tablets. These measures prevent the level of blood sugar from falling, and reduce the quantity of glucose that must be stored as glycogen. Some sufferers are treated surgically, by means of a newly developed technique. This involves diverting the portal vein, which carries carbohydrates from the intestines, so that it by-passes the liver, the main site of glycogen metabolism in the body.

Defects in amino acid metabolism give rise to three rare metabolic disorders: *phenylketonuria*, cystinuria and the Toni Fanconi syndrome. In cystinuria, an excessive amount of cystine, an amino acid *(p44)*, accumulates in the blood and is excreted in the urine. This leads to the formation of cystine stones in the kidneys, which may obstruct the flow of urine. In the Toni Fanconi syndrome, an affected child fails to grow after the age of six months, and suffers from bouts of vomiting and *fever* and a type of severe *rickets* that does not respond to vitamin D therapy. There may also be *acidosis*, polyuria—excessive excretion of urine—and *dehydration*. In adult life, sufferers develop *osteomalacia*. There is no effective treatment for the condition, which often progresses to *kidney failure* and death.

Disorders in the metabolism of fats cause the *lipid storage diseases* and a series of inherited conditions known as hyperlipidaemias. These cause obesity, *xanthomas*, and *atherosclerosis*. Hyperlipidaemias are controlled by means of a low-fat, low calorie diet.

METASTASIZE
The process by which cells from a tumour slough off into blood or lymph vessels and establish new

colonies elsewhere in the body.
See also cancer.

MIGRAINE

A severe recurrent headache, sometimes called a 'one-sided headache' because the pain tends to be confined to one side of the head. The headache is often accompanied by visual disturbances and by abdominal symptoms.

Surveys carried out recently by a number of migraine sufferers' associations have shown that at least one person in ten suffers from migraine. Of these, some have attacks once or twice a week and others as infrequently as once a year. There are no symptoms between attacks.

There are various different types of migraine. In classical migraine, the attack is usually preceded by an 'aura', a sensation that may be different for each sufferer. Typically, auras include numbness or weakness on one side of the body, bright, white or coloured shapes, spots or lines before the eyes, or problems such as double vision and blind spots in the vision; these signs may last for up to half an hour before the attack begins. When there is no aura, the condition is termed common migraine.

Migraine attacks may also be preceded and accompanied by various physical and psychological symptoms. Some patients feel extremely cheerful and energetic before an attack, but irritable and depressed once it begins; others feel extremely hungry before an attack, but are unable to eat once the headache begins. Some people develop an intense sensitivity to odours or sounds before and during an attack; while others gain weight because of fluid retention before an attack and urinate frequently afterwards, losing the weight gained. Other warning signs include: dizziness; hallucinations; nausea and vomiting; tingling sensations; alterations in mood; yawning; trembling; nervousness; difficulties in speaking; pains in the neck or shoulders; skin rashes or pallor; and frequency of urination.

An attack consists of an intense, throbbing headache. It is often accompanied by photophobia—that is, an inability to tolerate light—difficulty in focusing and, if the attack is severe, loss of appetite, nausea, vomiting, constipation or diarrhoea. These symptoms may last for only a few hours or several days, depending on the individual.

Migraines are caused by an excessive sensitivity of the blood vessels in the head. In the initial phase, arteries and capillaries within the skull and over the face and scalp contract, giving rise to the aura. Next, they dilate, or widen, causing pain by stretching the nerve endings in the walls of the arteries. Muscular contractions may exacerbate the pain.

The reasons why the blood vessels of the head react in this way are not fully understood. However, most migraine sufferers have at least one close relative who is also a sufferer, and the tendency to suffer from this complaint is thought to be hereditary. In addition, certain specific types of migraine can be distinguished, and have specific causes.

Migrainous neuralgia, for example, a type of migraine in which attacks occur in clusters, is exacerbated, and probably also induced by alcohol. This problem is most common in men and begins during the third or fourth decade of life. The sufferer is often awoken by an attack on a number of successive mornings. The pain usually centres at the back of one eye, which may become red, swollen and watery, and the nostril on that side may become congested.

Migraines can be triggered by a number of factors, which vary from person to person. Foods such as cheese, for example, that contain tyramine, a chemical known to widen blood vessels, are thought to bring about migraine attacks in certain people. The British Migraine Trust lists the following migraine triggers for susceptible people:
* Emotional upsets, including anxiety, worry, depression, shock and excitement
* Over-exertion, physical or mental fatigue, lifting heavy weights, bending and stooping
* A change of routine, including going on holiday, shift work, changing jobs or getting up late at the weekend or while on holiday
* Travel, a change of climate or changes in the weather, including high winds
* Glare, including bright sunlight, artificial light, or prolonged focusing on a screen
* Very hot baths
* Intense noise or penetrating odours
* Certain foods, including cheese, chocolate, dairy products, fruit, alcohol, fried, fatty foods, vegetables, tea and coffee, meat, particularly pork, sea food, pickled herrings and concentrated meat or yeast extracts
* Prolonged lack of food, including fasting, dieting and irregular meals
* Menstruation, oral contraceptives and the menopause
* High blood pressure
* Pain elsewhere in the body, especially in the teeth and neck
* Taking sleeping tablets.

Many people are incapacitated by a migraine attack and have to go to bed in a darkened room until the attack has passed. However, perhaps because a person suffering from migraine has no visible signs of illness, many people feel that they should try and carry on with their usual activities. Unfortunately, this can prolong or worsen the attack and sufferers usually find that if they take a painkiller as soon as an attack seems imminent, and sleep for a couple of hours, the attack passes. It is important, therefore, that sufferers should treat their migraine as an illness and explain it as such to their employers and colleagues.

A number of drugs can be used to treat a migraine attack. They include simple painkillers, such as aspirin, codeine and paracetamol, and combinations of these three drugs, preferably in a fast-acting soluble or effervescent form: *anti-emetics*, which reduce nausea and vomiting; *sedatives* that relax muscles; and drugs, such as ergotamine tartrate, that have been found to have a specific effect on migraine. Migrainous neuralgia can usually be prevented if an ergotamine tartrate suppository is inserted into the rectum before an attack is expected. Doctor and patient usually have to experiment, trying out different drugs and combinations of drugs, until they find the form of treatment most effective in reducing the severity or duration of an attack. In addition, acupuncture (p306) has proved effective in curing migraines and regular yoga appears to help reduce the frequency of attacks.

By keeping careful records of attacks and of activities, diet and other circumstances surrounding the occurrence of each attack, many migraine sufferers are able to isolate the factors that trigger attacks and take preventive measures. Many people learn to avoid migraine attacks altogether by eliminating cheese, chocolate, white wine or spirits from their diets. Alternatively, they may learn to ward off a threatened attack by becoming aware of warning signs and taking their medication before the attack begins.

The herbal remedy feverfew is used by many patients in the treatment of migraine and arthritis. A recent double-blind trial of feverfew carried out in the City of London Migraine Clinic showed that it was certainly effective, and there were few side effects (the patients were all using the medicine already). However, no studies on long-term use have yet been done.

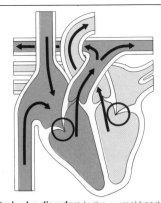 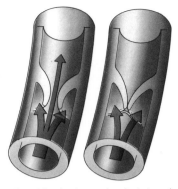 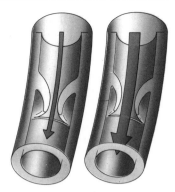

Mitral valve disorders In the normal heart *(left)* the mitral valve separates the left atrium and ventricle. It opens to allow blood to pass from the atrium to the ventricle, and then closes, so that blood cannot flow back into the atrium when the ventricle contracts. When the valve is weakened — a condition called mitral incompetence *(middle)* — the pumping action of the ventricle pushes blood back into the atrium, reducing the amount of

blood reaching the tissues. In mitral stenosis *(right)*, the valve is narrow and thick. The result is that not all the blood in the atrium can pass through it to the ventricle. This also reduces the amount of oxygenated blood reaching the tissues. The two problems often occur together. They are both usually the result of rhematic fever — though mitral incompetence can be present at birth — and both cause an enlargement of the heart. This

is because the heart muscle becomes larger and more powerful in an attempt to increase the flow of blood to the tissues by pumping harder. Eventually, the extra demands on the heart may lead to heart failure, and surgery may be necessary.

MISCARRIAGE—see Abortion

MITE
A minute insect of the Acarina family. Some species of mites are parasites and infest humans, while others are carriers of disease. The itch mite, for instance, causes *scabies* in humans, while harvest mites can transmit scrub *typhus* to humans. Mites of the Dermatophagoides family live in sugar, flour and other foodstuffs and cause forms of *dermatitis* in humans.

The house mite, which lives in the warm, damp conditions found in bedding, upholstery and carpets, is also a carrier of infection. *Rickettsiae* organisms living within the mites produce *antibodies* when they come into contact with human blood. In adults, the result is an *allergic* reaction, such as *asthma*,

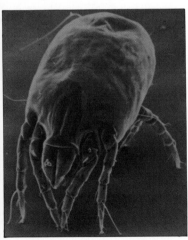

House-dust Mite The house-dust mite *(enlarged above)* lives in the dust and dirt of every house, inhabiting carpets, curtains, furniture and corners. People allergic to these mites develop a form of hay-fever called rhinitis, which has the characteristic symptoms of sneezing bouts and runny eyes.

breathlessness, a runny nose or mild dermatitis. In children, however, the infection can cause Kawasaki's disease, first recognized in Japan in the 1960s. Symptoms include prolonged *fever*, a sore mouth and tongue, a skin rash, swelling and **peeling of the skin of hands and** feet and swollen glands in the neck. In severely affected children, the arteries of the heart are affected, and this can lead to death in a small percentage of cases.

The disease is most common in Japan, the UK and USA. So far, no specific drug treatment has proved effective. As far as possible, therefore, people should avoid raising dust when children are present.

MITRAL INCOMPETENCE
A weakness of the mitral valve, which divides the left atrium and left ventricle in the heart—*see The Blood and Lymph Systems, p21*.

Mitral incompetence may either be present at birth—*see congenital heart defects*—or caused by a disorder that affects the heart tissues, such as *rheumatic fever*. As a result of the weakness of the valve, blood that has passed into the left ventricle tends to leak back into the left atrium. This means that the heart has to pump harder to force the normal amount of blood into the aorta and through the circulation. The heart often enlarges, in an attempt to do this. Eventually, however, the extra demands on the heart muscle may lead to congestive *heart failure* and breathlessness, as the backlog of blood causes a build-up of fluid in the lungs. Treatment may either be by drugs or surgery, depending on the severity of the problem—*see valvular heart disease*.

See also mitral stenosis.

MITRAL STENOSIS
A narrowing and thickening of the mitral valve, which separates the left atrium and left ventricle in the heart—*see The Blood and Lymph Systems, p21*.

Mitral stenosis commonly occurs in association with *mitral incompetence*, and is generally the result of scarring caused by *rheumatic fever*. As a result of the narrowing of the valve, blood tends to pool in the left atrium and lungs, and the muscles of the right ventricle have to work much harder to keep the blood circulating. Initially, this may only result in breathlessness, but as the heart muscle is weakened by the extra demands placed on it the supply of blood to the whole body falters. In this condition, called right-sided *heart failure*, the ankles become swollen and there is a general feeling of tiredness. There is also a risk that the muscles of the atria will start to contract spasmodically, in a condition called *atrial fibrillation*.

Eventually, surgery may be necessary to open up the valve—*see valvular heart disease*.

MOLLUSCUM CONTAGIOSUM
An infectious *viral* skin disease, in which globular, fluid-filled *benign tumours* appear on the skin. The areas usually affected are the face, eyelids, breasts, genitals and the inner surface of the thigh. The disease is transmitted by touch.

The tumours can grow to the size of peas. They can be treated by freezing with liquid nitrogen, or by pricking them with an orange stick coated with the corrosive chemical phenol. After treatment they waste away and fall off the body.

MONGOLISM—see Down's syndrome

MONILIA—see Candidiasis

MORNING SICKNESS—see Hyperemesis gravidarum

MOTOR NEURONE DISEASE

A rare progressive disorder of the nervous system (p32), in which the motor nerves gradually atrophy, causing wasting of the muscles they supply. The disease is rarely found in people under 40 and is most common in people over 60. It affects men more often than women.

The cause of motor neurone disease is unknown, though it may be the result of poisoning by a metal such as aluminium, an *auto-immune response*, or, most probably, a virus. The disease passes through several stages, each of which has its own name. In progressive bulbar palsy, for example, the first symptom is difficulty in articulating words. The sufferer also finds it hard to swallow and becomes hoarse. In the case of amyotrophic lateral sclerosis, the first sign is some loss of control over the movement of the limbs. This gives way to weakness and wasting of the muscles of the hands and arms and progresses to the legs. The sufferer eventually becomes paralysed. In progressive muscular atrophy, a loss of control of the foot is usually the first symptom, followed by weakness and wasting of the hands and limbs. In both amyotrophic lateral sclerosis and progressive muscular atrophy, the symptoms of progressive bulbar palsy may appear in the later stages.

Motor neurone disease is incurable and death from *pneumonia* and respiratory failure usually occurs some two and 10 years from its onset, depending on the course taken by the disease. Treatment is largely supportive—the provision of wheelchairs and walking aids, for instance—though drugs are prescribed to relieve the cramps and aches that occur in the wasting muscles. In the final stages of the disease, constant nursing may be required, as the patient frequently loses the use of his or her limbs, the ability to speak distinctly and to swallow.

MULTIPLE MYELOMA

A progressive disease, also known as myeloma and myelomatosis, in which multiple *malignant tumours* affect the plasma cells in the bone marrow. It is rare in people under 30, but the incidence increases with age; the condition is more common in men than in women and most common in black-skinned men over 60.

Changes in the blood can usually be detected many years before any

Multiple Sclerosis Many nerve fibres in the brain and spinal cord are sheathed with a fatty substance called myelin. This sheath *(below)* protects the axons of the nerves and speeds up the impulses along them. In multiple sclerosis, the sheaths of many nerves degenerate in the white matter of the central nervous system. The main areas affected are the optic nerves, the spinal cord and around or near the ventricles of the brain. A technique called nuclear magnetic resonance (NMR) is able to detect some lesions around the ventricles of the brain in the dark areas *(right)*.

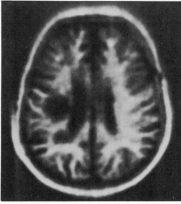

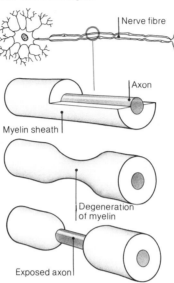

Nerve fibre

Axon

Myelin sheath

Degeneration of myelin

Exposed axon

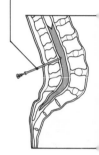

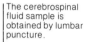

The insulating sheath of myelin *(left)* slowly degenerates, exposing the axon of the fibre and reducing the flow of impulses along it. As a result, muscles weaken and sensations are lost in some parts of the body. An analysis of the cerebrospinal fluid reveals a high gammaglobulin level. This is an important protein in the body's defence system.

The cerebrospinal fluid sample is obtained by lumbar puncture.

symptoms of multiple myeloma appear and are sometimes discovered in a blood test taken for another purpose. The disease eventually gives rise to a number of different symptoms. The first to appear are often either *anaemia*, internal bleeding and spontaneous fractures of the ribs, clavicle or pelvis, or *osteoporosis* of the spine and collapse of the vertebrae. Sometimes, however, the first symptom is an infection of the respiratory tract, or a kidney infection. As the tumour grows, the level of calcium in the blood increases. This causes nausea, vomiting, *dehydration, delirium*, lethargy, and, eventually, *kidney failure* and severe, exhausting pain in the bones.

The diagnosis of multiple myeloma is confirmed by means of blood tests and X-rays—*see Special Tests, p84*. The outlook is different for each individual. Some patients die soon after the onset of symptoms from kidney failure or infection. Others may survive for as long as 20 years, with or without treatment. This normally consists of *radiotherapy* and the use of *cytotoxic* drugs.

MULTIPLE SCLEROSIS

An incurable disease of the nervous system, in which the protective myelin sheaths that cover the nerves become inflamed and eventually

scarred—*see The Nervous System, p32*. The result is that the working of the nerves is affected, and this can lead to major disability. The symptoms of the disease vary, depending on which nerves are involved.

The causes of multiple sclerosis are unknown, though intensive research is being carried out in the attempt to discover them. It is thought, for instance, that the disease may be caused by a deficiency or abnormality of the fatty substance that makes up the myelin, a persistent viral infection, an *auto-immune disorder* or a combination of many factors. Multiple sclerosis is common in temperate climates— with an incidence rate of about one in 2,000—but very rare in tropical ones. This fact, too, may provide researchers with a clue as to the cause of the disease. It affects women twice as frequently as men and seems to be most prevalent among middle-income groups. Multiple sclerosis may occur more frequently among members of the same family than in the population as a whole, but there is no evidence to show that the disease is inherited.

Though the symptoms of the disease vary, its course is fixed in a pattern of relapses and periods of remission. The time spent in relapse and in remission varies: cases have been recorded in which people have stayed in remission for more than 20 years after the initial attack. Typically, the first attack occurs between the ages of 20 and 40. It is often difficult to diagnose, because symptoms are so variable, but characteristic signs include weakness of an arm or a leg, or pins and needles in a limb, and the disease should always be suspected when these complaints arise in young people. Because the optic nerves are frequently affected, there may be pain on moving the eyes and deterioration of sight, particularly in the centre of the field of vision. This can go hand in hand with double vision, or *diploplia*, and *nystagmus*. The optic disc becomes pale: this can be detected on examination with an ophthalmoscope, but is not always easy to spot.

Special tests to assess the speed at which the brain responds to various visual stimuli or sounds may help in diagnosis—*see Special Tests, p84*— while a sample of cerebrospinal fluid (*p32*), obtained by a lumbar puncture (*p84*), may also show the characteristic abnormalities associated with the disease. Other common features are *ataxia*, or poor balance, and *vertigo*, or spells of giddiness. Less common symptoms are *epilepsy*, facial *palsy*, facial pain and *hemiplegia*, or paralysis of one side of the body.

Sufferers usually recover completely within a few months of the initial attack, but inevitably there is a later recurrence. This is again followed by a further period of remission in the majority of cases, and then by another attack. The cycle repeats itself, the degree of improvement after each attack gradually diminishing over the years.

Occasionally, there is no remission and each relapse is followed by steadily increasing neurological deterioration and disability. About 50% of victims eventually lose the use of their lower limbs, becoming totally crippled; however, the other 50% are much less severely affected and may stay in almost permanent remission. Severely affected people may also find it difficult to speak clearly, suffer from muscular tremors and have bladder problems, finding it necessary to urinate frequently and being prone to urinary infections, or, conversely, becoming constipated. Fatigue is a universal symptom, and sufferers should 'give in' to this and make sure of adequate rest and sleep, and not push themselves, explaining to others that this fatigue is part of the illness. The majority of sufferers find that their symptoms become worse in hot weather, and that limb problems are exacerbated by hot baths.

Because the disease is incurable and can be progressively crippling, depression is a frequent psychological side-effect amongst all sufferers, though they may also experience bouts of euphoria for no known reason. There is usually no impairment of mental faculties until very late in the course of the disease.

Various treatments can be given to relieve symptoms and prolong the periods of remission. *Corticosteroids* are often used to treat an acute attack. However, these have troublesome side-effects, while there is no hard and fast evidence that prolonged courses of these powerful drugs give anything but temporary relief. Anti-spasticity drugs may be given to treat the limbs, while *physiotherapy* can help strengthen the muscles.

In addition to these established forms of treatment, considerable research is being directed towards discovering further therapies, two of which have shown promising initial results. The first of these, under trial in the USA, involves the stimulation of the body's immune system (*p52*) with snake venom injections, called PROven. *Interferon* can also be used. The second involves the addition of certain fatty acids to the diet, since it is known that the levels of such acids are lower in multiple sclerosis victims than in people in good health. These fatty acids are found in sunflower, safflower and evening primrose oils. Other recommendations include exclusion of gluten from the diet. However, there is no evidence to show that multiple sclerosis is caused by an allergy to gluten.

Because the course of the disease can vary so widely, it is difficult to assess the success rate of any therapy. Only a limited number of people are crippled; though many are left with minor disabilities, these do not prevent them leading near-

normal lives. Good signs include complete recovery after attacks and a long gap between the first attack and the subsequent relapse. Bad signs include a very early onset of the disease, poor recovery from its attacks and premature muscular disability. Men tend to be more at risk from the most severe effects of the disease than women.

The most important thing multiple sclerosis victims can do to help themselves is to try to come to terms with the disease and the limitations it may necessarily impose. The support and encouragement shown by doctors, nurses and family can be vital in achieving this.

MUMPS

An infectious disease, caused by a *virus*, that is spread by droplets released into the air when an infected person coughs or sneezes. People of any age or either sex can contract mumps, but children are most commonly affected.

The *incubation period* is between two and three weeks. After this the symptoms appear: they include swelling of the parotid glands on one or both sides of the face, *fever*, pain in the muscles of the jaw, ear and abdomen, and swelling of other glands. Vomiting is common, as the virus may also affect the pancreas, causing mild *pancreatitis*. One in four men who contract mumps after puberty also develop *orchitis*, a painful inflammation of the testicles that can sometimes lead to sterility.

Most cases of mumps are extremely mild, and so the disease is correspondingly difficult to diagnose. In cases of doubt, its presence can be confirmed by a blood test. Once a diagnosis of mumps has been confirmed, however, the patient is normally isolated, to prevent the spread of the infection, and confined to the house

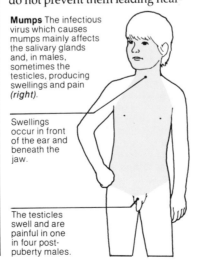

Mumps The infectious virus which causes mumps mainly affects the salivary glands and, in males, sometimes the testicles, producing swellings and pain *(right)*.

Swellings occur in front of the ear and beneath the jaw.

The testicles swell and are painful in one in four post-puberty males.

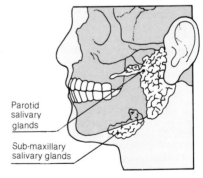

Parotid salivary glands

Sub-maxillary salivary glands

Pain in the jaws and ears are the main symptoms of mumps, because the virus infects the parotid and sub-maxillary salivary glands *(above)*. The parotid gland lies in front of and below the ear, while the sub-maxillary gland lies in front of the parotid and secretes its saliva below the tongue.

until the swollen glands have subsided—*see Home Nursing, p352*. Special treatment, other than for orchitis, is rarely necessary. Any pain or discomfort can usually be relieved with mild painkillers or sedatives. Staying in bed for at least 12 days seems to reduce the risk of orchitis developing.

Very rarely, sufferers from mumps develop serious complications. These may include *pancreatitis*, *meningitis* and *meningo-encephalitis*, *deafness*, facial *palsy*, *arthritis*, *rheumatic fever* and *thrombocytopenic purpura*. However, unlike the case of German measles— *see rubella*—there is usually no effect on the foetus when a pregnant woman contracts mumps.

A person who has had mumps is normally immune to the disease for life, though re-infection is possible in some cases. Vaccination is also available against the disease, though this is not routinely recommended. The effective life of the vaccine is five years, after which a booster must be given.

MUSCULAR DYSTROPHY
A group of serious, inherited disorders in which the muscles waste away.

The most common type of muscular dystrophy is called Duchenne dystrophy. This principally affects male children, because the *gene* carrying the disease is linked to the male X chromosome. Initially, the disease causes weakness of the pelvis and lower limbs, which spreads to the shoulders as the condition progresses. Duchenne dystrophy is suspected if a young child walks with a waddling gait and stands up by rolling on to his face, using the arms to lever himself up. Affected children gradually become more disabled, as the muscles shrink and become shortened. Death usually occurs between the ages of 10 and 20, either from infection of the respiratory tract or extreme weakness.

A second type of muscular dystrophy, called limb girdle dystrophy, affects both sexes and usually first appears in young adults in their 20s or 30s. The initial symptom is a weakness in either the pelvis or shoulder girdle; later this spreads to involve both areas. Limb girdle dystrophy usually progresses very slowly, but within 20 years the sufferer is often severely disabled and rarely survives into old age.

Facio-scapulo-humeral dystrophy can appear at any age, and may affect several children of the same family. It first attacks the muscles of the face and gradually spreads to the shoulder and pelvic girdles. This type of dystrophy progresses slowly, and periods of remission often delay the onset of serious disabilities. As a result, the life expectancy is much greater than that for other forms of dystrophy.

There is no cure for any of these three forms of muscular dystrophy, although the deformities caused by wasting and muscle shrinkage can now be prevented and counteracted to an extent by physiotherapy and orthopaedic techniques.

MYALGIC ENCEPHALOMYELITIS (ME)
A name applied to a particular syndrome, or group of symptoms, of unknown cause. Even its origins are mysterious. What may or may not have been the same disorder was first described in the 1950s, following an outbreak of a mysterious disease at the Royal Free Hospital in London; it was therefore called Royal Free Disease. The term Postviral Fatigue Syndrome has also been applied to more or less the same clinical picture. This confusion about what to call the condition reflects the considerable uncertainty that exists about ME.

A typical way for ME to begin is with a sore throat, running nose, and enlarged nodes (glands) in the neck. Most people would describe these symptoms as flu and, indeed, they are practically identical. In addition, there may be diarrhoea and vomiting, or sometimes giddiness and a fast pulse rate. At this stage, some sufferers complain of headaches and blurred and double vision. However, the worst symptom is usually severe muscular weakness, together with a feeling of intense physical and mental distress.

As time passes, both physical and mental debility persist, though they may vary in intensity from day to day, or even within the same 24-hour time span. Some patients are so badly affected that they become bed-ridden; if they get up, they may find that even the smallest household chore is too much for them, while going to work is out of the question. The muscles may be actually tender to the touch.

Memory is often affected. The ability to concentrate is impaired or lost, and patients may be more emotional than usual, being liable to bouts of crying, or outbursts of anger at things that would normally seem trivial. Sleep patterns may be disrupted. Other symptoms include cold hands and feet, extreme sensitivity to changes in temperature and weather, bouts of sweating, and palpitations. The patient may have to pass urine more frequently than normal.

As the months pass, these symptoms may diminish in intensity although without completely disappearing; patients can go back to work, but find that they are exhausted at the end of the day and have no energy for anything else. This may persist for months, or even years. A few more severely affected patients do not recover even to this limited extent, and have to spend most of their time in bed.

There is no agreement about what causes ME. At one extreme, some doctors regard it as a wholly psychological disorder, while others are convinced that it is due to a preceding viral infection. Probably there is some truth in both views. Some doctors believe that ME is caused by *hyperventilation*, but although this is certainly part of the clinical picture in a number of cases, the two disorders are probably not identical. It is likely that there is no single cause for ME; instead, it seems to be a group of symptoms that can be brought about in a number of different ways.

Treatment of ME is inevitably unsatisfactory, in view of the uncertainty about what causes it. Doctors who believe it is due to depression may prescribe antidepressant drugs, which help some patients. If, on the other hand, it is thought to be the result of a previous or persisting viral infection, there is little positive therapy that can be prescribed. This frustrates many doctors and can breed resentment in patients, who feel that no one has adequately recognized the seriousness of their condition.

MYELOMATOSIS—see Multiple myeloma

MYOCARDIAL INFARCTION
The death of an area of heart muscle occurring when the blood supply to that part of the heart is inadequate. A myocardial infarction is commonly called a heart attack, and is probably the most common cause of emergency admission to hospital. The amount of damage to the heart muscle varies widely; it can range from superficial damage, involving practically no pain or disability at one extreme to the destruction of large areas of heart muscle and sudden death at the other. Myocardial infarction may occur at any age but is rare under 30. Men used to be affected much more frequently than women, but this statistic is changing, since so many women now smoke cigarettes, a prime factor in the potential causes of the problem.

In a heart attack one of the three

Myocardial Infarction The muscles of the heart are supplied with blood by the two coronary arteries *(right)*. When one of the arteries, or one of their branches, is obstructed by a blood clot or thrombus, part of the muscle is deprived of blood. The result is a heart attack — what doctors call myocardial infarction or coronary thrombosis. The thrombus is more likely to form if an atheroma or plaque of fatty tissue builds up along the inner wall of the artery.

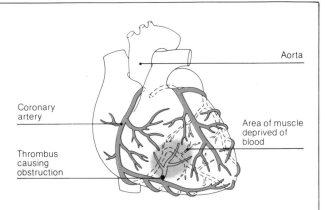

Aorta

Coronary artery

Thrombus causing obstruction

Area of muscle deprived of blood

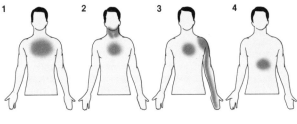

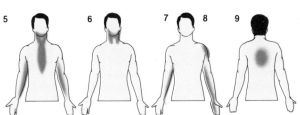

The pain caused by a heart attack can be very severe. The characteristic feelings of tightness and constriction can be felt in various parts of the body *(left)*. Pain can be localized in the breastbone or felt over the entire upper chest, **1**. It can be localized in the mid-chest, neck and jaw, **2**, or felt in the mid-chest, the left shoulder and along the inside of the arms, particularly the left arm, **3**. It can occur in the upper abdomen, **4**, and in the central chest region, in the neck, jaw and along the inside of both arms, **5**. The pain can spread from the centre of the lower neck to both sides of the upper neck and along the jaw from ear to ear, **6**, from the inside of the right arm to below the elbow, **7**, from the left shoulder and along the inside of the left arm to the hand, **8**. It can also be localized in the back between the shoulder blades, **9**.

main coronary arteries *(p21)* usually becomes occluded or blocked by atheroma, a fatty substance that is laid down in arteries, so narrowing them considerably and obstructing or cutting off the blood supply to the heart muscle. A blood clot, called a *thrombus*, may form around the atheroma. This is called a coronary thrombosis, a term also used to describe a heart attack.

The condition causing the build-up of fat in the coronary arteries is called *coronary artery disease*. Cigarette-smoking, high blood pressure, diabetes and abnormally high levels of fat in the blood all contribute to this. Coronary artery disease also causes a severe chest pain, called *angina pectoris*. Most victims experience this pain in the weeks prior to the attack. This is not always the case, however; a myocardial infarction can just as easily occur without warning.

Excruciating chest pain is the most common feature of a heart attack. The pain is central in position and constricting in character, and is accompanied by sweating and pallor. The victim may also show signs of shortness of breath and nausea. If a sizeable portion of the left ventricle is affected the blood pressure may fall, since the heart is unable to pump efficiently. The result may be collapse and loss of consciousness.

The blood pressure may also be affected by changes in the normal heart rhythm. Such changes are termed *arrythmias*. The most serious of these is ventricular *fibrillation*, a condition in which the heart muscles contract individually, without co-ordination, so reducing the ability of the heart to pump blood. No pulse can be felt at the radial site in the arm, or at the carotid site in the neck; the person loses consciousness and may die if the correct rhythm is not restored immediately. Sometimes this can be achieved in an emergency by a sharp blow to the chest over the breast bone—*see First Aid, p369*—but more often *defibrillation* is required. This involves giving the heart a short, sharp electric shock, using a defibrillating machine that delivers the current through two electrodes placed on the chest wall. Defibrillators are standard equipment in all casualty departments and intensive care units, and thus anyone who is unconsciousness and whose pulse is undetectable should be transferred to hospital immediately. Meanwhile, his or her life may be saved by cardiac massage and mouth-to-mouth respiration—*see First Aid, p369*.

Ventricular fibrillation is thought to account for the majority of deaths immediately after an attack. Other arrhythmias, including *heart block* and atrial fibrillation may also occur as a consequence of an infarct. These may also threaten life by causing low blood pressure and consequent *heart failure*. They are the chief reason for admission to specialized coronary care units, where heart rate and rhythm is continuously monitored by highly trained staff.

Hospital procedure in the case of a myocardial infarct or suspected infarct is routine. The victim is examined carefully, and given powerful painkillers directly into a vein, by means of a *drip*, to stop the dreadful pain and help relieve anxiety. An ECG—*see Special Tests, p84*—is carried out to confirm the suspected diagnosis, together with a chest X-ray to show the size of the heart and whether there is any fluid in the lungs, a condition called *pulmonary oedema*, due to failure of the left ventricle. Blood samples are taken to measure the level of enzymes released by the damaged heart muscle. Oxygen may be given if necessary and a drip is set up to provide a quick way of giving drugs.

This entire procedure is often carried out in a casualty department. The patient is then transferred to the coronary care unit, where he or she is attached to a heart monitor and may have a urinary catheter inserted into the bladder. Should the pain recur it is treated promptly with intravenous injections of morphine; other drugs may be prescribed to control any arrhythmias. Further drugs may also be given to treat low blood pressure and any pulmonary oedema.

The outlook for the patient depends very much upon the extent of the damage. Generally speaking, the prognosis improves dramatically after the person has survived for 24 hours, since it is during this period that three quarters of patients die, half of them in the first two hours alone.

The first couple of days of recovery are spent in bed in the coronary care unit and the next week or so sitting up in a chair, often in a conventional medical ward. Patients without complications are usually discharged on or about the tenth day after the attack. Thereafter the road back to full activity is slow and gentle. The heart muscle takes from 4-6 weeks to heal properly, so no strenuous exertion should be undertaken during this time. The victim can return to work from about two or three months after the initial attack. Long-term drug therapy may be prescribed to treat high blood pressure—*see hypertension*—or to reduce the risk of further myocardial infarction.

After discharge from hospital, the patient is usually advised to take light exercise, such as walking. Over the next few months or so, he or she should gradually build up to more strenuous exercise, taking care not to overdo things—*see Exercise, p316*. Full sexual activity can be resumed at this stage.

MYOMECTOMY

An operation to remove a *fibroid*, a benign growth in the muscle fibres in the wall of the uterus. Sometimes fibroids are treated by the removal of the whole womb in an operation called a *hysterectomy*. However, if the patient wishes to have more children, a myomectomy may be performed instead. In this case only the affected tissue is removed.

MYOPIA

The medical term for short-sightedness. The condition tends to run in families, usually developing during late adolescence and stabilizing by adulthood.

Myopia occurs when the lens of the eye is more convex than usual or when the axis of the eyeball is elongated. These defects cause the rays of light that enter the eye through the pupil to focus before they strike the retina *(p32)*. The lens is unable to adjust sufficiently to project light reflected by objects more than six metres (about 20 feet) away directly on to the retina. As a result, a person with short sight receives a blurred image of much of the visual field.

Myopia is easily corrected by spectacles with slightly concave lenses. The condition is unlikely to deteriorate, but, as a precaution, people with short sight should have their eyes tested by an optician every few years—*see Special Tests, p84*.

MYOSITIS

A group of diseases in which the muscles become inflamed. Myositis may develop as a result of the spread of a *bacterial* or *viral* infection in the neighbouring tissues, but can also be a symptom of disorders affecting the whole body.

There are three main types of myositis. Polymyositis, the most common type, usually affects people between the ages of 30 and 50, and occurs most frequently in women. It is associated with the group of diseases of connective tissue *(p16)* known as the *collagen-vascular disorders*. The first symptom of polymyositis may be difficulty in climbing stairs or rising from a sitting position. From this, the disease often progresses rapidly to severe weakness of the muscles of the pharynx and of the larynx *(p28)* and the respiratory muscles. This makes it difficult to speak and swallow, while respiratory failure can also occur. There is often a spontaneous remission of the disease, but in many sufferers the muscles eventually shorten, shrink and lose substance, causing *arthritis*.

Dermatomyositis, another form of myositis, is most common in women. It causes extreme weakness and pain in the muscles, generalized *oedema* and a rash on the upper eyelids. As the condition progresses, the sufferer loses weight and usually the rash spreads down the chest and along the limbs.

Inflammatory myositis occurs in people over the age of 40, most commonly in men. Symptoms similar to those of polymyositis and dermatomyositis develop gradually in association with a malignant growth. This may not become evident for two or three years and is usually a *cancer* of the bronchus, prostate, ovary, uterus, breast or colon. If the growth is surgically removed the myositis often disappears.

The symptoms of myositis are treated by dosages of *corticosteroid* drugs to induce a remission of the diseases, or with *immunosuppressive* drugs if steroids have no effect. The patient is advised to rest in bed, to avoid fatigue and cold, and to take frequent hot baths to relieve any pain and stiffness in the muscles. Splinting and physiotherapy may help to prevent the muscles from becoming deformed.

The younger the age at which symptoms first appear, the more likely it is that treatment will be successful in inducing long-term remission. Without treatment, however, the various forms of myositis are likely to progress to a chronic stage and in some patients to severe disability and death.

MYRINGOTOMY

A surgical operation carried out on patients with *otitis media*, an inflammation of the middle ear. In a myringotomy, an incision is made in the ear drum to enable fluid to drain out, thus relieving the pressure caused by the inflammation.

MYXOEDEMA

A disease caused by hypothyroidism, an underactivity of the thyroid gland, and a subsequent lack of thyroxine, the hormone that controls the rate of metabolism — *see The Endocrine System, p48*. Myxoedema affects mainly teenagers and adults, and is more common in women than men. The cause of the disease is unknown, although it is thought to involve an *auto-immune response* in a number of cases, and may follow the surgical removal of the thyroid gland. This operation is often performed in the treatment of *thyrotoxicosis*.

The first symptoms include tiredness, aches and pains, forgetfulness, sensitivity to cold, poor hearing, dryness of the hair and skin, constipation, weight gain and, in women, irregular periods.

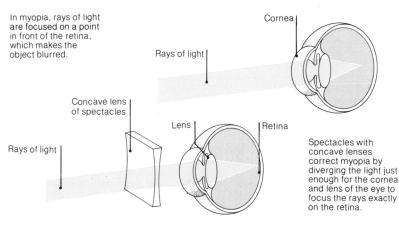

In myopia, rays of light are focused on a point in front of the retina, which makes the object blurred.

Cornea

Rays of light

Concave lens of spectacles

Lens | Retina

Rays of light

Spectacles with concave lenses correct myopia by diverging the light just enough for the cornea and lens of the eye to focus the rays exactly on the retina.

Myopia is a visual defect, in which sufferers cannot focus properly on objects more than about six metres away from them. This is because rays of light focus in front of the retina *(top)*, rather than on it, either because the eyeball is too long or because the focusing power of the cornea and lens is too strong. The defect can be corrected by wearing spectacles with concave lenses which focus exactly on the retina *(below)*.

Children may become apathetic, and their physical growth and intellectual progress may slow down.

As the disease progresses there may be tingling in the fingers and *anaemia*, and the face starts to look swollen, with puffy eyelids, lips and tongue. The skin of the body takes on a yellow tinge and flakes on rubbing, but the cheeks may be flushed. Both features and hair coarsen and speech becomes slow. Adults with severe hypothyroidism may show signs of *psychosis*, while affected infants may develop *cretinism*. If the condition is untreated the body's heat-regulating mechanism eventually fails and the sufferer develops *hypothermia* and sinks into a *coma*.

On examining a patient with myxoedema, a doctor will notice that the pulse is slow, as are the reflexes (*p32*), and the heart may be enlarged. Myxoedema is easily treated with tablets containing replacement thyroxine, which must be taken for life.

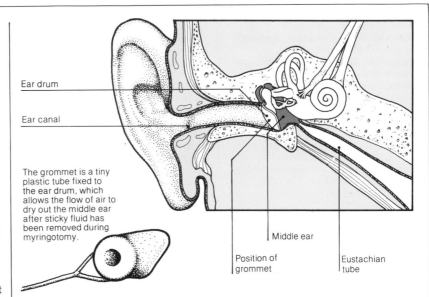

Ear drum

Ear canal

The grommet is a tiny plastic tube fixed to the ear drum, which allows the flow of air to dry out the middle ear after sticky fluid has been removed during myringotomy.

Middle ear

Position of grommet

Eustachian tube

Myringotomy Children who suffer from repeated attacks of otitis media may develop glue ear, in which the middle ear and Eustachian tube are blocked by a sticky fluid. Both conditions are usually treated by an operation called a myringotomy. Using a myringotomy knife, the surgeon makes a small incision in the ear drum and inserts a tiny syringe to draw out the fluid and then wash the middle ear. A minute plastic tube called a grommet is passed through the incision to allow air to dry out the middle ear. When the grommet is removed after several months, the ear drum heals of its own accord.

N

NAEVUS

A birthmark, or patch of discoloured skin, either present at birth or appearing soon afterwards. There are several types of naevus; some gradually disappear, while others remain for life.

The marks fall into two categories: vascular naevi and pigmented naevi. The former, sometimes called haemangiomas, are caused by the abnormal development of tiny blood vessels in the skin and can be either temporary or permanent. Pigmented naevi are caused by the abnormal development of the cells that produce skin pigment, or melanin. They appear either as light brown patches of skin or as moles, and are usually permanent.

The strawberry mark is one of the most common of the temporary vascular birthmarks. It is a bright red, slightly raised mark, usually no more than 4cm (1.5in) across. It often becomes larger as the child grows, before becoming patchy and eventually disappearing. A capillary naevus, sometimes called a 'stork's

bite' mark, is another common type of temporary birthmark. It is a pink or brownish area that nearly always fades and disappears within eighteen months.

The commonest permanent type of vascular naevus is a port-wine stain. This is a reddish or purple mark, covering a fairly extensive area on the scalp, face or neck. The mark may fade slightly as the child grows older, but rarely completely disappears.

If a permanent birthmark is unsightly, it can be covered with special cream, or removed by plastic surgery or *laser* therapy. Removal of a port-wine stain, however, usually leaves scar tissue that is sometimes as disfiguring as the mark itself.

Generally, birthmarks have no medical significance. The only exception is when a mole begins to grow, changes colour, becomes sore or itchy, or bleeds. These may be early signs of a *melanoma*, or skin tumour, which requires immediate treatment.

See also telangiectasis.

NAPPY RASH

A rash on a baby's buttocks, thighs and genitals. It can be caused by the ammonia content of the urine, bacteria in the faeces, or a soap or detergent residue that has been allowed to impregnate the nappies. It also occurs if nappies are not changed frequently, and it can be aggravated by waterproof pants. The affected area is moist and sore, with a red, spotty rash, and sometimes small, shallow ulcers. If the rash is caused by urine, there may also be a strong smell of ammonia.

Nappy rash is not a serious medical problem, although a boy's foreskin may become inflamed, causing pain and difficulty in passing urine. The affected area should be bathed with clean warm water, dried with a soft towel, and sprinkled lightly with talcum powder. Soothing cream should also be applied. The longer the area can be exposed to warm, dry air, the better. Prompt action is important, because, after about 24 hours, nappy rash becomes infected with thrush—*see candidiasis*—in which case an antifungal cream will be needed.

To avoid the problem, nappies should always be washed in detergent and rinsed well, and disposable nappies should be discarded after a short period of use. Sometimes a final rinse in a weak vinegar solution is helpful—about a tablespoon of vinegar to 4.5 litres (one gallon) of water. The baby should be changed frequently and plastic pants should not be used until the rash disappears.

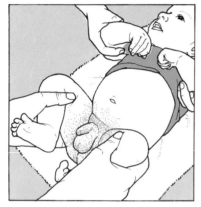

Nappy rash If a baby's nappies irritate and inflame the skin around the thighs, buttocks and groin, a rash will result. The irritation is exacerbated by the ammonia produced when faeces and urine react chemically together. The sore, moist skin may be treated with a zinc-based, soothing cream.

NARCOLEPSY
A disorder in which sufferers suddenly fall asleep without warning, but can easily be awakened.

Narcolepsy is associated with two other conditions: cataplexy, in which power is suddenly lost from the limbs while the person is wide awake; and sleep paralysis, in which the person is also awake, but unable to move. As with these conditions, narcolepsy usually has no apparent cause. There is usually no detectable abnormality in the nervous system, though occasionally the condition is associated with disease in the hypothalamic region of the brain (*p32*). In children, it may follow an attack of *encephalitis*.

The effects of a narcoleptic attack are temporary, but attacks tend to recur. The only area of risk stems from the sufferer's inability to predict when and where an attack will recur. For this reason, those suffering from narcolepsy should not drive. Drugs of the *amphetamine* group can be used to lessen the frequency of the attacks.

NARCOTICS
Any drug that produces narcosis, or dulling of the consciousness. The term is often used specifically to describe the drugs also known as *opiates*. These include opium and all its derivatives, which range from morphine, heroin and the artificial narcotics, pethidine and methadone—used in hospitals as part of anaesthesia—to codeine.

All narcotics relieve pain, induce sedation and impair mental awareness to a greater or lesser extent. Codeine, for instance, is much less addictive than other opiates, and is recognized as an extremely effective way of suppressing headaches and migraines. However, even codeine can become physically addictive—that is, after repeated dosages, most people who take them will suffer from pain and withdrawal symptoms if the regular dosage is not maintained. In cases of overdose or long-term regular use, all narcotics suppress the brain's control over vital functions, such as breathing. For this reason, their use should be carefully controlled.

NAUSEA
A feeling of sickness or queasiness, often accompanied by faintness and dizziness and followed by *vomiting*. It is frequently the result of stomach irritation, while it can also be a feature of early pregnancy—*see hyperemesis gravidarum*—and of *migraine*. Psychological causes include disgusting sights or smells. The act of vomiting usually relieves the pain.

Nausea can be controlled by the use of *antiemetic* drugs.

NEONATE
A new-born baby. Babies are referred to as neonates for the first four weeks of life.

NEOPLASM
A term meaning 'a new growth', that is applied to any type of *tumour*, whether it is benign or *malignant*. *See cancer.*

NEPHRECTOMY
The surgical removal of a kidney. A nephrectomy may become necessary in a variety of conditions—*see kidney disease.*

NEPHRITIS
A general term for an inflammation of the kidneys—*see glomerulonephritis; pyelonephritis.*

NEPHROSIS—see Nephrotic syndrome

NEPHROSTOMY
A surgical procedure in which a *catheter*, or plastic tube, is passed into a kidney through the skin in order to drain urine from it. A nephrostomy is often used as a temporary measure after an operation involving the kidney.

NEPHROTIC SYNDROME
A collection of symptoms caused by damage to the glomeruli (*p40*), the systems of tiny vessels inside the kidney in which blood is filtered. Any damage to the structure of the kidney is known as nephrosis; as a result, this term is sometimes used as an alternative to nephrotic syndrome.

In the first instance, the disruption to the filtering function of the glomeruli causes *proteinuria*, a loss of large quantities of protein in the urine. This disturbs the balance of *electrolytes* in the body. As a result, body fluids build up in the tissues, causing *oedema*. The outward signs are swelling and puffiness, especially of the face.

In around 80% of cases, the damage to the glomeruli is the result of *glomerulonephritis*. In such cases, the damage is not usually permanent, and after treatment most sufferers recover completely. However, the glomeruli may also be damaged by a number of other problems. These include: *malaria; diabetes; lupus erythematosus; amyloid disease; thrombosis* of the renal vein; poisoning with mercury; and large dosages of troxidone, a drug previously used in the treatment of *epilepsy*. In such cases, the damage is sometimes permanent and leads to *kidney failure*.

Treatment of the symptoms of nephrotic syndrome depends on the root cause of the problem. *Steroids* may be prescribed to suppress any immunological reaction that is contributing to the glomerulonephritis, as well as *antibiotics* to combat any infection. The electrolyte balance is restored by restricting the amount of salt and water in the diet and by giving *diuretics* to stimulate the excretion of excess fluid. Bed rest is usually necessary, together with a high-protein diet to restore the lost nutrients.

NERVE BLOCK
An interruption to the flow of impulses along nerve fibres, resulting in a loss of feeling in the affected region, and often accompanied by *paraesthesiae*, or 'pins and needles'.

Nerve block can be caused by cold, lack of oxygen, pressure or, less commonly, by a disorder affecting the nerves, such as *multiple sclerosis*. Pressure applied on the arm, for instance, may cause the hand to 'go to sleep'. The nerve fibres recover when the cause is removed, but nerve cell bodies in the central nervous system can be destroyed by pressure. However, this is rarely serious, unless excessive pressure continues for a long time.

A nerve block may also be induced by the injection of a local *anaesthetic*. This is often done before a minor surgical operation. Before a fractured bone is set, for example, the nerves supplying the affected area of bone may be blocked by an injection of anaesthetic to eliminate any pain.

NEURALGIA

A term often used generally to describe a pain originating in a nerve. The pain is usually intense and spasmodic; it may occur as a result of infection or damage to the nerve cells, or for no apparent reason.

Neuralgia is most commonly the result of an inflammation of a nerve. In this case the problem normally clears up on its own within a short time, and painkillers are the only treatment required. Occasionally, however, neuralgia is caused by other conditions, which may require treatment. These include *trigeminal neuralgia*, in which the facial nerve is affected; *sciatica*, in which spinal nerves are trapped between vertebrae; post-herpetic neuralgia, when *herpes zoster*, the virus that causes shingles, is responsible for pain at the site of a previous attack; and migrainous neuralgia—*see migraine*.

NEURITIS

An inflammation of a nerve. Neuritis is a vague term, often used as an alternative to *neuropathy*. Sometimes, however, it is used to denote an inflammation of a specific nerve, as in the case of optic neuritis.

In this condition, inflammation of the optic nerve *(p32)* causes pain in the eye, especially if moved. There is often a degree of visual disturbance, including blurred vision and sometimes images in the centre of the field of vision cannot be seen.

When the head of the optic nerve is involved, the condition is termed *papillitis*. In this case, the optic disc appears pale on examination with an ophthalmoscope—*see Special Tests, p84*. When the affected area lies behind the optic nerve, the disc appears normal and the condition is called retrobulbar neuritis.

Optic neuritis may be caused by a variety of conditions. These include: *multiple sclerosis*; *syphilis*; chemical poisoning; vitamin deficiencies—in particular, a deficiency of vitamin B12, *(p321)*; or raised intracranial pressure, normally the result of *hypertension* or a brain tumour. On such occasions, the condition is treated according to its cause. Sometimes, however, optic neuritis is caused by a small lesion in the nerve. In this case, the condition normally clears up spontaneously, and complete normal vision is restored.

NEUROFIBROMA—see Neuroma

NEUROFIBROMATOSIS

Also known as von Recklinghausen's disease, neurofibromatosis is a rare hereditary condition in which lumpy swellings develop in the tissue that surrounds nerves. Benign, or harmless, *tumours*, may also grow inside the bones, causing deformities and a pronounced curvature of the spine. Characteristically, tan-coloured blotches, known as 'café-au-lait spots', appear on the skin. These may be the size of a pin-head or of a large coin.

The disease progresses slowly, throughout the life of the sufferer, with the appearance of new tumours and the further growth of those that already exist. In severe cases, the deformities caused by neurofibromatosis are grotesque— the most well-known example being George Merrick, a 19th-century sufferer, who became famous as 'the Elephant Man'.

There is no treatment for the disease, other than surgery to attempt to correct disfiguring deformities. Occasionally, a tumour may show *malignant* changes, or impinge upon a nerve, in which case it is removed by surgery.

NEUROMA

A benign *tumour* that develops in the fibrous sheath covering a nerve; such a tumour may also be called a neurofibroma or a neurinoma.

Neuromas may affect any nerve in the body, and generally cause no symptoms. Occasionally, however, they may impinge on a nerve, disrupting its function and causing *neuralgia*. In such cases, neuromas are removed by surgery.

The most common example of this is when a neuroma compresses one of the eight cranial nerves in the brain *(p32)* which supply the ears. This condition is known as an acoustic neuroma. The first symptoms are *tinnitus*, or ringing in the ears, together with *vertigo*. Eventually, the tumour may cause deafness, and, if not removed by surgery, may cause pressure on other areas of the brain, with serious consequences.

NEUROPATHY

A general term used to describe any disruption of the structure or function of either a single nerve or all the nerves of the body. Neuropathy has a variety of causes.

When only one nerve is involved, the condition is termed mononeuropathy. The symptoms are confined to the area supplied by the affected nerve, and may include loss of sensation, reduction in muscular power and *paraesthesiae*, or pins and needles, in the skin. The most common cause of mononeuropathy is an injury; depending on the seriousness of the injury, the nerve may recover its function, with the help of *physiotherapy*, or may be permanently damaged. Another common cause of mononeuropathy is the compression of a nerve by pressure, either from the enlargement of a neighbouring organ or tissue, or a tumour—*see neuroma*. A good example is *carpal tunnel syndrome*, in which compression of the median nerve as it passes through the wrist eventually leads to loss of function in the thumb and first two fingers.

When a large number of nerves is involved, the condition is called polyneuropathy. Symptoms are often felt first in the hands and feet—doctors call this the 'glove and stocking' distribution. Initially, they may take the form of pins and needles and a loss of sensation, a condition known as peripheral neuropathy. The reflexes *(p32)* may be affected, and as the condition progresses, the muscles may begin to waste away, eventually leading to paralysis of the limbs. Some forms of neuropathy primarily affect the autonomic nervous system *(p32)*. When this is the case there may be *impotence, diarrhoea*, sweating, and problems with urination.

Polyneuropathy may be caused by a number of conditions, and is treated accordingly. They include: *vitamin deficiencies*—especially those of the vitamin B complex; poisons, such as lead, mercury and arsenic; *diabetes mellitus; liver diseases; leprosy;* certain *cancers; diphtheria;* connective tissue disorders *(p16)*, notably *rheumatoid arthritis* and *lupus erythematosus;* and, on rare occasions, certain drugs, such as *anticonvulsants. Alcoholism* is a common cause of polyneuropathy, because sufferers are often both deficient in vitamin B and affected by diseases of the liver. In this case, the neuropathy is called alcoholic neuropathy.

A specific form of neuropathy, called acute post-infective polyneuropathy, or Guillain-Barré syndrome, sometimes follows a viral infection. At first, there may be tingling in the limbs and muscular weakness. This rapidly progresses to paralysis, sometimes involving the facial muscles and the muscles of respiration *(p28)*. The condition is extremely serious. Sufferers require immediate treatment, and the use of an artificial *ventilator* to maintain breathing. If treatment is prompt, the majority of patients recover completely within two months, but about 5% die during the acute stage, and another 5% are left with a degree of paralysis.

NEUROSIS

A mental disorder that renders people exceptionally vulnerable to mental or emotional distress. It is often difficult to decide where normal behaviour ends and neurosis begins; one school of psychology states that, to a greater or lesser degree, we are all neurotic, and that there is no such thing as 'normal'. Certainly mild neuroses, such as depressions, obsessions and phobias are common.

In neurotic illness, unpleasant experiences or feelings tend to be more intense and of longer duration than usual. The neurotic not only worries excessively, but is aware of the fact, without being able to do anything about it.

The disease typically manifests itself in one of several ways. A person suffering from an obsessive neurosis may feel the need to repeat certain actions while being aware that this is unnecessary—to wash constantly, for example, or to check and recheck at night that the lights have been turned off. In a phobic neurosis, there is an irrational phobia, or fear, such as that of spiders, of heights, or of flying. People with an anxiety neurosis worry constantly about the possibility—but not the certainty—that a difficult or unpleasant situation will arise. In a depressive neurosis, an individual becomes unhappy to the point of depression, as a result of difficulties at work, for example, or problematic personal relationships.

Some neurotics are not unhappy; they are aware of their tendencies and can cope with them. A neurotic may need treatment when his or her condition becomes cyclic, or self-fulfilling: if someone worries about the risk of becoming unemployed to the extent that his or her performance at work suffers, he or she is more likely to find the worry fulfilled. Neurotics who cannot cope with their anxieties or fears may eventually be subject to severe *depression*, a debilitating and even dangerous illness.

Neurotics can be treated with drugs—*tranquillizers* or *antidepressants*—and with counselling and *behaviour therapy*.

NIEMANN-PICK DISEASE—see Lipid storage diseases

NIGHT SWEATS

Profuse sweating at night when there is no obvious cause, such as too many bedclothes. Night sweats may be a symptom of a *fever*, such as that caused by *malaria* or a *viral* infection, or of *depression*. They are also a common, and harmless, feature of the *menopause*. However, if there is no fever, night sweats may be an indication of a serious disease. Most commonly, this is *tuberculosis*, but the problem also occurs in cases of *Hodgkin's disease* and *leukaemia*.

NITROUS OXIDE

A general anaesthetic, often known as laughing gas. Pioneered in 1844 by Horace Wells, an American dentist, nitrous oxide was one of the first general anaesthetics to be used.

Today, nitrous oxide is often given in small dosages to give relief from pain during the first stage of labour *(p60)*. For this purpose it is combined with oxygen and is referred to as 'gas and air', or entonox.

NOCTURIA

Urinating at night. In most people, urine builds up in the bladder during the night because the sensory signals *(p32)* that inform the brain of the increasing quantities of urine stored are suppressed. Unless the build-up is excessive, it is ignored until the person wakes up in the morning.

In adults suffering from nocturia, this mechanism is disrupted, either by a physical or psychological problem—*see incontinence*. Children frequently suffer from nocturia, but in a different form, because they generally remain asleep, and wet the bed. This problem is known as nocturnal enuresis.

In young children, nocturnal enuresis is quite normal, because it takes several years to acquire full control of the bladder. Most children grow out of bed-wetting by about the age of four, but others do not. Sometimes this is due to an inbuilt abnormality in the urinary tract, but, more commonly, it is caused by late development or a behavioural problem, often the result of stress *(p332)*. If the problem persists, however, parents should consult a doctor

While bed-wetting is irritating for the parents, it is very important not to scold a child after a wet night, and to praise him or her after a dry one, since anger will only upset the child and reinforce the behaviour. It is often helpful to wake the child late in the evening to go to the lavatory. Other techniques include keeping a star chart and giving the child a star for each dry night.

In persistent cases, an alarm can be fitted to a pad in the bed. This wakes the child up as soon as urine is passed. In time, the child comes to associate waking up with urination, and eventually wakes up before urinating; this method is only suitable for children over seven. If all else fails, drugs, such as imipramine, may be prescribed.

Though there may be occasional relapses, especially at times of stress, nocturnal enuresis generally clears up by late adolescence.

NON-SPECIFIC URETHRITIS—see Urethritis

NON-STEROIDAL ANTI-INFLAMMATORY DRUG (NSAID)

One of a number of drugs belonging to a group used for the control of pain and inflammation, especially in rheumatoid arthritis and osteoarthritis. Many have been introduced in the last ten years, but several have been withdrawn because of side effects, which sometimes have been fatal. The main ones are worsening of an existing asthmatic condition and peptic ulcers. The drugs should therefore be avoided entirely by patients with an active ulcer, or a history of ulcers in the past, except under specific instructions from a doctor, who will take precautions to prevent complications. All patients should take their NSAIDS together with food or milk.

NOSEBLEEDS—see Epistaxis

NOTIFIABLE DISEASES

In virtually every country in the world, certain diseases must be reported to the health authorities, so that preventive measures can be taken to avoid the risk of an *epidemic*.

In the UK notifiable diseases must be reported to the local Medical Officer of Health, who makes a weekly return of information to the Department of Health and Social Security. In the case of any particularly serious disease, however, the DHSS is notified immediately, and an operation to trace all the contacts of any sufferer from the disease is set in motion.

At present, the following diseases are notifiable in Britain: *cholera, diphtheria, dysentery*, acute *encephalitis, food poisoning*, infective *jaundice, lassa fever, leptospirosis, malaria, green monkey disease* (also called Marburg disease), *measles,* acute *meningitis, ophthalmia neonatorum, Pasteurella pestis* (plague), acute *poliomyelitis* (both paralytic and non-paralytic), *rabies,* relapsing fever (caused by a bacterium transmitted by lice or ticks), *scarlet fever, smallpox, tetanus, tuberculosis, typhoid* and paratyphoid fever, *typhus fever* (spotted fever), viral haemorrhagic disease (which attacks the walls of blood vessels), *whooping cough* (pertussis), and *yellow fever.*

The list is subject to change, and is not necessarily the same in other countries. In addition, some diseases must be reported to the World Health Organization in Geneva. These are cholera, plague, relapsing fever, smallpox, typhus, and yellow fever.

NSU—see Urethritis

NUTRITIONAL DISORDERS

Any disorder that results from an inadequate or excessive intake, digestion or absorption of food.

A balanced diet is essential for good health. This should include sufficient fat, carbohydrate, protein, vitamins and minerals—*see Diet, p321.* Generally, nutritional disorders arise from a lack of one, some or all of these factors in the diet, though there are also several other causes. If a person eats too little—for psychological reasons, as in *anorexia nervosa,* or because of poverty—he or she may suffer from *malnutrition.* If, on the other hand, a person eats too much, he may suffer from *obesity,* or may be more likely to contract *diabetes mellitus.*

Sometimes, however, a clinical condition prevents the body from absorbing nutrients properly. *Diabetes, gastroenteritis* and *malabsorption syndrome,* for example, can all have this effect. *Alcoholism* may result in a deficiency of vitamin B, while *cirrhosis* of the liver, some forms of *cancer, kidney failure* and use of certain drugs may mean that, despite an adequate diet, food is not utilized correctly in the body.

NYSTAGMUS

Involuntary rapid, small movements of the eyeball, which may be vertical or horizontal. Nystagmus is sometimes a harmless, inborn condition. However, if the condition develops during life, it may be a caused by an overdose of drugs or alcohol, or be a sign of a serious disease affecting the brain or ear, or *multiple sclerosis.* Any person who suffers from nystagmus should consult a doctor.

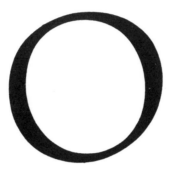

OBESITY

Obesity is an excess of body fat. This is usually estimated by weighing: comparing body weight in relation to height gives a reasonably accurate indication of the amount of fat in most cases, although in people who are unusually muscular, it may be misleading. Obesity is arbitrarily defined as a weight that is 20 per cent or more above the maximum ideal weight for that individual. The modern height/weight tables do not take account of frame size, since there is no objective way of measuring this.

Being overweight increases the chances of suffering from a number of diseases. These include high blood pressure, heart attacks, gall stones, osteoarthritis, diabetes mellitus, hiatus hernia, and varicose veins. There is an increased risk of death during surgery. Overall, life expectancy decreases as weight increases. (However, being underweight is also associated with decreased life expectancy).

There is no mystery about the immediate reason why people become overweight: it is because they take in more energy in food than they put out, though the reasons why this occurs are not always easy to unravel. However, there is no doubt about what must be done by those who want to lose weight: they must take in less energy than they put out. In practice, this means eating less food, taking more exercise, or both. Although exercise by itself does not use up a lot of calories, it is nevertheless an important component of any weight-losing regimen.

The kind of food that is eaten is important, as well as the amount. Fat intake should be reduced, since fat contains twice as many calories, weight for weight, as other sorts of food. The emphasis should be on carbohydrates (potatoes, beans, and other foods containing starches), which give a more sustained smoother rise in blood sugar levels. Contrary to what used to be believed, protein is not specially valuable to dieters, who should aim at a varied menu.

It is important to be realistic about the rate at which weight can be lost. A pound of fat is worth 4,000 kcal, so — given that the daily energy deficit to aim at is about 1,000 kcal — not more than two lbs will be lost a week. A loss of this size is easily masked by variations in the water content of the body, so it is unrealistic to expect to notice any real change in weight in less than a week. The diet should restrict energy intake to about half or two-thirds of what was being taken in previously. This usually means about 1,000 kcal daily for a woman, 1,500 kcal for a man.

As regards composition, the food should contain reduced amounts of fat, alcohol, and sugar. The dieter should take three meals a day. The meals should contain foods from each of the four major food groups: meat and fish, milk and cheese, bread and cereals, vegetables and fruit. Low-calorie foods, such as vegetables, can be used as snacks.

The psychological approach is important. Many obese patients do better if they are in a group. The best results of all seem to occur with *behaviour therapy,* in which patients are taught to record meticulously the circumstances associated with eating, so as to identify and then avoid the psychological triggers that make them eat. However, this requires a great deal of time from both the patients and the therapist.

Really obese patients present a considerable problem. Recently there has been a vogue for very-low-calorie diets in the treatment of such people, but such diets should not be implemented for more than three or four weeks without medical supervision. Moreover, they probably cause an undesirable loss of muscle in addition to fat, while they do little to modify long-term eating habits.

Drugs exist that can reduce appetite, but they are not very satisfactory for various reasons and should not be used for more than one to two months at a time. Substances that are intended to increase the bulk of the stomach contents and so prevent hunger do not work, nor do drugs that are supposed to prevent starch digestion.

Surgery is sometimes the last resort of the seriously overweight. Some patients have their jaws wired to reduce the amount they eat, but the weight is almost always regained when the wires are removed. The operation mainly used at present consists in stapling the stomach so as to reduce the amount it can hold.

A simple technique that is surprisingly effective in preventing weight gain after successful dieting is to tie a nylon cord round the waist, to serve as a reminder and to make it uncomfortable to overeat.

In general, the aim should be to prevent obesity or catch it early. Children and teenagers should not be allowed to become fat; the older the fat person is, the harder it becomes to treat him or her. However, children who are overweight should not be subjected to severe diets; instead, their food intake should be only moderately restricted with avoidance of foodstuffs containing what are termed empty calories (sugar, sweet drinks, crisps) and an increase in exercise.

In spite of the undoubted risks of being overweight, it is important to keep a sense of proportion about the matter. Minor degrees of overweightness do not make a large difference to health; for some people worrying about the situation can do more harm than the overweight itself. For middle-aged people, especially women, it is often better simply to accept things as they are and not to try to lose weight; simply avoid putting on any more.

There is some evidence to suggest that the distribution of fat is important, as well as the amount. For women, it seems to be better to have the fat around the hips than on the trunk, while for men it is a paunch, that is undesirable.

OBSESSION

A persistent idea, or compulsion to act in a certain way, which the patient knows is unnecessary, anti-social or even repulsive, but is unable to stop. Many normal people are preoccupied by their own habits and special interests; if these cross the boundary of obsession, however, the individual is dominated by them. Some people, for example, develop a hand-washing obsession; others find their life dominated by rituals, such as continually touching all four corners of every table at which they sit. At this point, treatment becomes necessary. This depends on the nature of the obsession, but is likely to involve *psychotherapy* and *behaviour therapy*.

See also neurosis.

OBSTRUCTION

A blockage or disturbance to the passage of material through an organ. Two key areas where obstruction may occur are the intestines and the urinary tract.

Doctors define the type of an obstruction according to its cause. In mechanical obstructions, the affected organ is actively blocked by tissue or physical matter, while in paralytic obstruction the organ becomes blocked because the force driving matter through it is interrupted or fails.

A mechanical intestinal obstruction occurs when the bowel is blocked, or constricted, by something pressing on it from outside, as in the case of an *adhesion* or a *hernia*. The risk of this type of obstruction increases in the elderly, since they are more prone to *volvulus*—a twist in the intestine—*impacted faeces*, or a *tumour* of the large intestine. In very young children, the cause may be *intussusception*, where part of the intestine is telescoped into the adjoining part.

In paralytic intestinal obstruction, *peristalsis* ceases—*see ileus paralyticus*. (Peristalsis is a sequence of rhythmic muscular contractions that pushes food through the intestines). This may be caused by an injury to the spine, *peritonitis*, *hypotension*—low blood pressure—or occur as a consequence of one of the forms of obstruction described above. It may also occur temporarily as a result of an abdominal operation.

Both types of obstruction produce intense pain in the region of the blockage. This pain is usually intermittent, like that of *colic*. Pain from a mechanical blockage is usually accompanied by 'stomach rumbles' and intermittent vomiting, whereas with a paralytic obstruction there is usually no sound, and less vomiting. The intestines are likely to be distended, although this may be visible only if the patient is thin.

Whatever the position or cause of the obstruction, one of the main effects will be loss of water and *electrolytes*, or salts, from the body, either through vomiting or loss of absorption from the gut. This may lead to *kidney failure*, particularly in the elderly. Where the intestine is trapped or twisted, as in a hernia or volvulus, there is a risk of strangulation, or interruption of the blood supply to the intestine, and a resulting danger of *gangrene* and perforation of the intestine. This can lead to peritonitis.

Prompt medical treatment is essential, whatever the cause of the blockage, and surgery is often necessary to remove the obstruction. Fluids and electrolytes must be replaced, by means of a *drip*, and the pressure relieved by pumping out the contents of the stomach.

The urinary tract may become obstructed at any part of its course: the kidney, ureter, bladder or urethra. It can be caused by a kidney stone—*see kidney disease*— a blood clot, or a *tumour*. Sometimes a section of the tract is compressed, as a result of a disorder of a nearby organ. Such disorders include *cervical cancer*, *fibrosis* of the tissues supporting the abdominal organs and, in men, enlargement of the prostate gland (p54).

Wherever any such blockage occurs, it eventually stops the flow of urine. The result is that the pressure in the tract rises, causing either the affected part, or sometimes the whole of the tract, to swell. The tissues of the kidney gradually degenerate, while the blockage leads to an infection.

If the blockage happens suddenly, the pain is acute, but, if it is gradual, the first symptom is usually an ache in the lower part of the back. If infection is present passing urine is painful, and the urine may be bloodstained. If the flow of urine is completely blocked, the bladder becomes distended, producing a visible swelling of the lower abdomen. Production of urine may stop altogether.

If the distension is severe, the first step may be to drain the build-up of urine. This can be done either by passing a tube called a *catheter* through the urethra into the bladder, or, in the case of kidney swelling—*hydronephrosis*—by positioning the tube directly in the pelvis of the kidney. This procedure is termed a *nephrostomy*. The next priority is to establish what is causing the obstruction and deal with it. In the case of infection, *antibiotics* are prescribed. If only one kidney is badly damaged it may be removed in an operation known as a *nephrectomy*. The body can survive using the other kidney. If both kidneys have been damaged, however, *dialysis* will be necessary for the rest of the patient's life—*see kidney failure*.

OBSTRUCTIVE AIRWAYS DISEASE

A disorder caused by the combined effects of chronic *bronchitis* and *emphysema*. One or the other may be the dominant factor, but the result always affects the flow of air to and from the lungs. Both conditions are referred to as chronic obstructive airways disease, or COAD, because they are at the most only partially reversible, through the use of bronchodilator drugs, which widen the air passages.

OCCUPATIONAL DISEASES—see Industrial diseases

OCCUPATIONAL THERAPY

Treatment for chronically ill and disabled people, and for those convalescing after a debilitating illness. All forms of occupational therapy are aimed at reviving or creating a skill or interest, thus helping the process of rehabilitation. The relief of boredom and feelings of uselessness is in itself an aid to recovery.

The overall aim is to prepare the patient, mentally and physically, to cope with life as independently as possible. For this reason occupational therapy may overlap with *psychotherapy*, *physiotherapy* and industrial training schemes.

OEDEMA

Swelling or puffiness of the tissues caused by retention of excess fluid. This may be generalized, or may affect only certain parts of the body. Oedema is often an obvious physical symptom of several different underlying disorders, including *kidney diseases*, *heart failure* and *cirrhosis* of the liver. In addition, changes in hormonal levels just before menstruation (p54), during pregnancy or through the use of oral contraceptives (p338) may also cause fluid retention. A number of other drugs have a similar effect, as do some nutritional deficiencies, such as a lack of vitamin B.

The direct cause of a build-up of fluid in the tissues is an imbalance between the amount of water pumped into them from the capillaries and the amount drawn back into them after fuel and chemicals have been delivered to the cells. Normally, very little protein is allowed to pass into the tissues; if too much is allowed through because the capillaries are damaged by infection or bruising, the excess will interfere with the reabsorption of fluid. The result is that excess water will be retained in the tissues. Similarly, if the protein level in the blood is too low, as in *nephrotic syndrome*, less water than normal is returned from the tissues.

Kidney disease often causes fluid retention since the excretory function of the kidneys is impaired. The fluid that is not excreted by the kidneys builds up in the body until it exceeds the capacity of the blood to absorb it. It is then displaced into the tissues, and oedema results. This process may be accelerated or aggravated by other factors, such as hypoproteinaemia—low protein levels in the blood—and salt retention.

Oedema is also caused by *heart failure*. In this condition, the blood tends to stagnate in the veins, **especially in the veins of the legs**. This congestion prevents the reabsorption of water from the tissues. The lungs may also be affected, in which case the condition is known as pulmonary oedema, causing shortness of breath.

The same thing may happen if muscles are immobile for long periods. The legs are particularly affected, especially when there is also a slight pressure on them. Sitting for hours without moving, as on a long air journey, causes the feet and ankles to swell, for example. Standing still for long periods of time has the same effect, although this is also due partly to gravity.

Treatment depends largely upon the cause of the oedema, but is based on restricting the intake of salt and water in the diet or removing them from the body with the help of *diuretics*.

OESOPHAGITIS

Inflammation of the oesophagus (p40), the tube running from the back of the throat to the stomach. The most frequent type is reflux oesophagitis, caused by an hiatus *hernia*—a protrusion of the stomach, at the point of its junction with the oesophagus, through the diaphragm. This causes stomach acid to be regurgitated into the lower part of the oesophagus. As the lining of the oesophagus is not designed to withstand this, it quickly becomes inflamed and may bleed.

Symptoms include dysphagia—difficulty in swallowing—flatulence, and heartburn. This is a burning pain deep in the chest which may be aggravated by bending over or lying down flat, allowing more stomach acid to run back up into the oesophagus. Preliminary diagnosis can be difficult, because the symptoms can be easily mistaken for those of coronary artery disease, or an ulcer. For this reason, a contrast X-ray, called a barium swallow and meal, is always taken for accurate diagnosis—*see Special Tests, p84*.

Drugs, careful control of diet, and changes in posture are all part of the treatment for this disease. Almost instant relief can often be obtained from antacid tablets. These not only neutralize the acids in the stomach but also provide the oesophagus with a temporary protective layer. Only small amounts of food should be eaten at a time; if swallowing is extremely difficult, a liquid diet is often recommended. Fatty foods and alcohol should also be avoided, since they aggravate the condition by increasing stomach acidity. Smoking should be cut down or stopped altogether, as it reduces the pressure of the muscular ring, or sphincter, at the junction of the oesophagus and stomach. Bending over should be avoided, while it is best to sleep with the upper part of the bed slightly raised. It may also help to loosen a tight belt and, if the patient is obese, he or she should lose weight. If the condition is severe, surgery may be necessary to deal with the hernia.

ONCHOCERCIASIS—see Blindness

OOPHORECTOMY

The surgical removal of an ovary (p54); the operation is also known as an ovariectomy.

An oophorectomy is generally performed to remove an ovarian *tumour* or a large *ovarian cyst*. However, in certain cases the operation is performed to control the spread of breast cancer—*see breast lumps*—and is sometimes carried out as part of a total *hysterectomy* when the patient has passed the menopause. In this case both ovaries are removed, and the operation is called a bilateral oophorectomy.

If an ovary has been removed from a pre-menopausal woman, the resulting deficiency in female sex hormones is made up by *hormone replacement therapy*. The operation has no effect on fertility unless it is bilateral, since it is perfectly possible for a woman to conceive a child when she has only one ovary.

OOPHORITIS

An inflammation of an ovary that sometimes develops when a pelvic infection, such as *salpingitis*, spreads up the Fallopian tubes (p54).

Treatment involves rest, pain-killers and *antibiotics* to fight the infection. Prompt diagnosis is important, since, if the condition is left untreated, an *abscess* may form in the tube or ovary. This damages the tissue and can cause infertility.

OPHTHALMIA NEONATORUM

Severe *conjunctivitis*, or superficial infection of the eye, in new-born babies, caused by diseases such as *gonorrhoea*, which affect the mother and are transmitted to the baby during the passage of the head through the vagina at birth.

In the West, most infections affecting pregnant women are detected at ante-natal examinations and treated with *antibiotics*. This considerably reduces the risk of infection of the baby before the birth, while antibiotic treatment of the baby quickly clears up any infection after birth. However, ophthalmia neonaturum is still a major problem in the underdeveloped countries, where it is a common cause of blindness.

OPIATES

Preparations or derivatives of opium, a drug obtained from a species of poppy called Papaver somniferum. All opiates are *narcotics*—that is, they dull the senses, induce drowsiness, relieve pain and anxiety, and become addictive if abused. They also depress the respiratory system and coughing mechanisms.

Opium has been used in medicine for thousands of years, to treat pain, *insomnia*, *anxiety* and *diarrhoea*. In modern times, a number of other chemicals, including morphine, heroin and codeine, have been refined from opium in an attempt to reduce its side-effects of *nausea* and *addiction*.

Morphine is used to relieve intense pain, such as post-operative pain and that caused by *cancer*. Codeine is much less powerful and is used in small quantities in headache and cough remedies. Heroin, in the form of a drug called diamorphine, may be used in the treatment of heart attacks and severe *pulmonary oedema*, and to relieve severe pain in terminal care—*see Coming to Terms with Death, p366*. Both heroin and morphine are abused for the euphoria and relief from anxiety they provide—*see Abuses of the Body, p328*. However, users quickly become tolerant of the drugs. In order to continue to experience their effects, the dosages have to be increased, resulting in addiction and eventually a fatal overdose.

The artificial opiates, pethedine and methadone, are also dangerous and addictive, but less so than heroin and morphine. Because of this, they are often used to wean addicts off the more dangerous drugs, in an attempt to treat their addiction.

OPTIC ATROPHY

A degeneration of, or loss of fibres in, the optic nerve (p32), ultimately resulting in loss of vision. It may be caused by injury, by interference to the blood supply to the optic nerve due to pressure from *glaucoma* or a *tumour*, by a *thrombus*, or a blood clot, in the central retinal artery, or by the spread of an infection such as *syphilis* to the central nervous system. Most frequently, however, it is caused by optic *neuritis*, an inflammation of the optic nerve.

Optic neuritis is often itself caused by *demyelinating diseases*, in which the nerve fibres lose their protective coating of myelin; the most common of these is *multiple sclerosis*. Optic neuritis is aggravated, or may be caused, by heavy tobacco smoking, as tobacco contains cyanide, which facilitates the nerve damage. Vitamin B12 is involved in the detoxification of the cyanide, therefore a deficiency in this vitamin is a significant contributory factor.

On examination with an ophthalmoscope—*see Special Tests, p84*—the optic disc appears very pale grey or white. The patient feels pain in the eye and its direct reaction to light is impaired. Treatment depends on the cause of the inflammation.

OPTIC NEURITIS—see Optic atrophy

ORCHIDECTOMY

The surgical removal of a testicle (p54); the operation is also known as an orchiectomy.

An orchidectomy may be performed for a variety of reasons. Most commonly, its purpose is to remove a testicular tumour, or *seminoma*. In this case, the operation is often bilateral—that is, both testicles are removed—because the cancer may have spread to involve other tissue in the scrotum. Orchidectomy may also be necessary when cancer of the prostate gland has spread to the testicles; when they have been seriously affected by an infection, such as *epididymitis* or *orchitis*; or when they have been damaged by an injury or by *torsion of the testis*.

An orchidectomy is occasionally performed as part of the treatment of cancer of the breast in men, and in cases where undescended testicles—

see cryptorchidism—have been diagnosed too late for them to be lowered surgically. This is because there is a tendency for testicles that have not descended to become *malignant*.

Orchidectomy of a single testicle does not necessarily have any effect on fertility or masculinity. Any shortfall in testosterone, the male sex hormone produced by the testicles, can be made up by hormone replacement therapy. Prosthetic testicles, made of plastic, can be placed in the scrotum to retain its normal appearance.

ORCHITIS

An inflammation of the testes, which become red, swollen, and extremely painful.

Orchitis is generally the result of a spread of infection down the vas deferens (p54). In this case, there is often *epididymitis* as well, and the condition is known as epididymo-orchitis.Orchitis may also be a complication of diseases such as *mumps, tuberculosis* and *gonorrhoea*. Of these, mumps orchitis is the most common. It affects one in four of all males who contract mumps after puberty—and may cause sterility if both testicles are involved.

Treatment is by painkillers and *antibiotics*, and, in the case of mumps orchitis, by *corticosteroid* drugs. A suspensory bandage is often used to give support to the swollen scrotum. Orchitis generally responds to treatment within a few days, but in serious cases, an *orchidectomy* may be necessary.

ORNITHOSIS

A disease of the respiratory system, caused by an organism called *Chlamydia*. Ornithosis can be transmitted to humans by birds, and is similar to *psittacosis*, or parrot disease.

The symptoms are similar to those caused by *pneumonia*: a cough, headaches, aches in the muscles, joint pains, and a *fever*. The condition responds well to treatment with *antibiotics*, such as tetracycline, but is highly infectious. When nursing a sufferer from ornithosis, care should be taken to prevent the spread of the infection through droplets coughed or sneezed into the air—*see Health and Hygiene, p334*.

ORTHOPNOEA

Breathlessness on lying flat, which is relieved by sitting up. Orthopnoea is a symptom of left-sided *heart failure*, in which fluid builds up in the lungs. When a sufferer from this condition lies flat, the fluid swamps the alveoli, the tiny pouches in which oxygen and carbon dioxide are exchanged. As a result, the body is deprived of oxygen, and the sufferer gasps for breath in an attempt to make up the shortfall. The breathlessness is often accompanied by a dry, repetitive cough.

OSTEITIS DEFORMANS—see Paget's disease

OSTEOARTHRITIS—see Arthritis

OSTEOCHONDRITIS

An inflammation of the cartilage and bone *(p16)*, leading to defective growth and deformity. There are two main types of the condition: osteochondritis deformans juvenilis and osteochondritis dessicans.

In osteochondritis deformans juvenilis, which affects children, there is a change in an epiphysis *(p16)*, the centre of a bone's growth. As a result, bone tissue degenerates or dies, and the affected bone grows abnormally. This causes a variety of deformities, depending on the bone involved. The most common bones to be affected are the head of the hip (Perthe's disease) and the vertebrae (Scheuermann's disease), causing lameness or a hunch back respectively. The tubercle of the tibia, below the knee, may also be affected (Osgood-Schlatter's disease), causing lameness. Osteochondritis deformans juvenilis cannot be treated, but the deformities that it causes can sometimes be corrected by surgery. However, sufferers are likely to suffer from forms of *arthritis* in later life.

Osteochondritis dessicans can develop at any age, but mainly affects young people. It is triggered by an injury in which a small piece of bone is broken off near a joint. Instead of healing, more particles of bone break away, forming separate clumps of bone that impede movement of the joint. The joints most commonly affected are the knee, ankle, shoulder and elbow. Treatment consists of either removing the loose clumps of bone by surgery, or pinning them to the parent bone in the hope that they will eventually fuse together.

OSTEOGENESIS IMPERFECTA

An *hereditary* condition in which a baby is born with abnormally fragile bones. Sometimes the condition is so serious that an affected baby dies during, or shortly after birth, as a result of multiple fractures received in the womb.

In less serious cases, the condition does not cause problems until the baby has grown sufficiently to be active. Then, even minor injuries tend to cause fractures. The bones normally become slightly stronger at adolescence, but by then there are often gross deformities, and sometimes *dwarfism*. Characteristically, children with osteogenesis imperfecta have blue sclerae, the parts of the eyes that are normally white.

There is no treatment for the condition, though the deformities it causes may occasionally be corrected by surgery.

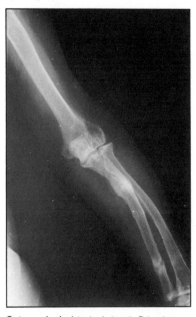

Osteomalacia A lack of vitamin D leads to a softening of the bones, called osteomalacia in adults and rickets in children. Bones lose their strength, bending and distorting under physical stress. The X-ray *(above)* shows how the radius and the ulna bones of the forearm have bowed outwards due to osteomalacia.

OSTEOMALACIA

A softening of the bones, caused by a deficiency in vitamin D *(p322)*. This vitamin plays a vital role in the deposition of calcium in bones. A deficiency causes a loss of bony substance and its replacement with softer tissues. In children, osteomalacia is known as *rickets*.

A vitamin D deficiency may have a number of causes. It is sometimes the result of an inadequate diet—the vitamin is found in dairy products, liver and fish oils, *see Diet, p322*—but this is uncommon in the West. It can also be caused by intestinal disorders, such as *malabsorption syndrome*, which interfere with the absorption of vitamin D by the bowel, and occasionally by chronic *kidney disease*.

There are three more causes of osteomalacia. The first is the long-term use of *anticonvulsants*, because these drugs break down calcium in the body. The second is pregnancy, in which the demands of the growing foetus for calcium may deplete the mother's resources unless supplements are taken. Finally, a lack of sunlight may cause osteomalacia. This is because vitamin D is synthesized in the body as a result of the exposure of the skin to sunlight, as well as being taken in the diet. Lack of sunlight is often a problem for people who have emigrated from countries with a sunny climate to colder areas. They tend to suffer from a degree of osteomalacia until they become acclimatized, because their bodies are accustomed to synthesizing a large proportion of their vitamin D requirements.

Symptoms of osteomalacia include tiredness, pain in the limbs, weakness and sometimes a waddling gait. If left untreated, the condition may result in deformities, such as bowing of the legs, and spontaneous fractures may occur in the weight-bearing bones such as the pelvis and long bones of the leg.

Osteomalacia is easily treated, however, by vitamin D and calcium supplements. Since vitamin D is poisonous in large quantities, the dosages must be carefully controlled.

OSTEOMYELITIS

An inflammation of the bone marrow, caused by *bacterial* infection.

Osteomyelitis occurs most commonly in children under 12. The infection normally sets in after a compound fracture, but sometimes the bacteria are carried to the site by the blood from an infection elsewhere in the body, such as a boil or septic throat. The inflammation causes a build-up of pus, which cannot escape into the tissues, and therefore spreads along the bone. This cuts off the blood supply to the bone, and not only prevents the antibodies produced by the body's defences *(p52)*, and drugs, from reaching the site of infection, but causes the death of bone tissue.

Symptoms of osteomyelitis include pain and tenderness at the site of the infection, and, in the later stages, fever and nausea. Treatment consists of draining the pus and the removal of any dead tissue by surgery. After the blood supply to the area has been re-established by this means, antibiotics are prescribed to clear up the infection, and to prevent it from spreading to other bones.

OSTEOPOROSIS

A change in the mass or texture of bone, caused by a depletion in the level of calcium it contains. As a result, the bones become weak.

Osteoporosis affects the majority of elderly people to some degree, and is a part of the natural process of ageing. It is exacerbated by a number of factors, including immobility, and deficiencies of the sex hormones, or of calcium and vitamin D. Younger people may also be affected if they suffer from these problems. Women develop osteoporosis more often than men, especially if they have passed the menopause, or had their ovaries removed. The disease may also be caused by various disorders of the endocrine glands, such as *Cushing's syndrome*, and is a side-effect of long-term treatment with *corticosteroid* drugs.

Osteoporosis may be symptomless, but there is sometimes pain in the back, trunk and limbs. When the condition is severe, it can cause compression of the vertebrae, resulting in spinal curvature and loss of height. The bones tend to fracture more easily, but heal normally.

There is no specific treatment for osteoporosis. *Hormone replacement therapy* may help to stop the progress of the disease, especially in post-menopausal women, as may a diet rich in calcium, vitamin D and protein and exercise to maintain mobility—*see Diet, p322; Exercise, p316.* Pain can be relieved by *analgesics*, but, once lost, bone mass cannot be restored.

OTITIS

An inflammation of the ear, named according to the part of the ear that is involved—*see The Nervous System, p32.* An inflammation of the outer ear is called otitis externa; of the middle ear, otitis media; and of the inner ear, otitis interna.

Otitis externa may be caused by an *allergic* reaction to a foreign body in the outer ear, or by a *bacterial* or *fungal* infection. Such infections are often contracted when swimming, because organisms can enter the ear from the water, and moisture provides an environment in which they can multiply. This can be avoided if the outer ear is kept dry and clean. If an infection sets in, it can be treated by *antibiotic* or fungicidal ear drops, depending on its nature.

In otitis media, bacteria or *viruses* from a throat infection enter the middle ear by means of the Eustachian tube, which connects the two. As the bacteria multiply, earache develops, and there may be a *fever*; children often experience abdominal pain. If untreated, pus builds up, causing deafness, and eventually the pressure may become so great that the eardrum is perforated. Sometimes, pus drains to the bone behind the ear, causing *mastoiditis*, and, very occasionally, enters the skull, causing an *abscess*. This is a serious condition, and requires immediate treatment.

Normal treatment is with *antibiotics* to clear up the infection and *antihistamines* to help relieve the pressure of pus. Generally, a perforated ear drum heals on its own within a few weeks.

Otitis interna, also called labyrinthitis, is more rare. It is caused by either a virus or bacteria from a throat infection that reaches the inner ear through a Eustachian tube. The labyrinth controls balance, and the result of an infection is a loss of balance, dizziness and *vertigo*. There may also be nausea, vomiting and *nystagmus*. Treatment consists of bed-rest for around a week, with certain *tranquillizers* to control giddiness and *antiemetics* to relieve nausea. Otitis interna normally clears up on its own within a few weeks.

OTOSCLEROSIS

A defect of the middle ear *(p32)* that usually develops in late adolescence and is hereditary in 50% of cases.

Otosclerosis causes a thickening of the tiny bones of the middle ear. These transmit vibrations to the middle ear, and are vital for hearing. When they become thickened, they are unable to transmit vibrations and deafness is the result. This may be partial or total, depending on the stage of disease. In about 80% of sufferers, both ears are affected. Other symptoms may include *tinnitus*, a constant ringing sound in the ears, and *vertigo*, a spinning sensation.

If hearing has been seriously affected, the bones of the middle ear may be replaced surgically by a synthetic graft. However, a hearing aid is often still necessary.
See also deafness.

OVARIAN CYST

A fluid-filled swelling that develops in the ovaries *(p54)*.

Ovarian cysts rarely cause any symptoms, and are often not discovered until they reach a size at which they can be felt on a routine vaginal examination. Occasionally, however, they may cause pain in the lower abdomen, and discomfort on intercourse. If they are not detected, the cysts may grow to such a size that the affected woman appears to be pregnant. If this happens, the cysts may twist and burst, leaking their contents into the abdomen and causing *peritonitis*.

For this reason, once ovarian cysts have been diagnosed, they are generally removed by surgery. Another reason is that, though ovarian cysts are normally benign—harmless—they may occasionally become *malignant*. If the cysts are small, it may be possible to excise them without removing the rest of the ovarian tissue. This operation is called an ovarian cystectomy. If the cysts are large, or malignant, the whole ovary is removed. This operation is called an *oophorectomy*.

Any deficiency in female sex hormones resulting from an oophorectomy can be made up by *hormone replacement therapy*. The operation has no effect on fertility.

Otitis Externa and Media
When the membrane lining the ear canal is damaged or left moist after bathing, there is a danger of infection by bacteria or fungi. The result is otitis externa, in which either a boil or abscess forms or the whole canal becomes inflamed. In each case, a discharge of pus may block the canal, leading to a loss of hearing.
In otitis media, the middle ear is infected by a virus or bacteria, which usually enters the ear from the throat via the Eustachian tube. Alternatively, the infection can enter through a ruptured eardrum. In a bacterial infection, the middle ear chamber and the Eustachian tube may be blocked by pus. If left untreated, the pus may spread to the air cells of the mastoid process or even perforate the eardrum.

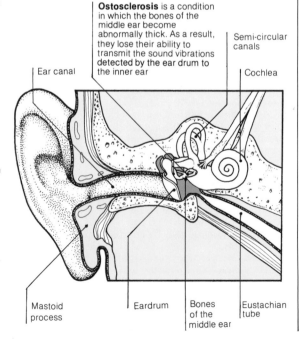

Ostosclerosis is a condition in which the bones of the middle ear become abnormally thick. As a result, they lose their ability to transmit the sound vibrations detected by the ear drum to the inner ear

Ear canal

Semi-circular canals

Cochlea

Mastoid process

Eardrum

Bones of the middle ear

Eustachian tube

P

PACEMAKER

The term used to describe the function of the sino-atrial node, an area of heart muscle located at the junction of the superior vena cava and the right atrium—*see The Blood and Lymph Systems, p21*. The node initiates the heartbeat through a series of regular electrical impulses, which stimulate the contraction of the muscular walls of the atria. The impulses are then transmitted to the ventricles, which contract as a result.

If the sino-atrial node is damaged, a *heart block* results. This means that the pacemaker is unable to regulate the heartbeat properly. In an emergency, an artificial pacemaker outside the body is used to regulate the heartbeat artificially. Wires from the pacemaker are passed to the right atrium and right ventricle via a catheter inserted into the subclavian or jugular veins.

If the pacemaker is permanently damaged, an artificial pacemaker is surgically implanted in the body to take over the node's functions. The procedure takes 30 minutes and is carried out under local anaesthetic. The pacemaker is normally implanted under the skin below the collar bone and the wires threaded along a vein into the right atrium, through the tricuspid valve and into the right ventricle.

Until recently, such pacemakers were battery-powered. The batteries lasted from three to five years, and were then replaced in another minor operation. Today, atomic pacemakers with a much longer life are normally used.

The outlook for patients with artificial pacemakers is excellent. They can lead a normal life, though the pacemaker must be checked every six months to ensure that it is working properly. They must check their pulses daily and contact their doctor if there are marked abnormalities. They should also avoid the electronic security devices found in airports, since these can affect the workings of certain types of pacemaker.

PAGET'S DISEASE

A bone disorder in which the skull, spine and long bones of the body

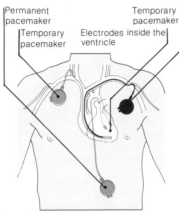

Pacemaker An artificial electric pacemaker is implanted in the body near the heart as a substitute for the heart's own failing pacemaker. Pacemakers can be either temporary or permanent — a temporary pacemaker is shown in the X-ray *(right)*. The

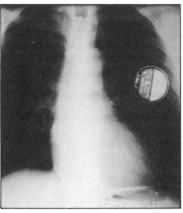

pacing wire, contained in a catheter, is inserted into the subclavian, external jugular, or basilic veins and then pushed forward through the right atrium into the right ventricle. The pulse source is a box strapped to the chest.

become softened, enlarged and bowed. Paget's disease, or osteitis deformans, mainly affects the elderly; it is more common in men than in women.

Normal bone—*see Bone and Muscle, p16*—consists of roughly equal proportions of osteoblasts, the cells that build up bone, and osteoclasts, the cells that destroy it. In Paget's disease, the osteoclasts outnumber the osteoblasts, so bringing about an increase in the number of blood vessels in the bone. This, together with the bone destruction that is taking place, causes the bones to soften and swell. Weakened bone also has a tendency to fracture easily.

The cause of Paget's disease is unknown. X-rays *(p84)* show that the affected bones are wider then normal and that their calcium content is lower. A blood test will detect a rise in the level of an enzyme called alkaline phosphatase. This normally occurs only in young children, whose bones are still developing. In rare cases, the calcium drained from the bone accumulates in the blood stream, especially in the bedridden. The bone often feels warm to the touch because of the increased volume of blood flowing through it.

In many people, Paget's disease causes no specific symptoms and the

presence of the disease may be discovered only accidentally during a routine X-ray. In some patients, however, it causes severe headaches, because certain cranial nerves *(p32)* may be trapped by the swelling skull at the point where they leave the brain. If the auditory nerve is trapped, *deafness* may occur, while, if the optic nerve is affected, vision is impaired. When the disease reaches an advanced stage, the weight of the body may cause the femur, or thigh bone, to become bowed. This makes the patient susceptible to osteoarthritis of the hip—*see arthritis. Paraplegia* and *sarcoma* are rare complications.

Paget's disease is not fatal and treatment is usually unnecessary, unless the pain is extremely severe. In such cases, calcitonin, a hormone *(p48)* that lowers the serum calcium level in the blood, is injected at regular intervals to relieve the pain. Before the injections are given, the patient is tested to ensure that he or she is not allergic to the replacement hormone. A course of treatment usually lasts for six months, and is repeated if the pain recurs.

PALPITATION

A general term used to describe either the sensation of an irregular heartbeat—often described as a 'missed' beat—or a sudden

245

awareness of a normal, fast or forceful heart beat.

Palpitations are very common, are usually harmless, and often go completely unnoticed. The 'missed beat' is not, in fact, a dropped beat, but is due to an *ectopic beat*, which occurs earlier than normal, so causing a longer, compensatory gap before the next beat. This gives the patient the impression that the heart has missed a beat. These extra beats are common in the elderly, in people suffering from *anxiety*, and when excessive amounts of stimulants, such as caffeine and nicotine, have been taken. After exertion, too, a pounding in the chest may be felt because the heart beat has speeded up and its force has increased.

The occasional palpitation is a normal occurrence. In persistent cases an electrocardiogram—*see Special Tests, p84*—can help to identify any underlying heart disorder.

PALSY
A general term for paralysis, frequently used by laymen to describe the paralysis that can occur as part of the effects of a stroke—*see cerebrovascular accident*. There are also various specific types, such as *Bell's palsy*, in which the facial nerve is paralysed for no known reason. *Erb's palsy* occurs when the nerve supply to the arm is slightly damaged at birth, the arm hanging oddly as a result. *Cerebral palsy* is a brain abnormality causing weakness and lack of co-ordination in the limbs.

PAN—see Polyarteritis nodosa

PANCREATIC CANCER
A malignant *tumour* of the pancreas *(p48)*, a gland in the abdomen that secretes gastric juices and insulin—the hormone responsible for maintaining the balance of glucose in the blood *(p44)*. The pancreas can be affected by *cancer* in three places—the head, where the pancreatic duct and the bile duct join to enter the duodenum; the tail; and the body.

Cancer of the head of the pancreas is the most serious of the three conditions. It can be diagnosed at an early stage if *jaundice* appears. This is the result of an accumulation of bile in the blood as a result of the blockage of the bile duct. Cancer in the tail of the pancreas, on the other hand, may cause no symptoms, and becomes apparent only when the tumour has spread to other organs. Sometimes, symptoms include pain in the upper abdomen or back. Similarly, cancer in the body of the pancreas is very hard to diagnose,

and there are often no symptoms until it is well advanced.

Treatment is by surgery, which becomes more complicated if the tumour is situated on or near the head of the pancreas. If the entire pancreas is removed, the digestive enzymes and insulin lost to the body as a result must be replaced by dietary supplements and daily injections respectively. Some patients recover completely after surgery, but 80% die within five years of diagnosis. This is because the cancer usually begins to spread before it is discovered.

PANCREATITIS
Inflammation of the pancreas *(p48)*, often caused by persistent heavy drinking. In pancreatitis, the duct carrying the digestive juices from the pancreas to the duodenum becomes inflamed. The resulting obstruction blocks the flow of juices, and, as a result, the pancreas begins to 'digest' itself. If the duct is blocked by a *gallstone*, the same process occurs. Pain may result if the pancreas has been damaged by alcohol, or if the duct is obstructed by an abnormal amount of mucus, as in *cystic fibrosis*.

There are two forms of the disease—acute and chronic. Acute pancreatitis causes agonizing abdominal pain, together with *vomiting* and *shock*. Chronic pancreatitis produces constant pain, often in the back, and may be accompanied by loss of weight. The lack of digestive juices in the duodenum interferes with the normal absorption of calcium, causing *osteomalacia*, a painful bone condition. It also causes surplus fat to be excreted in the faeces. Occasionally, the bile duct may be obstructed by swelling around the pancreas, with *jaundice* as the result.

Diagnosis can be difficult, as the symptoms of the condition closely resemble those of a peptic *ulcer*. In acute pancreatitis, there is an excessive level of the enzyme amylase in the blood, which can be detected by a blood test—*see Special Tests, p84*. However, the level of amylase may also rise in conditions such as bowel obstruction and perforated *ulcer*. Chronic pancreatitis is associated with increased calcium deposits in the pancreas. These can be detected by X-ray, as can gallstones.

Acute pancreatitis is treated by the intravenous replacement of the fluid lost through vomiting, and by drawing surplus fluid out of the stomach through a tube passed through the nose. Atropine injections reduce the volume of digestive juices produced. No food

is given by mouth, since solids cause the production of pancreatic juices. This form of pancreatitis has a mortality rate of about 5 per cent, but the majority of patients make a complete recovery.

Chronic pancreatitis is nearly always caused by heavy drinking, and can be relieved only if the patient gives up alcohol—*see Abuses of the Body, p328*. The damage done to the pancreas results in the permanent loss of some essential digestive enzymes; these are replaced by artificial substitutes sprinkled on food. In severe cases, *diabetes* develops because of a lack of insulin; this must be replaced by injection.

PAPILLOEDEMA
An eye disorder in which the optic nerve *(p32)* becomes swollen. Papilloedema is a symptom of a number of serious conditions, including *hypertension*, or high blood pressure, and a brain *tumour*.

Diagnosis is made by examining the patient's eye through an ophthalmoscope—*see Special Tests, p84*. Normally, the retina looks red and is covered with arteries and veins, all of which emerge from a pale, circular area, measuring about half a centimetre (one fifth of an inch) across. This is where the optic nerve, which transmits images to the brain in the form of electrical images, enters the eye. Usually, there is a distinct junction visible between the nerve and the retina. In papilloedema, however, the optic nerve is red, swollen and cannot be seen clearly.

The commonest cause of the condition is a rise in pressure within the skull. If this is due to severe *hypertension*, it is treated as a medical emergency with hypotensive drugs. Brain tumours—another potential cause—can be identified by a CAT scan—*see Special Tests, p84*. If possible, they are removed by surgery.

PARACETAMOL
A widely used drug for relief of pain and reduction of temperature in fever. It is similar in effectiveness to aspirin, but, unlike aspirin, it does not cause stomach problems and it is advised for fever in children in preference to aspirin because of the association between aspirin and *Reye's syndrome*. Care is required with paracetamol, however, because in over-dosage it can cause fatal liver damage which may not be apparent for several days. As little as 20 to 30 tablets can do this, so any patient who has swallowed an overdose of paracetamol should be taken to hospital immediately.

PARAESTHESIAE

The medical term for the tingling sensation of 'pins and needles'. This may be caused by pressure to the nerve root as it emerges from the spinal cord. However, paraesthesiae can also be a symptom of many serious diseases, such as *carpal tunnel syndrome*, *multiple sclerosis*, and vitamin B12 deficiency—*see vitamin deficiency diseases*.

PARALYSIS

The inability to move part of the body effectively, normally because the nerves which control the muscles involved have been damaged. Without *physiotherapy*, the muscles themselves become weak, and then atrophy through lack of use. The condition can affect any part of the body.

There are two main causes of paralysis. A stroke, or *cerebrovascular accident*, often causes hemiplegia, in which half the body is affected by paralysis to a greater or lesser extent. Paralysis from the waist downwards, caused by damage to the spinal cord, may be the result of a severe accident, or the pressure caused by a *tumour* or *abscess*. The victim is said to be paraplegic. Other causes of paralysis include *poliomyelitis* and *multiple sclerosis*.

In a stroke, the key areas of the brain responsible for movement may be damaged by *haemorrhage* or *thrombosis*. As a result, the affected parts of the body are paralyzed—that is, incapable of voluntary movement. In some cases, the muscles controlling speech and swallowing are paralyzed; this is called bulbar palsy, as it affects the part of the brain stem called the bulb from which the cranial nerves (p32) controlling swallowing emerge. Food tends to regurgitate through the nose, so solids may be easier to keep down than liquids. With physiotherapy, however, many stroke patients recover completely.

Although damage to the spinal cord and the brain is permanent, physiotherapy and occupational therapy can prevent the complete wasting away of the limbs. They can also prevent joint contractures in which patients become chair-shaped. Such therapies also help the disabled to come to terms with their paralysis. This is combined with the prescription of drugs to reduce the increased tone in the affected muscles in some cases.

PARAPLEGIA

Paralysis of the lower limbs, which may be the result of injury, spinal disease, or *multiple sclerosis*. Complications can arise, since the paralysis can lead to other medical problems, including pressure sores,

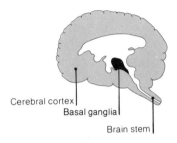

Parkinson's Disease The two main symptoms of Parkinson's disease are stiffness and tremor. The muscles of the face and limbs are difficult to control, either because they seem rigid or because they are trembling. Degeneration of the basal ganglia nerve cells in the brain stem *(below)* means that the supply of dopamine, a chemical neurotransmitter involved in initiating muscle movement, becomes random and uneven.

Cerebral cortex

Basal ganglia

Brain stem

urinary infections, kidney stones and bowel difficulties, especially intractable constipation.

Pressure sores may develop as a result of the circulatory problems that may arise if the patient is bedridden. In such cases, the patient should lie on a special rubber mattress, and have his or her position in bed changed every two to four hours—*see Home Nursing, p352*. The skin should be kept dry and clean. A suitable diet and laxatives will prevent constipation.

In some diseases, the paralysis becomes progressively worse. If, however, the degree of paralysis is stabilized, the patient may be able to learn to walk with the aid of calipers. In all cases, *physiotherapy* is important to prevent, or at least slow down, the wasting of muscular tissue.

PARKINSON'S DISEASE

A slowly progressive disease of the nervous system characterized by stiffness and shaking, mainly affecting the elderly, particularly men. It is also known as shaking palsy, paralysis agitans, or Parkinsonism. The disease is caused by degeneration of part of the nervous system, in particular the groups of brain cells known as the basal ganglia, which regulate voluntary movements—*see The Nervous System, p32*. The exact reason for this is unknown. Certain drugs, however, especially the major *tranquillizers* of the phenothiazine family, can cause Parkinsonism.

In Parkinson's disease, patients experience two main symptoms of varying severity. These are stiffness (paralysis) and tremor (agitans). These symptoms usually develop

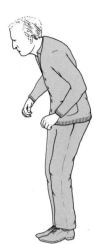

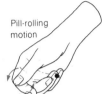

People with Parkinson's disease develop a stoop *(left)*, staring eyes, an expressionless face and a slow shuffling gait. Tremors and involuntary movements are common, such as the 'pill-rolling' habit of moving the thumb against the first two fingers *(below)*.

Pill-rolling motion

insidiously and may not become noticeable until the tremor is marked. In advanced cases, all the muscles are affected by constant stiffness. The sufferer finds it difficult to walk, other than in a tottering shuffle. Stiffness of the facial muscles results in a fixed expression, while stiffness of the tongue muscles impairs speech and the ability to swallow saliva, causing distressing dribbling. The tremor increases whenever the patient attempts to reach for and pick up an object. This makes it impossible to write legibly, to handle a knife and fork, or to drink from a glass or cup.

The most common form of treatment involves the use of the drug levodopa, or L-dopa, to lessen the tremor. The treatment replenishes the natural supply of dopamine, a chemical neurotransmitter normally manufactured by the brain, which is abnormally low in Parkinson's disease. The L-dopa, taken by mouth, is combined with other chemicals to lessen potentially harmful side-effects.

After a few years, both mental and physical disabilities may develop, including loss of memory, *anxiety*, and unsteadiness of gait. These symptoms may come and go quite suddenly, but they seem to become more pronounced in long-term L-dopa treatment. The patient stops taking the L-dopa for a few weeks so that, when the treatment is continued, he or she responds to the drug.

PAROTITIS

Inflammation of the parotid, or salivary, glands (p40). Parotitis is a symptom of *mumps*, though it can also be caused by bacterial infection of the glands, usually during *fever*.

Septic parotitis, in which an *abscess* forms in the glands, is a rare condition that is usually treated with penicillin. If this is ineffective, the abscess may be drained surgically and *antibiotics* given after this to clear up any remaining infection.

PASTEURELLA PESTIS

The organism that causes bubonic plague, spread by fleas from rats infected with the disease. It is extremely rare in temperate climates, but is still sometimes found in South-East Asia and East Africa. The incubation period is normally two to six days, and is characterized by high fever, *delirium* and swollen lymph glands. These make up a large lump called a bubo, which is located in the groin or armpit— hence the name bubonic plague.

In some cases, bleeding takes place under the skin, producing black patches which can develop into ulcers. If bacteria enter the blood stream, the condition is known as *septicaemic* plague; if the lungs become infected, it is called pneumonic plague. Both these conditions are usually fatal.

Bubonic plague can be treated by the *antibiotics* streptomycin or tetracycline in large dosages.

PATENT DUCTUS ARTERIOSUS—see Congenital heart disease

PATHOGEN

A small organism, such as a *bacterium*, that lives in a human or an animal and causes a disease.

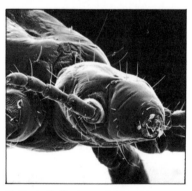

Pediculosis The human body louse (Pediculus humanus corporis) is a blood-sucking parasite which lives on human skin. Its mouth is specially adapted for piercing and sucking through skin, while each of its powerful legs is equipped with sharp, strong claws for digging. Its tiny white eggs, known as 'nits', are laid on body hair and among the fibres of clothing.

PEDICULOSIS

Infestation of the head or body with pediculus (lice). Three types of lice affect man: p. humanus capitis, the head louse; p. humanus corporis, the body louse; and phthirus pubis, the crab louse, which infests the pubic hair.

Lice are tiny insects that suck

blood from the skin. Their bites are extremely itchy. Head and body lice, often called nits, are frequently spread in schools. The eggs can usually be seen in the hair as small greyish white dots, which adhere firmly to it. Pubic lice are normally passed on by sexual contact.

Body lice can be treated by dusting with DDT powder, whereas head lice are destroyed by a special shampoo containing the chemical gamma benzene hexachloride. Pubic lice can similarly be dealt with by a suitable shampoo or a lotion.

PELVIC INFLAMMATORY DISEASE (PID)

A term used to describe long-standing infections of the pelvic organs in women.

Most of these organs share the same vascular system and lymphatic drainage—*see The Blood and Lymph Systems, p21*. They are also in direct contact with the outside of the body via the vagina, cervix, and uterine cavity. The three openings of the female genital tract—urethra, vagina and rectum (*p54*)—are all close together as well. This means that such infections are common, frequently affecting more than one organ.

Pelvic inflammatory disease is fairly frequently found in women of child-bearing age. It is more common among women who use the intra-uterine device as a contraceptive method—*see Sex and contraception, p338*—and among women with several sexual partners, since the latter are at greater risk of contracting *venereal disease*. Other infections, such as *tuberculosis*, can also reach the ovaries and Fallopian tubes to cause PID. A burst appendix may cause problems, because of its proximity to the right ovary and Fallopian tube, while an unsterile abortion is also a potential cause of PID.

In all cases, the severity of the symptoms depends on the nature of the infecting organism. The patient may be acutely ill, with high fever and severe pain; more commonly, there is intermittent pelvic pain, with vague symptoms of ill health. Sometimes PID is discovered during investigation of *infertility*. This is because, if *salpingitis* develops, the inflammation and pus produced may combine to block the Fallopian tubes.

Occasionally, large quantities of pus collect in the tubes, so distending them that, eventually, the tubes and ovaries on one or both sides are matted together with *adhesions*. As a result, a large *abscess* forms. Treatment is with bed rest and the appropriate antibiotics,

although surgical drainage may be necessary in the case of an abscess.

If pelvic inflammatory disease has contributed to infertility, careful surgery may correct this, but the outlook in such cases is generally poor.

PEMPHIGUS VULGARIS

A blistering disease that affects the mouth and skin. It is thought to be an *autoimmune* disorder. It usually begins in the mouth; both here and in the skin the blisters break easily, leaving a raw painful area exposed. It is one of the most dangerous skin diseases and used to have a very high death rate; however, corticosteroids are life-saving though they have to be given in very high dosage, which often produces side-effects.

Pemphigus needs to be distinguished from other causes of blistering, particularly *pemhigoid*, which is commoner than pemphigus and is less serious.

PENICILLIN

An *antibiotic* used to treat infections caused by a wide range of bacteria. Penicillin was one of the first antibiotics to be developed.

The drug is usually administered by injection, though it can be taken in tablet form. It has few potential side-effects, though some people are allergic to it. Symptoms of *allergy* include skin rashes, swelling of the throat and fever. For this reason, it is important that, if a patient is suffering from such an allergy, he or she always tells any doctor before antibiotic treatment is given.

PENILE DISCHARGE

The seepage of fluid from the end of the penis at times other than during urination or ejaculation. The discharge is usually yellowish or white in colour, and may be accompanied by *dysuria*, or pain on passing urine.

The condition is normally due to *urethritis*, or inflammation of the urethra. This, in turn, may be due to diseases such as *gonorrhoea*, or *Rieter's syndrome*, or conditions with no known cause, such as NSU—*see urethritis*.

The discharge is treated by dealing with the underlying cause. *Antibiotics* are normally prescribed, though, in Rieter's syndrome, these are combined with treatment for the *arthritis* and *iritis* associated with this condition.

PEPTIC ULCER—see Ulcer

PERIANAL HAEMATOMA—see Haematoma

PERICARDITIS

Inflammation of the *pericardium*, the membrane surrounding the heart—*see The Blood and Lymph Systems, p21*. Pericarditis is usually caused by a *viral* infection; it may also accompany certain *bacterial* infections, and can occur in conjunction with other diseases, such as *rheumatoid arthritis*. In addition, pericarditis can accompany *uraemia*, an effect of kidney failure, and is sometimes associated with an underlying *coronary thrombosis*.

Symptoms include central chest pain which may radiate up to the neck, the left shoulder and left arm. The pain is sharper in character than the pain of a heart attack, and may alter in intensity as the patient changes position in bed. It may also persist for weeks or even months—unlike the pain of a *myocardial infarction*, which usually lasts for only a few hours.

Because of its similarity to myocardial infarction, pericarditis can be difficult to diagnose. The chief diagnostic aid is an electrocardiogram—*see Special Tests, p84*—since the reading differs from the trace typical of a heart attack. If a bacterial cause is suspected, treatment is with rest, *analgesics*, and *antibiotics*. In other cases, anti-inflammatory drugs may give some relief.

Complications occur when quantities of fluid collect between the heart and the pericardium. This is called a pericardial effusion and severely impedes the heart's pumping action. The fluid is located with an echocardiogram—a specialized form of ultrasonic scanning (*p84*)—and is then drained away with a hollow needle inserted through the chest. Another complication is constrictive pericarditis, caused by long-term hardening and shrinking of the pericardium. This also interferes with the heart, so the affected pericardium may have to be removed surgically.

In most cases, however, full recovery follows treatment, with no permanent damage.

PERIODONTAL DISEASE

A disease of the gums, tooth ligaments and bone caused by the plaque, bacteria and food deposits that form round the base of the teeth. Gum disease is very common at all ages, and is the main cause of tooth loss. The condition may be caused by lack of dental hygiene, by ill-fitting dentures and by badly made crowns and fillings.

During the early stage of the disease, called *gingivitis*, the gums become swollen and infected and

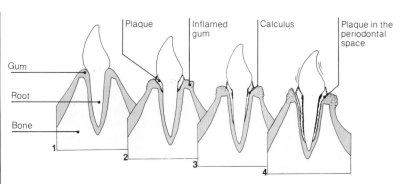

Periodontal Disease Healthy gums are pale pink and fit firmly around the tooth, **1**. When bacterial plaque forms between a gum and a tooth, the gum becomes red and inflamed and gingivitis sets in, **2**. The plaque is gradually deposited deeper and deeper into the periodontal space, forming a calculus on the tooth and weakening the gum, **3**. Untreated gingivitis progressively destroys the periodontal fibres that hold the tooth in place and allows pus to accumulate in the periodontal space, **4**. Finally, the tooth is loosened so much that it falls out.

bleed easily, especially when the teeth are brushed. At this stage a dentist or dental hygienist will remove the plaque, and teach the sufferer how to keep teeth and gums clean with dental floss. He or she may also advise the use of an antibacterial mouthwash and a disclosing agent, a mouthwash that discolours plaque so that it can be seen prior to cleaning the teeth.

If left untreated, the disease will spread to the tooth ligaments and bone. The bacteria eat into the bone and can eventually loosen the teeth until they fall out. The sufferer will have bad breath and aching gums.

The dentist will usually X-ray the mouth to find out whether the bone is affected. If the disease is far advanced, surgery on the gums—called gingivectomy—may be performed, either in the dentist's surgery or in a dental hospital.

The gums will be trimmed and a protective coating applied, usually of oil of cloves, zinc oxide and cotton wool, until the gums heal. If a tooth is loose, it may be held firmly in place with a periodontal splint, made of plastic or gold, which joins the tooth to others that surround it.

To a large extent, periodontal disease can be avoided if scrupulous dental hygiene is observed—*see Health and Hygiene, p334*.

PERITONEAL DIALYSIS—see Dialysis

PERITONITIS

An infection of the peritoneal cavity in the abdomen. The cavity is formed by a membrane called the peritoneum, which lines the abdomen and also surrounds the abdominal organs.

Peritonitis is usually the result of perforation of the intestines (*p40*). This may happen when the appendix ruptures, for example—*see appendicitis*—or be the result of a peptic *ulcer* or a ruptured diverticulum in the large bowel—*see diverticular disease*. The Fallopian tubes (*p54*) may also rupture if they are grossly infected, or stretched as the result of an *ectopic pregnancy*. In all such cases, bacteria and other material spill out into the abdomen, causing infection.

The infection may remain localized, as in the case of a ruptured appendix, which sometimes seals itself off to cause what doctors call an appendix mass in the right groin. Alternatively, the infection may spread through the abdomen. In such a case, the patient will be extremely ill, with high fever, abdominal pain and tenderness, and vomiting. If the condition is left untreated, the patient will become dehydrated and eventually die, as the infection overwhelms the body's natural defences against disease.

Treatment is with *antibiotics*, intravenous fluid replacement, and emergency surgery, if the patient's physical condition will stand immediate operation.

PERNICIOUS ANAEMIA

A form of anaemia caused by Vitamin B12 deficiency (*p322*). This vitamin is essential for healthy, productive bone marrow; without it, the numbers of red cells, white cells and platelets made in the bone marrow decrease (*p21*). The vitamin occurs naturally in meat, eggs and fish, raw liver being particularly rich in it.

The lack of Vitamin B12 stems from the body's failure to absorb enough of it from the intestine. This cannot take place unless the vitamin is first combined with a chemical, called intrinsic factor, secreted by the parietal cells in the stomach. Lack of this chemical means that absorption cannot occur, with pernicious anaemia as the consequence. This can happen for a number of reasons, from total *gastrectomy* to what is thought to be an *auto-immune* response in older women, and, very rarely, to a strict vegetarian diet with no meat or animal products.

Diagnosis is made by blood tests, which measure the B12 level—*see Special Tests, p84*. Most of the cells present are abnormally large. The diagnosis is confirmed by a Schilling test *(p84)*, in which the patient swallows a small amount of radioactive vitamin B12. This is then monitored to see how much of it has been absorbed.

Pernicious anaemia is treated by injections of vitamin B12 every one to three months for the rest of the patient's life.

PERSONALITY DISORDERS
Disorders of which the chief symptom is behaviour very different from that considered socially acceptable. In a personality disorder called kleptomania, for example, affected people compulsively steal articles of no great value. Other examples of such unacceptable behaviour include drug addiction and alcoholism—both drug addicts and alcoholics frequently suffer from personality disorders, though it is not clear-cut as to which is cause and which effect. In other cases, the sufferer is unaware of the problem, and it is relatives or friends who bring it to a doctor's attention. Personality disorders are treated by *psychotherapeutic* techniques such as *behaviour therapy*.

PERTUSSIS—see Whooping cough

PETIT MAL—see Epilepsy

PHAEOCHROMOCYTOMA
An uncommon *tumour* of the sympathetic nervous system *(p32)*, which is usually *benign*. The majority of such tumours are found in the adrenal glands *(p48)*. If left untreated, they cause severe high blood pressure—*see hypertension*—which may lead to *heart disease* and a stroke—*see cerebrovascular accident*.

Early symptoms include attacks of heavy sweating, during which the patient either becomes pale or flushes. The heart beats more intensely and the blood pressure usually rises. These attacks last from a few minutes to an hour or more. After some years the rise in blood pressure becomes sustained. This leads to enlargement of the heart, and the resulting damage to blood vessels increases the risk of coronary artery disease or strokes.

Diagnosis is made by testing the blood or urine for raised levels of adrenaline, a hormone produced by the adrenal glands. Normally, the

test is made on a sample of urine collected over 24 hours. CAT scans—*see Special Tests, p84*—can locate the site of the tumour, which is invariably removed by surgery. Large amounts of noradrenaline and adrenaline are sometimes discharged into the blood during the operation, and medication is given to counteract this. When the tumour has been removed, the patient's blood pressure usually returns to normal; in about 20 per cent of cases the pressure remains high and has to be treated with drugs. In about five per cent of cases the tumour recurs and further surgery is necessary.

PHARYNGITIS
Inflammation of the pharynx, the area of the throat between the back of the nose and the beginning of the trachea—*see The Respiratory System, p28*. This may be caused by *bacterial* or *viral* infection. An infection may also spread to the pharynx from the mouth, the sinuses, or the tonsils. Symptoms include hoarseness, difficulty in swallowing, fever and a sore throat. Treatment is with *antibiotics*.

See also upper respiratory tract infections.

PHENYLKETONURIA
A rare inherited condition which causes mental retardation. The condition is transmitted by a recessive *gene*. As a result of the condition, the child lacks the enzyme necessary to metabolize phenylalanine, a component of protein. The phenylalanine therefore accumulates in the body, affecting the function of the nervous system.

All new-born babies are screened for this disorder with the Guthrie test, in which a smear of blood is examined for the presence of the enzyme. The condition can also be detected soon after birth by a urine test. Treatment is by a special protein diet.

PHIMOSIS
Tightness of the foreskin, causing difficulty in drawing it back over the tip (glans) of the penis *(p54)*. In a new-born baby, the foreskin is not separated from the glans and normally no attempt should be made to withdraw it until at least the age of three. If, however, the baby finds it difficult to pass urine, treatment may be necessary.

Treatment is by a minor operation called *circumcision*, in which the foreskin is cut away, under general *anaesthetic*. Sometimes this becomes necessary in later life, when tightness of the foreskin causes a

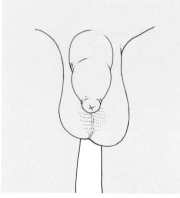

Phimosis is a tightness of the foreskin which prevents it from being drawn over the glans of the penis *(above)*. The condition cannot occur before the age of five, since the foreskin cannot be retracted before this. If phimosis persists and interferes with penile erection after puberty, the foreskin must be circumcised.

recurrent infection of the glans, called *balanitis*.

PHLEBITIS—see Thrombophlebitis

PHOBIA—see Neurosis

PHOTODERMATITIS
A *rash* caused by an *allergy*, often to soaps, detergents and shampoos. The skin is red, scaly and frequently itches, but the condition develops only when the affected area is exposed to sunlight.

The best treatment is to avoid the use of the substance causing the skin reaction. A patch test, in which suspected substances are applied to a small area of the skin, can be used to identify this. A *steroid* cream, and/or *antihistamine* tablets may be prescribed to control the allergic reaction.

PHYSIOTHERAPY
The term defining all the various physical therapies provided by trained physiotherapists to overcome the effects of various diseases and conditions. Examples of these include *arthritis, cerebrovascular accidents*—strokes—and *paralysis*.

In the course of their work, physiotherapists use special exercises, massage, manipulation, and modern scientific aids, such as infra-red lamps, to achieve a common aim. This is to encourage mobility, since, with any immobilizing condition, it is important not to let the muscles waste through lack of use. Often, such treatments are extremely successful; stroke patients, for instance, can often recover to a large degree.

PID—see Pelvic inflammatory disease

PILES—see Haemorrhoids

PILONIDAL SINUS

A skin cavity, called a sinus, containing hairs; the term literally means 'a nest of hairs'. The most common site for a pilonidal sinus is the hairy skin between the buttocks and at the base of the spine. The problem develops when a hair starts to grow inwards, carrying infection with it. Often, a large *abscess* develops, causing considerable pain. Treatment is with *antibiotics* to clear up the infection; minor surgery is often necessary to drain the pus and remove the hairs.

PINK EYE—see Conjunctivitis

PITTING OEDEMA

Swelling of the feet, legs, or ankles due to an excess of tissue fluid, which leaks out of adjacent blood vessels—*see oedema*. The condition is called pitting oedema because the pressure the swelling creates will leave a dimple or pit behind it when the pressure is removed.

Pitting oedema chiefly affects the elderly, particularly women. It may be caused by standing for protracted periods, or by wearing restrictive clothing, such as tight knee socks or garters. This can severely impede the blood flow and so cause swelling. The condition can also occur during pregnancy, as a complication of *varicose veins*, and be a symptom of *heart* or *liver disease*.

When the oedema is caused by poor venous return of blood from the legs as a result of long periods of standing, it is best treated by wearing support stockings, or by trying to exercise the legs as much as possible. Reducing salt levels by taking *diuretic* drugs may also help in treatment, as these promote the excretion of salt and water.

PITYRIASIS

A group of skin disorders in which a scaly *rash* is usually present.

Pityriasis rosea is a rash of itchy, oval-shaped red spots which gradually appear on the trunk and upper arms. The cause of the condition, which mostly affects children and young people, is unknown, though a *virus* is suspected. It generally disappears of its own accord, though *steroid* ointments may be prescribed if the rash is severe.

Pityriasis versicolor is a *fungal* infection in which pale or sometimes dark flaky skin patches appear on the trunk in dark-skinned people and darker patches appear on the skin of fair-skinned people. The condition is treated with antifungal ointment.

Pityriasis capitis is more commonly known as *dandruff*. It may be cured simply by using a good anti-dandruff shampoo, though, in some cases, a mildly acidic lotion or a steroid lotion.

PLACENTA PRAEVIA

A condition of pregnancy in which the placenta is situated extremely low down in the uterus—*see Pregnancy and Birth, p60*—and consequently lies in front of the baby's head. It may also overlap the cervix. The condition is often a dangerous one for both mother and baby. If it is not diagnosed before labour, the head of the foetus can compress the placenta as its descends into the pelvis, so cutting off its own blood supply. It is more usual, however, for the position of the placenta to prevent the head from descending and engaging in the pelvis.

Placenta praevia is now easy to diagnose and control, as the position of the placenta can be mapped on ultrasound—*see Special Tests, p84*—and checked at regular intervals if necessary. During pregnancy, the main risk is of a massive haemorrhage from the placenta, usually in the last three months. The haemorrhage may be initiated by strenuous sexual intercourse, or may begin spontaneously. As it occurs before labour, it is called ante-partum haemorrhage. Any substantial bleeding of more than a few spots in late pregnancy should be reported to a doctor. In cases where placenta praevia has been diagnosed, the mother is usually admitted to hospital at the 36th week of pregnancy and the baby delivered by *caesarian section*

PLANTAR RESPONSE

A reflex action of the big toe in response to stroking the side of the foot—*see The Nervous System, p32*. Movement of the big toe upwards, instead of downwards, indicates that the brain or spinal cord may have been damaged.

See also Babinski response.

PLANTAR WART—see Verruca

PLAQUE

A colourless, transparent layer of micro-organisms which grows on the crowns and spreads along the roots of teeth. If not removed by proper observance of dental hygiene—*see Health and Hygiene, p334*—it is the forerunner of dental *caries* and *periodontal disease*.

PLEURISY

Inflammation of the pleura, the sac-like membrane which surrounds the lungs—*see The Respiratory System, p28*—causing a sharp pain on taking a deep breath. The pain is caused by the two inflamed layers of pleura rubbing together. Pleurisy may be caused by a *viral* infection, or may be associated with a *bacterial* infection in the lungs.

Diagnosis can easily be made by listening to the chest with a stethoscope, since the creaking noise made by two layers rubbing together is clearly audible. The inflammation sometimes produces a surplus of pleural fluid, which collects between the two layers of pleura to cause a pleural effusion. This is painless, since the fluid protects the inflamed membrane against friction. Pleural effusion can be detected on physical examination—when the chest wall is tapped with the fingers, a dull note is produced—and by chest X-ray (*p84*).

In most cases, pleurisy is a fairly minor illness. If the cause is thought to be bacterial, the condition is treated with *antibiotics* and *analgesics*. In the case of viral infection, the patient should take aspirin, keep warm and if possible spend a few days in bed—*see Home Nursing, p352*. However, in a minority of cases, pleurisy may be a sign of a more serious disease, such as *pulmonary embolism* or *lung cancer*, while chronic pleurisy can be a symptom of *tuberculosis*.

PNEUMOCONIOSIS

A lung disease, caused by inhaling any one of several kinds of industrial dust over a long period of time. The irritating dust particles become lodged in the lungs and cause *fibrosis*. The chief symptom is progressive breathlessness. The disease is termed progressive; this means, after a certain stage, the fibrosis worsens regardless of whether or not the patient is exposed to dust.

There are various sub-classifications of the disease, depending on the dusts involved. Examples include *asbestosis*, caused by asbestos dust and fragments, and *silicosis*, caused by silica.

The main symptom is increasing breathlessness, which can force the sufferer to give up work. A cough and the production of excessive amounts of sputum are common—the spit may become blood-stained. Diagnosis is made by chest X-ray (*p84*), coupled with knowledge of the patient's work and the severity of symptoms. The outlook depends upon how far advanced the disease is at the time of diagnosis. At an advanced stage, the condition is fatal. For this reason, preventive measures are widespread. These

include the careful control of the dust content in industrial atmospheres, and regular chest X-rays for people at risk, so that action can be taken on the first sign of symptoms.
See also industrial diseases.

PNEUMONIA

An infection of the lung, usually caused by *viruses* or *bacteria*. These enter the lungs via the upper respiratory tract *(p28)*, their presence leading to inflammation of the lung tissue.

Pneumonia may affect a part of one lung—this is called lobar pneumonia—or both lungs—*bronchopneumonia*. The main symptom is a cough, together with *fever*, sweating and *rigors*. The patient may experience sudden chest pains and cough up yellow, green, or brown sputum. Sometimes the sputum is blood-stained.

Diagnosis is usually made by clinical examination and confirmed by chest X-ray *(p84)*. Treatment depends upon the cause of the disease. *Antibiotics* are not effective against viruses, though they are prescribed in the case of bacterial infection, Penicillin, however, is often avoided, since some bacteria are now penicillin-resistant. *Physiotherapy* is important to help clear the infection, while, in severe cases, oxygen may be necessary.

Young and middle-aged patients can be treated at home. Generally, recovery is quick, provided that they are reasonably physically fit. However, children, the old, and people with reduced resistance are more at risk from the disease.

PNEUMOTHORAX

Collapse of the lung due to air entering the pleural cavity between the two layers of pleura, one of which lines the chest wall and the other surrounds the lungs—*see The Respiratory System, p28*. The patient experiences a sudden, sharp pain in the chest, and may become breathless. Pain may also be felt on the tips of the shoulders.

The condition usually affects men in their late teens or early twenties. Treatment consists of passing a tube through the chest wall and into the air space under local anaesthetic. A special underwater seal apparatus allows the air to pass through a one-way valve, so that no further air can enter through the same tube. The lung can then expand fully again.

If the pneumothorax is small and the patient is young and otherwise fit, the lung gradually expands again of its own accord. Repeated collapse

is treated surgically. Talcum powder is introduced into the pleural cavity to help the lung adhere to the chest wall, so that it can expand normally.

POLIOMYELITIS

An infectious disease, sometimes resulting in paralysis. It can be caused by any one of three viruses, all of which damage the motor nerves running from the spinal cord to the muscles—*see The Nervous System, p32*. In about 50 per cent of cases, the result is permanent paralysis of some part of the body, particularly the legs. The extent of the paralysis is thought to depend upon the amount of physical exercise taken during the incubation period; the more vigorous the exercise, the more extensive the paralysis. Initially, symptoms are similar to those of *influenza*. A proportion of patients suffer no further symptoms. In some cases, however, they are followed by pain in the affected muscles and then paralysis.

There is no treatment for poliomyelitis. However, the disease is now extremely rare, at least in the Western world. It is now routine for children to be protected against the disease by *immunization*,—*see Health and Your Child, p348*.

POLYARTERITIS NODOSA (PAN)

A rare inflammatory disease of the arteries, which may occur anywhere in the body and occurs three times as often in men as in women. Nodules develop in the walls of the blood vessels, causing impaired circulation to nearby organs.

Symptoms include generalized pain, fever, sweating, localized *oedema*, and *hypertension*. If an organ suffers from *ischaemia*—or shortage of blood—other serious conditions may follow, such as *haematuria* if the kidneys are involved, or asthma-like symptoms if the lungs are affected. *Myocardial infarction, pericarditis,* or *angina pectoris* can occur if the heart is involved. The disease can occur in several places at once, so that these symptoms can occur in combination with one another.

Polyarteritis nodosa is thought to be a disorder of the immune system *(p52)*; many of the effects resemble those of *allergy*, but usually no cause can be found. It is a progressive disease, for which there is no cure, though *corticosteroid* drug therapy can help to control it in some cases. Furthermore, the large number of possible symptoms and side-effects make it difficult to diagnose and treat. Mild cases last for years and then resolve themselves, but in about half, patients die within five years of diagnosis.

POLYARTHRITIS—see Arthritis

POLYCYTHAEMIA

An abnormal increase in the number of red blood cells in the blood—*see The Blood and Lymph Systems, p21*. The increase is caused by insufficient oxygen reaching the blood cells; the bone marrow tries to compensate for this by increasing its production of red cells.

The condition most frequently occurs in heavy smokers, because the carbon monoxide in tobacco smoke combines with the red cells, so stopping them from carrying oxygen. Polycythaemia is also found among people living at high altitudes, where the atmosphere contains less oxygen. In chronic *bronchitis*, where lung damage 'reduces the oxygen supply, the increase in red cells may make the blood viscous and so clot more easily.

Polycythaemia is treated by the removal of a pint of blood from the body every month for six months. Sometimes the excessive production of new red cells is controlled by *radiotherapy* or drug therapy.

POLYMYALGIA RHEUMATICA

A inflammatory disease, causing aches and stiffness in the muscles of the hips and shoulders. The disease chiefly affects the elderly and is uncommon under the age of 50. *Corticosteroids* are the normal treatment. Though these normally relieve the symptoms quickly, they must be continued for a period of several years.

POLYMYOSITIS—see Myositis

POLYPS

Small tumours, which are almost always *benign*—harmless—attached to a mucous membrane by a stalk or 'foot'. They are also called polypi and can occur in the nose, larynx, cervix, and intestines.

Nasal polyps are swellings of the nasal membranes, caused by an *allergy*, such as hay fever, or by infection. They may interfere with breathing, or, if they block a passage to a sinus cavity, cause headaches. They are removed surgically.

The cause of other kinds of polyps is unknown, and often there are no symptoms. A polyp in the larynx may lead to hoarseness, while a cervical polyp may cause a watery, bloody discharge between periods, or after intercourse. Intestinal polyps may cause blood to appear in the faeces. In all three cases, the polyps are normally harmless, but are usually surgically removed by endoscopy—*see Special Tests, p84*—when discovered because they can burst, bleed and sometimes, in the case of intestinal polyps, cause obstruction. Cervical polyps, in particular, are examined carefully to ensure that they are benign.

POMPHOLYX

A type of *dermatitis* which appears on the palms of the hands and the soles of the feet. Blisters occur, and sometimes burst, while the skin may also crack and become infected. The condition is most common in young adults.

An attack usually lasts for two or three weeks. The rash can be caused by stress (p332), and there may be further attacks if this is not relieved. *Steroid* creams may be prescribed to relieve inflammation.

PORTAL HYPERTENSION

High blood pressure, or *hypertension*, in the network of veins carrying blood from the intestines and spleen to the liver—*see Metabolism, p44*. The condition may be caused by a blockage in the portal vein, which may be due to *thrombosis*, or compression by a hepatic *tumour*.

Probably the commonest cause of portal hypertension is *cirrhosis* of the liver. Cirrhosis obstructs the portal system, causing pressure to rise in the intestinal veins. As a result, a form of *varicose veins* called oesophageal *varices* develop at the lower end of the oesophagus, while *haemorrhoids* sometimes occur around the anus. These veins may rupture and cause massive bleeding—the most serious complication of portal hypertension. The spleen also swells—*see splenomegaly*—and may be felt beneath the ribs on the left side of the abdomen. Occasionally, fluid called *ascites* gathers in the abdominal cavity, in much the same way as it does around the ankles in *heart failure*.

If the patient is fit enough to withstand surgery, portal hypertension can be relieved by an operation called a portacaval anastomosis, or portacaval shunt. A connection is made between the portal vein and the inferior vena cava, allowing blood to bypass the liver. An alternative is to sew the splenic vein to the left renal vein. Both operations greatly reduce the risk of internal bleeding, though, because potentially poisonous substances normally detoxified by the liver can now reach the brain, there is the risk of *coma*. Protein-rich food is particularly dangerous, so a low protein diet must be followed for life after the operation.

Bleeding from oesophageal varices is a surgical emergency, which necessitates massive blood transfusions. It may sometimes be stopped by injecting a sclerosing agent into the veins though a gastroscope to harden them. Another form of treatment involves compressing the varices with a rubber balloon—*see varices*.

PORTACAVAL SHUNT—see Portal hypertension

POST-NATAL DEPRESSION

A term describing the feelings of *depression* experienced by some mothers after childbirth, also called post-partum depression. The feelings of depression vary in intensity. At one end of the scale, many women go through a short period—it may last only a day—of feeling depressed and tearful for no apparent reason, usually during the first week after the birth. They feel extremely vulnerable and are easily upset. This is commonly called 'post baby blues'.

More serious depression, however, can sometimes develop. This lasts much longer, and can be caused by a number of factors. The changing hormonal levels in the mother's body, associated with birth and breast-feeding, may be involved—*see Pregnancy and Birth, p60*. Compared to the excitement of birth, the first few weeks of motherhood may seem like an anti-climax, while, paradoxically, the enormous responsibilities created by the new baby may appear daunting. In addition, the mother may find it difficult to relax, as she is often exhausted through lack of sleep and through coping with the baby's constant needs and demands.

Sometimes, she may feel mentally and physically desperate as a result, both feelings being augmented by her inability to bring her problems into the open, since she sees being unable to cope with them as a personal failure. She may also suffer from physical discomfort, caused by soreness and breast engorgement, while possibly finding problems in establishing a breast-feeding routine.

The extreme of the condition is full-scale puerperal psychosis. This used to be regarded as a separate mental illness to which mothers were prone; it is now thought to be the natural result of the enormous physical and emotional stresses placed on a vulnerable personality by labour, delivery and the period immediately after birth. The classic symptom of this is complete detachment from the baby; the mother may go as far as to deny that the baby is hers.

Mild post-natal depression usually responds to explanation and reassurance. More severe depression may require treatment with *anti-depressants*. In extreme cases, puerperal psychosis may necessitate compulsory admission to a special psychiatric unit, where the patient can receive treatment and learn to care for her baby under supervision.

POST-PARTUM DEPRESSION—see Post-natal depression

POST-PARTUM HAEMORRHAGE

Excessive bleeding from the uterus after childbirth. Often this is caused by inadequate contraction of the uterine muscles, so that the bleeding produced by the placenta's separation from the uterus cannot be controlled—*see Pregnancy and Birth, p60*. The muscles may be weakened by an exhaustingly long labour, by stretching in a previous pregnancy, or by a sequence of pregnancies. Drugs may be administered to help the uterus to contract to avoid this problem, which must be treated as a surgical emergency.

PRE-ECLAMPSIA—see Eclampsia

PREMATURE EJACULATION—See Sex and Contraception, p338

PREGNANCY TEST

A simple test usually performed on an early morning urine specimen to detect pregnancy.

Approximately two weeks after the missed period—that is, six weeks after the last period, or four weeks after conception—the growing placenta secretes human chorionic gonadotrophin (HCG)—*see Pregnancy and Birth, p60*—in sufficient quantities to be detected in the urine by a simple agglutination test. The HCG can also be measured in the blood to confirm pregnancy, but the urine test is much more common. It can be carried out in the doctor's surgery, the microbiology laboratory, or by the patient with a self-diagnosis kit.

PREMATURITY

The birth of a baby before full term—*see Pregnancy and Birth, p60*. As there is often confusion about the date of the last menstrual period, prematurity is usually judged by the baby's weight. Babies weighing under 2,500g (5½lb) are said to be premature. Usually the cause of the prematurity is unknown.

Depending on the weight and other factors, the baby may be put into an *incubator* to keep it warm and given oxygen. It may be fed through a tube inserted through the mouth or noise into the stomach. Some premature babies may have difficulty breathing—*see respiratory distress syndrome*—or may be in danger of developing neonatal *jaundice*.

To a great extent, prematurity can be prevented by good ante-natal care. One important factor that should be remembered by all expectant mothers is the effect of smoking on baby weight. Babies born to mothers who smoke are often lighter than those born to those who do not.

PREMENSTRUAL TENSION
Physical and emotional changes which affect many women up to ten days before a menstrual period. More than 50 per cent of women experience some symptoms of PMT, which often becomes worse after the age of 35. Symptoms include irritability, depression, aggressiveness, headache, bloated stomach and tender breasts. Fluid retention usually occurs before a period, which may account for some of the symptoms, but PMT seems to be mainly due to hormonal changes prior to menstruation—*see Sex and Reproduction, p54.*

In severe cases *diuretics* and hormones may be prescribed to relieve symptoms. The hormone progestogen may be taken either in tablet form, or as a suppository before a period. Vitamin B6 therapy with pyridoxine is helpful in some cases, while painkillers may be given for headaches. If these forms of treatment are unsuccessful, mild *tranquillizers* may be prescribed for the worst days.

PRESBYOPIA
A condition in which the lens of the eye becomes less elastic, making it difficult to focus on objects at close range—*see The Nervous System, p32.* The condition is known as long-sightedness. It usually affects people over the age of 45, and the majority of people over 65. A sufferer may not be able to read a book normally, and can focus on it only at arm's length.

An optician will prescribe glasses with convex lenses to correct the fault. If glasses are already worn for other reasons, bifocals may be prescribed.

PRESENILE DEMENTIA—see Dementia

PRICKLY HEAT
A rash of red spots which can appear on the body or face during hot weather. Children, old people and the overweight are particularly susceptible to this condition. When the sufferer moves into the shade, the rash usually disappears in hours.

PROLAPSE
The displacement of an organ caused by weakness of the muscles and ligaments that support it. The uterus and vagina are the most common organs to be affected; if the muscles have been affected, such displacement can occur after childbirth, and the problem may affect older women, as the ligaments become slacker after the *menopause.*

If both the uterus and vagina prolapse, part, or all, of the cervix may be visible at the vulva, or even protrude completely from it. This is called a procedentia. In this case, symptoms may include a feeling of heaviness and discomfort, occasional backache, stress and incontinence. If untreated, the condition can lead to infection.

Pelvic exercises after childbirth help to prevent the prolapse occurring—*see Ante-natal and Post-natal Exercises, p320.* Dieting, together with exercises to strengthen the muscles of the pelvic floor, may be all that is needed to treat a minor prolapse. In more severe prolapses, a polythene ring may be used to keep the organs in place, the patient being examined every four months to check for tissue damage. If this is not successful, surgery may be necessary to support the uterus. In post-menopausal cases, the problem is sometimes treated by *hysterectomy.*

Occasionally, too, the rectum can

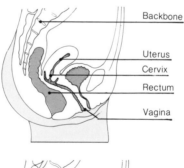

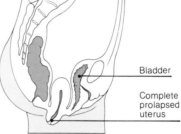

Prolapsed Womb The muscles and ligaments holding the uterus, cervix and vagina in place are normally strong and firm *(top)*. After childbirth or as a part of the ageing process, however, the muscles may weaken. This enables the uterus to prolapse, or fall, into the vagina, which sags and bulges as a result. In a complete prolapse of the womb, the uterus protrudes through the vaginal opening *(top)*. This is called a procedentia.

Image labels: Backbone, Uterus, Cervix, Rectum, Vagina, Bladder, Complete prolapsed uterus

prolapse and protrude as a result of excessive straining while defaecating. The prolapse is either manipulated back into position with a finger, or, if this fails, surgically replaced. A high-fibre diet helps prevents the problem—*see Diet, p322.*

PROLAPSED INTERVERTEBRAL DISC
The medical term for slipped disc. The intervertebral discs separate the vertebrae in the spinal column and act as shock absorbers between each pair of bones. Each disc is composed of two parts: an outer fibrous ring, which is firmly attached above and below to bone, surrounds an inner zone of jelly-like material called the *nucleus pulposus.* The disc cannot, in fact, slip; what happens is that a crack develops in the outer fibrous ring, which allows some or all of the nucleus pulposus to escape (prolapse) backwards into the vertebral canal. Here, it presses on the roots of spinal nerves or, sometimes on the spinal cord itself. The commonest site for this to happen is the lumbar region, but it can occur anywhere in the spinal column.

Disc prolapse is a very common condition; probably nearly half the population will experience it at some time in their lives. It can occur at any age but is commonest in middle life. Sometimes it follows a severe acute strain, such as lifting a heavy weight while twisting the back at the same time, but it can also come on after coughing, sneezing, stumbling, or for no apparent reason at all; in such cases the disc has been weakening progressively until at last even a small extra strain causes it to rupture.

If the prolapse occurs in the lumbar region, the result is usually an attack of pain in the lower back (lumbago). The onset can be immediately after the strain, or not for several hours or more. The pain is accompanied by a variable degree of spasm of the back muscles, which may prevent bending completely so that the sufferer cannot do up his shoelaces. After a few days, the pain in the back may ease, with the onset of pain going down one or other leg. This may be accompanied by pins and needles or loss of sensation and of reflexes in the leg, and is called *sciatica.* Most often the pain is felt down the back of the leg, possibly as far as the foot, but many other patterns occur. Occasionally there is inability to empty the bladder; this is an emergency, requiring urgent surgical treatment.

A prolapsed disc in the neck gives rise to pain in the neck and

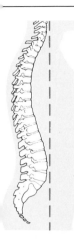

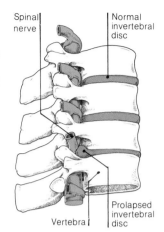

Prolapsed Invertebral Disc The individual vertebrae of the backbone *(left)* are separated by flexible discs of cartilage which act like shock absorbers when the back is moved. Undue strain on the back, particularly in the lumbar region, may rupture one of the invertebral discs, causing it to 'slip'. The prolapsed part of the disc *(right)* presses against a spinal nerve, causing pain in the area of the body served by the nerve.

Spinal nerve

Normal invertebral disc

Prolapsed invertebral disc

Vertebra

shoulder, with pain radiating down the arm, possibly as far as the hand.

Treatment for acute disc prolapse consists in giving drugs for pain relief and rest in bed. With this treatment most patients recover in about six weeks or less, though, for some, recovery takes longer—up to several months. Osteopathy or acupuncture are also sometimes used.

A few patients fail to recover and continue to suffer from lumbago and sciatica for years. In such cases surgery may be advised. Various surgical techniques are used, a common one being *laminectomy*, in which the spinal column is opened from behind and the prolapsed disc material is removed. Before an operation of this kind is undertaken a surgeon will carry out tests to establish whether a disc prolapse is in fact present and, if so, where it is; until recently a *myelogram*, in which fluid is injected to show up the discs on X ray, was the usual method, but nowadays a *CT scan* is sometimes performed instead.

PROSTATE DISORDERS

The general term for disorders of the male prostate gland—*see Sex and Reproduction, p54*—of which there are three main types. Prostatitis is the name given to the infection of the gland. The infection is usually caused by *bacteria* spreading to the prostate from the bladder and the result is pain on urination and, occasionally, blood in the urine. Treatment is with the appropriate *antibiotic*, depending on which bacterium is responsible for the condition.

Prostatic hypertrophy frequently occurs in elderly men. In it, the prostate gland becomes enlarged for no apparent reason, but, in doing so, compresses the urethra, which it surrounds. As a result, there is considerable pressure on both the bladder and urethra. Urine has to be passed frequently day and night—

see nocturia—the process being difficult to start and the flow being patchy, while afterwards there is often a terminal dribble. *Cystitis* is a possible complication, while, if the urethra is completely constricted, the bladder will be large, tender and distended, due to *retention of urine*.

To deal with the condition, it is usually necessary to remove part of the gland. This is done by means of a procedure called prostatectomy: either an incision is made in the abdominal wall, so the gland can be approached from the front, or a probe is passed up through the penis and pieces of the gland are removed by *diathermy*, rather like coring an apple.

Cancer of the prostate gland is the third most frequent form of cancer in men after *lung cancer* and *stomach cancer*. It tends to occur in men over the age of 60. It can cause frequent and difficult urination, as well as *haematuria*, the presence of blood in the urine. However, some cases are

symptomless, which makes the condition difficult to diagnose until the *tumour* has spread, or metastasized, to other parts of the body. Thus, it is often useless to remove the gland, since the cancer will have frequently spread from it.

Treatment is aimed at relieving any retention of urine, controlling any pain caused by the tumour and the associated secondary cancers, while hormone therapy is also given. The majority of patients improve when the hormone oestrogen is given, probably because it reduces the activity of the gonadotrophic hormones and the amount of androgens produced by the testes. If the therapy fails, the surgical removal of both testicles may reduce the size of the tumour—*see orchidectomy*.

PROSTATECTOMY—see Prostate disorders

PROTOZOA

A group of microscopically small animals, each consisting of a single cell, which may live as *parasites* in humans, causing disease. Examples include Plasmodium—*see malaria*—*Gardnella vaginalis*, and Trichomonas vaginalis—*see trichomoniasis*.

PROTEINURIA

The presence of protein in the urine. Occasionally, insignificant quantities of the protein albumin escape in the urine—especially after sleep, when the venous pressure in the kidneys is raised. This is called orthostatic proteinuria and is not indicative of any kidney disorder. Sometimes, during pregnancy, small amounts of protein are found in the urine. This

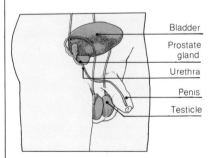

Bladder

Prostate gland

Urethra

Penis

Testicle

Prostatic Hypertrophy Every man has a prostate gland which surrounds the urethra as it leaves the bladder *(left and below)*. The gland contains tubules which make and secrete a fluid into the urethra during ejaculation. In prostatic hypertrophy, the gland is enlarged, so constricting the urethra, which runs through it. This, in turn, restricts the flow of urine. The bladder muscles enlarge as they try to force urine through the narrowed urethra *(below right)* and the bladder wall thickens. As a result, there is a frequent urge to urinate but only a small amount of urine is passed.

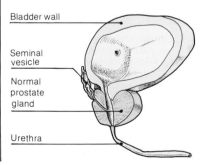

Bladder wall

Seminal vesicle

Normal prostate gland

Urethra

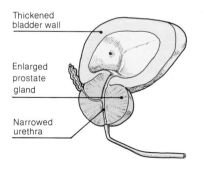

Thickened bladder wall

Enlarged prostate gland

Narrowed urethra

is because pregnancy can alter the sieve-like action of the kidneys. However, the amount of protein lost is minimal and ceases after childbirth. The loss of larger quantities during pregnancy may be an indication of pre-eclampsia—*see eclampsia*.

At other times, proteinuria is often a symptom of infections and inflammations of kidneys, bladder or urethra. Gross proteinuria is a feature of *nephrotic syndrome*, which is often caused by *glomerulonephritis*. The amount of protein in the urine can be roughly estimated in the doctor's surgery by means of specially coated dipsticks, and more precisely determined in the laboratory by special investigations—*see Special Tests, p84*.

PRURITUS

The medical term for itching. Pruritus is common in many skin conditions, but the term is usually applied specifically to itching when there is no visible cause for it in the skin. Pruritus may be localized, especially to the vulva or the anal region (where it is called pruritus ani); pruritus in these areas may be caused by fungal or other infections, or by lack of cleanliness; sometimes it has no apparent cause, in which case it is often due to psychological problems. These can produce intense localized itching in the skin without obvious cause.

Generalized pruritus is quite often seen in elderly patients in whom it is usually due to dryness of the skin; loneliness and depression make it worse. Generalized pruritus can occur as part of a number of systemic (internal) diseases—some kinds of jaundice, cancer, and kidney failure, for example. Anaemia can also cause pruritus, as can a lack of iron in the body.

If the cause of pruritus cannot be found or removed, the condition is treated by advising the patient to avoid overheating, alcohol, and hot drinks. Calamine lotion helps to cool the skin, which should be prevented from becoming too dry.

Antihistamines may reduce itching, as may ultraviolet light or sunlight.

PSITTACOSIS

A rare form of *pneumonia* caused by an infection carried by birds of the parrot family. The infection is spread in dust contaminated with faeces from an infected bird. The infecting organism was once thought to be a *virus*, but is now thought to be a small organism called *chlamydia*.

Psittacosis has an incubation period of between one and two weeks, after which symptoms of cough, *fever*, headache and general

malaise appear. In susceptible people, especially children and old people, the condition can be extremely serious. Diagnosis is by blood tests, and the disease is treated by the antibiotic *tetracycline*. This is usually successful, but a long period of convalescence may be necessary.

PSORIASIS

A common skin disorder that can affect any part of the body, in which itchy, red, flaky patches appear on the skin. The condition usually appears for the first time in adolescence.

The cause of psoriasis is not known, but various factors are thought to be connected with the condition: the disease tends to run in families; it is more common in cold, damp conditions than in the tropics; and it often appears for the first time after an acute illness, such as *tonsillitis*. Stress (*p332*) and anxiety may play a part in the development of psoriasis, and the condition often worsens at times of emotional or physical strain.

Large patches of psoriasis may occur on the scalp, knees, or elbows, while, in other types of psoriasis, the body is completely covered with red, scaly patches. Though there is no known cure, *steroid* creams seem to improve the disorder, though the psoriasis may increase again once application of the cream is stopped. Coal tar preparations and other ointments are often very effective, while ultra-violet treatment may also be recommended.

Severe psoriasis can be extremely debilitating in itself. It may occasionally also cause severe inflammation and tissue damage in the joints. This form of the condition, known as psoriatic arthropathy, leads to a particularly severe form of *arthritis*.

PSYCHOANALYSIS

A branch of psychiatry in which an analyst helps a person to understand and then come to terms with their problems by discussing past emotional experiences. In this way, present subconscious urges and worries are brought to the surface and acknowledged.

The precise way in which this is done varies according to which of the several schools of psychoanalyst the analyst subscribes. For example, some analysts subscribe to the Freudian school, named after the Austrian neurologist Sigmund Freud, in which the patient is asked to recall his or her dreams and fantasies. They believe that many psychological problems are the result of repressed, painful emotional experiences that

permanently affect the subconscious mind.

The main use of psychoanalysis is to treat neuroses—*see affective disorders*—rather than the *psychoses*, in which the mental state is often too altered to benefit from the technique.

PSYCHOSIS

Serious mental and behavioural disturbances, which make normal life impossible. Whether psychosis is an extreme form of *neurosis* or a completely different type of condition is controversial. Some experts believe the difference between the two is simply a matter of degree, while others think psychosis is a completely different disorder, caused by physiological changes in the nervous system. A patient is usually labelled a psychotic if he or she has withdrawn into a fantasy world, has delusions and hallucinations, or is unable to respond to the outside world.

Psychoses are classified into two groups. Organic psychoses are the result of damage to the central nervous system. Some of the conditions that can produce such damage and hence psychotic symptoms include head injuries, hardening of the arteries and lead poisoning.

Functional psychoses are thought to be caused by psychological factors, although biological causes may be involved. The most common psychoses are *schizophrenia*, in which hallucination and delusions are common; manic-depressive psychosis—*see affective disorders*—in which the sufferer is alternately very depressed and hyperactive and swings from one mood to the other in cycles of days, weeks or months.

Psychotic illnesses usually require hospitalization. Treatment is usually by drug therapy, often involving the use of major *tranquillizers*, though other forms of treatment, including *psychotherapy* and *group therapy*, may be prescribed. Unfortunately, however, the latter techniques are not often effective.

PSYCHOSOMATIC

A term used to describe a symptom that is not directly caused by disease or a physical problem, but is the result of emotional or psychological difficulties. A large proportion of the aches and pains about which patients consult their doctor are thought to be, in fact, psychosomatic in origin—pains such as headaches, dizziness and backache, particularly, are often psychosomatic. Nevertheless, to the patient such pains may be very real—*see The Doctor, The Patient and Disease, p70*.

PSYCHOTHERAPY

A form of treatment of minor mental disorders, which involves discussing the patient's problems rather than using drugs to treat them. Patients are encouraged to talk with a therapist, either singly in a one-to-one relationship, or in groups of people sharing similar problems.

From session to session, patients hope to gain a gradual and greater understanding of their problems and find support. Eventually, the aim is to help them solve their problems by themselves, and avoid similar ones in the future. The process is often protracted, involving many sessions stretching over a period of months and even years.

Therapists are not necessarily doctors. They have great experience in *counselling* and various techniques which encourage their patients to face up to problems.

PTOSIS

The drooping of one or both eyelids, caused by muscular weakness. Ptosis is a common symptom of *myaesthenia gravis*, for instance. Even if the muscle which lifts the eyelid is undamaged, it can be affected by disorders of either the main nerve supplying the eyelid, or part of the sympathetic nervous system *(p32)*.

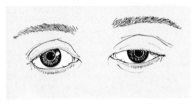

Ptosis In ptosis, the muscle that raises and lowers the eyelid is weakened, the eyelid droops and either partly or completely covers the eye . People may be born with this condition or develop it as a result of damage to the nerve or muscle controlling the movement of the eyelid, though it can occur naturally in old age, when all body muscles weaken. Both eyelids can be affected.

PUERPERAL FEVER

An infection of the vagina or womb which can lead to *septicaemia*—blood poisoning—usually contracted within two weeks of childbirth. The condition is now extremely rare and can be easily treated with *antibiotics*.

PUERPERAL PSYCHOSIS—see post-natal depression

PULMONARY ABSCESS—see Lung abscess

PULMONARY EMBOLISM

A sudden obstruction by a blood clot of the pulmonary artery or one of its branches. The clot usually starts as a *thrombosis* in the deep leg veins. This becomes detached, passes through the right side of the heart and then

Pulmonary Embolism The lungs have the ability to fragment small blood clots and to dissolve them. Such clots normally travel from veins elsewhere in the body, especially the deep veins of the leg *(below)*. However, when the blood clot is a large one, or when a large clot breaks up into a shower of small

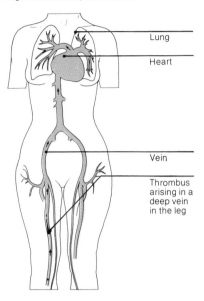

Lung
Heart
Vein
Thrombus arising in a deep vein in the leg

becomes trapped in the lungs, causing *ischaemia* in the part of the lung supplied by the affected artery.

Unless surgery is performed quickly or the clot dissolved, a large pulmonary embolism can cause sudden death. The patient suddenly becomes breathless and cyanosed; he or she may experience pain in the chest and become severely shocked. A small pulmonary embolism, however, may cause no symptoms, although, when at the periphery of the lungs, it may irritate the pleura and so cause pain. Preliminary diagnosis is made by chest X-ray and electrocardiogram and the findings confirmed by an angiogram—*see Special Tests, p84*.

Deep venous thrombosis is most likely to occur immediately after major surgery, when the patient has been confined to bed and the blood stagnates in the veins. It may also occur after childbirth, because the weight of the baby in the womb causes some obstruction of the pelvic veins. The risk of deep vein thrombosis is one of the reasons why patients are encouraged to get out of bed as soon as possible after an operation or childbirth. If the patient is confined to bed, simple leg exercises and special support stockings help.

Emergency treatment of a large pulmonary embolism can include cardiac massage, artificial respiration, and the administration of thrombolytic drugs to try to dissolve the clot.

Smaller pulmonary embolisms are

ones called emboli, the lungs are unable to cope. Consequently the blood clot lodges in the pulmonary artery, or in one of its branches, causing a pulmonary embolism. As a result, an area of the affected lung is deprived of blood *(below)* which causes pain, coughing, breathlessness and cyanosis.

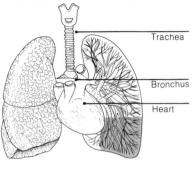

Trachea
Bronchus
Heart

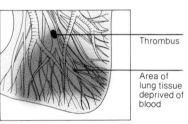

Thrombus
Area of lung tissue deprived of blood

treated with *anti-coagulant* drugs, which slow down the normal clotting time of blood. Frequent blood tests are carried out to ensure that the dosage is correct, as an overdose can lead to internal bleeding—*see Special Tests, p84*. In some cases, the treatment can last for a year or more, as the condition may recur. Most patients however, recover completely and can stop the drugs after six months.

See also embolism.

PULMONARY HYPERTENSION

A chronic rise in the pressure of blood circulating through the lungs—*see The Respiratory System, p28*—which can be caused by a number of factors. These include *mitral stenosis*—the narrowing of the mitral valve in the heart—chronic *bronchitis* and *pulmonary embolism*.

Pulmonary hypertension gives rise to *pulmonary oedema*—an accumulation of fluid in the lungs—which, in turn causes breathlessness, the main symptom of the condition. The sputum may also be tinged with blood. Diagnosis is by chest X-ray *(p84)* and the measurement of the pressure in the pulmonary blood vessels by passing a catheter along a vein through the right side of the heart, into the pulmonary artery. Pulmonary hypertension is treated according to its cause. Mitral stenosis, for example, may be repaired by surgery; recurrent pulmonary emboli are treated by *anti-coagulants*.

PULMONARY OEDEMA

An accumulation of fluid in the lungs—*see oedema*—caused by the stagnation of blood in the lungs, as occurs in left-sided *heart failure*, or by an increase in the pressure of blood in the lungs—*see pulmonary hypertension*.

Pulmonary oedema causes breathlessness, especially when lying down. Treatment is according to the cause of the problem, and *diuretics* are given to directly reduce the fluid level in the body.

PULMONARY STENOSIS—see Congenital heart defects

PUPILLARY REFLEX

The automatic contraction of the pupil—*see The Nervous System, p32*—when light is shone into the eye, called the direct light reflex, and also the contraction of the pupil of the opposite eye, called the consensual reflex. This reflex is an important aid when diagnosing and assessing the extent of head injuries. When the sensory part of the reflex is paralysed, for instance, this is an indication of serious bleeding inside the skull.

PURPURA

A purple spotted skin rash caused by bleeding from the capillaries. The spots can be anything from the size of a pin head to 2.5cm (1in) in diameter. The condition is a symptom of disease rather than a disease in itself. It can be a symptom of *leukaemia*, for example, or can be caused by a rare allergic reaction. The problem sometimes occurs in elderly people, when it is termed senile purpura. In this, the rash commonly appears on the hands.

PYELONEPHRITIS

An inflammation of the kidney, usually caused by a bacterial infection. When the condition is confined to the pelvis of the kidney—the point where the urethra joins the kidney—it is known as pyelitis. Both diseases can be acute or chronic; they have the same cause, symptoms and treatment.

Pyelonephritis may accompany an obstruction of part of the urinary tract, which causes the urine to stagnate and so predisposes to infection. In men, the obstruction may be due to an enlarged prostate gland—*see prostate disorders*—or a stone in the ureter or kidney. In pregnant women, the weight of the womb may cause an obstruction. In children, pyelonephritis is usually associated with a bladder, kidney or urethral abnormality.

The disease may also occur in the absence of such an obstruction. Kidney infections are fairly common in *diabetes*, for instance. The infection may spread from the rectum to the urethra and then to the bladder and up the ureters to the kidneys. The proximity of the urethra and rectum in women probably accounts for the number of adult women who suffer from pyelonephritis, and emphasizes the necessity of good hygiene—*see Health and Hygiene, p334*.

Symptoms include *fever*, hot sweats, low backache, and *rigors*. The patient may also frequently pass small amounts of cloudy urine, while the act of passing urine causes pain and a stinging sensation. This is due to *cystitis*, which is usually associated with the disease.

Diagnosis is made by examining the small of the back for tenderness,

and by bacteriological examination of a specimen of urine—*see Special Tests, p84*. Treatment is by *antibiotics*.

Recurrent pyelonephritis, or inadequate treatment, may lead to chronic pyelonephritis, *hypertension* and, in extreme cases, *kidney failure*. It is vital that the infection is treated without delay, and that a urine specimen is examined after antibiotic treatment has finished to ensure all the bacteria have been killed.

After treatment of an acute infection, an intravenous pyelogram—*see Special Tests, p84*—is usually performed to detect any possible obstruction in the urinary tract. If an obstruction is discovered, it is usually removed surgically.

See also kidney disorders.

PYLORIC STENOSIS

A narrowing of the outlet of the stomach to the duodenum—*see The Digestive System, p40*—that usually affects children, being more common in boys than in girls. It may be present from birth, or else appear in adulthood as a result of peptic *ulcer*.

The symptoms of congenital pyloric stenosis usually begin in the second or third week after birth. The main symptom is violent, or 'projectile', vomiting. At first, the baby only vomits occasionally after a meal, but, after a while, he vomits after every feed. The vomit usually contains milk curds, but no bile. As food fails to reach the intestine, the baby does not put on sufficient weight and is constipated.

In some instances, the condition is treated with drugs to relax the affected muscle. Generally, an operation is required,

PYREXIA—see Fever

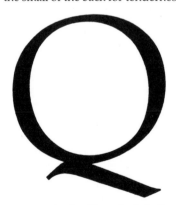

Q FEVER

An infectious disease caused by Coxiella burneti, a parasitic micro-organism of the *Rickettsiae* family. The organism is found in wild animals and sheep, cows and goats and is carried from one animal to another by ticks. Humans become infected by drinking contaminated,

unpasteurized milk, or by inhaling infected dust.

Q fever has an *incubation period* of between one and three weeks, after which symptoms similar to those of *influenza* appear. There may be a severe headache, tiredness and a *fever*, usually with a cough and pain in the chest; a chest X-ray (p84) may

show areas of inflammation. Occasionally, other organs are involved and there may be *hepatitis*, *endcocarditis* or *meningitis*. The disease is treated with *antibiotics*.

QUADRIPLEGIA

The paralysis of all four limbs. The most common cause of quadriplegia is injury to the spinal cord caused by road traffic accidents or sporting injuries. The condition is usually permanent, but after physiotherapy and rehabilitation in special centres, many quadriplegics learn to be completely independent in their wheelchairs; if a house has been specially adapted and special equipment is available they may be able to live at home—*see Looking After Disabled People, p358.*

See also *paraplegia*.

QUARANTINE
A period of enforced *isolation* during the infectious phase of a *contagious* disease. The quarantine periods of different diseases are listed in the table. *See immunization*.

QUINSY
An *abscess*, or infected swelling, of the tissue that surrounds the tonsils *(p21)*, which often follows a severe attack of *tonsillitis*

The abscess causes pain and swelling in the neck as well as difficulty in swallowing. There is usually a *fever* with aching limbs, and the sufferer often feels extremely ill.

The doctor will be able to diagnose quinsy easily by an examination of the throat. The abscess usually ruptures spontaneously and clears up without treatment. However, *antibiotics* are prescribed to prevent the infection from spreading to the ears and sinuses.

If the abscess does not burst spontaneously it may be lanced by a doctor, under local anaesthetic, to allow the pus to drain away. Hot salt mouthwashes and a course of antibiotics are given to ensure complete healing.

Quinsy is much less common these days as tonsillitis is usually treated quickly and effectively with antibiotics. However, some children suffer from recurrent attacks of quinsy, and in these cases the tonsils may be removed.

R

RABIES
A serious, usually fatal, viral disease that is transmitted to humans by animals. This can happen as a result of a bite from an infected animal, or through the contact of infected saliva on a cut or graze.

The incubation period is usually between 30 and 70 days, although it may be as short as nine days or take several months. This is because the time it takes for the virus to reach the spinal cord and brain varies, depending on the site of the original infection. However, not everyone who is bitten by an infected animal develops rabies.

The first symptoms are a slight *fever*, accompanied by pain or pins and needles at the site of the infection and, in many cases, *anxiety*. The next stage is a high fever and powerful spasms of the throat muscles. These spasms are triggered by the sight, sound or even mention of water—hence the old name for the disease, hydrophobia. Later, the patient suffers from periods of *delusions* and *hallucinations*, during which spitting and biting are common. These are punctuated by lucid spells. Generally, *paralysis* and death follow within a week.

There is no treatment for rabies, though the symptoms can be relieved by sedation, and once the illness has developed rabies is invariably fatal. However, its development may sometimes be prevented during the incubation period. After a bite from an animal suspected of having rabies, immediate hospital admission is essential. The wound is thoroughly cleansed, and the patient is then given an *antiserum*. A new serum called human rabies immune globin may be injected around the wound and into the nearby muscles. This is a much safer method of treatment than the one offered by the most widely available of the older serums, since these caused paralysis in one in 1,600 recipients, and severe pain in the majority. Injections are given at regular intervals for a period of three months from the day of the bite.

Rabies is rare in the UK, but the disease is *endemic* in Europe. Vaccines are available to protect vets, farmers and other people whose occupations put them at risk from the disease. A specific vaccine is also available for domestic animals. In the UK, however, animals can be vaccinated against rabies only if leaving the country.

Unfortunately, rabies has spread westwards from eastern Europe during the last few years and has now reached northern France. The UK's stringent quarantine laws have so far prevented the reintroduction of the disease into the country.

RADIATION SICKNESS
An illness caused by excessive exposure to radioactivity, such as that contained in X-rays, gamma rays, plutonium and other radioactive elements. Excessive exposure to radiation may be the result of the explosion of an atomic weapon, a leak of radiation from a nuclear power plant, or of *radiotherapy* treatment for *cancer*.

High dosages of radiation destroy parts of the nervous system, and people exposed to such dosages normally die within hours. Low, but repeated, dosages of radiation can cause acute *vomiting* and *diarrhoea*, followed a week or so later by hair loss and internal bleeding, with blood appearing in the faeces. These symptoms cause serious *dehydration*, and are likely to prove fatal unless controlled.

Survival, therefore, depends on the level of radiation to which a sufferer is exposed. However, radiation also has long-term effects. The risk of contracting *leukaemia* and a variety of *cancers* has been shown to be much greater in survivors of the Hiroshima and Nagasaki explosions of 1945 than in the population as a whole. In addition, since growing cells are particularly sensitive to radiation, there may be permanent damage to the gonads—*see Sex and Reproduction, p54*—causing sterility. For the same reason, women who are pregnant at the time of exposure stand an increased risk of giving birth to a malformed baby—*see congenital abnormalities.*

RADIOTHERAPY
The use of radiation to treat *malignant* disease. During the many

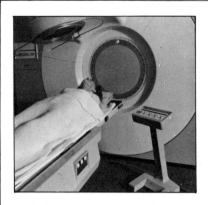

Radiotherapy Over the years, radiotherapy has become a major method of treatment for cancer. Carefully-controlled dosages of radiation are used to destroy the malignant cells of cancerous tumours. These can be given in either of two ways — either by irradiating the area of the tumour externally *(above)*, or by implanting radioactive material in the tumour in the form of a pellet or needle.

years in which X-rays were used solely in the diagnosis of disease, it was observed that radiation could kill growing cells. As scientists began to understand the mechanism of *cancer*, it was realized that carefully judged dosages of radiation could be used to destroy the rapidly growing cells of malignant tumours. Radiotherapy techniques have been refined, with the result that the effect of radiation on healthy tissues can now be minimized.

Radiation may be applied to a tumour in either of two ways, depending on its size and position. Normally, the radioactive material is housed in a special machine, which directs controlled amounts of radiation at the tumour. In other cases, the radioactive material is implanted in the tumour, in the form of controlled-release needles or pellets. Since healthy tissues may be affected by the radiation to a greater or lesser extent, radiotherapy may be cause unpleasant side-effects—*see radiation sickness*. These effects may include nausea and vomiting, hair loss and a general feeling of tiredness and ill-health.

Radiotherapy treatment is given over a period of time, often combined with chemotherapy, in which *cytotoxic* drugs are given. Some types of tumour—the lymphomas associated with Hodgkin's disease, for example—are known to be more sensitive to radiotherapy than others; such tumours often rapidly shrink in response to treatment.

RASH

A discoloration of the skin. There are many different types of rash, but most are temporary: the result of an illness or skin disorder. Rashes may be localized, confined to one part of

the body, or generalized, covering the whole body.

A rash may consist of a red, blotchy discolored area—as in some forms of *dermatitis*, for example—or of widespread collections of tiny red spots, which merge together to give a blotchy appearance—as in *measles*. Sometimes the spots are larger, as in *chickenpox*, and contain a blob of fluid. Such spots are known as vesicles; in time, they break down, forming scabs.

Certain illnesses are characterized by their rashes. Such illnesses include *chickenpox, measles* and *rubella*. In each case the rash begins in a particular place, spreads in a well known pattern and lasts for a certain length of time before disappearing.

Most rashes fade away in time, without leaving any scars—unless, in the case of chicken pox, they have been scratched. Itchiness associated with a rash can be relieved by the application of soothing lotions, such as calamine. However, if a rash does not clear up within a few days, a doctor should be consulted. He or she may prescribe *antihistamine* tablets to relieve the itching if an *allergic reaction* is responsible, or initiate appropriate treatment if the rash has a different cause.

See also nappy rash.

RAYNAUD'S DISEASE

A disorder in which the arteries of the fingers, and sometimes of the toes, contract in spasm. As a result, the affected areas turn white and numb, then blue and finally red. They may be painful, tingling and burning.

In Raynaud's disease, this happens as a response to cold, and mainly affects young women. Why this happens is not known. In Raynaud's phenomenon, sometimes called Raynaud's syndrome, the changes have a more serious cause. They may be symptoms of a disease affecting the circulation, such as *atherosclerosis*, or of a connective tissue *(p16)* disorder, such as *scleroderma* or *lupus erythematosus*. Raynaud's phenomenon is also a hazard for people whose hands are subject to constant vibration, as a result, for example, of operating a pneumatic drill.

Raynaud's disease is rarely a serious problem, and usually improves with age. It is difficult, however, to distinguish Raynaud's disease from Raynaud's phenomenon. The latter may have serious effects. These include endarteritis, an inflammation of the arteries of the fingers and toes which

may lead to the formation of a blood clot, called a *thrombus*. If untreated, this may cause *gangrene*, and necessitate amputation of the affected part.

When Raynaud's phenomenon is caused by disease, the symptoms usually improve as soon as the disease is treated; if the cause is occupational hazard, sufferers are advised to take time off work. Regardless of the cause, however, the hands and feet should be kept warm and protected from cold. Sufferers who smoke are advised to give up—*see Abuses of the Body, p328*—since smoking exacerbates the problem.

Such measures are often successful in preventing the problem from affecting the toes. Raynaud's phenomenon in the fingers, however, is more intractable. Should the condition become chronic, an operation called a *sympathectomy* may be necessary. In this, the sympathetic nervous supply to the limbs is removed, so that the arteries no longer have the ability to contract—*see The Nervous System, p32*

REFERRED PAIN

A pain that occurs in a part of the body apparently unaffected by the original disorder or injury. Pain from the digestive tract, for example, may be at a specific point some distance from the site of the problem. This may happen because nerves from different parts of the body share the same pathways in the spinal cord, and impulses are exchanged between them—*see The Nervous System, p32*.

REHABILITATION

The process by which a person recovering from a disease or disability is helped to return, as far as possible, to a normal life, and to come to terms with any limitations in activity. A team of health workers is involved, including doctors, a *physiotherapist, occupational therapist* and *speech therapist*. Social workers and the district nurse continue the process of rehabilitation at the patient's own home—*see Looking After Disabled People, p358*.

REITER'S SYNDROME

An illness resembling *gonorrhoea* that affects men but not women. In the classic form, non-specific *urethritis* (NSU), *conjunctivitis* and inflammatory *arthritis* are combined, but variants occur in which only one or two of these symptoms are present. Reiter's syndrome is thought to be caused by a *viral* infection; most commonly, it is transmitted by sexual activity, but it can follow a bout of bacterial *dysentery*.

The first symptoms usually appear suddenly, around three weeks after the original infection, but may vary widely, making diagnosis difficult. Sometimes, there is a *fever*, with pain and swelling in the joints, some soreness in the urethra and *conjunctivitis*. Other patients feel pain in the heels, the Achilles tendons or the feet, together with *balanitis* and a *rash* on the hands, feet, scalp or trunk.

Initially, treatment consists of bed-rest and painkillers. In most patients the conjunctivitis is mild, and clears up without treatment within a month. In some cases, however, a serious eye inflammation—*see iritis*—occurs from the outset of the disease. This requires immediate treatment with *corticosteroid* drugs. The NSU usually responds to *antibiotics*. Serious arthritic pains may require treatment with *anti-inflammatory* drugs, but mild pains usually disappear spontaneously within two to three months. However, Reiter's syndrome may have complications. These include back pain and stiffness, caused by a *sacroileitis*, spondylitis—a degeneration of the spinal joints—and meningo-*encephalitis*, peripheral *neuropathy*, *pericarditis* and *pleurisy*.

The syndrome has an unfortunate tendency to recur; 10 per cent of patients experience recurrences as many as 20 years after the first attack, even if they have not been exposed to further infection. Sufferers should abstain from sexual activity while symptoms are in evidence.

REMISSION
A period during the course of a long-standing and progressive disease in which the patient's condition temporarily improves, and the progress of the disease is halted. Periods of remission may last for anything from days to 20 or more years—*see multiple sclerosis*; they may be induced by treatment, or occur spontaneously.

RENAL FAILURE—see Kidney disorders

RESECTION
The surgical removal of body tissue. A diseased or malfunctioning part of the intestine, for example, may be resected and the remaining healthy tissue joined together to restore normal function.

RESPIRATORY DISTRESS SYNDROME (RDS)
A serious and sometimes fatal condition affecting the respiration of premature babies. The precise cause of respiratory distress syndrome is not known, but a number of factors contribute towards it. These include an inadequate supply of oxygen to the foetus while it is in the womb; *diabetes* in the mother; and, since RDS rarely affects full-term babies, low birth weight and immaturity.

The lungs of a full-term baby contain *surfactant*, a substance secreted by the cells of the alveoli—*see The Respiratory System, p28*. The function of surfactant is to reduce surface tension and prevent the walls of the alveoli from sticking together. Surfactant is absent, or much reduced, in babies suffering from RDS, and, as a result, air cannot inflate the alveoli. Breathing becomes difficult, and the baby suffers from a lack of oxygen—*see hypoxia*.

Eventually, a thin membrane forms in the lungs, exacerbating the problem—this is called a hyaline membrane because its composition is similar to that of hyaline cartilage.

The new-born baby is too breathless to suck at the breast, takes on a bluish colour—*see cyanosis*—and, characteristically, grunts as he or she strives to breathe. The lower part of the breast bone and ribs often appear to be drawn inwards. Diagnosis is confirmed by a chest X-ray—*see Special Tests, p84*.

The main aim of treatment is to keep the baby alive until the lungs have matured sufficiently to secrete surfactant. This is done by nursing the baby in an incubator, giving oxygen when necessary, and sometimes by the use of a *ventilator*. However, the risk of a premature birth, and so of RDS, can be reduced by regular attendance at ante-natal classes and clinics—*see Pregnancy and Birth, p60*.

RESTLESS LEGS SYNDROME (EKBOM'S SYNDROME)
A common disorder, in which the patient feels intense discomfort in the legs, but only at rest. The sensations are of pins and needles, burning, or actual pain, and are relieved only briefly by change in position. Some patients cannot sleep because of the discomfort.

In many patients, especially women, the cause is anaemia. In this case, giving iron by mouth relieves the symptoms completely.

RETARDATION—see Mental subnormality

RETENTION OF URINE
The inability to empty the bladder of urine. This commonly affects elderly men, in whom there is a tendency for the prostate gland to enlarge and constrict the urethra, the outlet from the bladder to the penis—*see prostatic disorders*. Occasionally, retention of urine is caused by a disorder affecting the nervous system, such as *multiple sclerosis*, or by a blood clot or *tumour* that compresses the spinal cord and affects the nerve supply to the bladder. In women, the most common cause of retention of urine is inflammation of the urethra caused by severe cystitis.

Sometimes the problem develops suddenly, with the result that urination becomes impossible and the bladder swells, becoming extremely tender and painful. Usually, however, the process is more gradual. In such cases, there is frequent urination during the day, with only a small amount of urine passed on each occasion, and leakage at night—*see incontinence*. Most of the urine is retained, however, and the bladder gradually enlarges over a period. Eventually, it may sometimes be seen and felt as a large round swelling that reaches as high as the umbilicus—the appearance is similar to that of mid-pregnancy.

The retained urine stagnates, predisposing to infection. This infected urine may reflux through the ureters, causing *kidney* infections. The increased pressure of fluid in the bladder may also be transmitted to the kidneys through the ureters. This process, called *hydronephrosis*, may result in enlargement of the kidneys and serious damage to their tissues.

For these reasons, it is important that the build-up of urine is released as soon as possible. This is done by inserting a catheter into the bladder. An operation to remove the enlarged prostate gland may be necessary at a later date—*see transurethral resection (TUR)*.

RETINOPATHY
A degeneration of the retina of the eye—*see The Nervous System, p32*. Retinopathy is sometimes the result of high blood pressure—*see hypertension*. The most common cause, however, is *diabetes*. In this case, the condition is known as diabetic retinopathy.

Diabetic retinopathy is the most common cause of *blindness* in middle-aged people. Diabetes causes the formation of *aneurysms*, or swellings, in the walls of the arteries feeding the retina, and twists in the retinal veins. This results in tiny *haemorrhages* and the degeneration and death of areas of retinal tissue. New blood vessels develop, but these are fragile and easily leak and rupture.

Without treatment, the disease progresses and the retina becomes covered with fibrous tissue, resulting in total blindness. If the condition is diagnosed by retinoscopy—*see Special Tests, p84*—at an early stage, however, it can often be treated successfully by a technique known as photocoagulation. In this, a laser is used to destroy the abnormal, fragile vessels of the retina and to hasten the absorption of the fluid that has leaked into the eye. Nevertheless, the diabetes must be carefully controlled to prevent the condition from recurring; once retinopathy has progressed to the later stages it may be impossible to prevent blindness.

REYE'S SYNDROME

A rare, but serious children's disease affecting the brain and liver, that may be precipitated by giving aspirin to reduce a temperature. It was first described in the 1960s, and most of the reported cases have been in the USA. It starts with an apparently trivial infection, such as a cold or gastrointestinal upset. After about three days, there is a sudden worsening, with repeated vomiting and neurological signs, including impairment of consciousness and fits. At this time the liver is abnormal, containing excessive amounts of fat, and the brain is swollen.

When Reye's syndrome was first recognized, over 80 per cent of patients either died or suffered severe brain damage. Now, if the children are treated by specialists, the results are much better, with up to 75 per cent making a complete recovery. Because the condition is now known to be precipitated by aspirin, children should never be given aspirin to bring down a fever; paracetamol should be used instead.

RHESUS MISMATCH—see Haemolytic disease of the newborn

RHEUMATIC FEVER

A serious illness whose precise cause is unknown. Rheumatic fever is often preceded by an attack of *tonsillitis, pharyngitis,* or other *upper respiratory tract infection,* and is thought to be caused by a reaction to the *streptococcal* bacterium. The illness was once common among children and adolescents in the West, but now occurs mainly in Asia, Africa and eastern Europe. The condition is most common among people whose housing and sanitation are inadequate.

The onset of rheumatic fever may be gradual, with loss of weight and a general feeling of tiredness and ill-health. More often, however, it begins suddenly, with a *fever* in which the affected child sweats profusely, refuses food and becomes constipated. The fever is often accompanied by a racing pulse, pain, swelling and stiffness in the joints; in some children, the limbs may jerk and twitch involuntarily—*see chorea.*

In the majority of cases, the pericardium, the membrane surrounding the heart, and the endocardium, the lining of the heart and heart valves, become infected—*see pericarditis; endocarditis.* In the short term, this may cause a heart *murmur,* but in around 50% of cases the long-term result may be damage to the heart valves—*see valvular heart disease.* (This problem is sometimes known as rheumatic heart disease).In severe cases, small lumps, called rheumatic nodules, appear under the skin of the elbows, knees, shoulder blades, the back of the head and the spine; in others a red, crescent-shaped rash with a white centre may form on the chest.

Treatment consists of bed-rest, aspirin to help to reduce inflammation and pain, and *antibiotics* to fight the infection; in severe cases *steroids* are administered to control inflammation of the heart and joints. The symptoms usually subside after a few weeks, but a long period of convalescence may be needed before the sufferer can resume normal activity. During this period, an ECG (electrocardiogram)—*see Special Tests, p84*—may be performed to establish whether the heart has been affected. Because there is a danger that serious damage to the heart valves will ensue if there is a recurrence of rheumatic fever, sufferers often have to take *antibiotics* as a preventive measure for many years.

RHEUMATIC HEART DISEASE—see Rheumatic fever

RHEUMATOID ARTHRITIS

A chronic, inflammatory form of arthritis that affects people of all ages, but most commonly arises between the ages of 30 and 50 and affects women more often than men. The precise cause of rheumatoid arthritis is unknown. One theory states that it is caused by an infecting organism, but most of the available evidence suggests that it may be caused by an inherited *auto-immune* disorder.

Rheumatoid arthritis may take a number of forms. Most commonly, however, the first sign is swelling, stiffness, inflammation and pain in the small joints of the fingers and toes. This often occurs after rest, especially on waking in the morning. The symptoms gradually spread, involving the joints of the wrists, elbows, shoulders, feet, and ankles. There is often pain in the neck and spine, and in the most severe cases, the hip joint is involved. The symptoms are sometimes experienced in sudden, severe attacks, lasting for a few hours and affecting only one part of the body. In a small proportion of cases, however, pain simultaneously affects a number of joints, and is accompanied by *fever,* weight loss and extreme tiredness. This form of the condition is known as polyarthritis.

Rheumatoid arthritis is a progressive disease, and eventually the inflammation leads to a gradual deterioration of the affected joints, and spasm in the related muscles causes disability and deformity. Flexion contractures—shrinking of the muscles—in the fingers, hands, toes and feet are common, with the result that the sufferer loses the use of his or her hands and feet. Since the disease affects the entire body, other disorders, including *Raynaud's phenomenon, lymphadenopathy; osteoporosis,* muscle weakness and wasting, *keratoconjunctivitis, pleurisy* and *neuropathy,* may occur as complications.

Treatment is directed towards relieving symptoms, arresting the progress of the disease and preserving, as much as possible, the function of the affected joints. The earlier the disease is diagnosed the more effective the treatment is likely to be. A combination of measures are used. *Anti-inflammatory drugs; rest,* to repair severely affected joints and *physiotherapy* are all vital. If necessary, contractures can be treated by surgery, and particularly painful joints can be splinted until the worst symptoms subside.

If the symptoms are mild, the sufferer is advised to rest in a bed for two or three weeks to induce a remission of the symptoms. The bed should have a hard mattress and a back rest, but few pillows. To prevent deformities from developing, an hour each day should be spent lying flat—a simple measure to prevent the development of flexion contractures of the hips—and a exercise programme followed to keep the affected parts of the body mobile—*see Exercise, p316.*

Several drugs have proved helpful in the treatment of rheumatoid arthritis. These include *corticosteroids; analgesics,* especially aspirin; drugs of the chloroquine family, used in the treatment of *malaria;* penicillamine (a drug that binds metals); gold; and *immunosuppressive* drugs. In addition, the sufferer may be prescribed specific drugs to treat any complications that may arise, together with minerals, such as iron, and vitamins, to improve overall health.

Many special diets have been devised, both by doctors and by sufferers, to help reduce the effects of rheumatoid arthritis. Most of these are based on foods low in acids. Although some sufferers claim that such diets bring about prolonged periods of remission or spectacular improvement, low acid diets do not appear to be effective in the majority of cases. However, research is being carried out to see if any dietary factor can be identified as causing or exacerbating the disease.

Orthopaedic surgery is often suggested when drugs and physiotherapy fail to relieve pain effectively, or recommended to arrest the progress of the disease. For example, a synovectomy—the removal of the synovial membrane in a joint— may help to relieve painful pressure. Reconstructive surgery can sometimes help a sufferer to regain the use of a limb, hand or finger in cases where tendons, cartilage and bone have drastically deteriorated.

Sufferers from rheumatoid arthritis can call upon a large team of health workers to help them adapt to problems caused by the disease and prevent its progress. The team includes doctors, nurses, physiotherapists, orthopaedic surgeons, *occupational therapists*, counsellors and housing and social services officials—*see Looking After Disabled People, p358*. With dedicated care and treatment, more than 65% of sufferers are able to live normal daily lives, unaffected by severe disability.

RHINITIS—see Hay fever

RICKETS

A form of *osteomalacia*, occurring in children as a result of a deficiency of vitamin D (*p322*). In adults, a vitamin D deficiency prevents the bones from properly absorbing the calcium and phosphorus obtained in the diet, with the result that the bones become soft and lose their substance. In children, the same process inhibits the growth of bone substance necessary for physical development.

Children suffering from rickets are normally restless and pale. Often, they have a distended abdomen, and sweat on the head. Babies fail to grow at the normal rate, and do not sit, stand, crawl and walk at the usual ages—*see Health and Your Child, p348*; the teeth may also may appear later than usual. If the disease is not treated by the age of

three, deformities may appear. These include *kyphosis*, 'knock knees' and 'bow legs'. In addition, there may be spasm of the facial muscles, and, in some cases, *epilepsy*.

Rickets is diagnosed by X-rays—*see Special Tests, p84*—which show characteristic changes in the bones. The condition is easily treated by regular dosages of vitamin D, often in the form of halibut oil, plus at least half a litre (.88pt) of milk or other calcium-rich drink each day. Once severe deformities have developed, however, they are rarely corrected by such treatment.

RICKETTSIA

A family of micro-organisms that share some of the characteristics of both *viruses* and *bacteria*. Rickettsia organisms live in lice, fleas, mites and ticks, and are transmitted to humans by the bites of these insects.

In humans, Rickettsiae live and multiply in the arteries and veins. They can cause a variety of diseases, all of which involve a rash and a high *fever*. These include the various types of *typhus* and Q *fever*. Rickettsia infections are treated by the *antibiotics* tetracycline and chloramphenicol. Since the organisms are highly infectious, sufferers are de-infested with special powders. Infested clothing and bedding is destroyed.

RIGOR

A sudden attack of shivering and chill, accompanied by a raised temperature. This often precedes the onset of a *fever*. Since the chill is usually followed by a period of heat and perspiration, rigor is sometimes described as the cold stage of a fever.

RISK REGISTER—see Battered baby syndrome

RODENT ULCER—see Basal cell carcinoma

ROSACEA—see Acne

ROSEOLA INFANTUM

A non-infectious *viral* illness that affects babies.

The first symptoms of roseola infantum appear after an incubation period of ten to l5 days. These consist of a sore throat and *fever*, with a sudden rise in temperature to between 39°C and 40.5°C (l02°F-l05°F). The spleen, liver and glands of the neck may also become enlarged.

These symptoms last for two or three days, after which a characteristic pink rash develops, usually on the skin of the trunk. The

rash sometimes spreads to the face, neck and limbs, but normally disappears within another two days.

There is no specific treatment for roseola infantum, but the disease is rarely serious.

RUBELLA

An infectious viral disease, commonly called German measles. Rubella most often affects children and adolescents, but can also be caught by adults. It is spread by the droplets coughed or sneezed into the air by an infected person—*see Health and Hygiene, p334*.

The first symptoms appear after an incubation period of between 10 and 21 days. These are usually mild aches and pains, and a rash, consisting of pink spots, which appears behind the ears and then spreads to the forehead chest and limbs. The eyes often appear bloodshot and the lymph glands in the neck and other parts of the body may become enlarged and slightly tender. In children, there may be a mild *fever*, but often this is scarcely noticeable. In older adolescents and adults, however, the illness is sometimes more serious, with a high fever.

There is no treatment for rubella, which normally subsides after a few days. Bed-rest and plenty of fluids are all that is needed—*see Home Nursing, p352*. Complications are uncommon and rarely persist, but may include *encephalomyelitis* and *thrombocytopaenia*.

The main danger of rubella is the effect it has on an unborn foetus. Depending on the stage of foetal development at which the mother contracts rubella, the foetus may be born with *cataracts*, *deafness*, *congenital heart defects* and *mental subnormality*. The highest risk of such foetal damage occurs during the first 16 weeks of pregnancy.

As a result, adolescent girls are routinely offered *immunization* against the disease. Older women who attended school before the vaccination programme had been initiated are advised to consult their doctor to check that they have immunity to rubella before becoming pregnant. For the same reason, pregnant women should avoid all contact with sufferers from rubella—sufferers are infectious from one week before the appearance of the rash, and for three weeks afterwards. Pregnant women who have been exposed to rubella are eligible for a termination of pregnancy.

RUPTURE—see Hernia

S

SABIN VACCINE
A vaccine used for *immunization* against *poliomyelitis*. The vaccine is 'live'—that is, it contains a weakened strain of the virus—and is administered by mouth, often on a sugar lump. It works by stimulating the production of *antibodies* against the disease. Sabin vaccine is now the most widely used poliomyelitis vaccine, and has replaced the *Salk vaccine*, which must be given by an injection.

SACROILEIITIS
An inflammation of the sacroiliac joint, which links the hip-bone and the sacrum, at the bottom end of the spine *(p16)*. Sacroileiitis often occurs during the course of diseases involving inflammation of the joints, such as *ankylosing spondylitis*, *Reiter's syndrome* and psoriatic *arthritis*. It causes pain and stiffness in the lower part of the back, and is treated with bed rest and painkillers.

SADISM
A psychosexual disorder in which sexual pleasure is derived from inflicting physical or mental pain upon another person. Sadism is usually a deep-rooted disorder and can only be treated by long-term psychotherapy, which may include *behaviour therapy*.

ST VITUS'S DANCE—see Sydenham's chorea

SALBUTAMOL
A drug prescribed to widen the bronchi—*see bronchodilator*—without stimulating the heart in cases of *asthma* and chronic *bronchitis*.

SALINE
A weak solution of sodium chloride—salt—in water, given directly into a vein by means of a *drip* to maintain the balance of fluids in the body *(p21)*. The salt in the solution makes up for the salt lost to the body through abnormal sweating, *vomiting* or *diarrhoea*, all of which may cause *dehydration*. Saline is also given after operations, to replace any fluids that have been lost during surgery.

SALK VACCINE
The first successful vaccine to be produced for *immunization* against *poliomyelitis*. It contains three different types of poliomyelitis virus that have been treated with formalin, a chemical that renders them harmless but still capable of stimulating the production of *antibodies*. Salk vaccine, which is administered by injection, has now largely been replaced by the *Sabin vaccine*, which is taken by mouth.

SALMONELLA INFECTIONS
Infections caused by a variety of *bacteria* of the Salmonella family. Strains of Salmonella bacteria sometimes cause *food-poisoning*, with ensuing *gastroenteritis*; Salmonella typhi and a close relative, Salmonella paratyphi, respectively cause *typhoid fever* and paratyphoid fever. Salmonella infections are treated with *antibiotics*.

SALPINGECTOMY
The removal of one or both Fallopian tubes *(p54)*. The operation may be performed to treat conditions such as *salpingitis* and *pelvic inflammatory disease*, in which the Fallopian tubes become badly infected and blocked, or when the tubes have become enlarged and distorted by an accumulation of fluid. The operation is usually also necessary in cases of an *ectopic* or tubal *pregnancy*, when the foetus develops in the Fallopian tube, rather than in the womb. It may also be undertaken as part of a total *hysterectomy*.

Women can usually leave hospital between a week and ten days after a salpingectomy, and resume a normal sex life within a month. As the ovaries are left in place, there is no reduction in the level of female hormones *(p54)* in the body. However, it is impossible for a woman to conceive by normal methods if both Fallopian tubes have been removed—*see infertility*.

SALPINGITIS
An inflammation of the Fallopian tubes *(p54)*, usually the result of *bacterial* infection. It is thought that, in some cases, intra-uterine devices (IUDs) may predispose users to pelvic infection, and, hence, to salpingitis—*see Sex and Contraception, p338*.

The infection may be carried in the bloodstream, but more often it spreads to the Fallopian tubes from the uterus or vagina. In *acute* cases, salpingitis causes severe pain in the lower abdomen, *fever* and *vomiting*, together with irregular menstrual periods. Prompt diagnosis and treatment are important, because, if these are delayed, the Fallopian tubes may become badly inflamed and blocked by scar tissue. If such a blockage occurs in both tubes, conception is impossible. Normal treatment is by a course of *antibiotics* to clear up the infection. In severe cases, however, an *abscess*, known as a pyosalpinx, may be formed, in which case surgery may be necessary—*see salpingectomy*. Occasionally the tubes are enlarged by the production of large quantities of fluid. Such cases are also treated surgically.

SARCOIDOSIS
A rare disease in which small areas of inflammation appear in the lymph nodes, lungs, liver, spleen, skin, eyes and parotid glands at the angle of the jaw. The cause of the condition is unknown, but it is thought to be an *auto-immune disease*—the result of a malfunction of the body's defences against infection.

Sarcoidosis generally causes few symptoms other than the enlargement of the lymph nodes in the lungs, which are sometimes detected on examination of a routine X-ray *(p84)*. In such cases, treatment is unusually unnecessary. However, the disease may also occur in a more serious form, in which the organs involved can be permanently damaged. In the lungs, sarcoidosis may lead to the deposition of fibrous tissue, pulmonary *hypertension* and shortness of breath. Rarely, heart problems such as *cor pulmonale*, *arrhythmias* and *cardiomyopathy* occur. *Lesions* in the eye may cause *iritis* and lead to *blindness* if untreated.

If a *biopsy* of an area of inflamed skin confirms a diagnosis of chronic sarcoidosis, the disease is treated with *corticosteroid drugs*, taken over a period of years.

SARCOMA

A *malignant tumour* that can occur in the muscles, the bones, or any part of the body's connective tissue (the material that protects and supports the organs within the body).

Sarcomas are described according to the tissue in which they occur. For example, a sarcoma in bone tissue is an osteosarcoma. *See cancer.*

SCABIES

A skin disease caused by the *mite* Sarcoptes scabiei, or itch mite. The main symptom is intense itching, particularly at night. The areas usually affected are the sides of the fingers, the elbows, the groin, the buttocks, the nipples and, in men, the penis. The face is not usually affected in adults, but it may be in children.

The female mite burrows under the skin and lays eggs that hatch in three to four days. The mites, which reach adult form in about 14 days, mate on the skin, and the life cycle thus continues. If left untreated, the infection may spread to the rest of the body.

Scabies is extremely infectious. It can be transmitted by physical contact, or through infected bedding, clothes, or towels. For this reason, other members of the sufferer's household are normally checked to see if they are infested.

Scabies is treated by applying benzyl benzoate solution all over the body from the neck downwards, at least once a day after a bath. The treatment must be repeated for three or more days to kill the mites. Infected clothing and bedding should be washed thoroughly.

SCARLET FEVER

An infectious *notifiable* disease, also known as scarlatina, that occurs mainly in childhood. It is caused by a strain of *Streptococcal bacteria*, spread in droplets in the breath, coughs and sneezes of an infected person. The disease is highly contagious, with an incubation period of anything from a day to a week. During its course, a patient should be kept in bed and away from other children.

The bacteria produce a toxin that circulates in the blood, causing a sore throat, *fever* and *vomiting*. The glands in the neck are usually greatly enlarged, and a yellow membrane forms on the tonsils. The face may be flushed, but there is a pale area around the mouth. After about two days a *rash* of tiny red spots appears behind the ears and spreads all over the body, lasting for about a week. The tongue is covered with a white fur that later peels off, leaving it looking clean and red. Protruding red *papillae* give the tongue the appearance of a strawberry—hence the traditional description 'strawberry tongue'.

Before the discovery of *antibiotics*, scarlet fever was an extremely serious illness. Nowadays, however, treatment with these drugs is swift and effective. Complications are extremely rare, but can include *rheumatic fever* and a form of *nephritis*, or inflammation of the kidneys. Scarlet fever itself does not usually recur, since the body develops an immunity to the disease as a result of the initial infection.

SCHISTOSOMIASIS

A disease, also called bilharziasis, caused by an infestation of worms of the Schistosoma family. These worms are also known as Bilharzia worms, trematode worms, and blood-flukes. Schistosomiasis is contracted by skin contact with water contaminated by the urine or faeces of a sufferer. After penetrating the skin, immature worms develop as they travel through the lungs, diaphragm *(p28)* and liver, finally lodging in the portal vein *(p44)*. After about a month, they move to blood vessels in the pelvis, and produce eggs which pass into the large intestine, rectum or bladder. The eggs are then excreted in urine and faeces.

There are three different types of schistosomiasis, according to the precise type of schistosoma worm involved. The first symptoms are similar in all cases, however: there is sometimes itching at the site at which the worms have penetrated the skin, and sometimes a serious *allergic* reaction develops. The symptoms subside within a few weeks, and thereafter the course of schistosomiasis varies.

Schistosoma haematobium, *endemic* in Egypt and East Africa, and common in the Middle East, primarily affects the urinary tract in later life. The worm may cause inflammation of the kidneys *(p40)*, ureters, bladder, and, in men, the prostate gland, a common outward symptom being *haematuria*—blood in the urine.

Schistosoma mansoni, common in Africa, the Middle East and South America, primarily affects the large intestine, the symptoms appearing several months after the original infestation. The eggs cause inflammation, *ulceration* and bleeding in the large intestine, resulting in diarrhoea with stools containing blood and mucus. In addition, the eggs may travel to the lungs, causing *pulmonary hypertension*, and the liver, causing *portal hypertension*. If untreated, this can prove fatal. On occasions, the eggs also compress the spinal cord, causing paralysis.

Schistosoma japonicum, the third type of schistosoma worm, is common in the Far East. An infestation takes the same form as that with schistosoma mansoni, but tends to be more serious. This is because S. japonicum produces many more eggs than the other varieties of worm.

Schistosomiasis is diagnosed by examination of the urine and faeces for the presence of eggs, and, if necessary, by examination of the bladder and large intestine by endoscopy—*see Special Tests, p84*. Treatment is by a drug called niridazole, which kills the worm. This is highly effective in the case of infestations by S. haematobium and S. mansoni, but less effective in the case of S. japonicum.

SCHIZOPHRENIA

One of the major mental illnesses, affecting some 30 per cent of patients admitted to psychiatric hospitals.

The word 'schizophrenic' means, literally, 'split mind', and this has given rise to the misconception that the schizophrenic has a dual personality. The 'split mind' in fact refers to the schizophrenic's dissociation of himself or herself from reality. Normally, a person sorts out a mass of impressions and decides which are important, or 'real'; but to a schizophrenic, everything is a jumble. A symptom of this dissociation is that the patient frequently refers to himself in the third person, rather than as 'I'.

The causes of schizophrenia are not understood. Since the symptoms can be precipitated or reduced by various drugs, there is a theory that it is caused by chemical abnormalities in the brain, but the evidence for this is slight. Some psychiatrists believe that the tendency to develop schizophrenic illness at moments of stress can be inherited; studies on identical twins show that if one twin develops the disorder, the other twin is likely to do so, even if they have been brought up in entirely different environments.

There is a great deal of evidence to suggest that the existing tendency to develop schizophrenia is exacerbated by family problems in childhood. Schizophrenia is a disorder that occurs most commonly in adolescents and young adults, and is rare in childhood, but records show that many schizophrenic patients have grown up in an environment in which family relationships are governed by distrust, dislike or hostility.

Schizophrenics exhibit many of the symptoms commonly associated with the popular idea of madness. They become withdrawn from reality, substituting a day-dream existence for relationships with the outside world. Disordered judgement and thought blocks—interruption of thought or speech—are common. Symptoms of depersonalization, a detached and terrible loneliness, can be very frightening for the sufferer; other patients regress into infantile behaviour, throwing violent tantrums for the slightest reason.

Patients with schizophrenia were once classified according to their most important symptoms into two main categories: process schizophrenia, the most common, and reactive schizophrenia. Nowadays, however, the division of schizophrenia into process and reactive types is generally considered to be artificial, having little relationship to the course of the disease or its treatment.

The treatment of schizophrenia is still at an experimental stage, and results are often disappointing. Some l0% of patients recover spontaneously, and about 40% respond to therapy if it is begun early enough in the course of the disease. In the other 50%, the schizophrenia cannot be cured, but can be controlled.

Treatment begins with control of acute and frightening symptoms, using *tranquillizers* and, in extreme cases, *ECT* (electroconvulsive therapy). Some patients require long-term medical treatment, such as injections every two to four weeks of long-acting major *tranquillizers*; others may need to be treated only during acute attacks.

Many schizophrenics, however, have to be hospitalized from time to time when their symptoms become extreme, either for their own safety or for that of other people. Unfortunately, *institutionalization* may worsen the patient's condition, precisely because he is shut off from social stimuli. Hospital staff therefore try to encourage patients to take part in organized activities. Some patients can be treated in hospital during acute episodes and as out-patients after the symptoms have improved.

SCIATICA
An intense pain in the lower back that is sometimes also felt in the buttocks, radiating down the outside of the thigh, calf and foot. It is exacerbated by coughing or sneezing, and it is often accompanied or preceded by *lumbago*. It may also be accompanied by pins and needles, and numbness.

Sciatica is a symptom, usually of a slipped disc—*see prolapsed invertebral disc*—that is, a disc that has become displaced and is pressing on a nerve. It often follows strenuous lifting of heavy weights, twisting of the spine, or childbirth. Sciatica may also be caused by a *tumour* of the spine, *ankylosing spondylitis, malignant* diseases of the pelvis and *tuberculosis* of the spine or sacroiliac joint *(p16)*, all of which result in pressure on the sciatic nerve.

Complete rest is the best form of treatment, together with *analgesics* to relieve any severe pain. The patient should lie on his or her back on a bed with a firm mattress supported by boards, for about two weeks. The rest must be total; if, during this period, the patient does as little as sitting up in bed or walking to the bathroom, the treatment may fail. The period of bed rest is usually followed by *physiotherapy*, consisting of back-strengthening exercises.

Should this treatment be ineffective or the condition recur, surgery may be necessary to relieve the pressure on the sciatic nerve.

SCLERODERMA
A rare disorder of the connective tissue, the material that supports, separates and protects the organs of the body *(p16)*. The disease is also called progressive systemic sclerosis. Its cause is unknown, but it is thought to have an *auto-immune* basis. In general, it is three to four times more common in women than in men and commonly occurs between the ages of 30 and 40.

Raynaud's disease is sometimes the first sign of scleroderma. In this, the small arteries, particularly in the fingers and toes, are abnormally sensitive to cold. The condition can affect the patient for many years before other symptoms appear. Eventually, however, the fingers may begin to swell, becoming sausage-shaped and difficult to move. Later, their skin becomes shiny and thin, and the fingertips may become ulcerated. There may also be pain and stiffness in the finger joints.

As the disease progresses, patches of skin over the affected areas become pigmented, thickened and tight, making movement difficult and uncomfortable. The face looks taut and mask-like, and the skin around the mouth may pucker. Though at first only one part of the body may be involved, the disease often spreads to the oesophagus, making swallowing difficult. Sections of bowel can become dilated. This causes pain, constipation and swelling of the abdomen. Pulmonary *fibrosis, cardiomyopathy, heart block, valvular heart disease* and *pericarditis* sometimes occur, with kidney failure being a common cause of death.

There is no effective treatment for scleroderma, although *corticosteroid* drug therapy may help control its symptoms. The patient should be protected as much as possible from cold and infections, while *hypertension* and respiratory, gastrointestinal and kidney complaints should be treated as they arise. However, scleroderma is usually fatal; about 70 per cent of patients survive for only five years

SCOLIOSIS
A curvature of the spine to the side. Most commonly, scoliosis develops in people whose legs are of unequal length, and results from the posture adopted to compensate for this problem. In such cases, scoliosis can be avoided if sufferers hang by their hands from a bar for a few minutes each day.

Other causes of scoliosis include *congenital deformities*, such as *spina bifida* and an absence or failure to fuse of some of the vertebrae *(p16)*. The condition may also develop during life as a result of the paralysis of the muscles on one side of the body. This, in turn, may be caused by a disease, such as *poliomyelitis*, or by a stroke—*see cerebrovascular accident*.

Children born with scoliosis are given *physiotherapy* to help correct the deformity. In severe cases, special plaster jackets and splints may also be used to correct the curvature. However, orthopaedic surgery may be necessary during adolescence to fully correct the problem.

SCURVY
A disease caused by insufficient vitamin C in the diet *(p322)*. The intake of the vitamin has to be grossly deficient for about six months before symptoms appear.

The main symptoms of scurvy are a general feeling of tiredness and weakness, with stiff limbs, bleeding gums, loose teeth—which, in severe cases, may fall out—and coarsening of the skin. Bruises may appear for no apparent reason, first on the lower limbs and then all over the body. Resistance to infection is lowered and wounds may fail to heal. Death from heart failure may occur suddenly.

Nowadays scurvy is rare, but it is still occasionally found in infants as a result of poverty or neglect, in old people with poor diets, and in alcoholics and vagrants. Scurvy may develop in patients who need more vitamin C than other people; examples include people who have been severely burned; who have undergone major surgery; who are being treated with certain drugs, such as *steroids*, indomethacin and tetracycline; and people who smoke or drink heavily.

Scurvy can be easily treated by taking vitamin C tablets. Recovery is usually rapid and total.

SEDATIVE
A drug used to soothe people, that allays fear, over-excitement and anxiety. Sedatives are also known as anti-anxiety drugs, anxiolytics, or minor *tranquillizers*.

SEPTAL DEFECT—see Congenital heart defects

SEPTICAEMIA
The spread of infection through the body, caused by the circulation and multiplication in the blood of bacteria or other infecting micro-organisms, with possible eventual damage to the bone, liver, brain or heart valves. The popular name for the condition is blood poisoning.

Normally, the white blood cells *(p21)* are able to destroy any harmful bacteria and the toxins they release. However, illness inevitably means that the natural resistance to infection is weakened. Septicaemia, therefore, may follow any serious infection, such as a *lung abscess*. Symptoms include sudden *hypothermia*, a slowing of the heartbeat and *thrombocytopenia*. Immediate treatment with *antibiotics* is essential, since the condition can be fatal.

SERUM HEPATITIS—see Hepatitis

SERUM SICKNESS
A condition brought about by an *allergic* reaction to the serum used in certain types of *immunization* and in the preparation of certain drugs. (Serum is blood plasma that separates from the blood after clotting; it is a clear yellowish fluid). Serum sickness is an *iatrogenic* condition—that is, it is brought about by treatment.

About a week after the injection of serum, antibodies form in the blood—*see Natural Defences Against Disease, p52*—and react. Symptoms include *fever*, a *rash*, pain, stiffness and swelling in some joints. In rare cases the patient may develop low blood pressure— *see*

hypertension —and *shock*. The duration of the reaction varies, but usually lasts for only a few days.

SEX CHROMOSOMES—see Chromosomes

SEXUALLY TRANSMITTED DISEASES
A number of diseases and infections transmitted from person to person by sexual activity. The STDs include: *AIDS, chancroid,* genital *herpes*, genital *warts, gonorrhoea,* non-specific *urethritis* (NSU), *pediculosis*—commonly called crabs—serum *hepatitis* and *syphilis*.

Sexually transmitted diseases, or STDs, are no longer generally termed venereal diseases by doctors; this is because the term venereal disease, or VD, carried implications of immorality. In fact, a number of the STDs can also be transmitted by physical contact other than sexual contact. Examples of such problems include NSU and genital herpes.

See also Routine Health Checks, p346; Sex and Contraception, p338.

SHINGLES—see Herpes

SHOCK
In medical terms, shock is a serious condition in which the blood pressure falls sharply, causing a reduction in the amount of blood reaching the tissues and, in particular, the brain. Shock is often a cause of death in cases of major injury or acute illness.

Shock may occur for several reasons. After an injury to the heart—caused, for example, by a coronary *thrombosis*—the blood pressure falls dramatically. The same thing can happen when there is serious bleeding from a wound. If only a small quantity of blood is lost, the blood vessels can contract to maintain the normal blood pressure, but if the bleeding is serious this is not possible. Another cause of a drop in blood pressure is a reduction in body fluids, as may happen in severe *diarrhoea*, or *vomiting*. In this case, the fluid content of the blood falls, reducing its volume, and so its pressure. Infection, extreme allergic reaction or injury may cause blood vessels to dilate or widen, so that although the quantity of blood remains the same, it is not sufficient to maintain adequate pressure within the increased area through which it must flow.

When the blood pressure falls for any reason, a vicious circle develops, because a decrease in the supply of blood will make the heart short of oxygen. This will reduce the pumping-action of the heart, causing a further drop in blood

pressure. Once this happens, the body is unable to recover spontaneously and the condition will be fatal unless it is treated.

Symptoms of shock may appear without warning. They include sweating, faintness, nausea and irregular breathing. The patient will probably have a weak but rapid pulse rate, and will be pale, with a damp, clammy skin. As the supply of blood to the brain lessens, the patient may become drowsy and confused, eventually losing consciousness.

Swift, specialized medical treatment is vital in all cases. Help should be summoned immediately. For emergency action—*see p369*.

SHORT SIGHT—see Myopia

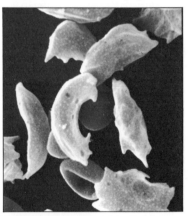

Sickle-cell Anaemia is an inherited disease in which the red blood cells take on a sickle shape *(above)*, magnified 12,000 times. In sickle-cell anaemia, red cell deformities are caused by abnormal haemoglobin molecules, especially when there is a shortage of oxygen. Sickle cells prevent the smooth flow of blood and may obstruct tiny capillaries. The body's cells become anoxic, or short of oxygen, as a result.

SICKLE-CELL ANAEMIA
A hereditary form of *anaemia* found in people of African descent. Its name is derived from the fact that the disease causes the red blood cells to become crescent- or sickle-shaped. It is caused by an abnormal constituent of the haemoglobin in the blood, and is incurable.

In parts of Africa almost half the population are *carriers* of sickle-cell anaemia—*see genes*—and are said to have sickle-cell trait. This means that they are usually unaffected by the disease, but may transmit it to their children.

Carriers usually lead normal lives, but they may become ill when demands on the circulatory system increase: at high altitudes where the air is thin, for example, or in case of emergency surgery without blood *transfusions*. If two carriers have offspring, one out of four of their children is likely to be entirely normal, two may be carriers—that is, they may have sickle-cell trait—and the fourth may have sickle-cell anaemia.

Not only are the red blood cells distorted into a sickle shape in sickle-cell anaemia, but they are also more fragile, so that they disintegrate more quickly than new ones can be formed. The sickled cells obstruct the smooth flow of blood through the capillaries or small blood vessels, thus preventing blood from reaching the tissues. This, in turn, reduces the concentration of oxygen in the blood, which may trigger more cells to become sickled.

The blood clots, or *thrombi*, that result from blockages in the capillaries, eventually cause the death of areas of tissue. The problem is exacerbated by any infection that affects the body, and is known as a 'sickle-cell crisis'. Pain may be extremely severe during the first 24 hours and there may be swelling and tenderness in the affected area of tissue. The reduced blood flow may also cause damage to the organs, and death may result from heart or kidney failure.

The first symptoms of sickle-cell anaemia are usually seen during the fourth month after birth, when the baby develops severe anaemia. Growth may be retarded and puberty may occur later than normal. The child may be physically weak and susceptible to *jaundice*, infections, stomach pains and bouts of swelling and pain in the muscles and joints.

Without medical care, which treats the symptoms rather than the disease, children with sickle-cell anaemia usually die before reaching adulthood. With care, affected children may live almost normal lives, but are unlikely to survive to old age.

Patients should avoid becoming chilled or *dehydrated*, and any infections should be treated immediately. Oral contraceptives may increase the risk of blood clotting, therefore likely sufferers should not use the contraceptive pill unless they have had a sickle-cell test—*see Special Tests, p84*. The disease may also cause problems during pregnancy, due to the increased demands on the blood circulation. People who have a history of sickle-cell anaemia should ask for a test in any case, since they risk transmitting the disease to their children.

SIDS—see Cot death

SILICOSIS
An incurable lung disease, caused by inhalation of air polluted with silica dust. Silica is a hard, glassy, insoluble, non-metallic mineral, found in mines, foundries, potteries, and anywhere metals are ground or sharpened.

The disease is caused by the deposition of fine particles of the dust in the lungs. This irritates the lung tissues and eventually leads to irreversible scarring of them. The process may take many years; in the early stages there are often no symptoms, but eventually symptoms similar to those of *bronchitis* and *asthma* occur. There is shortness of breath and large quantities of phlegm are coughed up.

Because of the danger of permanent lung damage, it is important that people at risk should have regular chest X-rays. If there is any sign of disease, the patient should change jobs at once. There is no treatment for the silicosis, but the associated symptoms or complications can be treated.

Preventive measures, such as dust control, provision of adequate ventilation and the wearing of face masks, are now usually required by law in places where employees are at risk from silicosis. Compensation and special benefits are available for those who have been disabled by the disease—*see industrial diseases*.

SINUSITIS
An inflammation of the mucous membranes lining one or more of the sinuses, the air-filled cavities in the bones of the face and skull.

Symptoms of sinusitis include loss of the sense of smell, headache, pain resembling toothache, tenderness over the sinuses, and pain between and behind the eyes. The sufferer may feel ill and feverish while the inflammation lasts, and the face may ache and swell. Attacks often clear up spontaneously, though a course of *antibiotics* may be advisable in acute cases.

The most common causes of sinusitis include the common cold, an infection of the respiratory tract, such as *influenza*, an *abscess* on a tooth, and foreign bodies in the nose. Since the sinuses communicate with the nose, any infections there are likely to spread back to attack the sinuses.

Some people have a tendency to recurrent sinusitis, so that the condition becomes *chronic*; in such cases it may be necessary to drain the sinuses surgically to remove any pus that has accumulated.

SKIN CANCER—see Basal cell carcinoma; Melanoma

SLEEPING SICKNESS—see Trypanosomiasis

SLIPPED DISC—see Prolapsed intervertebral disc

SMALLPOX
A highly infectious tropical disease that has now been almost totally eradicated, world-wide. Smallpox is caused by a virus, of which there three types. The most virulent of these, called variola major, causes a serious disease that is often fatal, and the second type, called variola minor, causes a mild form of the disease; the third type of variola virus is harmless, and is used in *immunization* against smallpox.

Smallpox proves fatal in around 25% of cases. Those who survive are often grotesquely scarred by pock marks. There is no effective treatment, though *antibiotics* may be given to prevent the scabs from becoming infected. Since the disease is highly infectious—the scabs which fall off the spots contain live variola viruses—patients are nursed in strict isolation.

The almost total eradication of the disease has been achieved by a programme of mass immunization, developed by the World Health Organization. Children are routinely immunized against the disease—*see Health and Your Child, p346*—and hospital workers at risk of infection receive regular booster injections.

SMEAR—see Special Tests, p84

SNORING
Although usually spoken of as if it were a joke, snoring can cause considerable marital disharmony; recently, moreover, it has been discovered to have surprising medical significance.

Snoring is due to vibration of the soft palate, which tends to occur when the snorer is lying on his back with the mouth open. In this position the muscles of the throat are relaxed, and the soft palate can fall back, partially blocking the airway and setting up vibration.

Snoring is commoner in men than in women. It is made worse by obesity, alcohol, and smoking. In some people it is associated with *sleep apnoea*, in which the sleeper stops breathing for a minute or more and the oxygen concentration in his blood falls. There is increasing and current medical concern about sleep apnoea, which appears to contribute to arterial disease and heart disease and to interfere with efficiency during the day.

Folk remedies for snoring include getting the sufferer to sleep on a side, rather than the back, or sewing a hard object, such as a cotton reel,

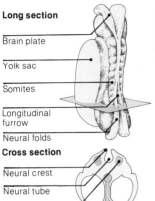

Long section

Brain plate

Yolk sac

Somites

Longitudinal furrow

Neural folds

Cross section

Neural crest

Neural tube

Somite

During the first weeks of a foetus' life, a longitudinal furrow forms on its back, bordered by a series of paired blocks of tissue, called somites. The tissues *(top)* either side of the furrow fold up and over it, enclosing the neural tube *(below)*.

Spina Bifida is a disorder of the spinal column which results from incomplete development of the backbone during gestation *(left)*. The spines or neural arches on the vertebrae in the lumbar or sacral regions *(top right)* fail to form properly and leave the spinal cord exposed. In spina bifida occulta, neither the spinal cord nor the meninges — the three layers of membrane surrounding the cord — protrude from the back. Instead, there is only a pigmented area of skin or a patch of hair over the affected area. In the meningocele and meningo-myelocele forms of the disease, the meninges surrounding the cord expand with cerebrospinal fluid and form a balloon above the affected area *(bottom right)*. In these cases, there is either partial or complete paralysis of the spinal nerves in that area. This causes a loss of control and sensation in the legs, bladder and bowels.

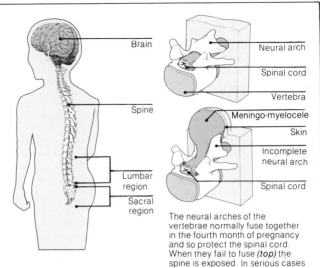

Brain

Spine

Lumbar region

Sacral region

Neural arch

Spinal cord

Vertebra

Meningo-myelocele

Skin

Incomplete neural arch

Spinal cord

The neural arches of the vertebrae normally fuse together in the fourth month of pregnancy and so protect the spinal cord. When they fail to fuse *(top)* the spine is exposed. In serious cases of spina bifida, the meninges swell and form a meningo-myelocele, a small balloon of cerebrospinal fluid *(below)*.

into the back of the snorer's pyjamas; when he turns on his back the pressure wakes him. More sophisticated modern devices include electronic apparatus that detects the sound of the snore and wakes the sleeper. However, none of these are dramatically effective. Really severe snoring can be cured by surgery to the soft palate and the walls of the throat, but this is seldom undertaken.

SOLVENT ABUSE
A form of drug abuse that occurs almost exclusively among children and young people. The incidence is increasing at present and there have been a number of deaths. Many industrial products and household substances contain solvents: they include glues, thinners, dry cleaning solutions, paint strippers, nail varnish, and petrol and lighter fuels. When inhaled they can cause hallucinations and elation at first, followed by drowsiness and finally unconsciousness. The affected person may stagger, and have dilated pupils. Eventually, liver and kidney damage may result.

Signs that can alert adults to the fact that a child is inhaling solvents include the smell of the solvent on the breath, personality changes, and signs of irritation round the nose and mouth.

If someone is found suffering from the effects of inhaling vapour, urgent action is needed. If they are conscious, they should be kept under observation and a doctor should be called. If they have become unconscious, remove the source of the vapour, open doors and windows, and, if they are not breathing, apply artificial respiration. Once they are breathing again, they should be put in the recovery position. Throughout, remember that most solvents are highly flammable.

Even if the child has apparently recovered, he or she should still be seen in hospital or by a doctor because of the risk of liver and kidney damage.

SORE THROAT—see Upper respiratory tract infection

SPASTIC COLON—see Irritable bowel syndrome

SPASTIC PARALYSIS
A type of paralysis caused by damage to nerve cells in the brain and spinal cord—*see The Nervous System, p32*. This damage causes loss of conscious control of the affected muscles and involuntary spasms in them, most commonly in the limbs.

Spastic paralysis may be a *congenital abnormality*, or occur as a result of damage to the foetus in the womb, in which case the condition is called *cerebral palsy* or spastic diplegia. It may also be caused by accidental damage, such as forceps damage during delivery. Later in life spastic paralysis may be caused by a stroke—*see cerebrovascular accident*—a *tumour* of the brain, or by *poliomyelitis* or *multiple sclerosis*.

Spastic paralysis is not a progressive disease, but it is irreversible and incurable. However, its effects vary considerably. Some children are born paralysed in all limbs, with speech defects, *deafness* and *mental subnormality*, but in many cases, only the arms or legs are affected, and the child's intelligence is normal. Remedial therapies can be of considerable help in improving a sufferer's condition. Surgery and *physiotherapy*, for example, can help to improve the mobility of the limbs, and braces can be used to help support them. Antispasmodic drugs can be given to counteract exaggerated reflex movements. Speech defects may be improved by *speech therapy* and hearing aids can help to restore some degree of hearing.

SPEECH THERAPY
A form of therapy used to help people overcome speech defects. Such problems can be extremely varied, but the aim of the therapist is always to teach people to speak as clearly as possible, whatever the underlying cause.

The most common use of speech therapy is probably in helping deaf people to speak; they may have great difficulty in this, not only because they cannot hear the speech of others in order to imitate it, but also because they cannot hear themselves. They are taught to control the volume and tone of their speech, and to enunciate clearly.

Another common problem is a *stammer*. Stammering is usually involved with nervousness, but, paradoxically, the stammerer may forget to be nervous if he or she is taught by speech therapy to concentrate on the mechanical aspects of speaking.

Other major speech problems are caused by physical defects, such as a *cleft palate*, in which speech is totally nasal. A *laryngectomy*, the removal of the larynx, usually as a treatment for *cancer*, means that the patient has to learn how to speak intelligibly through a hole in the throat, using a method of controlling swallowed air or an electric vibrator that is held against the neck to produce intelligible speech. Patients suffering the after-effects of a stroke—*see cerebrovascular accident*—may need speech therapy if their speech is slurred, or if they have difficulty in finding the right word.

Children may suffer from speech defects for several reasons. These may be the result of an overall delay in development, caused by a problem such as *cerebral palsy*, or the delay may be specific, caused by lack of verbal communication from those around them. Treatment in such cases involves counselling of the parents as well as specific vocal exercises and stimulation for the affected child.

SPINA BIFIDA

A congenital abnormality of the spinal cord, caused by a defect in the neural tube, the precursor of the spinal cord in the embryo—*see Embryology, p12.*

In serious cases, the baby is born with its spinal cord and meninges exposed and bulging through an opening in the back, and the unprotected spinal nerves are defective. This condition is usually accompanied by mental retardation and paralysis. It is caused by the failure of one or more neural arches, the hind parts of the vertebrae that protect the spinal cord *(p16)*, to fuse together. The vertebrae in the lower part of the backbone are most commonly affected. The disease is commonly accompanied by *hydrocephalus*, a condition in which cerebrospinal fluid accumulates in the brain.

Spina bifida meningocele and spina bifida meningo-myelocele are the most serious forms of the condition. In the severe cases, the baby may be stillborn, or live for only a few hours. Babies who survive may be *mentally subnormal* and are often at least partially paralysed, some having only an area of numbness, while others have a complete lack of bodily control from the waist down.

The cause of spina bifida is unknown, but statistically, a woman who has given birth to one affected infant runs an increased risk of the same thing happening again. In general, older women are more at risk; a women over 37 is usually offered an amniocentesis—*see Special Tests, p84*—which can reveal spina bifida during pregnancy. Should abnormalities be detected, a decision can be made as to whether to terminate the pregnancy.

One form of spina bifida is much less serious. This is spina bifida occulta, in which the neural arches may be partially fused and the spinal

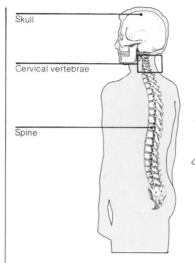

Skull
Cervical vertebrae
Spine

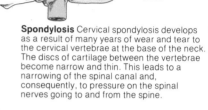

Spinal cord
Cervical vertebra
Spinal nerves
Narrow and thin intervertebral discs

Spondylosis Cervical spondylosis develops as a result of many years of wear and tear to the cervical vertebrae at the base of the neck. The discs of cartilage between the vertebrae become narrow and thin. This leads to a narrowing of the spinal canal and, consequently, to pressure on the spinal nerves going to and from the spine.

cord undamaged. There are often no adverse effects, and the area of incomplete fusion may be marked only by a pigmented area of skin or a patch of hair.

The physical defects spina bifida causes can be repaired to some extent, and modern surgical methods have enabled many babies to survive and lead reasonably normal lives. However, there has been much controversy over the practice of operating to save the lives of seriously affected children who may be mentally subnormal, as well as paralysed and incontinent, throughout their lives.

SPLENECTOMY

Removal of the spleen, an organ situated below the ribs on the left side of the body. The spleen acts as a filter for the blood, and destroys red blood cells at the end of their life span *(p21)*.

The most usual reason for the removal of the spleen is accidental damage to it. Such damage may occur as a consequence of blows to the stomach or as part of more widespread injuries received in an accident. In car accidents, for example, the spleen is often damaged through impact with the steering wheel. Diseases that affect the spleen, such as *Hodgkin's disease* or *spherocytosis*, may also necessitate its removal.

In adults the operation to remove the spleen is fairly major, but comparatively safe. There are no after-effects, since the spleen's functions are taken over by other parts of the body. However, in small children the operation is generally avoided if possible, since it may lead to a reduction in a child's immunity to infection.

SPONDYLOSIS

A disorder of the spine in which the discs of cartilage that separate the

vertebrae gradually disintegrate and may also become displaced—*see prolapsed invertebral disc.* Either condition may compress the spinal nerves, causing pain and stiffness in the affected part of the spine.

Spondylosis can occur at any age, but is most likely between 60 and 70. It most commonly affects the disc between the sixth and seventh cervical vertebrae in the neck, but several discs may be affected; when the neck is affected the disorder is known as cervical spondylosis. The condition is diagnosed by an X-ray *(p84)*, which usually shows protruding discs, a narrowing of the spaces they occupy and irregular growths of bony tissue around the joints. Osteoarthritis—*see arthritis*—often develops in the affected vertebrae.

Cervical spondylosis may cause pain in the shoulders and arms as well as the neck, while spondylosis of the lumbar region of the spine may cause pain and weakness in the legs. These symptoms may occur suddenly, often after a minor accident to the spine caused, for example, by a sudden twisting of the body, or by lifting a heavy weight. This form of *acute* spondylosis is treated by complete bed rest or by physiotherapy. In cases of cervical spondylosis the neck may be supported for some time in a special collar to rest the muscles and relieve any pain, while a patient with severe lumbar spondylosis may have to wear a surgical belt. Severe or *chronic* cases may fail to respond to such treatment; in these cases surgery may be necessary to relieve the pressure on the affected nerves.

SPRAIN

The general term for an injury to a joint that results in damage to the ligaments around it. A sprain causes immediate, intense pain;

tenderness, swelling and bruising of the skin soon develops around the affected area.

A sprained joint should be rested, so as not to hinder the natural process of healing, and treated with a cold compress— see First Aid, p369—to reduce the swelling. The joint may be supported with an elastic bandage while it is still painful. A sprain usually heals of its own accord over a few weeks.

If an apparent sprain causes considerable pain it should be examined by a doctor to rule out the possibility that a bone has been fractured.

SPRUE—see Tropical sprue

SQUINT—see Strabismus

STAMMER
A speech disorder in which a person finds it difficult to articulate certain sounds. While stammering, the affected person may move his or her mouth in the correct fashion, yet be momentarily unable to produce the sound; alternatively, he or she may repeat one sound or syllable over and over again before being able to go on to the next.

Stammering (or stuttering, as it is also called, particularly in America) is not caused by any abnormality of the organs of speech or of the part of the brain that controls speech. It is the result of a lack of co-ordination between the chest, larynx, tongue, palate and lips—the parts of the body that must work together to produce speech. This is often associated with anxiety and nervousness. A stammer is more common in men than in women and seems to be more prevalent in left-handed or ambidextrous people.

Many children grow out of the habit, but in more severe cases speech therapy may be required to teach the sufferer the correct way of controlling and co-ordinating the parts of the body that produce speech.

STAPHYLOCOCCUS
A group of bacteria causing infection in humans. Staphylococci live harmlessly on the skin and in the noses of healthy people, who, therefore, are carriers of staphylococcal infection. In sensitive people, however, they may cause infections such as boils, impetigo and abscesses; the bacteria are especially dangerous in surgical wards in hospitals, where they may cause wounds to become infected.

Wound infections and abscesses are treated with the antibiotic, penicillin. Unfortunately, many strains of staphylococcal bacteria are now resistant to this drug, and other, less-effective antibiotics are prescribed instead. Skin infections can often be successfully treated by antibiotic creams.

STEATORRHOEA
The excretion in the faeces of undigested fat, which is normally absorbed in the intestines. In steatorrhoea the stools are pale, and they tend to float and look greasy. The condition also causes the loss of calcium, which may ultimately lead to a painful disorder of bone called osteomalacia.

Steatorrhoea is a symptom of malabsorption, and may be caused by pancreatitis, tropical sprue or by coeliac disease. Diagnosis is made by collecting samples of stools for three days and weighing the amount of fat present. Normally, people lose no more than five grams (less than two ounces) of fat in the stools each day.

The condition clears up when the problem causing it is treated.

STERILITY—see Infertility

STERILIZATION—see Tubal ligation; vasectomy

STEROIDS
A group of chemicals which have a similar structure and occur naturally in the body. The steroids include: cholesterol; the bile salts (p40); the forerunner of vitamin D (p322)—converted into the vitamin in the skin by the action of sunlight; and hydrocortisone, aldosterone—see The Endocrine System, p48—and the sex hormones—see Sex and Reproduction, p54. All these chemicals have an important function in the body. They can either be replaced in cases of deficiency, or their natural effects reinforced as part of the treatment of a disease, by synthetic steroids given as drugs.

The most important natural steroids are those produced by the cortex of the adrenal glands (p48). They are known by two names: corticosteroids, because of the site of their production, and glucocorticoids, because they increase the level of glucose in the blood, and increase the breakdown of proteins. Their synthetic counterparts are known as corticosteroid, or corticoid, drugs.

The main corticosteroid is called hydrocortisone, or cortisol. A synthetic precursor of hydrocortisone called cortisone is sometimes given as a drug; it is converted into hydrocortisone by the liver. Hydrocortisone is a potent anti-inflammatory agent, and also depresses allergic reactions; as a result it is used in the treatment of conditions that involve inflammation, such as rheumatoid arthritis and dermatitis, and of allergies, such as asthma.

The second group of steroids comprises the hormones known as mineralocorticoids. The most important of these is aldosterone. This affects the retention of water and salt, and the excretion of potassium, and so the body's fluid balance. Synthetic aldosterone is given to patients suffering from Addison's Disease, in which there is a lack of the hormone.

The third group of steroids comprises the sex hormones. The male sex hormones, or androgens, are secreted by cells in the testes, and are necessary for sperm production and for the development of male secondary sexual characteristics. As these characteristics include the growth of muscles, by a process called anabolism in which protein is built up, androgens are taken by some athletes to increase their muscular development. The use of these chemicals, called anabolic steroids, is controversial. This is not only because such athletes have an unfair advantage in competition, but because they are likely to suffer from permanent side-effects. However, testosterone, the main androgen, is occasionally used to treat impotence.

Oestrogens, the female sex hormones, are also steroids, and are secreted by the ovaries. They are used in the combined contraceptive pill—see Sex and Contraception, p338—and in hormone replacement therapy to relieve the side-effects of the menopause. Both testosterone and oestrogen are occasionally used in the treatment of hormone-dependent cancers.

Steroids may be administered in a variety of ways—in the form of pills, by injection into a vein or muscle, in an aerosol in the treatment of asthma, or in the form of a suppository in the treatment of inflammatory proctitis. Steroid creams may be used in the treatment of eczema and other skin conditions that cause inflammation.

The use of every synthetic steroid is carefully controlled and monitored because of the risk of potentially harmful side-effects in long-term use. These include osteoporosis, or thinning of the bones. This means that even minor injuries may cause fractures or the collapse of a vertebra. Peptic ulceration may be a problem, as steroids irritate the stomach lining; the chances of this are reduced if they are prescribed in the form of sugar-coated pills, so that they dissolve gradually further down the digestive tract. Other side-effects include the deposition of fat on the abdomen and shoulders and weakness of the underlying muscles, and acne on the face and back. The face may become moon-shaped—one of the symptoms of *Cushing's disease*. Sometimes steroids cause mental disturbances, such as *depression* or *euphoria*. Occasionally a *psychosis* is induced, usually with feelings of *paranoia*.

Doctors try to minimize the possibility of adverse affects by giving steroids in short courses, rather than long-term. This is important, because, after a short time, the natural functions of the adrenal glands tend to be suppressed by the drugs, so they must be stopped gradually to allow the glands to recover. Patients taking steroids should always carry a card saying so and recording the dosage. This is because it is vital to know that steroids have been prescribed in many cases of medical emergency. The list of side-effects is daunting, but steroids, nevertheless, are extremely potent and effective drugs. In many cases, they are the only drugs that have any effect upon a condition, and they improve the quality of a sufferer's life to such an extent that their benefits outweigh their possible side-effects.

STILLBIRTH
The birth of a foetus that died within the womb in or after the 28th week after conception (p60). Before this time, the birth of the foetus is known as a miscarriage, or spontaneous *abortion*.

The first sign that the foetus has died is usually the mother's realization that the foetus has stopped moving inside her; should a mother say that she can no longer feel movement for any length of time after *quickening*, she will usually be admitted to hospital for further investigations, such as an ultrasound examination (p84). If the foetus is found to be dead, labour is normally *induced*.

A foetus may survive the full term of pregnancy but die during labour, unable to withstand the strain of birth. However, modern techniques, including careful monitoring of the foetus and delivery by *caesarian section* if there are signs of *foetal distress*, have made this a rare occurrence.

STOKES-ADAMS ATTACK
Sudden unconsciousness, due to a disturbance of the normal heart rhythm (p21). This is usually caused by a *heart block*, or by aortic stenosis, the abnormal narrowing of the aortic valve—*see valvular heart disease*. During an attack, the patient turns pale and collapses, and no pulse can

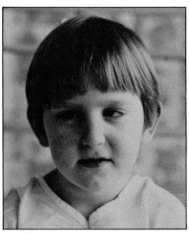

Strabismus is the medical term for squinting, in which the two eyes do not look in the same direction at once *(above)*. The movements of the eyeballs are controlled by six muscles, four of them straight and two of them oblique. Two of the straight muscles turn the eyeball from side to side *(top right)*. In adults, a disorder elsewhere in the body can affect the nerves controlling these muscles to produce either an inward or an outward squint.

be detected. The sufferer usually recovers after a few seconds, but if this is not the case emergency treatment is essential, involving immediate mouth-to-mouth resuscitation—*see First Aid p369*—and admission to hospital.

Once diagnosed by electrocardiography—*see Special Tests, p84*—the condition is treated by the insertion of an artificial *pacemaker* to maintain the normal heart rhythm.

STOMACH CANCER
A *malignant* disease affecting the stomach. Stomach cancer is the third most common form of cancer in Britain, after *lung cancer* and cancer of the breasts—*see breast lumps*. Stomach cancer can affect people of any age and either sex, but tends to occur most frequently in people who suffer from *pernicious anaemia*; its incidence is highest in the Far East.

Stomach cancer causes a variety of symptoms, making diagnosis difficult. The most common symptoms, however, are pain in the upper abdomen and loss of appetite. As the *tumour* grows, there may be loss of weight and vomiting of blood, and blood may be passed in the stools. Diagnosis is by barium meal X-rays, and gastroscopy, in which a biopsy is taken—*see Special Tests, p84*.

Treatment is by surgery, in which the whole stomach is removed and the oesophagus joined to the remainder of the small intestine—*see gastrectomy*. However, even with gastrectomy the outlook for victims of stomach cancer is poor.

See also cancer.

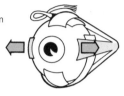

Muscles which turn the eye from side to side

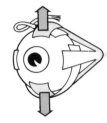

Muscles which move the eye up and down

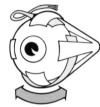

Muscles which turn the eye to oblique positions

STOMATITIS
An inflammation of any natural opening in the body, such as the lips and mouth, or of any artificial opening in the body, whether temporary or permanent. The term is therefore used to describe an inflammation of the opening created when the colon or ileum is brought to the surface of the abdomen, in a *colostomy* or *ileostomy*. Stomatitis can be avoided if the stoma is kept scrupulously clean and the surrounding skin kept dry, and protected by various special creams and sealants.

STRABISMUS
The medical name for squint, a condition in which each eye looks in a slightly different direction, instead of both eyes working together, so that they both focus on the same object at the same time. It can sometimes be accompanied by double vision.

Various forms of squint can arise. Most squints are concomitant; that is, the angle of divergence between the eyes remains the same regardless of which way they are looking and which eye is focusing. In a divergent squint, one eye looks outwards; in a convergent squint, one looks inwards. Squints in which one eye looks up or down are rare.

There are several possible causes. In children, these are usually physical problems in the eye itself; a defect in the structure of the cornea, lens, retina, nerves or, most frequently, the muscles of the eye (p32) can cause squinting. In adults a squint is usually the result of a disease elsewhere in the body that affects the eye muscles, or the nerves linking eye and brain. Examples of such diseases include *encephalitis, meningitis, septicaemia, syphilis, poliomyelitis* and various physical brain disorders, together with poisons, such as lead, carbon dioxide and alcohol, and toxic *bacterial* infections.

In children, a squint is often the result of congenital *hypermetropia*, or long-sightedness. Usually only one eye is affected; the condition becomes apparent after about three months, by which time a baby has normally learned how to use its eyes correctly. If the condition is left untreated, the brain reacts by ignoring the signals it receives from the affected eye, which becomes 'lazy' until eventually it may cease to function.

Treatment for a squint in children should begin as early as possible and certainly before the age of seven, after which the chances that the eye will be permanently affected increase substantially. Usually, the non-squinting eye is covered with a patch, to force the other eye to work and to force the brain to process the images from it. If focusing has become affected, the child may be taught a series of special eye exercises to correct the problem. In severe cases, surgery to shorten one or more of the eye muscles may be carried out.

Adult treatment is broadly similar, though here the doctor will look for an underlying cause, and treat that as well as the squint.

STREPTOCOCCUS

A genus of *bacteria*, certain species of which can be extremely dangerous to humans.

Streptococcus pyogenes, for

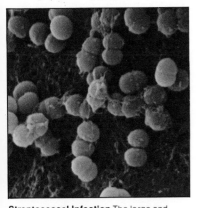

Streptococcal Infection The large and varied group of streptococcal bacteria, one of which is shown magnified 25,600 times *(above)*, is responsible for a number of diseases. Some streptococci are normally found in the mouth and throat, while others inhabit the intestine. Normally, their action is kept in check by the body's own defences, but when resistance is low they may cause disease.

example, which some people carry in the mouth and throat, is responsible for the infection of wounds, and can cause *scarlet fever, tonsillitis* and *impetigo*. It can cause infections in the lymphatic system, and the toxins it produces are responsible for *erysipelas* and other inflammations. S. faecalis, which inhabits the intestine, may cause *pyelonephritis*, and either S. faecalis or S. viridans, which normally inhabit the mouth and throat, can cause *endocarditis*, while other streptococci can cause liver *abscesses* and pulmonary infections. All these varieties of streptococcal bacteria can cause *septicaemia*, or blood poisoning.

Fortunately, streptococci are normally destroyed without difficulty by the body's natural defences (*p52*). When they cause infection, for example in cases where the body's resistance is lowered by another disease, streptococci are highly susceptible to treatment with *penicillin* and other *antibiotics*.

STRETCH MARKS—see Stria

STRIA

A line or streak that appears on the surface of the skin. Striae may be raised above or depressed below the level of the surrounding tissue, and are often a slightly different colour to the skin. They often appear on the thighs, abdomen, buttocks and breasts in *obesity* and on skin that has been stretched by a *tumour* or *oedema*. The 'stretch marks' that appear during pregnancy are known as striae gravidarum. Striae often appear as a side-effect of long term treatment with *steroid* drugs.

Striae are caused by two factors—an accelerated production of hormones, and a weight increase that is rapid enough to stretch the skin. The idea that some people have a type of skin that is more prone to stretch marks than others is not medically proven, but, if true, would account for the fact that some people develop striae while others do not.

Striae gravidarum usually appear suddenly, as the growth of the breasts and abdomen accelerates after the l6th week of pregnancy. They first occur as pink lines on or just under the surface of the skin, and over several months very gradually subside to form a silvery pattern. The reason for their appearance is that the skin has been stretched to the point where its fibres have been broken; once formed, the striae will never disappear and the skin will not regain its former elasticity.

Stretch marks can be prevented

only by careful control of weight gain by means of diet and exercise. Teenagers and people prone to obesity should not allow their weight to increase beyond the optimum for their age and height— *see Diet, p320*. Pregnant women should gain no more than 13kg (28.6lb) during their pregnancy, or l7kg (37.4lb) if carrying twins.

Despite popular belief, massaging the abdomen with oil during pregnancy does not prevent stretch marks, though it may appear to do so if oil is used in combination with careful control of the weight gained and exercise—*see Exercise, p320*.

STROKE—see Cerebrovascular accident

STUTTER—see Stammer

STYE—see Chalazion

SUBARACHNOID HAEMORRHAGE

Bleeding into the subarachnoid space surrounding the brain (*p32*). This is usually caused by the rupture of an *aneurysm*, a swelling in the wall of an artery. Occasionally, it is the result of bleeding from a congenital malformation of a blood vessel, a seepage of blood into the subarachnoid space from a haemorrhage in an adjacent area of the brain or a bleeding brain *tumour*.

A subarachnoid haemorrhage is a form of *cerebrovascular accident*, or stroke. The bleeding causes a severe headache that may be followed by loss of consciousness. When consciousness is regained there may be a stiff neck, double vision, *hemiplegia*, or a paralysis of one side of the body, and *aphasia*.

A patient with a suspected subarachnoid haemorrhage is given a lumbar puncture—*see Special Tests p84*—because the presence of blood in the cerebrospinal fluid confirms the diagnosis. A CAT scan—*see Special Tests, p84*—may then be performed, to pinpoint the site of the bleeding and see if it is possible to tie off the leaking blood vessel by surgery. However, even if this can be done, the damage that has been caused is irreversible. If the victim does not regain consciousness, *coma* and death is likely.

SUBNORMALITY—see Mental handicap

SUDDEN INFANT DEATH SYNDROME—see Cot death

SULPHONAMIDES

A group of antibiotics which were first used in 1936 in the treatment of *puerperal fever*, an infection which often affected the mother after childbirth and was frequently fatal. The drugs work by competing with *bacteria* for supplies of a chemical in the body necessary for the bacteria to multiply. As their only action is to prevent the multiplication of bacteria, sulphonamides are called bacteriostatic drugs, as opposed to bacteriocidal drugs, such as *penicillin*, which actually kill the bacteria.

However, sulphonamides are less used today than they were previously, because many bacteria quickly develop resistance to them, and many more suitable alternatives are now available. A sulphonamide called sulphamethoxazole is still widely used in combination with another antibacterial drug in the treatment of *cystitis* and other urinary tract infections; the combination is called co-trimoxazole.

Sulphonamides have several side-effects. The most common are skin rashes, but very occasionally they cause *kidney failure* and *agranulocytosis*.

SUPPOSITORY

A drug combined with soap, glycerinated gelatine or cocoa butter that is moulded into a shape convenient for insertion into the rectum, urethra or vagina. The base material of a suppository is solid at normal room temperatures but liquid at body temperatures, so that it dissolves when inserted.

In Britain and America, suppositories are generally used only to release a drug near to the site of its intended action—for example, a suppository may contain substances to relieve the discomfort of piles—or as an enema, to cause evacuation of the bowels before surgery or to treat constipation. However, in some countries, particularly France, suppositories are used to administer a wide range of drugs.

SYDENHAM'S CHOREA

A symptom of some *fevers*, especially of *rheumatic fever*, in which the jerky, unco-ordinated movements are made with the arms and legs. Sydenham's chorea, sometimes known as St Vitus' Dance, is thought to be due to an involvement of the brain in the disease process.

Treatment is the same as that for the underlying fever, involving bed rest and aspirin—*see Home Nursing*, *p352*. Sometimes a mild sedative is prescribed to control restlessness.

SYMPATHECTOMY

An operation to cut specific sympathetic nerves (*p32*) at the point where they leave the spinal cord. Which nerves are cut depends on which facet of sympathetic nervous activity the operation is intended to reduce. It is sometimes performed in an attempt to improve the blood supply to the legs in case of severe intermittent *claudication*—in which case the reduced sympathetic activity widens the relevant blood vessels. Sometimes, a sympathectomy is performed to inhibit excessive perspiration or to relieve photophobia, a hypersensitivity to light caused by abnormal dilation of the pupil of the eye.

The alternative to surgery is the use of drugs, such as *beta blockers*, that inhibit of the activity of the sympathetic nervous system. These drugs are non-specific, however, and may have effects other than those required.

SYMPATHOMIMETIC

A drug that mimics the effects of the natural substances, adrenaline and noradrenaline (*p48*), which stimulate the sympathetic nervous system. Synthetic adrenaline and noradrenaline are used as sympathomimetics, as well as similar drugs that have been isolated from related compounds found in animals and plants.

The various sympathomimetics work in three different ways: some act directly on the parasympathetic nervous system (*p32*); some stimulate the release of adrenaline and noradrenaline by the body; and others do both. They have a number of uses: to control superficial bleeding from the skin, because they can constrict blood vessels; to alter the rate of the heartbeat; and as muscle relaxants and nasal decongestants.

SYNCOPE

A temporary loss of consciousness, due to an inadequate supply of blood to the brain.

Fainting is the most common and least serious form of syncope. It may be brought about by pain, fear, heat, an unpleasant sight or smell, or any condition from which the body needs temporary relief. Faints are also called vaso-vagal episodes, because the mechanism that causes them involves stimulation of the vagus nerve (*p32*), which slows the heart rate and causes peripheral vasodilatation—that is, a reduction in the volume of blood returning to the heart. Both these factors lower the blood pressure suddenly. The brain is the first organ to be affected by this, since it is located at the top of the body. The faint and subsequent fall to the ground are thus a protective mechanism which attempts to place the head on the same level as the heart.

Certain drugs such as methyl dopa, which is used to treat *hypertension*, may also predispose people to fainting by causing postural hypotension—a fall in blood pressure while standing—as a side-effect. The same thing can happen in long-standing *diabetes mellitus*, when it is due to *neuropathy*, or degeneration of the nerves, involving the autonomous nervous system (*p32*).

Cough syncope is caused by coughing vigorously; the pressure changes in the chest slow the return of blood to the heart. Similarly, micturition syncope sometimes occurs when elderly people strain to open the bowels or pass urine.

More serious causes of syncope include *heart block* and *Stokes Adams attacks*. In both of these, the heartbeat is slowed because of disease of the conducting nerves in the heart (*p21*). If the normal heart rhythm is restored, the patient usually regains consciousness. Similarly, consciousness is often lost after a *myocardial infarction*. These examples of syncope are due to heart disease of one type or another, and are unrelated to ordinary fainting.

Other causes of temporary loss of consciousness include *hypoglycaemia*, a low level of sugar in the blood, and *hypoxia*, or lack of oxygen from any cause. If these factors are reversed, the patient regains consciousness, though there may be brain damage if the syncope is prolonged.

Simple faints are treated by slackening tight clothing, ensuring that the airway is free so that the patient can breathe, and raising the feet above the level of the heart, so as to assist the return of blood to the heart—*see also First Aid, p369*.

The investigation of fainting, particularly in an older person, includes measurement of blood pressure both standing and lying down, and an ECG test, or electrocardiogram—*see Special Tests, p84*.

SYNOVITIS

An inflammation of the synovium, the membrane that lines a joint. A joint affected by synovitis is usually painful and swollen, since synovial fluid seeps into the synovial sac surrounding the joint (*p16*).

Synovitis may be caused by a wound, by an injury such as a *sprain*, or by a chronic inflammatory disease, such as *rheumatoid arthritis*. In the case of a sprain, no treatment, other than resting the affected joint, is normally necessary. The joint usually heals spontaneously, the pain lessening and the swelling subsiding as the fluid and blood in the sac are absorbed. However, if a large amount of fluid remains in the cavity, the synovitis may become chronic. The membrane becomes permanently thickened by the formation of fibrous tissue. The joint becomes weakened, difficult to move and particularly painful. This condition can be alleviated to some extent by drawing off the fluid with a special needle, and by the use of *anti-inflammatory* drugs.

SYPHILIS

A *sexually transmitted disease* caused by the bacterium Treponema pallidum, a member of the family of bacteria known as spirochaetes. The bacteria may enter the body during sexual intercourse via the penis, vagina, anus or mouth; but they may also pass through an open cut or graze elsewhere on the body. They may infect a foetus in the womb via the placenta, in the condition known as congenital syphilis.

Acquired syphilis (as opposed to congenital syphilis) has three distinct phases. The primary stage usually occurs after an incubation period of between nine and 90 days, when a small, pink ulcer, called a chancre, appears at the site of the infection. The chancre usually secretes a thin discharge, and the lymph nodes *(p21)* in the area often become enlarged. The chancre normally lasts for several weeks, and then disappears. It is painless, and it may be mistaken for a sore caused by abrasion, or it may be so small that it passes unnoticed.

The secondary stage usually begins from six to eight weeks after the appearance of the chancre, when signs of systemic infection, such as *malaise*, headache, and intermittent *fever* may appear. A red rash breaks out in about 75% of patients, while others may develop small, superficial ulcers in the mouth, or broad, flat wart-like growths known as condylomata. These appear on the mucous membranes of the

genitals. They are highly infectious because they contain large numbers of bacteria which can be transmitted by kissing or sexual intercourse. *Lymphadenopathy* is a common symptom during this stage of the disease.

The second stage is commonly followed by a long period in which the disease is latent—that is, it shows no symptoms and seems to have disappeared. This can last for two to ten years, or even longer. Then, in the tertiary stage, the disease may begin to attack the skin and subcutaneous tissues, mucous membranes and long bones. It eventually spreads to the nervous system, causing degeneration of the brain and spinal cord.

At this stage, however, the symptoms of syphilis may resemble any one of a number of diseases—hence its medical nickname of 'the great imitator'. Small, painless *tumours* called gummas, which take a long time to heal, spread throughout the body. If located in the brain, they may be mistaken for slowly developing *tumours* of the brain. Infection of the meninges—the membranes enclosing the brain and spinal cord—may damage the cranial nerves *(p32)*, causing headaches, fits and cranial nerve paralysis, while degeneration of the brain's cortex leads in some cases to general paralysis of the insane between five and 15 years after infection. In this condition, sufferers become *demented* and experience paralysis in the limbs.

In some patients, tertiary syphilis takes another form, affecting the nerves which serve the lower back. This condition, called tabes dorsalis, develops between five and 20 years after infection. Symptoms include pain in the lower abdomen, legs and feet, *ataxia* and *incontinence*.

In addition to the damage to the nervous system, the sufferer may develop heart disease. Inflammation of the linings of the arteries may lead to *thrombosis*, or the blockage of a blood vessel by a clot. Some patients develop syphilitic *aortitis* between 15 and 20 years after infection; this is a

condition in which inflammation causes dilatation of the aorta. These conditions may be fatal.

In congenital syphilis there is no primary stage. If a foetus is infected with syphilis, a spontaneous abortion may occur, or the child may be stillborn. Babies who are born with the disease may have skin eruptions at birth, or may appear normal, but develop a rash and characteristic signs of disease of the bone or internal organs soon after birth. Sometimes, however, the child may survive for several years without symptoms, but later develop deformities of the bones and teeth, *iritis, keratitis,* or signs of nervous disease.

Acquired syphilis is diagnosed by blood tests—*see STS, Special Tests, p84.* Such tests are routinely performed on expectant mothers to rule out the possibility that she will pass the disease on to her child. In the first two stages, the disease can be cured by large injections of penicillin. In the third stage, however, it is possible only to arrest its progress. Any damage to the tissues or nerves that may have occurred cannot be repaired. Congenital syphilis is also cured by early injections of penicillin.

The destructive symptoms that occur in the later stages are now fairly rare; congenital syphilis is even more rare, due to improved ante-natal care. During the last 15 years, however, the incidence of syphilis has been increasing, particularly among male homosexuals. Anyone with the slightest suspicion that they may have contracted the disease should contact a doctor immediately and should refrain from close bodily contact with another person until pronounced free of it.

SYRINGOMYELIA

A disease caused by a cavity within the spinal cord. There have recently been considerable advances in medical knowledge of this condition; it is now believed that in most cases it is due to a congenital abnormality of the brain that causes partial obstruction to the flow of cerebrospinal fluid. The pressure of the fluid increases inside the spinal cord and makes it dilate. When such an abnormality is present it can sometimes be helped, at least partially, by surgery.

The symptoms of syringomyelia usually first appear in early adult life. They take the form of weakness and muscle wasting of the hands; the ability to feel pain is lost and consequently patients burn themselves without realizing it. Sensitivity to touch, however, is

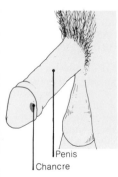

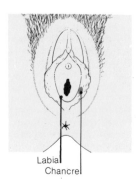

Syphilis is a disease which progresses through three stages. In the first, a sore called a chancre grows where the bacterium, Treponema pallidum, enters the body. In a man, this sore usually develops on the penis **(left)** or on the anus in homosexuals. In a woman, it usually grows on one of the labia of the vulva **(right)**.

Penis
Chancre

Labia
Chancre

usually preserved. The legs may also be affected. The symptoms are made worse by coughing or sneezing. In some patients the disease remains stationary, but usually it becomes progressively worse unless surgical treatment is successful.

SYSTEMIC

An adjective describing a disease that affects the body as a whole, as opposed to a localized disease that affects only an area of the body. Similarly, a drug may have a local effect, acting on a particular system or part of the body, or a systemic effect, on the whole body.

SYSTEMIC LUPUS ERYTHEMATOSUS—see Lupus erythematosus

SYSTEMIC SCLEROSIS—see Scleroderma.

SYSTOLE

The period during the heartbeat—*see The Blood and Lymph System, p21*—during which the chambers of the heart contract. Atrial systole occurs when the muscles of the atria contract, forcing blood into the ventricles—these are in a state known as diastole. The atria then go into diastole, filling with blood, while the ventricles contract to pump blood . *See also diastole.*

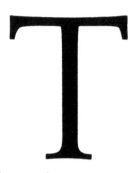

TABES DORSALIS—see Syphilis

TACHYCARDIA

A fast heart beat, giving rise to a pulse rate of more than 80 beats a minute. Tachycardia can have a number of causes. It may be a temporary response to the body's increased demands for blood in exercise, or to *anxiety*, a *fever* or the use of *amphetamine* drugs. Tachycardia may also be a symptom of specific illnesses and conditions, such as *thyrotoxicosis*, and *shock* caused by bleeding, in which the heart has to beat faster to make up for a sudden drop in blood pressure. Treatment of tachycardia is according to its cause; when this is anxiety, for example, *beta blockers* may be prescribed.

TALIPES

A *congenital deformity* of the foot and ankle, commonly known as club foot.

The precise cause of talipes is not known, but the condition is thought to be caused by compression of the foot while the foetus is in the womb. Very large babies, for example, tend to be slightly squashed in a small womb. In serious cases, talipes is associated with *spina bifida* or deformities elsewhere in the body.

The condition may affect one or both feet. There are two varieties: the foot may point upwards or downwards. In either case, the foot may point inwards or outwards. The most common type of talipes, however, is known as calcaneo valgus. In this, the feet point upwards and outwards, but the degree of deformity is often so slight that the feet appear almost normal.

In the second most common type, known as talipes equinovarus, the feet point downwards and inwards.

In mild cases, treatment is by gentle *physiotherapy* and stretching exercises. The child's relatives are taught how to perform these, so that treatment can continue at home. Such treatment is often successful, and no permanent disability results. In more serious cases, a series of different plaster casts and special splints may be required to coax the affected feet back into position. On rare occasions, an orthopaedic operation may be necessary.

TAMPONADE

A condition in which external pressure on the heart affects its ability to pump. The result is that blood pressure *(p21)* drops, leading to serious *shock*.

The most common cause of the increase in pressure is an *effusion* from the pericardium, the membrane surrounding the heart, into the pericardial cavity. This may be the result of *pericarditis*, an inflammation of the membrane, which is occasionally due to *tuberculosis*. Sometimes, also as a result of tuberculosis, the pericardium may shrink, increasing the pressure still further.

Cardiac tamponade is diagnosed by a chest X-ray—*see Special Tests, p84*—and by measuring the patient's blood pressure. This suddenly falls as he or she takes a breath, due to the further constriction of the heart by the expanding lungs. The condition is treated as an emergency. A needle is passed into the pericardial cavity through the patient's chest, and the fluid is

withdrawn, relieving the pressure on the heart. After this, treatment is according to the cause of the increase in pressure.

TAPEWORM—see Worms

TEMPORAL ARTERITIS (GIANT CELL ARTERITIS)

A form of arterial inflammation (arteritis), usually seen in older patients. It is fairly common and affects women more than men. It is related to polymyalgia rheumatica, which is defined as muscular aching and stiffness, especially in the morning, and lasting for more than a month.

The cause of temporal arteritis is unknown. Its chief importance is that it is a preventable cause of blindness. Onset is gradual or sudden. The sedimentation rate is nearly always very high. In typical cases the temporal artery at the side of the head is obviously swollen and tender, but sometimes the symptoms are much less obvious. Headache and sensitivity of the scalp are common. Disturbance of vision is found in about half the patients, and blindness, which may develop suddenly, has been reported in about 10 per cent of cases. The diagnosis is usually made by taking a *biopsy* of the temporal artery.

Corticosteroids relieve the syptoms dramatically and prevent blindness. Recovery after six months to two years is usual, though relapses often occur. Because of the danger of blindness, steroids are started immediately, without waiting for the biopsy result, if there is any suspicion of temporal arteritis.

TENNIS ELBOW

A painful condition thought to involve inflammation of the tendons of the muscles of the forearm at the point where they join the bone of the upper arm—see Bone and Muscle, p16. As a result of the inflammation, the elbow becomes painful, especially when the arm is straightened and the wrist rotated. The condition occurs spontaneously as a result of repeated movements of the forearm and wrist, as may be made, for example, by someone playing tennis or squash.

Tennis elbow usually clears up without treatment after a few days. In severe cases, relief can be obtained by the injection of hydrocortisone—see steroids—around the elbow joint.

TERATOGEN

Any agent that causes abnormal development in an embryo—see Embryology, p12.

There are a large number of teratogens, including the rubella virus and exposure to radiation—see radiation sickness; Special Tests, p84. Perhaps the best-known, however, is thalidomide. This drug, an anti-emetic prescribed to large numbers of pregnant women between 1959 and 1961, caused severe malformations to the limbs of thousands of foetuses.

Since the effects of thalidomide have been understood, all new drugs have had to pass rigorous tests before being licensed for use. Nevertheless, most doctors prefer not to prescribe drugs to pregnant women unless they are absolutely essential. By the same token, women who suspect that they may be pregnant should inform their doctor before continuing existing treatment or starting a new course of drugs.

It is now realized that alcohol and nicotine are also harmful to the foetus, even in small quantities. Consequently, women are strongly advised to give up smoking and alcohol altogether, as soon as they start a baby.

TERMINAL ILEITIS—see Crohn's disease

TESTICULAR TUMOUR

An abnormal growth in a testis, one of the two male sex glands—see Sex and Reproduction, p54.

Testicular tumours, are rare, accounting for around 2% of all cancers in men, but are important for two reasons. Firstly, such tumours tend to affect young adults, unlike most other cancers; secondly, testicular tumours are generally malignant. Tumours often develop in undescended testicles—see cryptorchidism—and, for this reason, testicles that cannot be moved to their correct position are usually removed by surgery.

There are two main types of testicular tumour: seminomas and teratomas. Occasionally, both types develop simultaneously. Seminomas, which develop in the tissues of the seminiferous tubules, account for around 40% of testicular tumours and mainly affect men between the ages of 30 and 40. Teratomas mainly affect men in their 20s, and arise from primitive cells that often contain elements of all three basic embryological tissues—see Embryology, p12.

The first sign of a testicular tumour is usually the enlargement of the scrotum. In around a third of all cases, there is no pain. As a result, the first noticeable signs may occur when the tumour has spread to other parts of the body, forming secondary growths.

Treatment is by surgical removal of the tumour—see orchidectomy—followed by radiotherapy and chemotherapy. The outlook depends on how much the tumour has grown before diagnosis. If secondary cancers have formed, the condition is likely to prove fatal. For this reason, any enlargement of the scrotum should be reported to a doctor.

TETANUS

A potentially fatal disease, also called lockjaw, caused by a toxin produced by the bacterium Clostridium tetani. Clostridia bacteria live in the intestines of both animals and humans and, as a result of faecal contamination, in soil and dirt. The bacteria enter the bloodstream through a scratch or graze and multiply in the infected wound.

The first symptoms appear after the bacterial toxin has spread through the blood to the nervous system; this takes between one day and two weeks, depending on the site of the infection. The toxin causes the voluntary muscles (p32) to contract in agonizingly painful spasms. The muscles of the jaw are the first to be affected. The spasms, called trismus, cause difficulty in opening the mouth—hence lockjaw, the common name for tetanus.

The muscular spasms rapidly spread, giving the face a fixed smile known to doctors as risus sardonicus. The muscles used in swallowing and those of the neck and back may also be involved, so that the whole body arches backwards. A severely affected patient may experience sudden violent spasms of the muscles of the upper part of the body, lasting up to three or four seconds. These may occur more and more frequently and violently, until the patient dies from exhaustion, or, if the respiratory muscles are affected, from suffocation.

A mild form of tetanus exists, but is much more rare. In this, there is stiffness or minor spasms around the site of infection, and sometimes mild convulsions. These begin about a week after the first signs of stiffness, and then die away.

Diagnosis of tetanus is difficult until the spasms start, since the bacteria are rarely found in the wound. As a result, treatment is routinely given to anyone who has an unclean wound, especially when the person is at risk by the nature of his or her occupation—a veterinary surgeon, farm worker or gardener, for example. The wound is cleaned and, if necessary, drained of pus or fluid, and an antiserum containing an antitoxin known as tetanus toxoid is injected near the site. Human antiserum is preferred, but this is expensive and not always available; antiserum taken from horses is an effective substitute, but occasionally causes a serious allergic reaction in some people. The injection is followed by a course of antibiotics.

If symptoms have already appeared, however, the sufferer is admitted to hospital, and nursed in a darkened, quiet room. The bed clothes are supported by a metal cage and the patient handled gently, because any pressure, noise or light may trigger spasms. These are controlled by diazepam, a drug used as a tranquillizer, or, in more severe cases, by curare, a muscle relaxant. Such treatment is usually successful, but death results in around ten per cent of cases.

Tetanus is rare in the Western world, though several people in Britain die as a result of the disease each year. In the underdeveloped countries, however, the condition is common. It often affects newborn babies, who contract the disease when they are born in dirty conditions. In such cases, tetanus is nearly always fatal.

A prime factor in the rarity of tetanus in the West is the success of immunization as a preventive measure. Children are vaccinated against tetanus on three occasions during childhood—see Health and Your Child, p 348—and all adults should ask their doctor for a booster injection every five years.

TETANY

A condition in which the peripheral nerves become abnormally excitable—that is, they transmit nerve impulses for no apparent cause, or in response to minor stimuli. As a result, pins and needles—see *paraesthesiae*,—are felt in hands and feet. Spasms, known as carpopedal spasms also occur in the hands and feet; the hands, in particular, tend to bend forwards at the wrist and knuckles while the fingers remain straight.

The direct cause of tetany is a biochemical change in which there is a reduced level of calcium in the blood. This chemical plays a vital part in controlling the excitability of nerves. The problem, known as hypocalcaemia, may be caused by a number of factors. These include a vitamin D deficiency, often the result of *malabsorption syndrome*, in which case tetany is associated with *rickets* and *osteomalacia*; underactivity, or removal, of the parathyroid glands (p48), which normally secrete parathormone, a hormone that controls the level of blood calcium; and *alkalosis*, in which the acid-base balance of the body is disturbed as a result of vomiting, taking an excessive amount of *antacids* or milk, or *hyperventilation*.

Treatment of tetany depends on its cause. Rickets, osteomalacia and malabsorption syndrome are treated by calcium and vitamin D supplements. Sufferers from alkalosis should stop taking antacids and milk; an aspirin overdose is treated with forced diuresis—that is, giving the victim large quantities of fluid and *diuretics* to increase the rate of the drug's excretion in the urine; and hyperventilation by making the patient breathe in and out of a paper bag to increase the level of carbon dioxide in the blood and restore the acid-base balance— see *The Respiratory System, p28*. In severe cases of tetany, however, emergency treatment may be necessary. This consists of injecting a calcium salt at a slow, controlled rate, into a vein or a muscle.

TETRACYCLINE

An *antibiotic* drug. Tetracycline does not kill *bacteria*, but neutralizes their activity and stops them from reproducing by preventing them from making proteins. As a result, it is known as a bacteriostatic antibiotic. Tetracycline is also effective against other disease organisms, such as *rickettsiae*.

THALASSAEMIA

An inherited abnormality of the haemoglobin in the red blood cells— see *The Blood and Lymph Systems, p21*. As a result of the abnormality, the spleen tends to destroy red blood cells before the end of their natural life-cycle, causing *anaemia*. Thalassaemia, also known as Cooley's *anaemia*, is particularly common among Mediterranean peoples and their descendants.

The two different chains of molecules within globin, the protein constituent of haemoglobin, are alpha and beta chains. Two different types of thalassaemia exist, depending on which of these chains is abnormal. Alpha chain thalassaemia is uncommon, and tends to be confined to South-East Asia. In serious cases, an affected foetus may be stillborn. Beta chain thalassaemia is more common, however, and may vary in severity according to the way in which it is inherited—see *genes*.

If the beta abnormality is inherited from only one parent, the resultant *anaemia* is mild; this condition is known as thalassaemia trait or thalassaemia minor. It is rarely a serious problem, and often goes unnoticed. If an abnormal beta gene is inherited from each parent, however, the result is more serious. In this condition, known as thalassaemia major, large numbers of red cells are destroyed by the spleen. The result is a severe, debilitating anaemia, with enlargement of the liver, spleen, and, sometimes, the heart. The extra load on the heart may result in death.

Affected children are normal at birth, but start to show symptoms of anaemia within three or four months. Without treatment, growth and development are retarded and survival for more than a few years is unlikely. Diagnosis is made through examination of a sample of blood— see *Special Tests, p84*—and treatment consists of regular *transfusion* and folic acid supplements (p322). The spleen is removed in serious cases— see *splenectomy*—reducing the need for transfusion; this, however, may cause accelerated enlargement of the liver.

THREADWORM—see Worms

THROMBO-ANGIITIS OBLITERANS—see Buerger's disease

THROMBOCYTHAEMIA

An increase in the number of platelets, also medically termed thrombocytes, circulating in the blood—see *The Blood and Lymph Systems, p21*. The direct cause of this is an increase in the number of specialized bone marrow cells that produce platelets. The mechanism is not fully understood, but is thought to resemble that of cancer of the bone marrow.

Thrombocythaemia may cause two different sets of symptoms; both are the result of the importance of platelets to the process by which blood clots (p21). Sometimes, sufferers tend to bleed, either spontaneously or after minor bumps and bangs. There may be bleeding from the digestive tract or the womb, and bruises may form in the skin. Alternatively, the platelets may clump together, forming small blood clots. These may be carried through the bloodstream—see *embolisms*— and lodge in small arteries. The consequences can be serious. If the central retinal artery is blocked, for example, there may be sudden loss of vision. In the brain, the platelet clumps may cause *transient ischaemic attacks* (TIAs), minor, short-lived strokes. If clumps lodge in the small arteries of the fingers and toes, the result may be *ischaemia*, and, later, *gangrene*.

In the majority of cases, the only outward sign of thrombocythaemia is an enlarged spleen. Diagnosis is by examination of blood and bone marrow samples, which show the increased number of platelets and platelet-producing cells—see *Special Tests, p84*. Treatment is with radioactive phosphorus or bulsulphan, a drug that depresses the production of new cells in the bone marrow. This may control the symptoms, but is unlikely to completely cure the disease. There is a risk that death may suddenly occur from a stroke—see *cerebrovascular accident*—or that the condition of the bone marrow may deteriorate, causing a form of *leukaemia*.

THROMBOCYTOPAENIA

A reduction in the normal number of platelets, also called thrombocytes, circulating in the blood—see *The Blood and Lymph Systems, p21*. Since platelets are essential for the clotting of blood, the main symptom of thrombocytopaenia is excessive bleeding. This may be into the skin—small, red dots, called petechiae, which join together to form *purpura*, a feature of the condition—or in the form of nosebleeds—see *epistaxis*—heavy menstrual periods—see *menorrhagia*—or from the digestive tract. This loss of blood may cause a serious *anaemia*.

There are a number of causes of thrombocytopaenia. Several drugs may interfere with the production of platelets in the bone marrow. Such drugs include the *antibiotics* chloramphenicol and *tetracycline*, and phenylbutazone, an *anti-inflammatory* agent. Diseases affecting the bone marrow, such as *leukaemia* and *cancer*, may also have this effect.

Alternatively, the platelets circulating in the blood may be destroyed by an *auto-immune* reaction which may, in turn, be due to sensitivity to a specific drug. In this case the concentration of platelets in the blood returns to normal once the drug is stopped. The number of platelets in the blood may also be reduced by an *acute* infection, especially *typhoid* and glandular fever—*see infectious mononucleosis*. Sometimes the level of platelets drops for no apparent cause, in which case the condition is known as idiopathic thrombocytopaenic purpura.

Diagnosis is by examination of the numbers of platelets in a blood sample—*see Special Tests, p84*. Treatment of the condition depends on its cause. The first step is usually to re-evaluate any drug therapy, and, if possible, to prescribe alternative drugs. If this does not work, *transfusions* may be necessary to replaces blood loss, *Steroid* drugs are prescribed, in high dosages at first, until the platelet count approaches normal levels. If these measures fail and the platelet count does not rise, *splenectomy*, removal of the spleen, may be effective. This is because platelets naturally tend to become trapped in the spleen.

A small proportion of patients do not respond to any treatment. Such people usually live relatively normal lives, without serious complications. They may experience minor episodes of bleeding into the skin, and there is a danger that blood vessels inside the brain may bleed, causing a stroke—*see cerebrovascular accident*. However, the danger is less than that associated with long-term steroid therapy.

THROMBOPHLEBITIS

An inflammation of the superficial veins—that is, those closest to the skin—most commonly affecting the legs. Thrombophlebitis is caused by tiny blood clots, which irritate and damage the smooth lining of the veins, allowing inflammation to set in. The condition sometimes follows surgery to the legs.

Symptoms include considerable pain in the affected area. Since the damaged vessels tend to leak fluid into the tissues, the area may also be slightly swollen—*see oedema*. The condition is usually short-lived, however, and rarely spreads to involve other veins.

Treatment is with *anti-inflammatory* drugs. Sufferers are advised to take gentle exercise if possible; this is also recommended as a preventive measure after surgery. When lying down the legs should be elevated to keep the blood

from lying stagnant in the legs—*see varicose veins*—and elastic support stockings can be worn to keep gentle pressure on the veins. *Antibiotics* may be necessary if there is marked infection or associated ulceration of the skin—*see ulcer*.

THROMBOSIS

The formation of a blood clot, called a thrombus, in a blood vessel. Clots most commonly form around atheromas, fatty deposits that build up on the walls of blood vessels as a result of *atherosclerosis*. Thrombosis may occur in either arteries or veins, with different consequences in each case.

In an arterial thrombosis, the part of the body supplied by the affected artery is deprived of blood and becomes *ischaemic*. When this occurs in a limb, for example, the tissues beyond the blood clot become pale, swollen, and extremely painful. When a coronary artery is blocked by a thrombus, an area of heart muscle is deprived of blood. The result may be a heart attack—*see myocardial infarction; coronary artery disease*. Thrombosis in the blood vessels of the brain may cause a stroke—*see cerebrovascular accident*—or a *transient ischaemic attack*. Treatment of arterial thrombosis depends on the cause and site of the thrombus.

Thrombosis in the veins may have equally serious consequences. Most commonly, thrombi form in the deep veins of the legs. This condition is known as deep vein thrombosis (DVT). Thrombosis in the superficial veins is less serious, but may cause *thrombophlebitis*.

A number of factors predispose to deep vein thrombosis. These include *obesity*; immobility, especially after surgery; pregnancy; and certain drugs, such as the contraceptive pill—*see Sex and Contraception, p338*. The affected leg becomes swollen, slightly reddish and warm, and so painful that walking is impossible. There is a danger that a deep vein thrombus may become dislodged and be carried to another part of the body by the bloodstream; when this happens, the thrombus is known as an *embolism*. If the embolism lodges in the lungs, the result is an extremely serious condition called a *pulmonary embolism*.

Diagnosis is confirmed by X-rays—*see Special Tests, p84*. Treatment begins with bed rest, supportive bandages, elevation of the affected limb and *anticoagulant* drugs to prevent the formation of further thromboses. At first, these drugs are given by injection, directly into a vein. Later, a course of *warfarin* tablets is prescribed, lasting

for around three months. During this period, the other veins of the affected leg become gradually wider, establishing alternative pathways for the blood.

The development of post-operative venous thrombosis is made less likely by maintaining the circulation in the legs during and immediately after surgery. This can be achieved by wearing elastic stockings that compress the veins and help to stop the blood from pooling and stagnating in the lower limbs; and by *physiotherapy*, which may include leg exercises, and getting patients up and walking around as soon as possible after surgery. Patients at greatest risk of deep venous thrombosis following surgery, such as the elderly and the obese, may be treated with anticoagulants.

THROMBUS—see Thrombosis

THRUSH—see Candidiasis

THUMB-SUCKING

A normal activity in babies and small children. Usually it disappears spontaneously by the age of five or six years; if it persists, mothers sometimes become worried about it and try to stop it. This is a mistake. Thumb-sucking is completely harmless. If it persists or recurs in a child of school age, it may be an indication that something is bothering him or her; perhaps the strain of going to a new school, or some change in the home environment. Parents should never threaten or punish a child for sucking his thumb, since this can only make matters worse by increasing the tension; instead, look for anything that may be causing it. However, no reason may be apparent; there is probably no single cause for persistent thumb-sucking.

Thumb-sucking does not force the teeth out of position, and indeed there is some evidence that children who suck their thumbs actually have less tooth decay than others, though the reason for this is unknown. The sucked thumb may acquire a hard patch of skin (callus), but this is not important and will disappear when the child eventually stops sucking it.

If parents dislike seeing a baby sucking its thumb they can provide a dummy; this needs to be kept clean, and sterilized.

THYROID DISEASE—see Thyrotoxicosis; Myxoedema; Thyroiditis

THYROIDECTOMY

An operation to remove part or all of the thyroid gland—*see The Endocrine*

System, p48. A subtotal thyroidectomy, in which a part of the gland is removed, may be necessary to treat *thyrotoxicosis*; the whole gland may be removed to treat a *thyroid tumour*. In this case, thyroxine, the hormone normally produced by the gland, must be replaced. This is done by thyroxine tablets, which must be taken for life. Since it is extremely difficult to remove the thyroid without affecting the parathyroid glands embedded in it, a substitute for parathormone may also be necessary. This is calciferol, a vitamin D2 compound *(p322)*. Pre-operatively, iodine is often given, to help shrink the gland. The operation leaves a barely noticeable hairline scar.

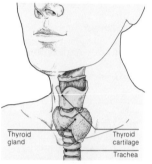

Thyroid gland | Thyroid cartilage | Trachea

Thyroid Gland The two lobes of the thyroid gland lie below the thyroid cartilage of the larynx and either side of the trachea *(above)*. The principal role of the gland is to secrete the thyroid hormone which contains iodine and is important in the regulation of the rate of the body's metabolism.

THYROIDITIS
The collective name for a number of conditions in which the thyroid gland becomes inflamed—*see The Endocrine System, p48*. These conditions include acute suppurative thyroiditis; Hashimoto's thyroiditis; De Quervain's thyroiditis; and Reidel's thyroiditis.

The most common cause of thyroiditis is a defect in the immune response—*see auto-immune disease*. In this condition, known as Hashimoto's thyroiditis, the body either forms antibodies against thyroglobulin, a protein found in the gland, or against the glandular tissue itself. Hashimoto's thyroiditis is most common in middle-aged women. It causes *goitre*, an enlargement of the gland; an ache in the neck and *dysphagia*, or difficulty in swallowing. Some patients also suffer from underactivity of the gland—*see myxoedema*. If the condition occurs in adolescents, it may spontaneously clear up after a course of tablets containing thyroxine, the hormone secreted by the thyroid gland. When the condition occurs in adults, however, the thyroxine treatment must be continued for life.

De Quervain's thyroiditis, also known as subacute thyroiditis and giant cell thyroidism, is a painful condition, thought to be caused by a *virus*. The cells of the thyroid gland enlarge, resulting in goitre, an enlargement of the gland itself. The condition sometimes clears up on its own, but can persist. It generally responds to daily thyroxine treatment, but a course of *corticosteroid* drugs may also be necessary.

The two other forms of thyroiditis are more rare. Acute suppurative thyroiditis may either be caused by *bacterial* infection, *sarcoidosis*, *tuberculosis* or *syphilis*. It is treated according to its cause, generally with *antibiotics*. The least common form of thyroiditis is known as Reidel's thyroiditis, or struma. The cause of this condition is unknown, but it results in enlargment and hardening of the gland, and, eventually, *myxoedema*. The hardening of the gland may put pressure on the laryngeal nerve, causing hoarseness and noisy breathing. Reidel's thyroiditis is difficult to diagnose, because the symptoms are very similar to those caused by a *thyroid tumour*. The two conditions can be distinguished, however, by a biopsy—*see Special Tests, p84*.

A *thyroidectomy*, the surgical removal of the thyroid gland, would be the ideal form of treatment. This is impossible in Reidel's thyroiditis, however, since the glandular tissues adhere firmly to the other structures in the neck. Surgery is therefore confined to relieving the pressure on the laryngeal nerve, and, if necessary, the condition is treated with daily dosages of thyroxine.

THYROTOXICOSIS
A condition in which overactivity of the thyroid gland causes the production of excessive amounts of thyroxine, the thyroid hormone—*see The Endocrine System, p48*. Thyrotoxicosis is also known as hyperthyroidism, and Graves' disease.

Since thyroxine controls the metabolic rate—the rate at which the body uses energy, *see Metabolism, p44*—the symptoms of thyrotoxicosis are all related to an increase in this rate. They include weight loss, hunger, a rapid pulse, and excessive heat production, causing sweating at night and a preference for cool conditions. The muscles tend to waste, especially around the shoulders and hips. The strain on the heart muscle may cause atrial *fibrillation*, an irregularity of the heart beat, and, in the elderly, *heart failure*. There may also be a fine tremor of the outstretched hands, diarrhoea

and scanty or absent menstrual periods. The eyes tend to bulge and the eyelids are retracted, so that the white can be seen all around the iris—this symptom is termed exophthalmos. The thyroid gland can often be felt as a lump.

Treatment depends upon the patient's age. The most effective treatment is by radioactive iodine. This is given either in tablet form or in a drink, and taken up by the thyroid gland, which uses iodine in the formation of thyroxine; the dosage is carefully controlled so that only the desired amount of glandular tissue is destroyed. However, this treatment is not suitable for women of childbearing age, and men who still wish to have children, because there is a slight risk that the radioactivity will cause mutations in the male and female sex cells—*see Sex and Reproduction, p54*. Ordinary iodine, in tablet form, may also have the effect of temporarily reducing thyroid output. Sometimes the period of remission produced in this way lasts for a long time; however, around half of patients treated with ordinary iodine quickly suffer a relapse.

A partial *thyroidectomy*—surgical removal of a part of the thyroid gland—is sometimes the only effective form of treatment. Often, however, this causes *myxoedema*, an underproduction of thyroxine, with the result that replacement thyroid hormone must be taken for the rest of life. This may also occur as a result of radioactive iodine treatment.

TIA—see Transient ischaemic attack

TICS
Sudden, abrupt, purposeless, involuntary muscular contractions. They may take the form of blinking, head shaking, shoulder shrugging, or indeed any sudden gesture of the limbs or face. Often they are a response to stress. Tics should be distinguished from *chorea* and also from the involuntary twitching of the eyelid that affects many normal people at times, especially if they are tired. Minor tics are also common in normal people. If they are severe or persistent, however, they require psychiatric treatment.

A rare, but dramatic, form of the tic is called Gilles de la Tourette's syndrome, which is thought to be a disease of the central nervous system. It begins in childhood and is characterized by facial twitching and an irresistible compulsion to shout out swear words and obscenities. Many patients have an involuntary tendency to repeat words or sentences that they have just heard, or to imitate other people's movements. In a few cases the symptoms improve after adolescence, but in most it lasts for the whole of the patient's life. Mentally these patients are normal. Drugs that can relieve the symptoms exist, but they have possible serious side effects, and since they must be continued indefinitely, it may often be better not to treat the condition.

TINEA
A group of skin infections also known as ringworm. This name is misleading, because the infections are not caused by a worm, but by a group of related *fungi*. In some cases, however, the fungus causes inflammation of a ring-shaped patch of skin, and the raised outer edge of the ring looks worm-like. This type of tinea is known as tinea circinata. In other cases, there is no clearly defined outer edge; the inflamed skin becomes spongy and eventually flakes and peels. Both types of tinea cause an intense itchiness that comes and goes.

Tinea fungi can attack any area of the skin, but the damp, warm parts of the body are the most vulnerable. The form of tinea that affects the groin is called tinea cruris, or dhobie itch; tinea capitis affects the scalp; and tinea barbae, sometimes known as barber's rash, affects the beard. The most common form, however, is tinea pedis. Also known as athlete's foot, this attacks the warm, moist areas between the toes. When tinea affects other areas of the skin, the condition is known as tinea corporis.

Tinea is highly infectious, and spreads from person to person through close physical contact. To a large extent the problem can be avoided if people use only their own towels, especially if living in large communities, where the risk of infection is high, and thoroughly dry themselves after washing—*see Health and Hygiene, p334.*

Treatment of tinea depends on its site and type. Tinea of the groin and feet is treated with antifungal cream, for example, and tinea circinata is treated with twice-daily applications of benzoic acid compound ointment. An antifungal drug called griseofulvin may be given in tablet form for the treatment of tinea of the scalp and beard.

A number of self-help measures also aid healing, and prevent the spread of infection. People suffering from athlete's foot, for example, should dry their feet with a separate towel and avoid wearing shoes and socks made from synthetic materials. These do not allow the feet to breathe, or the air to circulate,

and create the warm, damp conditions in which fungi flourish. For the same reason, people with tinea cruris should wear cotton underwear. Socks and underwear should be changed daily, and thoroughly washed.

TINNITUS
A condition in which sounds are heard in the ear for no apparent reason. Usually, the sounds are inaudible to others, though in rare cases they can be heard; generally they seem extremely loud to the sufferer. They may take the form of buzzing, whistling, ringing or a series of clicks, and occur either continuously or intermittently. The condition is normally a symptom of an underlying disorder, such as *otosclerosis, otitis interna, Mèniére's disease,* or, less seriously, the presence of wax in the ear—*see cerumen.* Occasionally, it is caused by long-term exposure to loud noises, such as industrial noise, gunfire and loud music.

There are two types of tinnitus: subjective and objective. Subjective tinnitus is the more common, and affects people with normal hearing as well as those with impaired hearing. The sounds are generated inside the ear and can only be heard by the sufferer. This type of tinnitus is described as subjective because it takes different forms in different people, making treatment extremely difficult.

Objective tinnitus is more rare, and the sounds caused by it can sometimes be heard by other people, often as a series of faint clicks. These may be caused by rhythmic contractions of the muscles of the palate, by grating of the jaw bones at the joint beneath the ear, or by irregular surges of blood through the arteries serving the ear.

Tinnitus cannot be cured. It may, however, be relieved by treatment for any underlying disorder, and can sometimes be masked. A device that generates a continuous, gentle tone, similar to that caused by the tinnitus, is placed in the ear. After a time, the brain becomes so accustomed to the noise that it ignores it, filtering the nerve signals out of the subconscious mind. This is not always successful, but has relieved the distress of a number of tinnitus sufferers.

Since tinnitus takes such varied forms, individual sufferers have to experiment to discover the most appropriate form of treatment. Cleaning wax from the ears, abstaining from alcohol, tea, coffee, smoking or certain foods may all help to alleviate the condition, and some sufferers have found relief

through yoga and acupuncture—*see Alternative Medicine, p305.* By contrast, aspirin and loud noises exacerbate the problem in many sufferers. The British Tinnitus Association exists to help tinnitus sufferers, and advise on developments in treatment.

TONSILLITIS
An inflammation of the tonsils, two collections of lymph tissue at the back of the throat—*see The Blood and Lymph Systems, p21.*

Tonsillitis may be caused by either a *bacterial* or *viral* infection. Recurrent infections are common during childhood, but the condition is rarely seen in adults. Symptoms include a sore throat, a general feeling of tiredness and ill-health, and, in some cases, a *fever.* The *adenoids,* nodules of lymph tissue at the back of the nose, may also become infected and inflamed. In some cases, a serious bacterial infection may set in, causing the formation of an *abscess* around the tonsils. This condition is known as *quinsy.*

Diagnosis is made by examination of the throat. The red, enlarged tonsils can be seen protruding behind folds, known as fauces, at the back of the mouth. Sometimes, flecks of pus can be clearly seen on their surfaces.

Treatment is by *antibiotics* to clear up any bacterial infection, and aspirin to control any fever. With this treatment, and bed-rest—*see Home Nursing, p352*—the symptoms usually subside within a few days. At one time, recurrent tonsillitis was routinely treated by the surgical removal of the tonsils. This operation, called a tonsillectomy, was often performed with an adenoidectomy. It has now been realized that this was largely unnecessary, since recurrent tonsillitis generally clears up during adolescence. Today, the operation is performed only in serious, persistent cases.

TORSION OF THE TESTIS
An uncommon condition in which the spermatic cord becomes twisted inside the scrotum—*see Sex and Reproduction p54.*

Torsion of the testicle most commonly occurs during adolescence, though it can affect males of all ages. It is usually associated with some minor abnormality of the testes, such as looseness of the outer protective layer that attaches the body of the testis to the spermatic cord. The result of torsion is swelling of the scrotum and considerable pain; the testis often appears to have been drawn up towards the body. There may also be nausea and vomiting.

Immediate surgery is necessary, as the twists in the cord may trap blood vessels, cutting off the blood supply to the testis. This may result in *ischaemia* and death of the tissue. The scrotum is opened, the cord is untwisted, and the testicle fixed in the scrotum, so that it is unable to twist again. If there has been a delay in diagnosis and treatment, *orchidectomy*—the surgical removal of the testicle—may be necessary.

TORTICOLLIS

Acute torticollis in adults may occur for no obvious reason, though it is thought that at least in some cases it is due to a prolapsed intervertebral disc in the neck. Other cases may be due to the development of trigger points in the neck muscles. Acute torticollis often improves spontaneously in a few days, but if not, *acupuncture* or *physiotherapy* may be helpful.

Spasmodic torticollis is quite a different condition. In this, there are prolonged involuntary contractions of the muscles of the neck, leading to slow twisting, turning movements of the head. The head assumes an abnormal position, usually turned to one side, and this may be sustained for long periods. Sometimes the face or arm is involved as well. Spasmodic torticollis can develop at any age, though usually it appears during middle life.

There is no satisfactory treatment, although in severe cases surgery has been tried; the affected muscles or their nerves may be cut, or an operation on the brain itself may be performed. Injection of botulinum toxin has also been tried.

TOXAEMIA OF PREGNANCY

A group of disorders which were once thought to be caused by a toxin, a poisonous chemical, circulating in the blood during pregnancy. However, since no such toxin has ever been identified, the term is no longer generally used. The disorders include *eclampsia*, *nephritis* and essential *hypertension* in pregnancy, and give rise to similar symptoms, such as *oedema* and *proteinuria*.

TOXIC SHOCK SYNDROME

A recently discovered condition of extreme seriousness, thought to be caused by the bacterium, *Staphylococcus aureus*.

Toxic shock syndrome was first described in 1978, when seven children, both boys and girls, were reported to have suddenly contracted a serious infection; subsequently, one of the victims

died. The initial symptoms were a sore throat, a high *fever*, a rash and redness of the skin. Within a short time, *conjunctivitis*, muscle pains and diarrhoea developed, and the blood pressure became dangerously low, leading to *kidney failure*. One to two weeks after the onset, during the convalescent period, the skin peeled from the hands and soles of the feet.

At the time, the cause of the disease was not known. In 1980, however, a variant form of toxic shock syndrome was described in America. The symptoms and course of this form of the disease were the same, but it seemed to primarily affect menstruating women. Since then, more has been discovered about the disease. In America, there were 1,200 cases up to the middle of 1982, of which 90 proved fatal. Patients' ages varied greatly, but the average age was 23. In the vast majority of cases, those affected were previously healthy women who used tampons, and the symptoms appeared at, or around, the time of menstruation. (The precise statistics are a matter of dispute between certain doctors and the tampon manufacturers). In the majority, but not in all, cases, Staphylococcus aureus was found to be present, in the vagina in women, or in skin abscesses in men.

Reports in the media have emphasized the connection between the use of tampons and toxic shock syndrome. Women using tampons made by all five of the major manufacturers have been affected, but 75% of such women had used a tampon called Rely. This brand was sold only in the USA, and was voluntarily withdrawn by its manufacturers, Proctor & Gamble, in September 1980. Since cases of toxic shock syndrome have been reported in men and in post-menopausal women, doctors now believe that the bacteria responsible may enter the body through a

wound, or by absorption through the vaginal membrane when a tampon contaminated by dirty fingers has been inserted. Because of this, women should observe scrupulous hygiene before inserting a tampon, and change tampons frequently.

Once inside the body, Staphylococcus aureus is thought to produce a unique toxin, to which the body has little resistance. The symptoms are treated by broad-spectrum *antibiotics* of the penicillin family, and the patient is given *saline* and nutrients through an intravenous *drip*. If the diagnosis is made early, this treatment is usually successful.

TOXOCARIASIS—see Worms

TRACHEITIS

An acute inflammation of the trachea—*see The Respiratory System, p28*. Tracheitis may be either caused by a *viral* or a *bacterial* infection, and causes soreness behind the breastbone and a cough.

The condition is often associated with an infection elsewhere in the respiratory tract, such as *influenza* and *bronchitis*. In small children tracheitis may develop as a complication of *laryngitis*, and spread to infect the bronchi of the lungs. This condition, known as laryngotracheobronchitis, can become serious if the walls of the airway swell, interrupting breathing.

Treatment is by *antibiotics*. In mild cases, however, this may not be necessary, since the symptoms may be relieved by a number of simple measures. These include steam inhalations, clean air, unpolluted by cigarette smoke, and the use of a linctus to suppress the irritating cough.

TRACHEOTOMY

An operation performed to allow breathing to continue when the

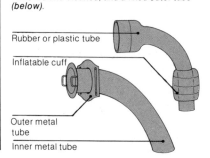

Tracheotomy When an incision is made in the throat and a tube inserted, the procedure is called a tracheotomy **(right)**. Rubber or polythene tubes have an inflatable cuff so that a respirator can be fitted.
Metal tubes have an inner tube, which can be removed and cleaned, and a fixed outer tube **(below)**.

Rubber or plastic tube

Inflatable cuff

Outer metal tube

Inner metal tube

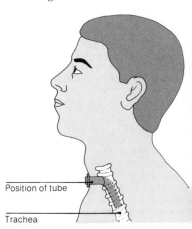

Position of tube

Trachea

upper respiratory tract is obstructed—see *The Respiratory System, p28.*

A temporary tracheotomy may be performed as an emergency, using local *anaesthesia* if possible, if breathing is so difficult that there is a danger of suffocation. A 2.5cm (1in) incision is made just below the Adam's apple between the rings of cartilage. A tube is pushed through the incision to prevent it from closing and to permit the passage of air.

A temporary tracheotomy may become necessary in a number of conditions. These include *diphtheria*, when the larynx becomes seriously inflamed and swollen; paralysis or damage to the nerves that control breathing, as in *barbiturate* poisoning, *tetanus*, bulbar *poliomyelitis*, or serious head injuries; and the obstruction of the windpipe by a foreign body.

It may be necessary to fashion a permanent tracheotomy when a part of the upper airway has been removed, in the treatment of *cancer* of the larynx, for example. Speech is usually impossible after such an operation, but sufferers can be taught to use some of the surviving muscles to produce recognizable sound. However, this process may take several years of intensive *speech therapy.*

TRACHOMA
A severe and progressive form of *conjunctivitis* caused by Chlamydia trachomitis, an organism with characteristics of both *viruses* and *bacteria—see chlamydia.*

The first symptoms of trachoma are an inflammation of the membrane lining the eyelids, which results in the formation of nodules. As the condition progresses, the eyelashes turn inwards, irritating the cornea *(p32).* In response, a hazy film containing blood vessels develops over the cornea, protecting it, but causing *blindness.*

In underdeveloped countries, trachoma is one of the most common causes of blindness. The condition is easily treated, however, being completely cured in its early stages by a combination of *antibiotic* eye-drops and *sulphonamide* tablets. In the later stages a corneal transplant—*see keratoplasty*—successfully reverses the condition.

TRACTION
The application of force, by means of weights, ropes and pulleys, to counteract the natural tension in tissues surrounding a broken or dislocated bone, which tend to pull them apart. Traction may be necessary in the early stages of

healing to ensure that bone fragments are aligned properly, particularly in the case of fracture of long bones, such as the femur—*see Bone and Muscle, pl6.*

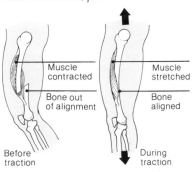

Traction is an essential part of treatment for a fractured femur. This is because the femur is buried among the large muscles of the thigh, which contract when the bone is fractured. This means that a plaster or a splint cannot be applied to hold the bone in place. Instead, a traction system of heavy weights and pulleys is attached to the foot to stretch the muscles and pull the femur back into position.

TRANQUILLIZERS
A group of drugs used to mildly sedate and relax a patient, without affecting his or her level of consciousness, or causing drowsiness.

The drugs fall into two main groups: the minor and the major tranquillizers. The minor tranquillizers are more commonly used; they are prescribed in the treatment of *anxiety* and stress—*see The Problem of Stress, p332.* Valium, a brand name for diazepam, is the best-known member of this family. This drug also has a muscle-relaxant action, and is sometimes given by injection in the emergency treatment of status epilepticus—*see epilepsy*—and before dental treatment.

What some people regard as the over-prescription of these drugs has recently aroused considerable controversy. It is argued, on one hand, that some doctors use such drugs as placebos, rather than spend the time talking to the patient to try to get to the root of the actual problem. On the other hand, tranquillizers are known to be of major assistance in helping people cope with the strains and stresses of modern life, which they simply find impossible to tackle on their own.

What is essential is that the use of such drugs is properly controlled, and that medical instructions are always followed. One problem which is hard to avoid is the rebound heightening of anxiety when the drugs are stopped. The patient may then feel just as bad as before. The danger is that this may lead to psychological dependence on the drugs. In addition, recent

research studies indicate that some patients may develop a physical addiction to tranquillizers after long-term use; some doctors believe that long-term use of tranquillizers may lead to brain damage, *See also Abuses of the Body, p328.* In the short term—for a few months—however, tranquillizers are extremely useful.

TRANSCUTANEOUS ELECTRICAL NERVE STIMULATION (TENS)
A method of relieving pain, in which a pulsed electrical current is applied to nerves via the skin. The current is produced by a small portable battery-powered machine and is applied to the skin via a pair of conducting rubber electrodes, which are strapped in place. The frequency of the current is usually about 80 pulses per second, and the patient adjusts the intensity of the stimulation to produce a sensation of tingling that is perceptible but not unpleasant. The rubber pads are placed on either side of the painful area, or else over a major nerve leading to the area.

If the treatment works, pain relief is often experienced as soon as the machine is switched on and lasts for as long as it is running. There is often a variable period of relief after the machine is switched off. Usually relief is not permanent.

TRANSFUSION
The replacement of blood or body fluids that have been depleted as a result of injury or disease. The replacement fluid is introduced directly into a vein, at a controlled rate, by means of a *drip.*

Saline transfusions are given in cases of *dehydration* or serious burns—*see First Aid, p369.* Blood transfusions are given in cases where blood has been lost as a result of bleeding—either from a wound or during surgery—or when the existing blood is in some way deficient, as, for example, in the case of *sickle cell anaemia.* In extreme cases, for example when a baby suffers from *haemolytic disease of the new-born,* the blood is completely replaced. This is known as an *exchange transfusion.*

In Britain, all blood used for transfusions is taken from volunteer donors. Giving blood is painless and harmless. A blood sample from the donor is tested to ensure no disease organisms are present, and then around 500ml (0.88pt) is taken through a needle attached to a vein in the arm. (An average person has 5 litres, 8.5pts, of blood). The blood is then stored in a blood bank, according to its blood group—*see The Blood and Lymph Systems, p21.*

TRANSIENT ISCHAEMIC ATTACK (TIA)

A minor stroke—see *cerebrovascular accident*—in which there may be temporary loss of vision, difficulty with speech, dizziness and, sometimes, loss of consciousness.

A transient ischaemic attack (TIA) is caused by a temporary disruption to the blood supply of a small area of the brain. As a result, the affected area becomes *ischaemic* and ceases to function. The blockage is often caused by a tiny clot of blood, called a *thrombus*, and is more likely to occur in elderly people whose arteries have become narrowed by *arteriosclerosis*, part of the natural process of ageing. The effects of a TIA are temporary because the thrombus quickly moves away from the blood vessel or becomes dispersed, with the result that the blood supply to the brain is only briefly interrupted. As a result, the damage is not permanent, in contrast to that caused by a stroke.

Though TIAs are not serious in themselves, they may be an indication of an underlying disorder, such as *atherosclerosis*, *hypertension* and *arteriosclerosis*, and the forerunner of a serious stroke. This can often be prevented if *anticoagulants* are given to prevent thrombi from forming, and any underlying disorder is treated. This may involve controlled exercise, a low-fat diet and giving up smoking—see *Exercise, p316; Diet, p322; and Abuses of the Body, p328.*

TRANSPLANTATION

The surgical replacement of a faulty organ or tissue. The tissue to be transplanted is called a graft, and may be taken from a live donor or from someone who has just died.

Together with corneal grafting—see *keratoplasty*—kidney transplants are the most commonly performed transplant operations, and now have a high degree of success—see *kidney disease*. The most publicized type of transplant, however, is the heart transplant. At present, the operation is only performed at a few specialized centres, and has had varying degrees of success. The maximum survival period after a heart transplant is so far only a few years. However, this is partly because of the damage that heart disease, or the factors which contribute to the disease, such as smoking, has already done to other parts of the body. Liver transplants are now possible, though extremely difficult—see *liver disease*—and research continues into the possibility of lung transplants.

Whichever organs are involved, transplant surgery is beset with problems. The first of these is concerned with the selection of the donor tissue. It is important that this resembles the recipient's own tissues as closely as possible; tissues can be identified and typed according to a number of characteristics. The similarity helps to minimize the second major problem, the risk of tissue rejection. When the body recognizes foreign tissue, it mobilizes its defences to destroy that tissue—see *Natural Defences Against Disease, p52*. To avoid rejection, the transplanted tissue must either be so similar to that of the body that the defence systems do not recognize it as foreign, or the defence system must be neutralized. Kidney transplants have a particularly high success rate, because the replacement organ is often donated by a close relative and is not always recognized as foreign. In other cases, however, the body's defences must be artificially lowered by *steroid* and other *immunosuppressive drugs.*

The risk of post-operative infection is another problem of transplantation surgery. This is always a danger after major surgery, but in transplant operations the risk is greatly increased, because natural immunity to infection is suppressed by the drugs given to prevent rejection. As a result, the patient is much less able to fight off infection in the usual way, and is vulnerable to minor infections.

As well as medical problems, the question of transplant surgery has aroused considerable moral and ethical concern. Some people fear that, in order to secure healthy organs for transplantation, the rules regarding the medical and legal definition of death have sometimes been relaxed. This has led to a rigorous definition and a wide acceptance of the concept of *brain death*.

TRANSSEXUALISM

A condition in which a person who appears to belong to one sex wishes to become a member of the opposite sex, and assume what is termed a new gender identity. This is not the same as *transvestitism*, a condition in which a person simply enjoys or derives sexual pleasure from dressing in clothes associated with the opposite sex.

Transsexuals often live as a member of the desired sex rather than conforming to their own gender identity. They may dress and behave so convincingly that casual observers are convinced that they are what they seem to be. They often feel that, at heart, they have been trapped in a body belonging to the wrong sex. Since some transsexuals have an unusual configuration of the sex chromosomes, or hormonal abnormalities, this feeling is often justified—see *intersex*.

In many cases, transsexuals are sure enough of their true gender identity to wish to make their outward body conform to their inner feelings. This can be done by means of a gender reassignment operation, often called a sex change. The operation is only available at special gender identity clinics. It is preceded by extensive psychiatric counselling, and the patient is required to live, dress and work in the desired gender role for several years before an operation is considered.

Male transsexuals, for instance, have to show that they can live comfortably as women before they are offered surgery. They are also given long-term hormone therapy to encourage the development of feminine *secondary sexual characteristics* and to inhibit the growth of facial hair.

Surgery involves the removal of the external genitalia and the construction of new organs. Thus a male transsexual may have silicone implants as well as oestrogen therapy to enlarge the breasts. The penis and testes are removed, and a vagina constructed out of the remaining tissue.

Gender reassignment operations for women are far less common and much more difficult. Male secondary sexual characteristics can be induced and female ones subdued by hormone therapy; this also has the effect of enlarging the clitoris—see *Sex and Reproduction, p54*. The labia of the vagina are joined to form a scrotum and prosthetic testes implanted. Tissue can be implanted into the enlarged clitoris to give the appearance of a penis, but this cannot become erect.

In neither case does a gender reassignment operation allow a transsexual to enjoy completely normal sexual activity. The disadvantages of this, however, are outweighed by the psychological satisfaction the transsexual derives from possessing external genitals and a body that conforms to what he or she feels to be the correct gender.

TRANS URETHRAL RESECTION

An operation performed if an enlargement of the prostate gland—see *prostate disorders*—in men obstructs the urethra passing through it, causing the *retention of urine* in the bladder.

Trans urethral resection takes place under *general anaesthesia*. A narrow metal tube is inserted into the urethra at the end of the penis and pushed upwards to the section of the urethra that passes through the prostate. A portion of the gland is then removed by cutting away small pieces at a time with *diathermy*. This utilizes a high-frequency electric current to generate sufficient heat to destroy tissues bloodlessly. The procedure is rather like coring an apple.

Afterwards, a *catheter* is placed in the bladder to restore the continuity of the urethra. The patient is encouraged to drink large quantities of water to keep up the flow of urine and to discourage formation of blood clots which may block the urethra once more.

TRANSVESTISM

Wearing the clothes of the opposite sex, also called cross-dressing. In practice, it always refers to men dressing as women. Transvestism must be distinguished from *transsexualism*, which is the desire to change sex. Transvestites are not transsexuals, nor are they homosexual. They do not pose any danger to children or to anyone else. There is no tendency for transvestism to be inherited.

The reason why some men wish to dress as women is unknown; it probably varies from person to person. Some men find it sexually stimulating, while others feel more relaxed when dressed in this way. The practice may begin before puberty, or only later, after marriage.

Although transvestism is perfectly harmless, it can cause anxiety to the man himself and his partner. It is unlikely that a transvestite will be able to give up the practice completely, and therefore he and his wife, if he is married, need to try to come to terms with it. Some women find this very difficult, in which case they should ask for help from their family doctor. The doctor can refer the man to a psychiatrist, who will try to find reasons for anxiety in the man's life that may be driving him to seek comfort in cross-dressing. However, the man must actively want help if he is to derive benefit from psychiatry, and even so it is unlikely that he will be fully cured. However, the compulsion may diminish in middle age.

TRAVEL SICKNESS

A condition in which nausea and vomiting are caused by the motion of a car, an aeroplane or a ship.

Doctors believe that travel sickness results when motion disturbs the delicate mechanisms controlling balance—*see The Nervous System, p32*. Though travel sickness is not an indication of any serious disorder, the symptoms are similar to those caused by mild forms of conditions affecting the balance organs, such as *labyrinthitis*.

Many folk remedies are claimed to provide cures for travel sickness. The most effective preventive measure, however, is to take *antihistamine* drugs shortly before travelling. Such drugs can be prescribed by a doctor, or purchased from a chemist; they are the basis of a number of proprietary travel sickness pills. However, drivers should not take anti-histamines, since these drugs have a number of side-effects, including drowsiness. Many sufferers also find it helpful to distract themselves from the motion by concentrating on something, the road ahead, for instance. Plenty of fresh air also helps.

TREMOR

An involuntary shaking of any part of the body. The condition often occurs in elderly people for no apparent reason, and a tendency to tremors runs in families. In younger people tremors may be harmless symptoms of *anxiety* or tiredness. However, a tremor may be a symptom of any of a number of disorders.

A tremor is a feature of *Parkinson's disease*, for example. A so-called intention tremor is seen in some diseases of the cerebellum, the part of the brain that controls muscular movement—*see The Nervous System, p32*. This is an uncontrollable shaking of the hands when a sufferer reaches for an object. A mild

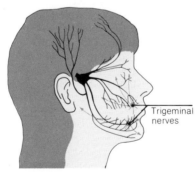

Trigeminal Neuralgia The two trigeminal nerves, one on each side of the head, are the major sensory nerves of the face. They carry sensations from the teeth, cheeks, mouth, tongue and nose and motor nerve fibres which control the movements of the jaw When, for some reason, one of the trigeminal nerves is compressed or inflamed, severe pain is felt on that side of the face.

tremor may be caused by *thyrotoxicosis*, an overactivity of the thyroid gland.

Tremors also appear as one of the symptoms of withdrawal for drug addiction. Alcoholics, for example, often experience a tremor when they have not had a drink for some time. In non-alcoholics, tremors may follow a heavy bout of drinking. In this case, however, the tremor subsides after about a day.

Since, in some cases, a persistent tremor may be a symptom of disease, people suffering from the problem should consult a doctor.

TRICHINOSIS—see Worms

TRICHOMONIASIS

An infection of the genital tract by the *protozoan* Trichomonas vaginalis. Trichomoniasis primarily affects women; the organism lives in the vagina, causing soreness and an offensive yellow discharge—*see vaginitis*. However, Trichomonas can be transmitted to men during sexual intercourse. In men, the infection causes *urethritis*. The infection can be successfully treated by a drug called metronidazole.

TRICUSPID VALVE DISORDERS—see Valvular heart disorders

TRIGEMINAL NEURALGIA

A severe pain, also known as tic douloureux, felt in the area of the face supplied by the trigeminal (5th cranial) nerve—*see The Nervous System, p32*.

Sufferers experience sharp spasms of intense pain on one side of the face, usually in front of the ear and around the jaw. The cause of trigeminal neuralgia is not fully understood. Occasionally, it is due to compression of the nerve by a brain tumour, but this is rare. Often, an attack is initiated when a 'trigger zone' on the affected side of the face is touched, or the hair on that side of the face is brushed.

Trigeminal neuralgia tends to affect older people, and can be extremely disabling, causing serious *depression*. In younger people, a pain with the characteristics of trigeminal neuralgia may, occasionally, be caused by *multiple sclerosis*.

Treatment is with a drug called carbamezepine, sometimes in combination with the *anticonvulsant* drug, phenytoin. Dosages are steadily increased until the pain is relieved. Occasionally, neither of these drugs is successful. In this case, alcohol is injected into the trigeminal nerve. This destroys the pain fibres in the nerve, but the sensory fibres are also damaged, with the result that all sensation in the affected side of the face is lost.

TRYPANOSOMIASIS

A tropical disease, also known as sleeping sickness, caused by microorganisms called trypanosomes. Trypanosomiasis is spread by the bite of the Tsetse fly, and is *endemic* in parts of equatorial Africa.

When an infected Tsetse fly bites a human, it leaves saliva containing trypanosomes inside the skin. These multiply, and reach the bloodstream a few weeks later. Over a period of several months, depending on the site of the bite, the trypanosomes travel to the brain, where they disrupt the function of the nerve tissue. The result is symptoms including headaches, abnormal behaviour and extreme tiredness.

If the disease is not promptly diagnosed, and treated with drugs that kill the trypanosomes, the sufferer may sink into a *coma* and die.

TUBAL LIGATION
Female sterilization, in which the Fallopian tubes are sealed off so that eggs can no longer travel from the ovary to the womb—*see Sex and Reproduction, p54.*

The Fallopian tubes may be sealed off in a number of ways. They may be cut and tied off with sutures, squeezed shut by small clips, or interrupted and sealed off by the application of heat—*see cautery.* The patient is given a general *anaesthetic*, and a laparoscope—*see Special Tests, p84*—containing a cautery probe or surgical tool is pushed through the incision. The surgeon can keep a constant visual check on the position of the instrument through the laparoscope. Usually, an overnight stay in hospital is all that is necessary. There is little post-operative pain, though the abdomen may feel uncomfortable and distended for a few days.

The tubes may be cut and tied off by surgery after a birth by *caesarian section* if a mother has decided that she does not wish to have any more children.

The operation has no effect on hormone production, libido or the menopause. There is only one side-effect: many women find that their periods become slightly heavier after the operation. The procedure is not, however, reversible. Because of this, doctors prefer that the woman and her partner attend several sessions of explanation and *counselling* before the operation is performed.

See also Sex and Contraception, p338.

TUBAL PREGNANCY—see Ectopic pregnancy

TUBERCULOSIS
An infectious disease, usually called TB, caused by three species of bacteria: Mycobacterium tuberculosis, which causes most infections in humans; M. bovis, which causes the disease in cattle;

and an unnamed and variable mycobacterium that causes a rare form of the disease that affects the lymph nodes of children and the lungs of adults.

Tuberculosis is *endemic* throughout the world, but its incidence in Europe and the USA has been rapidly decreasing for some decades. (Recently, this trend has been reversed in Britain, due to the high incidence of TB among Asian immigrants). Throughout the world, it most commonly occurs in poor people, whose housing, diet, medical care and sanitation are predisposing factors to the disease.

Tuberculosis once seemed to affect mainly young people, especially young women. Today, however, most sufferers in the West are male, and over 45. Certain diseases, including *diabetes mellitus* and *silicosis*, tend to predispose to tuberculosis, as do operations to remove all or part of the stomach—*see gastrectomy*—and treatment with *corticosteroid* and *immunosuppressive* drugs.

The infecting bacteria can enter the body through the digestive tract, often in unpasteurized milk from infected cows—one of the reasons for the decreasing incidence of TB in industrialized countries is legislation requiring strict inspection of dairy herds and heat treatment of milk. The disease can also be spread by droplet-infection from saliva—*see Health and Hygiene, p334.* The lungs are generally the first organs to be affected, although a primary infection may also occur in the tonsils or digestive tract.

In the first instance, the infection causes a primary tubercle, a *lesion* filled with a cheese-like substance, to form at the site. Normally, this heals after a short time, and rarely causes any noticeable symptoms. However, it leaves a characteristic scar that can be seen on an X-ray—*see Special Tests, p84.* Sometimes, especially in adolescents and young adults, the lesion does not heal, but leads to progressive pulmonary tuberculosis—the wasting disease that used to be known as 'consumption'. This form of TB may progress slowly for many years, fluctuating with variations in the sufferer's natural resistance. In its active phases, it causes loss of appetite, *fever*, night sweats, fatigue, considerable loss of weight and coughing, with the production of blood-stained sputum. Sufferers may be infectious during the latent, as well as the active, phases of the disease.

Once TB has become established, the disease can cause a number of additional problems. If the bacilli—

the medical name for the sausage-shaped bacteria responsible for TB—first affect the lymph nodes (*p21*), the resulting swelling may compress a bronchus, causing collapse of the lungs. This, in turn, may lead to *pleurisy* or *pericarditis*. Infection of the tonsils or digestive tract may cause the formation of *abscesses* in the neck or in the abdominal cavity—a condition known as tuberculous *peritonitis*.

The bacilli may spread through the blood stream to a variety of sites. Sometimes they infect the lymph nodes of the abdomen, causing *peritonitis*; they may also travel to the brain, causing *meningitis*, to the skin, causing tuberculous *ulcers*, or to the kidneys, intestines, bones or sex glands. Secondary infections may also occur in the larynx, causing hoarseness and difficulty with swallowing; in the testicles, causing swelling; the Fallopian tubes, causing *salpingitis* and abscesses; the adrenal glands, causing *Addison's disease*; and in the eyes, causing *keratoconjunctivitis*.

Diagnosis of pulmonary TB is by a chest X-ray, and by culturing a sample of sputum—*see Special Tests, p84.* Tuberculosis affecting other parts of the body is diagnosed by recognition of clinical symptoms and detection of the infecting bacilli in the tissue culture.

A combination of *antibiotics* is used to destroy the highly resistant TB bacilli. Usually, three antibiotics are administered together for about six weeks, and treatment with two is continued for approximately nine months. In the USA many doctors prefer to continue with the two drugs for as long as two years. With such treatment, it is no longer necessary to keep TB patients in hospital. After a few days or weeks of medication, the bacilli disappear from the sputum and the patient is no longer infectious. It is essential, however, that the patient completes the full course of drugs. The patient's close contacts are usually examined to see if they have contracted the infection.

Apart from the legislation governing milk-production, the main reason for the declining incidence of TB is widespread *immunization* against the disease. The degree of a person's immunity against TB can be tested by means of a Heaf or Mantoux test—*see Special Tests, p84.* If no immunity is found, this can given by a *BCG* vaccine, usually at around the age of 11—*see Health and Your Child, p348.*

TUMOUR
An abnormal growth of cells, which may occur anywhere in the body. A

tumour may either be harmless—*benign*—or *malignant*, showing the uncontrolled growth of *cancerous* cells.

Tumours are classified according to the type of tissue in which they arise. An *adenoma*, for example, is a tumour occurring in glandular tissue. Malignant tumours have the suffix '-carcinoma', so a malignant tumour of glandular tissue is known as an adenocarcinoma. Tumours occurring in connective tissue—*see Bone and Muscle, p16*—are named according to the specific tissues they affect. A benign bone tumour, for example, is called an osteoma, and a malignant bone tumour is known as an osteosarcoma. Similarly, a fibromyoma is a benign tumour of fibro-muscular tissue, of which the womb is composed—*see fibroid*. Tumours are treated in a variety of ways, according to their site and whether they are benign or malignant. If the diagnosis is certain, benign tumours are often left alone. Exceptions include cases where the large size of the growth causes problems, or where the tumour is of a type that tends to become malignant in time. For the treatment of malignant tumours, *see cancer*.

TYPHOID FEVER

An acute, highly infectious disease affecting the digestive tract, caused by the bacterium *Salmonella* typhi. Paratyphoid fever is a similar, but milder and more short-lived infection caused by a related bacterium, Salmonella paratyphi. The two diseases are collectively known as the enteric fevers.

Both typhoid and paratyphoid are most commonly contracted through contaminated food and drink—generally water, milk or shellfish. The disease is common in countries with poor sanitation, where flies carry the disease from human excrement to food and water.

The first symptoms appear after an incubation period of between seven and 14 days. These include a headache, aching in the limbs and a general feeling of tiredness. A *fever* develops, rising to a peak that lasts for four or five days. The fever then subsides, only to return a few days later. During the periods of fever the patient usually suffers from *constipation* and exhaustion; mental confusion is common. After a week to ten days the patient begins to suffer from diarrhoea, with distension of the abdomen, and red spots, called rose spots, appear on the chest and abdomen. *Bronchitis* is sometimes a complication.

Without treatment, the sufferer becomes increasingly ill. Lesions, known as Peyer's patches, develop in the intestinal lining. These may *ulcerate*, and perforate the intestinal wall, causing internal bleeding. Many *complications* are possible, including *pneumonia, meningitis* and *cholecystitis*. Severely affected patients may fall into a *coma*, and die after two to three weeks.

Diagnosis of both typhoid and paratyphoid is confirmed by examining samples of the patient's blood and faeces for the infecting bacteria. The patient is then isolated in hospital, and special care is taken to ensure that he or she does not become *dehydrated*. Both diseases are successfully treated with *antibiotics*; a second course is prescribed after the patient has recovered, both to prevent a relapse and to prevent him or her from becoming a *carrier*. (Carriers can also be detected by a blood test, and treated with the antibiotic co-trimoxazole).

Immunization against typhoid and paratyphoid is available—*see Health and Your Child, p348*. This gives protection for several years, but people travelling to countries in which the disease is rife should ask their doctor for a booster injection before departing.

TYPHUS FEVER

A group of infectious diseases found mainly in tropical countries where there is overcrowding and poor sanitation. Typhus is caused by *rickettsiae*, micro-organisms that share some of the characteristics of both viruses and bacteria.

The form of typhus known as epidemic typhus fever is caused by Rickettsia prowazeki, an organism primarily transmitted to humans by the body louse. The disease is highly contagious, however, and infection may enter the body through a scratch, graze or cut, or by inhalation. Symptoms usually appear suddenly, after an incubation period of just under two weeks. They include *fever*, chills, pains in the forehead, back and limbs, constipation and *bronchitis*. The patient may appear confused, with a flushed face and *cyanosis*. A rash, closely resembling that of *measles*, appears, usually in the armpits, and spreads along the arms and down the trunk. During the second week of illness the symptoms worsen, the tongue shrinks, becoming dry and brown, the pulse weakens and the patient may sink into a stupor and become *delirious*. This is the critical point: either the victim begins to gradually recover, or deteriorates, dying as a result of *heart failure, kidney failure* or *pneumonia*.

A similar but milder form of epidemic typhus fever is transmitted to humans by fleas. This condition is caused by Rickettsia mooseri, and known as endemic typhus fever. Rocky mountain spotted fever, caused by R. rickettsi, is transmitted through the bites of hard ticks of the genus Ixodidae. It is most common in North and South America. After an incubation period of about seven days, symptoms similar to those of epidemic typhus fever appear. In this case, however, the rash spreads over the body over a period of several days. In serious attacks, there may be bleeding from the genitals, ears, fingers and toes, resulting in *gangrene*. Mild cases often occur, but the disease can be rapidly fatal. Forms of tick-borne typhus fever also occur in other parts of the world.

Scrub typhus fever, endemic in the Far East and Australasia, is caused by R. tsutsugamushi and transmitted by mites. After an incubation period of about nine days a severe headache, fever, sweating, a cough and sometimes diarrhoea appear suddenly, and the patient may collapse. The characteristic rash appears after a week. In severe cases the patient may develop pneumonia and *deafness*, show signs of confusion and eventually die from heart or kidney failure. Patients who recover require a long period of convalescence, and show signs of a fast heart beat—*see Tachycardia*—for some weeks.

Typhus fever can usually be diagnosed from the symptoms alone, especially by the appearance of the characteristic rash. Sufferers are nursed in isolation in hospital, and given fluids and nutrients by means of a *drip*. Rickettsial diseases respond to daily treatment with *antibiotics* such as *tetracycline* and chloramphenicol. These cause the fever to subside rapidly, but, in order to prevent a relapse, treatment must be continued for about a week after the temperature has returned to normal. While the antibiotics are taking effect the patient is given *analgesics* to relieve the headache, and sedatives if there is delirium.

To prevent reinfection, measures are taken to kill the lice, fleas or ticks that are responsible for transmitting the fever, and their eggs. The patient is washed and treated with an insecticide, and his or her clothes and bedcovers must be destroyed or disinfected. Subsequently, scrupulous hygiene is necessary to prevent re-infection—*see Health and Hygiene, p334*.

Immunization is available to protect people at risk from infection with R. prowazeki, R. mooseri and R. rickettsi, but no vaccine has so far been developed to protect against mite-borne forms of typhus fever.

U

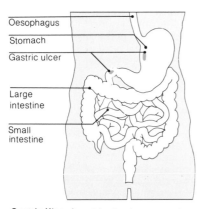

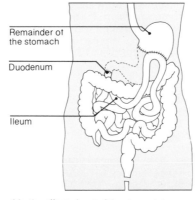

Gastric Ulcer A gastric ulcer is a raw spot that develops in the lining of the stomach. Prompt diagnosis is important, because of the intense, intermittent bouts of burning pain the ulcer causes throughout the upper abdomen. If a gastric ulcer fails to respond to medical treatment, or if it perforates, an operation called a partial gastrectomy is performed. In

this, the affected part of the stomach is removed and the remaining part is joined up to the small intestine between the duodenum and the ileum *(above)*. Gastric ulcers can develop for a variety of reasons, including continual irritation of the stomach lining by acid and pepsin, eating and drinking too much, stress and tension.

ULCER

A persistent sore on the skin, or on the surface of a membrane inside the body. There are a number of different types of ulcer, classified according to the part of the body that they affect.

The part of the body most commonly affected by ulcers is the inside of the mouth. There are two types of mouth ulcer, both extremely painful. Aphthous ulcers tend to develop when people feel run down, or under stress; in women, they often appear just before a period. Traumatic ulcers form on the site of an injury to the inside of the mouth. Both types of ulcer have a yellowish-white inside and an outer ring of red inflammation, though traumatic ulcers are normally single and large, while aphthous ulcers are small and develop in clusters.

Mouth ulcers usually heal on their own within a few weeks of their appearance. The pain they cause can be relieved by sucking lozenges, available from a chemist, that contain a mild anaesthetic. However, if mouth ulcers persist, treatment may be necessary, usually in the form of *steroid* ointments.

Ulcers that form on the skin persist for considerably longer than mouth ulcers, sometimes for several

years. They are uncomfortable and unpleasant, but rarely serious. The exception is a rodent ulcer, caused by the growth of a tumour—*see basal cell carcinoma*. Generally, however, skin ulcers are the result of a cut or a graze on the skin. Normally, these heal as new tissue is formed on the surface and at the edges. When the cut is constantly irritated—by rubbing, for example, or by *bacterial* infection—or when the blood supply, which carries substances vital to healing, is reduced, an ulcer will form. The loss of blood supply is the prime factor in the formation of a type of skin ulcer called a *bedsore*.

A skin ulcer is usually red, and it may be depressed below the level of the surrounding skin. A bluish line marks the edge of the surrounding healthy tissue. The ulcer may discharge a sticky white fluid, or pus if there is also a bacterial infection, and tends to be painful and to bleed readily. It may become crusted, and have an offensive smell.

People who suffer from *varicose veins* often develop skin ulcers, which in this case are called varicose ulcers. This is because varicose veins are themselves a result of poor circulation of blood. The reduction in blood supply to the skin causes an itchy *dermatitis*, which the sufferer

scratches, and ulcers form on the grazes that result. If varicose ulcers persist there is a danger that they may eat through the skin, causing bleeding from the veins beneath. The cure is bed rest, which helps the circulation by taking the weight off the legs. A soothing lotion, such as calamine, can be used to relieve the itching.

Ulcers may also attack the cornea, the transparent tissue at the front of the eye *(p32)*. There are two possible causes of a corneal ulcer. Most commonly, an ulcer forms as a result of bacterial infection of a graze caused by a foreign body in the eye. Occasionally, however, a corneal ulcer is the result of infection by a virus, *herpes simplex*. In this case, it is known as a dendritic ulcer.

A corneal ulcer is a serious problem, because, if untreated, it may result in permanent damage to the cornea, leading to blindness. Treatment is by *antibiotic* eye drops, if the cause is a bacterial infection, and by anti-viral eye drops in the case of a dendritic ulcer. If the cornea has already been damaged, a corneal transplant, called a *keratoplasty*, may be necessary. A dendritic ulcer, however, may recur, since the virus can lie dormant in the tissues for several years.

Ulcers of the internal membranes of the digestive tract *(p40)* are known as gastrointestinal, or peptic ulcers. They most commonly occur in the stomach, in which case they are called gastric ulcers, and in the duodenum; more rarely they develop in the lower oesophagus, associated with reflux *oesophagitis* and a hiatus *hernia*, and in the jejunum, usually as a result of *Zollinger-Ellison syndrome*. All are the result of the erosion of the internal membranes by acid and pepsin, two of the constituents of the digestive juices.

Acid and pepsin, an enzyme that breaks down proteins, are secreted by specialized cells in the lining of the stomach as part of the normal process of digestion—*see The Digestive System, p40*. Usually, they do no harm, but, if the strength or quantity of the secretions increases,

Oesophagus
Stomach
Gastric ulcer
Large intestine
Small intestine

Remainder of the stomach
Duodenum
Ileum

or the protective coating of the intestinal wall becomes weak, an ulcer is likely to form. Some people suffering from a peptic ulcer secrete an unusually strong acid and the production of pepsin is raised; others secrete abnormally large amounts of acid. This may be the result of continual irritation of the stomach, through eating spicy foods, drinking too much alcohol or smoking—*see Abuses of the Body, p328.* In a third group, the alkaline mucus which lines and protects the stomach and intestinal walls may be deficient, often as a result of a reduced supply of blood.

A number of other factors contribute to the formation of ulcers. Gastric ulcers and duodenal ulcers tend to run in families, for example, and are more common in people with blood group O and in men. Physical and mental stress is also a contributory factor in some cases— *see Stress, p332.*

Peptic ulcers may also be symptoms of disease. The bacteria responsible for *typhoid* fever, for example, may cause large, deep bleeding ulcers to form in the intestine. These normally disappear as the disease clears up, but usually leave a scar behind them. Ulcers may also form in the lining of the large bowel as a result of *ulcerative colitis.*

Ulcers in the digestive tract may be acute, having a sudden onset, or chronic, developing slowly. In either case they are often preceded by a period of intermittent indigestion that gradually becomes a permanent condition. Pain may be felt in the chest or back, and is sometimes accompanied by *nausea* and *heartburn.* This usually occurs after meals in cases of gastric ulcer, but sufferers from a duodenal ulcer may feel pain both before meals and in the early hours of the morning. The pain is relieved by vomiting, by taking antacid pills, or, in the case of the duodenal ulcer, by eating. The patient can usually feel some tenderness in the region of the ulcer—that is, in the epigastrium, the central, upper part of the abdomen.

Patients complaining of these symptoms are usually referred to hospital for special tests. These may include an internal examination called an endoscopy, and a barium X-ray—*see Special Tests, p84.* A sample of the ulcerated tissue may be taken at the same time, by a biopsy (*p84*). This is done to rule out the possibility of any *malignant* changes in the stomach tissue, since the symptoms of stomach *cancer* can be similar to those of a gastric ulcer. For the same reason, the faeces may

be tested for the presence of blood.

Bed-rest and complete abstinence from alcohol and spicy foods usually relieve the symptoms of an acute ulcer within a few days. The diet should be bland to ensure that the stomach is not irritated: soft, mild foods such as soups, milk puddings and puréed vegetables, are the most suitable. Antacids, such as magnesium and aluminium hydroxide, are prescribed to relieve pain, and drugs such as cimetidine are given to reduce the amount of acid secreted.

Long-term treatment involves the use of drugs. Two fairly recent additions are cimetidine and ranitidine, both of which act by reducing the amount of acid secreted by the stomach. Other drugs based on bismuth or aluminium have been introduced, while drugs derived from liquorice are still in use. With all of these, the problem is that the ulcers tend to recur once the treatment is stopped.

If an ulcer persists, and is chronic, further treatment is required. This is because there is a possibility that the ulcer will start to bleed, causing *anaemia,* and eventually perforate the wall of the digestive tract. If this happens, the tract's contents will leak into the abdominal cavity. The result is a serious, and sometimes fatal, condition called acute *peritonitis.* Occasionally, the perforation heals on its own, but, more often, surgery is necessary to repair it.

An operation may be necessary to prevent a chronic ulcer from perforating. If the ulcer is in the stomach, a partial *gastrectomy* is performed. In this, the affected part of the stomach is removed, along the area that contains the majority of the acid-producing cells. The remainder is connected to the duodenum by a technique called gastroenterostomy.

A partial gastrectomy is the only effective surgical treatment for a stomach ulcer, and may also be used to treat a duodenal ulcer. In the latter case, however, an operation called a highly selective vagotomy is more common, because it carries slightly less risk. In this, the surgeon cuts the fibres of the vagus nerve, a parasympathetic nerve that stimulates the production of acid by the stomach—*see The Nervous System, p32;* the ulcer heals on its own once the level of acid is reduced. Unfortunately, the operation also affects the speed with which the stomach releases food, causing side-effects such as diarrhoea. To avoid this, the pyloric sphincter, the lower opening of the stomach, is widened by a technique known as pyloroplasty.

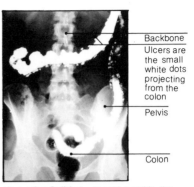

Backbone
Ulcers are the small white dots projecting from the colon
Pelvis
Colon

Ulcerative Colitis In ulcerative colitis, the lining of the colon becomes inflamed and ulcerated. The length of colon affected varies, but the rectum is almost always involved as well. The condition is detected by means of an abdominal X-ray *(above left),* a barium enema having been given prior to radiography.

ULCERATIVE COLITIS

A chronic inflammation of the large intestine, in which its lining becomes ulcerated. The condition tends to run in families, and mainly affects people in their 20s and 30s. Its cause is unknown, but the condition is thought by doctors to be associated with an *auto-immune* response, and, in some cases, an *allergic* response to certain foods. Since ulcerative colitis often occurs in people who tend to be anxious, a psychological factor is also thought to be involved.

Ulcerative colitis can affect any part of the large intestine, but the most common site is the rectum. In this case, the condition is known as ulcerative proctitis. First, the mucous membrane lining the intestine becomes swollen and inflamed and may bleed slightly. Later, ulcers form at the site of the inflammation, and sometimes bleed profusely. In severe cases, the mucous membrane may be stripped off, with the result that the ulcers attack the tissues of the intestinal wall, causing permanent damage.

Ulcerative colitis is suspected by a doctor if a patient complains of frequently passing loose stools accompanied by blood and mucus. The sufferer's abdomen may be tender, and, in severe cases, the profuse diarrhoea may cause *dehydration.* Bleeding from the ulcers can lead to *anaemia* and a general feeling of tiredness and ill health. Sometimes, the large intestine becomes twisted and distended, and may even perforate, causing acute *peritonitis.* A number of complications may also affect sufferers from ulcerative colitis. These include *cancer* of the colon, *arthritis, iritis* and *erythema nodosum.*

Diagnosis is confirmed by a sigmoidoscopy, in which the lower bowel is examined through a hollow

by drugs such as codeine phosphate in mild cases, and by the use of *steroids* applied directly to the site of inflammation, by means of an enema, in more serious cases. Steroids may also be given in tablet form for several months to suppress the inflammation, and a *sulphonamide* drug called sulphasalazine prescribed to control any bacterial infection.

In severe cases, however, this treatment may prove ineffective. Surgery is then required to prevent the condition progressing to involve serious bleeding, perforation of the intestines and the risk that malignant changes will occur.

ULTRAVIOLET RADIATION

Ultraviolet radiation is invisible, but has powerful effects on the skin. This is now very much in the news because of the reported thinning of the protective ozone layer in the atmosphere, caused by industrial pollution, which threatens to increase the amount of ultraviolet light reaching the earth's surface considerably.

Repeated exposure to sunlight damages the elastic fibres in the skin and causes other changes that age it. The surface of the skin becomes yellow-brown and thicker, and bleeds easily when scratched; this is called solar keratosis and predisposes the skin to cancer. If cancer does develop, it may be a basal cell carcinoma or a squamous epithelioma; fortunately these are not likely to spread to other areas (*metastasize*) and can be readily cured by surgery or X rays. Malignant melanoma, the other main form of cancer caused by ultraviolet light, is more serious, since it does metastasize.

In general, unnecessary exposure to sunlight is to be avoided; a tanned skin is not a sign of health. To minimize the risk of malignant melanoma, avoid getting sunburnt. Exposure to the sun should be gradual and progressive, and an effective sun screen should be applied by those liable to sunburn. People with a family history of malignant melanoma, or who have many moles, should avoid exposure to the sun altogether, or use a sun screen that gives complete protection. About half the cases arise in a previously existing mole, so these should be watched for any change. The things to look out for are increase in size, change in colour, the developemt of itching or soreness, and bleeding or crusting; if any of these are seen a doctor should be consulted. Large size, variation in pigment density, and an irregular margin are also danger signs.

URAEMIA

A condition in which the toxic waste products usually excreted in the urine accumulate in the blood. The cause of uraemia is *kidney failure*, which may, in turn, be the result of a number of other conditions. These include disease of the kidneys themselves, and loss of blood, tissue fluid—*see The Blood and Lymph Systems, p21*—or electrolytes, as a result of serious bleeding, burns or vomiting. The reduction in blood pressure this causes damages the tissues of the kidney, leading to kidney failure.

The kidney tissues may also be damaged by long-standing obstruction of the urinary tract by kidney stones or by a tumour, the result being kidney failure.

Uraemia may be either *acute*, developing suddenly, or *chronic*, progressing slowly. In acute uraemia, there is nausea, vomiting and confusion, leading to convulsions and loss of consciousness. This condition is extremely serious, and prompt treatment is required to save life. This may involve surgery.

In chronic uraemia, symptoms include nausea, headache, diarrhoea, loss of appetite, drowsiness during the day and sleeplessness at night. Some patients also become short of breath when lying down. If untreated, the symptoms become gradually worse and eventually the condition becomes acute.

If the kidney tissues have been seriously damaged, chronic uraemia is unlikely to be reversible. The symptoms, however, can be relieved by restricting the fluid intake or by giving *diuretics*, depending on the stage the condition has reached, and by giving a low-protein diet (p322). Sometimes, however, the toxic wastes can only be filtered from the blood by long-term *dialysis*.

URETHRAL STRICTURE

A narrowing of the urethra, the tube running from the bladder through which urine is excreted.

A urethral stricture, which is more common in men, may either be partial or complete. A partial stricture makes it difficult and painful to pass water, and the stream of urine is unusually thin and weak. A complete stricture makes urination impossible, and causes *retention of urine*, with the result that infection quickly sets in. If this is untreated, the infection may spread to the kidneys and prove fatal.

The urethra may become partially constricted as a result of swelling of the urethral wall. This usually only lasts for a few hours, and is caused

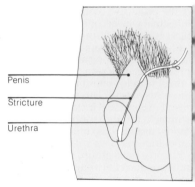

Urethral Stricture When the urethra narrows abruptly in one or more places, urination is painful and erection of the penis is awkward. The stricture is caused by the natural shrinking of scar tissue which has resulted from injury or inflammation of the urethra.

by a number of different factors. These include vigorous exercise, especially in the cold, an attack of *urethritis*, excessive consumption of alcohol or an operation or injury involving the urethra. Normally, the problem clears up without treatment on its own, but the pain caused can be relieved by rest and the application of a warm hot-water bottle to the lower back. If the pain is intense, the urine accumulated in the bladder and upper urethra can be drawn off through a *catheter*. If possible, sufferers should avoid drinking fluids while the stricture lasts.

A permanent stricture may be caused by scarring of the urethral wall. This is normally caused by a disease that affects the area, such as *gonorrhoea*, tuberculosis or chronic non-specific *urethritis* (NSU). The scarring develops gradually, but as the blockage becomes complete the bladder may be seriously distended, causing considerable pain. To avoid exacerbating the condition, sufferers should avoid alcohol and energetic sports, especially cycling or horse-riding, because these irritate the urethra, causing it to contract in spasms.

Permanent urethral strictures are treated by surgery. There are two methods: urethral dilatation, in which the urethra is widened under local *anaesthesia* with an instrument called a bougie; and urethrotomy. This procedure involves cutting out the stricture and reconstructing the urethra; it is only used in serious cases. Since urethrotomy may itself cause urethral spasms or strictures, dilatation is also required, the dilatation procedure being repeated at regular intervals for some months.

URETHRITIS

An inflammation of the urethra, the tube running from the bladder through which urine is excreted.

When the inflammation can be attributed to a specific cause, it is simply known as urethritis; when no cause can be established, the condition is known as NSU, or non-specific urethritis.

In women, urethritis is usually associated with an infection of the bladder, since the urethra is only a few inches long. It is difficult to distinguish between the two conditions, whose symptoms, causes and treatment are similar— see cystitis. A form of urethritis, known as 'honeymoon cystitis' is caused by bruising of the urethra during sexual intercourse. This problem is generally confined to women who have recently started to have intercourse, and can easily be relieved by changing the position adopted for love-making and by using a lubricating jelly—see Sex and Contraception, p338. In men, the main symptoms of urethritis are a discharge from the end of the penis and pain on urination, called dysuria.

In men, urethritis may be a symptom of a number of diseases. Most commonly, these include gonorrhoea, trichomoniasis and Reiter's syndrome—a condition in which urethritis, arthritis, conjunctivitis, iritis, and diarrhoea occur together. More rarely, urethritis may be caused in both sexes by an allergy, by congestion of blood in the urethra, or by infection of the urethral glands—see Sex and Reproduction, p54.

Gonococcal urethritis is treated by the antibiotic penicillin, and trichomoniasis urethritis by a different antibiotic, flagyl. Sufferers should abstain from alcohol, which interferes with the action of these drugs, and from sex. This is for two reasons: firstly, because the infection may be sexually transmitted; secondly, to allow the tissues time to heal.

When urethritis cannot be attributed to any of these problems, the condition is called NSU. Non-specific urethritis has become very common in recent years, and is believed by doctors to be a sexually transmitted disease. However, there is still doubt about its precise cause. Viruses and certain bacteria have been suspected, but recently the Chlamydia organisms—which have characteristics of both viruses and bacteria—have been found to be implicated, in both male and female patients.

The symptoms of NSU are slightly different from those of ordinary urethritis. In men, the first signs are difficulty and pain on urination and a clear, milky or yellow discharge, which is most apparent in the

mornings. In women, the symptoms are similar to those of cystitis, with a frequent desire to urinate. Occasionally, traces of pus are found in the urine.

These symptoms appear around two weeks after infection. In many cases, however, they are very mild, and as a result the disease often goes unnoticed for several months. Symptoms may become obvious for the first time or be exacerbated by a bout of heavy drinking, or by sexual intercourse. They may disappear for long periods and reappear spontaneously, even after treatment.

NSU is highly infectious and sufferers should abstain entirely from sex, from the first appearance of symptoms until treatment is complete. The disease is difficult to cure and often recurs; it responds only to therapy with the antibiotics tetracycline and erythromycin.

URTI—see Upper respiratory tract infection

URTICARIA
An allergy, also known as hives or nettle rash, that produces a skin eruption in people of all ages.

The reaction causes a rash of pale, itchy weals, similar to those caused by a nettle sting, to appear on the skin. Sometimes the whole body is affected, but the rash usually disappears within a few days, without treatment.

Urticaria may have a number of different causes. Sometimes it is a reaction to an allergy found in food, commonly in milk, eggs, wheat, nuts, chocolate, strawberries and shellfish. However, the allergy may also be to the venom in an insect sting, to a vaccine, shock or cold. Some people develop a form of urticaria when their skin is exposed to water or sunlight.

Treatment is not normally required, although soothing lotions, such as calamine, may help to relieve any irritation. In serious cases, antihistamine and corticosteroid drugs are prescribed to subdue the allergic reaction. However, the urticaria will recur unless its cause is identified and eliminated—see allergy.

UTERINE CANCER
The presence of a malignant tumour in the womb—see Sex and Reproduction, p54. Tumours of the neck, called the cervix, and the body of the womb account for around 85% of all cancers of the female reproductive system, the other main sites being the ovaries. Of these, 70% affect the cervix and 30% affect the body of the uterus.

Cervical cancer is one of the most common types of cancer, affecting around two out of every 100 women at some time in their lives. The condition appears to be more common in women who first had intercourse at an early age; its incidence increases with the number of sexual partners; and it is less common in women whose partners have been circumcised. However, with regular screening by means of a cervical smear—see Routine Checks, p338—cervical cancer can be diagnosed early, and usually treated successfully. This is because the smear test can detect pre-cancerous abnormalities in cervical cells.

Regular screening is especially important because there are no obvious symptoms in the early stages of cervical cancer. Sometimes, but by no means always, there is bleeding between periods, after intercourse or after the menopause, and a blood-stained, watery, vaginal discharge, which smells offensive. As the tumour grows, it may spread in a number of different directions: upwards into the body of the womb, downwards into the vagina, or to the bladder. In this case, it may compress the ureters—the tubes running from the kidneys to the bladder—causing kidney failure. Eventually, the tumour spreads throughout the pelvis, sloughs off cells to form secondary cancers at other sites in the body, and causes death.

If the tumour is detected in its precancerous state, or before it has spread, the tissue in which it lies can be surgically removed. In such cases, the outlook is generally good. When the cancer has reached the stage at which it causes symptoms, however, the chances of a complete recovery are cut by half. Treatment involves removing the womb, and often the ovaries, by a total hysterectomy. This is followed by radiotherapy and chemotherapy.

The most common type of cancer of the body of the uterus affects the endometrium—the lining of the womb—and is sometimes known as endometrial cancer. The endometrium contains glandular tissue, and the tumour is of the type known as an adenocarcinoma.

Endometrial cancer tends to affect an older age group than cervical cancer—mainly post-menopausal women who have never had children. It may occur in association with fibroids, and there is some evidence to suggest that it may be caused by oestrogen therapy in post-menopausal women. (This can be avoided by giving oestrogen for only three out of every four weeks, and adding progesterone to the treatment—*see hormone replacement therapy*.

The main symptom of endometrial cancer is irregular bleeding. This may be difficult to distinguish from the normal menstrual irregularities of the change of life. Sometimes, there is also an offensive, watery discharge that may be blood-stained. The diagnosis cannot be made by examination of the uterus, because this is not always enlarged, so a *D & C* is usually required. Treatment depends on the tumour's size and rate of growth. If the tumour has been diagnosed early, radiotherapy and chemotherapy may be given. In severe cases, however, a total hysterectomy is performed, and the ovaries are also removed, in an operation called an *oophorectomy*.

UTERINE PROLAPSE—see Prolapse

UVEITIS — see Iritis

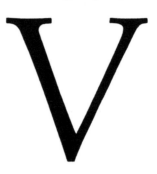

VACCINATION
The injection into the skin of a vaccine, a preparation containing modified forms of the organism that causes a specific disease. As a result, the body's natural defences manufacture antibodies against that disease—*see Natural Defences Against Disease, p52*. This process, which is also called inoculation, protects the body from future infections by the disease, by giving immunity against it. How this works is explained in the entry for *immunization*.

The technique of vaccination was pioneered in England in the late 18th century by Sir Edward Jenner, who noticed that milkmaids who had been exposed to cowpox were immune to the similar, but much more dangerous, *smallpox*. At that time no one knew how or why the technique worked, but the term 'vaccination' was coined to describe it, because the medical name for cowpox is 'vaccinia'.

VACCINE, VACCINIA—see Vaccination

VACUUM EXTRACTION—see Ventouse

VAGINAL DISCHARGE
The gradual excretion of fluid from the vagina. A certain amount of vaginal discharge is quite normal and healthy.

Fluid is always present in the vagina. It lubricates the delicate vaginal walls and protects the female reproductive system against infection—*see Natural Defences Against Disease, p52*. However, the fluid may change in quantity and consistency during a woman's reproductive life. It tends to be more copious during ovulation and the days immediately before and after menstruation, and gradually ceases after the *menopause*. At times when it is most copious, the fluid may leak from the vagina as a discharge of clear, slightly viscous, vaginal mucus.

During puberty, before the start of the menstrual periods, there may be a creamy discharge with a grainy appearance. This is caused by the shedding of the cells of the vaginal wall. The discharge disappears once the periods have settled down after the *menarche*.

During ovulation (*p54*), the normal mucus discharge from the vagina is increased by the production of the more watery cervical mucus. Its function is to make the womb more congenial to sperm. At times of sexual arousal, the discharge is increased by copious quantities of clear, watery fluid from the Bartholin's glands (*p54*) and the cervix. This lubricates the vagina to make penetration by the penis easier.

As the ovaries stop producing the hormone oestrogen, around the time of the menopause, the vagina secretes less and less mucus, and discharges are rare. There is also a change in the pattern of vaginal discharges during pregnancy. In the early months, there is very little discharge, but this increases as pregnancy progresses. A brownish discharge—the *lochia*—appears during the first few weeks after the birth of the child, and then gradually dries up.

Abnormal discharges, which are usually copious, itchy and have an offensive smell, are caused by vaginal infections. The most common is probably thrush—*see candidiasis*. This causes an intensely irritating white discharge that is sometimes said to look like cottage cheese. Similar, though less-irritating, discharges may be caused by a form of *vulvovaginitis* caused by *bacterial* infection. An offensive yellowish discharge accompanied by soreness of the vagina is generally either due to a micro-organism, such as Trichomonas vaginalis, *Chlamydia trachomatis* or *Gardnerella vaginalis*, or to *gonorrhoea*. The most unpleasant of all discharges, however, are caused by the presence of foreign bodies, such as a forgotten tampon, in the vagina.

All abnormal discharges should be reported to a doctor. This is especially important if the discharge is blood-stained. Such discharges may well be caused by *breakthrough bleeding*, but they can be caused by serious gynaecological problems, such as *uterine cancer*. Doctors can identify the cause of a vaginal infection by taking a swab from the top of the vagina and culturing it to see which organisms are present.

Vaginal deodorants and douches should not be used, either routinely or in attempt to treat a vaginal discharge. They are likely to make the problem worse, because they disturb the acid mucus of the vagina, weakening the area's natural defences—*see Natural Defences Against Disease, p52*.

VAGINISMUS
A form of *dyspareunia*—pain on sexual intercourse—in which the muscles of the lower vagina tighten spasmodically. This makes penetration by the penis difficult, and sometimes impossible. In extreme cases the spasm may involve the muscles of the pelvic floor and thigh, and may even occur when the vagina is examined by a doctor.

Vaginismus is usually a

psychosomatic disorder brought about by a negative attitude to sex. It occurs most frequently among a number of different groups: women who are deeply committed to religions whose teachings frown upon sexual freedom; women for whom sex has been a traumatic or intimidating experience; women with latent homosexual tendencies; and women whose knowledge of sex is limited or faulty.

Sometimes vaginismus can be a response to a physical problem that makes intercourse painful. Examples of such problems include abnormal dryness of the vagina, a *lesion* at the entrance to the vagina or on its wall, and *vaginitis*. In these cases treatment of the physical problem usually relieves the condition. Vaginismus may persist, however, if a strong association has developed between intercourse and pain.

If vaginismus is due to psychological factors, or persists after a physical problem, it must be treated by psychosexual *counselling*. This aims to relieve the underlying fear or guilt. The first task of the counsellor is to establish rapport with the patient, so that she can eventually undergo a vaginal examination without anxiety. This is often an important part of the treatment, because she may have to overcome her deepest inhibitions in order to permit such an examination. She will then be taught to flex her thigh muscles to relax the pelvic muscles, and be advised how to use a lubricant to help penetration before intercourse.

These techniques are normally successful. If vaginismus persists, however, more extensive *psychotherapy* may be necessary.
See also Sex and Contraception, p338.

VAGINITIS
An inflammation of the vagina, causing redness, swelling, itching and an offensive discharge. When the vulva, the entrance to the vagina, is also affected, the condition is known as vulvovaginitis.

The most common cause of vaginitis is an infection of the vagina by micro-organisms such as Candida albicans, a fungus—*see candidiasis*—and Trichomonas vaginalis, a protozoan—*see trichomoniasis.* Candidiasis is a particular hazard for sufferers from *diabetes*, since the fungus flourishes in the sugary environment caused by the presence of glucose in the urine of diabetics. Vaginitis may also be caused by a *bacterial* infection. Often, however, the precise type of bacterium cannot be identified, and in such cases the condition is known as non-specific

vaginitis. Both the vulva and vagina are normally affected, and there is a whitish, irritating discharge.

There are a number of causes of bacterial vaginitis. The most common is simple lack of hygiene, and infrequent washing of the genitals—*see Hygiene, p334.* Sometimes, however, the condition may be caused by over-scrupulous washing of the vagina, and the use of vaginal douches and deodorants. These kill naturally occurring bacteria called Lactobacilli acidolphus, which form an essential part of the vagina's natural defences—*see Natural Defences Against Disease, p52.* In their absence, hostile bacteria can flourish and cause infection.

Generally, the condition improves with frequent washing of the external genitals. Underwear should be regularly changed, and preferably made of cotton, through which air can pass. *Antibiotic* creams may be prescribed in persistent cases. They are not normally used, however, because of the risk that they, too, will kill Lactobacilli. Recently, experiments in re-infecting the vagina with beneficial bacteria have proved successful as a cure for vaginitis, and may, in the future, become the standard form of treatment.

Two other forms of vaginitis may occur, but both are easily treated. The first, known as irritant vaginitis, is the result of irritation of the tissues by a chemical, usually a spermicidal jelly. This usually clears up if an alternative brand of jelly is used. The second is senile vaginitis. This condition affects post-menopausal women, and is caused by changes in the mucous lining of the vagina due to a reduction in the level of oestrogen hormones in the blood

(p54). Senile vaginitis is easily treated by oestrogen creams or pessaries, or by *hormone replacement therapy.*

VAGOTOMY—see Ulcer

VALVOTOMY—see Valvular heart disorders

VALVULAR HEART DISORDERS
A group of disorders affecting one or more of the valves of the heart—*see The Blood and Lymph Systems, p21.*

There are several different types of disorder, but all affect the efficiency of the heart to a greater or lesser extent. Valves may become either stenosed or incompetent. A stenosed valve has an abnormally narrow opening, and thick, rigid walls; an incompetent valve, also known as a regurgitant valve, is unable to close properly.

As a result of the former condition, the muscle that pumps blood through the valve must work harder than normal to be effective. An incompetent valve allows blood to flow back, or regurgitate, into the chamber from which it has been pumped. Again, the heart muscle must work harder to pump efficiently. Both conditions increase the strain on the heart muscle and *heart failure* may be the result. The precise nature of the heart failure depends on the specific valve involved.

Disorders of the aortic and mitral valves, in the left side of the heart, may either be inborn—*see congenital heart defects*—or the result of *endocarditis.* This is an infection of the lining of the heart, usually caused by *rheumatic fever.* Disorders of the pulmonary valve are generally inborn, often as a part of Fallot's tetralogy—*see congenital heart defects.*

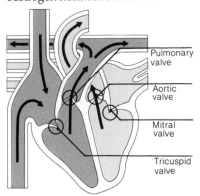

Valvular heart disease. The four valves of the heart *(above)* prevent the backward flow of blood. If a valve is affected by a disease, such as rheumatic fever, or is abnormal, as a result of a congenital defect, the heart becomes a less efficient pump. Its attempts to make up for this by working harder may lead to heart failure. If the valve becomes seriously weakened, it can be replaced by an artificial substitute *(right).*

Labels on figure:
Pulmonary valve
Aortic valve
Mitral valve
Tricuspid valve

Artificial valves

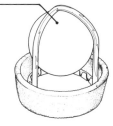

A ball valve, made of plastic, moves up with the flow of blood, then falls back to prevent any backward flow.

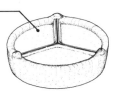

A flap valve, made of human or animal tissue, opens to allow blood to flow through it, then closes to prevent blood from leaking back.

The tricuspid valve is less frequently affected, and the results of damage to it are usually obscured by the greater damage sustained by other valves.

Many people suffering from valvular heart disorders live normal lives, and notice no ill-effects. They may be advised, however, to avoid strenuous activity and to visit their doctors for regular check-ups. Sufferers are particularly susceptible to *bacterial* infections of the heart and heart valves, such as *endocarditis*. To prevent these, people with damaged valves should inform the doctor or dentist of their condition before any procedure involving the possibility of surgery, however minor. They will usually be given *antibiotics* before, during and after treatment.

Surgery may be necessary in serious cases, where heart failure has developed. Stenosed valves can often be opened by cutting through the thickened walls of the valve, in an operation called a valvotomy. However, if the valve is too damaged for this type of surgery to be effective, it may be replaced by a prosthetic substitute.

VARICELLA—see Chickenpox

VARICOSE ECZEMA

A type of *dermatitis* that develops as a result of the sluggish circulation of blood to an area of skin. Varicose eczema most commonly affects the legs, in association with *varicose veins*. The skin becomes dry, shiny and itchy, and may break down if it is scratched, forming varicose *ulcers*.

Treatment consists of a long period of rest, with the legs supported on a footstool. The itching skin should not be scratched; instead, a soothing cream, such as zinc oxide paste, should be applied to relieve the irritation. When the eczema has healed, the sufferer should walk for at least an hour a day to improve the circulation, following this with a period of rest with the legs up. This helps to prevent the recurrence of varicose eczema and improves varicose veins.

VARICOSE VEINS

A condition in which veins become distended and twisted. Veins may become varicose in several parts of the body, including the rectum—where they are known as *haemorrhoids*—and the oesophagus—where they are called *varices*. Most commonly, however, the term varicose veins is used to describe distension and twisting of the saphenous vein of the leg—*see The Blood and Lymph Systems, p21*.

The direct cause of varicose veins is stagnation and pooling of the blood, which enlarges and distorts the thin walls of the veins at points of pressure or weakness. This happens as a result of a deficiency in the circulation. Normally, blood returns to the heart through the leg veins with the help of the muscle pump in the calves. As the muscles contract, they squeeze the blood upwards through a system of valves which prevents it from returning—*see The Blood and Lymph Systems, p21*. However, if the muscles do not contract for long periods—as when standing still, for example—the blood has only the pumping pressure of the heart to push it up the legs against the force of gravity. If this is insufficient, the blood tends to stagnate, and varicose veins may form.

There may be several reasons for this. Otherwise healthy people may develop varicose veins because they stand upright, without movement, for long periods. Some people may be born with slightly defective valves in the veins—this is often an inherited tendency; in others a deep vein *thrombosis* may predispose to varicose veins. Pregnancy may cause varicose veins because the growing foetus sometimes compresses the lymph vessels *(p21)* that drain tissue fluid from the legs and presses on the inferior vena cava *(p21)*; the increased volume of the intestines in *constipation* may have the same effect. Varicose veins are more common in people who are overweight because the weight of the body when standing upright increases the pressure exerted on the walls and valves of the veins.

The first symptoms of varicose veins are an ache in the legs and swollen, painful ankles or feet after standing for several hours. If the condition is not treated, standing becomes increasingly painful and the ache persists for several hours. Eventually, the swollen vein can be

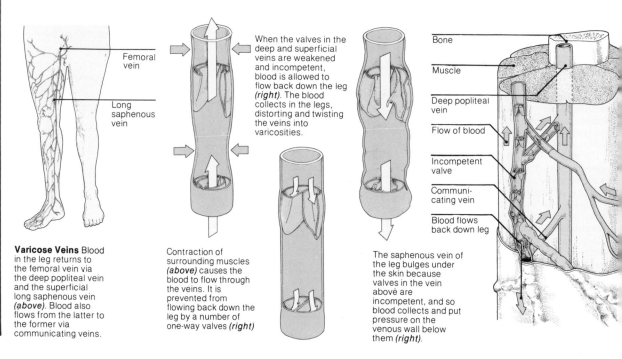

Varicose Veins Blood in the leg returns to the femoral vein via the deep popliteal vein and the superficial long saphenous vein *(above)*. Blood also flows from the latter to the former via communicating veins.

Femoral vein

Long saphenous vein

Contraction of surrounding muscles *(above)* causes the blood to flow through the veins. It is prevented from flowing back down the leg by a number of one-way valves *(right)*

When the valves in the deep and superficial veins are weakened and incompetent, blood is allowed to flow back down the leg *(right)*. The blood collects in the legs, distorting and twisting the veins into varicosities.

The saphenous vein of the leg bulges under the skin because valves in the vein above are incompetent, and so blood collects and put pressure on the venous wall below them *(right)*.

Bone

Muscle

Deep popliteal vein

Flow of blood

Incompetent valve

Communicating vein

Blood flows back down leg

clearly seen as a meandering line of purple, knotty protuberances just under the surface of the skin of the leg. The line often extends from the thigh to the ankle, and is especially pronounced around the sides of the knee and the back of the calf. The leg may swell and *varicose eczema* may develop. In extreme cases varicose *ulcers* appear on the skin; as these grow they may eat into the vein, causing bleeding. There is also a danger that the superficial veins will be affected by *thrombophlebitis* , and that a painful clot of blood, called a *thrombosis*, will form.

Treatment may take several different forms. When serious varicosities have not yet appeared, the problem often clears up with treatment of the cause. Varicose veins associated with obesity and constipation, for example, often clear up after weight is lost, or the bowel movements become regular; varicosities caused by pregnancy generally improve after the birth of the child. Thereafter, a few simple rules should be followed. These help to prevent varicose veins from recurring, and make them less likely to occur in people who have a tendency to developing the condition because of their occupation or inborn characteristics.

Anyone whose job involves long periods of standing should try to relieve the pressure on the legs as often as possible. In many countries, health regulations require that chairs are available for this purpose in shops, cafeterias and restaurants. If possible, the legs should be supported above the level of the head when lying down. Medically approved support tights or stockings should be worn to help prevent distension of the veins. However, for full effectiveness these should be put on first thing in the morning, before the veins have filled with stagnating blood.

Steady walking causes the muscles of the legs to contract, squeezing the veins of the legs and encouraging efficient circulation. Sufferers should therefore take every opportunity to walk and take gentle exercise—*see Exercise, p316*. If incipient varicose veins do not respond to these preventive measures, serious varicosities may develop, making further treatment necessary. This usually consists of injections of a chemical called sodium tetradecyl sulphate at intervals along the course of the affected vein. The treatment has the effect of closing and solidifying the vein and its contents, forcing the blood to flow back to the heart through deeper, less vulnerable, veins. After this procedure, preventive measures are resumed, but with greater emphasis on exercise. This is in order to restore the muscle pump to full efficiency, and to widen the alternative blood channels.

Injection treatment is usually successful. In serious cases, however, especially when there is an inborn defect of the valves in the veins, surgery may be necessary. The technique is called stripping. The affected vein is severed under general *anaesthesia* and tied off at top and bottom and then stripped away from the tissues and the smaller branches. Tight bandages are immediately applied, and on the following day the patient is encouraged to get up and walk about. As with injection treatment, an exercise programme should be started as soon as the patient leaves hospital.

VASECTOMY
Male sterilization. The operation consists of removing part of the vas deferens and tying off the severed ends. The vas deferens connect the testes to the seminal vesicles and carry sperm to the urethra—*see Sex and Reproduction, p54.*

Vasectomy is a simple operation and can be performed under local anaesthesia in a family doctor's surgery. The procedure takes around 30 minutes. Some doctors, however, prefer that the patient is treated in hospital under general anaesthesia; this may involve an overnight stay. The operation is not usually reversible and should be considered final; attempts are sometimes made to untie and rejoin the severed ends, but these are only successful in around 5% of cases. For this reason, doctors normally explain the implications of the procedure in detail before vasectomy.

The operation has few complications. However, in rare cases, blood may accumulate in the scrotum, causing discomfort. The blood can easily be drained in a minor surgical procedure. The scrotum is usually bruised and tender after a vasectomy, but any pain dies away after a few days.

Sexual activity can be resumed at any time, but it is important that either the man or his partner use contraception for around four months. This is because sperm stored in the seminal vesicles may persist for some time. Patients are advised to take a sample of semen to the hospital each month; when two consecutive samples have been shown to contain no sperm, other contraceptive methods can be abandoned.

Vasectomy has no effect on sex drive, performance or masculinity. Ejaculation is unaffected, because the major part of the ejaculate comes from the prostate and urethral glands. Sperm is still produced by the testes, but harmlessly reabsorbed into the tissues.
See also Sex and Contraception, p338.

VASOMOTOR RHINITIS
A term applied to rhinitis not caused by an allergy or an infection. It is common; about half the cases of chronic perennial rhinitis are of this kind. Like allergic rhinitis, vasomotor rhinitis causes blockage of the nose and a water discharge, but itching and sneezing are less prominent.

As the name implies, most cases of vasomotor rhinitis are probably caused by an imbalance in the way the autonomic nervous system controls the lining of the nose. Some, however, seem to be due to an abnormality of the nasal lining; this varient is called eosinophilic rhinitis because there is an increase in the number of eosinophils in the nose. Patients in both groups, but especially those suffering from eosinophilic rhinitis, tend to have asthma and nasal polyps.

Eosinophilic rhinitis can be effectively and safely treated with corticosteroids applied locally to the nose. This can also help to shrink nasal polyps and to prevent them from recurring after surgery. The non-eosinophilic form is harder to treat, though it may respond to drugs that mimic the action of adrenaline. Nasal sprays that shrink the lining of the nose are harmful if continued for a long time and should not be used. Surgery is used in severe cases, but the results are often disappointing.

VASOVAGAL ATTACK—see Syncope

VENEREAL DISEASE—see Sexually Transmitted Disease

VENTILATOR
A machine, also called an artificial lung, used to maintain respiration in a patient who cannot breathe as a result of paralysis of the respiratory muscles—*see The Respiratory System, p28.* This may occur as a result of a drug overdose, a *myocardial infarction* or general *anaesthesia*.

A ventilator consists of a tube and pump. The tube is placed in the trachea *(p28)*, and air pumped through it into the lungs. If it is necessary to use the ventilator for more than a few days, the tube is normally placed directly in the windpipe, by means of a *tracheotomy*.

VENTOUSE EXTRACTION

A method of delivering babies by vacuum extraction, introduced in the 1950s as an alternative to the use of *forceps—See Pregnancy and Birth, p60.*

Ventouse extraction, like forceps, is only used when it becomes obvious that intervention is necessary to ensure the safe delivery of the baby. During the second stage of pregnancy, a large cup, attached to a handle and a pump, is fixed to the head of the emerging foetus. The air is slowly pumped out of the cup, creating a vacuum, so that the cup adheres to the baby's scalp. The baby is then gently pulled out of the birth canal.

Delivery by this method is relatively slow, taking up to 30 minutes, and occasionally causes bruising of the baby's head. However, the risk of serious damage to the foetus and mother is generally less than that incurred by a forceps delivery.

VENTRICULAR FIBRILLATION— see Fibrillation

VENTRICULAR SEPTAL DEFECT—see Congenital heart defects

VERRUCA

A wart—a small, hard, usually discoloured growth that forms on the skin, often in clusters. Warts are highly infectious, but harmless, tumours. They are caused by a *virus,* and occur most commonly on the face, arms and hands, legs and feet and the genitals.

There are several different types of wart. Common warts, called verrucae vulgaris, consist of a bundle of fibres, surrounded and capped by thickened skin cells. Dirt often becomes trapped between the fibres, giving the wart a brownish colour. If the horny cap is knocked off, the wart may bleed.

Common warts usually appear on the backs of the hands and the knees of children and adolescents. Other types of wart have similar characteristics to common warts, but vary in details. Juvenile warts, for example, are similar to common warts, but smaller, often arising on the faces of children. Plane warts have flat tops and occur on the face and the backs of the hands. Soft warts, small nipple-shaped growths, occur on areas subject to continual irritation, such as the neck, chest, ears and eyelids. Seborrhoeic or senile warts occur in old people, usually on the face.

Present-day sexual freedom has brought about a serious increase in genital or venereal warts, also known as condyloma accuminata. This complaint is now one of the most common genito-urinary infections in male patients. Genital warts tend to occur in groups and have a cauliflower-like appearance. They may appear around the anus or on the foreskin of the penis in men, and on the cervix, the vagina and around the vulva in women.

Plantar warts are raised patches of white, hardened skin, usually with a dark centre, that appear on the soles of the feet. (These are the warts commonly known as verrucas). They most often appear in older children and young adults, and are often contracted as a result of walking bare-foot in changing-rooms or swimming pools. Since walking on plantar warts is painful, they are usually removed as soon as they develop.

Warts are normally harmless. However, there is a slight risk that a wart may become malignant. To guard against this possibility, a doctor should be consulted as soon as a wart appears. This is especially important if a wart darkens in colour, enlarges and spreads or begins to bleed around the edges. All these may be signs of *malignant* changes.

Warts of all types normally disappear in time, without treatment. However, the virus causing warts usually lies dormant, with the result that they may recur. This cannot be prevented, although recurrences respond much better to treatment than the original outbreak. Treatment consists of removing the growth with a solvent, such as formalin or solid carbon dioxide. This dissolves the hard cap of the wart, which then dries up and drops off, so that the deep-rooted fibres inside can be scraped away. Large, persistent warts can be cut out, burnt out by *cautery* or frozen out by *cryosurgery* after the surrounding area has been numbed by a local *anaesthetic.*

Since plantar warts are highly infectious, sufferers should make sure that their feet are always covered. Sufferers from genital warts should abstain from sex until two weeks after the warts have disappeared.

VERTEBRO-BASILAR INSUFFICIENCY

A deficiency of the supply of blood to the back of the brain caused by a blockage in either the vertebral or basilar arteries—*see The Nervous System, p32.*

Vertebro-basilar insufficiency may give rise to *transient ischaemic attacks.* During such an attack, there may be nausea, *vertigo, ataxia,* double-vision, numbness on one side of the head and, sometimes, temporary loss of consciousness. The symptoms normally develop gradually over a period of 48 hours, but may appear intermittently. Usually, they disappear spontaneously. The direct cause is often the blockage of the small capillaries by tiny *emboli,* consisting of fatty material and clumped platelets—*see The Blood and Lymph Systems, p21.*

Vertebro-basilar insufficiency is treated by bed-rest and *anticoagulants.* The aim is to prevent the arteries from becoming permanently blocked by clumped platelets, and so a serious stroke. Patients usually recover completely after this treatment, but may have to take anticoagulants for the rest of their lives to prevent a recurrence. *See also transient ischaemic attack.*

VERTIGO

A feeling that the surroundings are spinning or moving sideways, or that the brain is moving within the skull. Vertigo is often accompanied by symptoms such as nausea, vomiting, pallor and cold sweats.

Unlike giddiness and dizziness, vertigo is usually caused by a serious disturbance to the mechanism that controls balance. This may affect either the control centres in the brain stem or the organs of balance in the middle ear—*see The Nervous System, p32.* Both may be affected by a number of conditions: the brain stem, for example, by *multiple sclerosis,* alcohol or drug intoxication; the middle ear by *labyrinthitis.* Vertigo also is a symptom of *Ménière's disease.* Vertigo is treated according to its cause.

VESICLE

A fluid-filled swelling arising in the skin. Vesicles are usually round, with a maximum diameter of 1cm (0.25in), and either transparent, if filled with blood serum, or opaque if they contain blood.

Vesicles form in a number of conditions, including the types of *dermatitis* caused by stinging nettles and poison ivy; a cold sore, caused by the *herpes simplex* virus; heat rashes and *impetigo.* They are also symptoms of diseases such as *chicken pox* and *smallpox.*

Vesicles are extremely fragile, and are often ruptured by the pressure of clothes. They rupture spontaneously as the infection causing them progresses, forming a crust that dries up and heals.

VIRILISM

The appearance in a woman of male secondary sexual characteristics.

These may include hair on the face and trunk; an increase in muscular development; deepening of the voice; enlargement of the clitoris; a loss of periods, called *amenorrhoea*; and a receding hairline.

Virilism can have a variety of causes. It is sometimes congenital, as in the case of congenital *adrenal hyperplasia and intersex*, but can also develop later in life. In this case it may be due to *hypogonadism*, when the small amount of male sex hormone normally produced by the female adrenal glands *(p48)* has a disproportionate effect on the body, or to *Cushing's syndrome*. Virilism may also be caused by an excessive production of male sex hormones. This may either be the result of a *tumour* of an adrenal gland or of an ovary.

Virilism is treated according to its cause. Female sex hormones can be prescribed to reverse the effects of the condition, but cosmetic surgery may also be necessary in some cases.

VIRUS
A micro-organism between 0.0000l to 0.00005 millimetres long, which can only be seen through an electron microscope. Viruses consist of little more than molecules of the nucleic acids, DNA and RNA—*see chromosomes*—the fundamental chemicals of life. They are entirely inert until they lodge in a living animal or plant cell. Then, viruses can feed, grow and reproduce, forming exact replicas of themselves.

Different viruses attack different types of cells, damaging or destroying them in the process. More than 300 different viruses have been identified. They are classified in various ways: according to their chemical composition, the biological classification of their hosts, their method of transportation, the sites in which they are located in their host, and the diseases they cause.

Although many viruses are harmless to humans, others cause diseases. These range in severity from common, relatively innocent infections to debilitating, serious diseases. Viral diseases include coryza, the common *cold*; *influenza*; childhood diseases, such as *measles*, *chicken pox* and *mumps*; *poliomyelitis*; *yellow fever*; and *smallpox*.

Viruses are also thought to be responsible for the generalized *fevers* and gastrointestinal upsets that affect everybody from time to time, though the specific viruses have not yet been identified. Certain viruses have been shown to cause specific *cancers* in laboratory animals, but, as yet, there is as no evidence that viruses cause cancer in humans. Similarly, certain symptoms of

multiple sclerosis resemble damage typically caused by viruses, but there is no other evidence of viral activity in this disease.

So far, few drugs have proved effective against viruses. Anti-viral agents are available, but they tend to be so powerful and dangerous that they cannot be given in tablet form, or allowed to enter the blood stream. Such drugs are only used in local applications. Anti-viral eye-drops, for example, may be used to treat a dendritic *ulcer*, and anti-viral lotions may be painted on to the skin blisters caused by *herpes zoster*.

The result is that treatment of viral infections consists largely of relieving their symptoms. Contrary to popular belief, *antibiotics* are ineffective against viral diseases. However, they may be prescribed during the course of a viral infection to prevent *bacteria* from taking advantage of the body's lowered resistance.

Fortunately, the human body has defences of its own against viruses. These consist of antibodies and the immune response—*see Natural Defences Against Disease, p52*—and the principles they involve can be utilized in treatment. Certain viral diseases, for example, can be treated by an injection of *gammaglobulins* extracted from the blood of a person with *immunity* to the virus—*see antiserum*. Gammaglobulin injections are also used to *immunize* people against certain viruses, such as those responsible for infectious *hepatitis*.

Unfortunately, however, viruses are capable of mutation. Resistant strains constantly appear, producing diseases that may differ slightly from those already known to doctors; new strains of influenza, for example, appear every year. This makes treatment of the infection difficult and the *vaccination* of susceptible individuals almost impossible.

VITAMIN DEFICIENCY DISEASES
A group of disorders and diseases caused by inadequate or irregular supplies of one or more vitamins— *see Diet, p322*.

There are a number of serious vitamin deficiency diseases, caused by a correspondingly serious deficiency of a vitamin over a long period. Such diseases include *xerophthalmia*, caused by vitamin A deficiency; *beriberi*, the result of lack of vitamin B1 (thiamine); *pernicious anaemia*, caused by a deficiency of vitamin B12; *scurvy*, an insufficiency of vitamin C; and *rickets* and *osteomalacia*, caused by vitamin D deficiency.

Less serious vitamin deficiencies,

caused by minor inadequacies in the diet, may also cause symptoms. *Dermatitis*, for example, is commonly caused by a deficiency of vitamin A or of some of the B vitamins. Lack of vitamin B2 (niacin) may lead to *pellagra*, with headaches, weakness, dermatitis and mental disturbances. Vitamin B6 (pyridoxine) deficiency may cause wasting of the cells of the outer layer of the skin, the hair follicles and the sebaceous glands, as well as *neuritis*, an inflammation of the peripheral nerves. It is now known that vitamin E has a special role in pregnancy, since a deficiency can lead to a miscarriage—*see abortion*. A deficiency of vitamin K, a chemical essential to the clotting mechanism of the blood, may slow blood clotting and cause internal bleeding.

In children, inadequate quantities of certain vitamins in the diet may have other effects. Vitamin A deficiency, for example, causes defective development of the teeth; and insufficient vitamin B6 causes weight loss and *anaemia*, and may on rare occasions cause *infantile convulsions*.

All vitamin deficiency diseases can be treated by supplements of the appropriate vitamin, and avoided by taking a sensible, adequate diet—*see Diet, p322*.

VITILIGO
A condition in which round, white patches appear on the skin, giving the sufferer a piebald appearance. The patches usually occur on the face, neck, backs of the hands and arms, armpits and genitals; they are the result of a destruction of melanocytes, the cells containing the melanin pigment that gives the skin its colour.

The white patches often begin as small spots and grow to the size of a small coin. They are especially sensitive to sunburn and susceptible to the development of skin *cancer*. In rare cases the patches spread until the entire body is depigmented.

The cause of vitiligo is not known, and there is no effective cure. The problem sometimes occurs in people who contract *diabetes mellitus* late in life, and may develop in conjunction with conditions such as *pernicious anaemia, Addison's disease, thyrotoxicosis* and *cancer* of the stomach. To date, no detailed studies have been made of vitiligo, but it appears to run in families and may have a genetic origin—*see genes*.

VOLVULUS
A twist in the intestines, causing an obstruction to the passage of digested food. Volvuli most often occur in the part of the colon that

runs through the pelvis—*see The Digestive System, p40*, especially when the mesentery, the tissue that supports the intestines, is unusually long. The most common cause is chronic *constipation*, but a volvulus may also be caused by an infestation of *worms*, by an *ulcer* or by a *tumour*.

The first symptoms of a volvulus may be a rumbling stomach and a protracted feeling of fullness after eating, together with chronic constipation; the abdomen may be painful and distended. In *acute* cases there is violent retching and vomiting, followed by pain and swelling in the abdomen.

A volvulus causes inflammation as well as obstruction, and the intestines are distended with gas and faeces. As a result, doctors often find it difficult to distinguish a volvulus from other conditions that cause intestinal obstruction, such as a *hernia*, and to identify the precise site of the twist. A contrast X-ray—*see Special Tests, p84*—is not usually performed, because it tends to make the condition worse.

Initially, therefore, the aim of treatment is to relieve the inflammation so that surgery can be attempted. This is done by *antibiotics* and *sulphonamide* drugs, the patient being nourished by means of an intravenous *drip* to avoid putting pressure on the intestines. An exploratory operation, called a *laparotomy*, is performed. If the volvulus is mild, the loop of intestine will be untwisted and attached to the back wall of the abdomen to prevent the problem from recurring. When the twist is serious, however, there is a risk that the blood supply to the loop will be cut off, so allowing *gangrene* to set in. In this case, the affected loop of intestine is removed and the two ends are joined. This causes no permanent disability, but it may be necessary to construct a temporary *colostomy* to allow the intestine time to heal.

VOMITING

The process by which the contents of the stomach are expelled through the mouth. Vomiting is most commonly a reaction to the presence of noxious substances in the stomach, as, for example, in the case of *food poisoning* or a bout of heavy drinking. Sometimes, however, it is a symptom of illness or disease.

In children, vomiting can be a symptom of *fevers* and a wide variety of conditions, including *tonsillitis*, *otitis media* and *meningitis*; it is also caused by *pyloric stenosis*, a rare condition affecting first-born male babies. However, many young babies bring up small quantities of milk after feeding. This is known as 'possetting', and has no medical significance so long as the baby appears well and continues to gain weight. Vomiting in adults can follow *gastrectomy*, an operation to remove part or all of the stomach, and be a symptom of a large number of diseases. These include conditions that cause a fever, and gastrointestinal disorders, such as peptic *ulcers*, hiatus *hernia*, acute *appendicitis* and intestinal *obstruction*. In both children and adults, vomiting may be the result of *travel sickness* or a *migraine*. Women may vomit in the mornings for the first few months of pregnancy—*see hyperemesis gravidarum*.

Vomiting can be extremely dangerous when it occurs in small children, because they may quickly become *dehydrated*. This is less of a problem in older people. A person who is vomiting should not be left unattended, however, since there is a risk that the vomit will be inhaled. This may block the windpipe, causing suffocation—*see First Aid, p369*; alternatively, vomit may be inhaled into the lungs, causing infection.

Vomiting can be treated by *anti-emetic* drugs, given either in tablet form, or, in serious cases, by injection. The vomiting in morning sickness is an exception; anti-emetics are not given, since there is a risk that they may harm the foetus. All sufferers from vomiting should drink plenty of clear fluids, and avoid milk and solid foods until the stomach has settled.

VON RECKLINGHAUSEN'S SYNDROME—see Neurofibromatosis

VULVO VAGINITIS—see Vaginitis

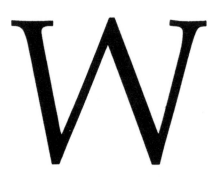

WARFARIN—see Anticoagulants

WART—see Verruca

WATERBRASH—see Dyspepsia

WEAL

A raised mark on the skin, first appearing as a red swelling, similar to the injury caused by a whip. The swelling subsides within a few hours, leaving a white centre and red edges.

Weals may develop as a result of injuries, stings, bites, *allergies*, such as *urticaria*, or irritations of the skin that have been exacerbated by rubbing or scratching—all these cause the release of *histamine* into the tissues. Weals usually clear up on their own after a few days, but anti-histamine creams may help to speed healing.

WEIL'S DISEASE—see Leptospirosis

WERNICKE'S ENCEPHALOPATHY—see Beriberi

WHIPLASH INJURY

An injury to the neck or cervical region of the spine, caused by the head being jerked backwards, as in the sudden braking of a motor car to avoid an accident. The chances of sustaining such an injury can be considerably reduced if seatbelts are worn, by the driver and passengers alike.

In serious cases, a whiplash injury is extremely painful, and may cause paralysis, either of the legs—*see paraplegia*—or of all the limbs—*see quadriplegia*. Generally, however, the symptoms are less severe. There may be pain in the neck and shoulders, and pins and needles in fingertips as a result of the minor injuries sustained by the spinal cord.

In cases where the spinal cord is

not seriously damaged the symptoms usually clear up after a few weeks. *Analgesics* are normally prescribed to relieve the pain, and a soft collar fitted to support the neck. A course of *physiotherapy* may be necessary to restore full movement to the head and neck.

WHIPPLE'S DISEASE—see Malabsorption syndrome

WHITLOW

A small *abscess* at the edge of a fingernail. Whitlows develop when *bacteria* enter the finger through a small cut or tear near the cuticle of a nail. Infection sets in, and pus collects in a pocket, putting pressure on the sensitive nerves around the fingernail and causing considerable pain.

Treatment consists of placing a poultice around the abscess to encourage it to come to a head and burst. *Antibiotics* may also be used, especially if the infection starts to spread up the finger; sometimes the whitlow is lanced with a sharp blade to allow the pus to drain away.

WHOOPING COUGH

An infectious disease of the upper respiratory tract, also called pertussis. It is named after the characteristic 'whoop' that sometimes follows a spasm of coughing.

Whooping cough is one of the most serious childhood illnesses, and is extremely distressing for both parents and child. In the first half of 1982, 45,000 cases of whooping cough were reported in the UK. Around one in every 3,000 sufferers died, usually from complications, such as *bronchopneumonia* and, less commonly, *encephalitis*; a slightly larger group sustained permanent brain or lung damage. The risk of fatalities is highest in children under six months

The disease is a *bacterial* infection, and is spread by droplets sneezed or coughed by a sufferer. The incubation period—the time between contact with the disease and the first sign of illness—varies from seven to 21 days. *Epidemics* of whooping cough occur roughly every four years—the figures given above are of epidemic proportions; their incidence appears to be linked to the degree of immunity in the population.

The first symptoms are cough, runny nose and *conjunctivitis*, in which the eyes are sore, pink and runny. At this stage, the illness is often thought to be merely a cold. However, after a week or so, the cough becomes paroxysmal, occurring in frightening spasms that

last for several minutes. During this time the affected child is unable to draw breath and may turn blue in the face.

The characteristic whoop follows a coughing spasm, and is made by a sharp blast of air rushing through the half-open epiglottis (*p28*), as the child tries to fill his lungs with air as quickly as possible. Doctors believe that whooping is a technique which is learned, in an attempt to draw air into the lungs efficiently; very young children often do not learn to whoop. The absence of the whoop makes diagnosis difficult.

Vomiting commonly occurs after the cough. This may be distressing to parents; however, it often clears congested mucus from the chest and upper respiratory tract, making breathing easier. This phase of whooping cough lasts for anything from two weeks to two months, although the cough may persist for several weeks more. The disease is infectious for a month from the appearance of the first symptoms, and affected children must be kept away from others for this time. An attack of whooping cough generally confers *immunity* for life, though occasional exceptions to this have been recorded.

Treatment is with *antibiotics*. Small babies may require oxygen, and special feeding to combat the *dehydration* that may result from vomiting.

In many other contagious diseases, immunity is passed from mother to child and lasts for some time after birth. Little or no immunity to whooping cough is conferred this way, however. As a result, it is the new born child who is most at risk. Immunity is given by *immunization*, usually as part of the triple vaccine given at three, five and nine months—*see Routine Checks, p346*.

Considerable controversy surrounds whooping cough vaccination, since the vaccine may itself cause encephalitis. However, this is extremely rare, and the risk is three times less than that of encephalitis occurring as a complication of whooping cough. In Britain, three in every 100,000 children contract encephalitis as a complication of whooping cough, compared to one per 100,000 as a complication of vaccination. Deaths from vaccination are extremely rare, and vaccination is therefore recommended for children—except where there is a history of *convulsions*, from any cause, in close relatives. In the past, *asthma* and *eczema* were considered to be reasons to avoid vaccination, because there was a risk that the child would have

an *allergic* reaction to constituents of the vaccine. However, the composition of modern vaccines has been changed to remove this risk.

Doctors believe that the 1982 whooping cough epidemic in Britain was a direct result of the refusal by many parents, influenced by adverse publicity, to have their children vaccinated against the disease. Over several years, this reduces the degree of immunity in the population, giving rise to the conditions in which an epidemic can develop. Parents should discuss the implications of vaccinating their child with the family doctor. If there are no special risks, vaccination is probably in the best interests of the child.

WILSON'S DISEASE

A rare hereditary disease caused by a defect in the metabolism of copper. In Wilson's disease, excess copper is absorbed from the intestines. Since it is not metabolized, some is excreted in the urine, but the rest is stored in the tissues. The brain, liver and eyes are the most common sites, and the copper can cause serious damage in these areas.

Though the disease is an inherited disorder, symptoms do not appear until adolescence. The first outward sign is the appearance of a characteristic coloured halo around the iris of the eye. By this time, however, the brain and liver have normally already suffered damage, due to the deposition of copper. The liver damage causes symptoms similar to those of *cirrhosis*, while copper deposits in the brain damage the basal ganglia (*p32*), causing symptoms similar to those of *Parkinson's disease*. There may be considerable *dementia*, loss of emotional control and peculiar writhing movements of the face and body. The excretion of abnormally large amounts of copper may also damage the kidneys.

Wilson's disease was once fatal but can now be treated with drugs called chelating agents. These remove copper from the tissues. If the diagnosis is made early in the course of the disease, serious damage may be prevented. However, drug treatment must continue for the rest of life.

WITHDRAWAL—see Addiction

WOMB CANCER—see Uterine cancer

WORMS

A group of primitive organisms, of which the flukes, tapeworms, threadworms, roundworms and hookworms can live as parasites in humans, causing disease. In medical terminology, worms in general are known as helminths.

The most common parasitic worm in Britain is the Enterobius vermicularis, the threadworm. Fortunately, it is also the least harmful of the parasitic worms. Threadworms, also called pinworms, are spread by the oral-faecal route—*see Hygiene, p334.* Small children often become infected when they suck objects, or their fingers, that have been contaminated by the worm's eggs. The eggs pass into the intestines, where the worms hatch and reproduce. The female worms lay eggs around the anus, and these cause an intense itching—the worms, around 10mm (0.5in) long, can sometimes be seen in the faeces or around the anus. Scratching the anus to relieve the irritation causes the eggs to be transferred to the fingers. From these, the eggs can be transferred to clothes, bed clothes and toys; the cycle of infection will be completed if such articles are sucked or touched by another child.

Threadworms cause few symptoms, other than the intense itching around the anus. Occasionally, however, they may be responsible for abdominal pain, slight *malnutrition* in an underfed child and mild *vaginitis* in young girls. The infestation can easily be cured by anti-helminthic drugs, which may be prescribed for the whole family as a precautionary measure. Many such drugs can be bought without prescription from a chemist. The itchiness around the anus is relieved with ointments. It is often impossible to effectively guard a child from becoming infected with threadworms, but scrupulous hygiene should be observed at home to prevent the spread of the infestation.

The other types of parasitic worm are rarely seen in Britain, though infestations occur from time to time. However, they are common in other countries. Such worms include the flukes, tapeworms, roundworms and filarial worms.

Flukes are parasitic flatworms. They can infest humans during the various stages of their life cycle, causing a number of diseases, depending on the species involved and the part of the body that they invade. Such diseases include *schistosomiasis*, a major problem in tropical areas, and, in Asia and the Middle East, serious disorders of the blood, lungs and intestines.

One species, Fasciola hepatica, the river fluke, is found in Europe. It spends part of its life cycle in the snail, which, in its turn, may contaminate vegetables, especially watercress, and water. The river fluke lodges in the liver, causing *fever*, tenderness of the liver, mild *hepatitis* and diarrhoea. The condition may be fatal, unless treated by anti-helminthic drugs.

Visitors to countries in which flukes are widespread should ensure, as far as possible, that all water, fruit and other food has been properly prepared. Water should be boiled, fruit washed in boiled or purified water and food thoroughly cooked.

Tapeworms, or Taeniae, are long, flat worms divided into segments. There are two main species, Taenis solium, the pork tapeworm, and Taenia saginata, the beef tapeworm. The former is now rare in Britain, though common in Europe, Asia and parts of Africa; the latter occurs throughout the world, including Britain.

Depending on their type, tapeworms may grow as long as 12 metres (40ft). They enter the body in an immature form in inadequately cooked meat, and attach themselves to the intestinal wall by means of rings of suckers or hooks. After maturing, the worms lay eggs, which are excreted with the faeces. These may cause an infestation in others by the oral-faecal route.

Tapeworms may cause no symptoms, though segments can sometimes be seen in the faeces or on underclothes. In the case of the pork tapeworm, however, immature forms may lodge in the muscles, and sometimes the brain, forming cysts. The cysts usually calcify after a few years, and the immature worms die without causing symptoms. Sometimes, however, they may cause *convulsions*.

A tapeworm infestation is treated by anti-helminthic drugs and purgatives; the faeces of the patient must be carefully examined for the heads of the worms, for if these are not completely expelled the worms may grow again. Preventive measures consist of observing strict hygiene—washing the hands before eating, for example, especially after working with animals— and ensuring that all meat is adequately cooked.

Most tapeworms are more of a nuisance than a serious problem. However a serious condition called hydatid disease may be caused by Taenia echninococcus, a species of very small tapeworm whose eggs hatch inside the body. This condition is rare in the UK, but common in Australia. The immature worm burrows through the intestinal wall and is carried in the blood to either the liver, the lungs or the brain, where it forms a cyst. Several years may pass before the symptoms appear, and these depend on which organ is involved. A hydatid cyst in the liver—the most common site—causes liver enlargment and *hepatitis*; there is shortness of breath when the lungs are affected; and blindness or *epilepsy* if the cyst has formed in the brain. If a cyst should burst, *fever* and *anaphylactic* shock may be the result. Hydatid cysts are removed by surgery.

Four varieties of roundworm may cause serious disease in humans: Ascaris lumbricoides, causing ascariasis; Trichinella spiralis, which causes trichinosis; Toxocara canis, causing toxicariasis; and Ancylostoma duodenale, the hookworm, which causes ancylostomiasis. In addition, Trichuris trichuria, the whipworm, may cause a mild, but persistent diarrhoea in children. Whipworms are around 4cm (1.5in) long and resemble a whip; they are found in insanitary conditions throughout the world, and transmitted by the oral-faecal route of infection. Infestations are easily cured by anti-helminthic drugs.

Ascaris, a long, pale-yellow worm, enters the body when contaminated food is eaten, or through the oral-faecal route. It is most commonly found in the tropics. The worm hatches in the duodenum, and is carried in the blood to the lungs. It then travels up the airways to the mouth, and is swallowed. The worm matures in the intestines, growing as long as 35cm (14in). The worm may cause serious lung infections, and *obstruction* of the intestines. Treatment is by anti-helminthic drugs, but surgery may be necessary to clear any intestinal obstruction.

Trichinosis is a serious disease caused by trichinella spiralis, a parasite of pigs found throughout the world. The worm is transmitted to humans in infected pork that has been inadequately cooked. The symptoms of *food-poisoning* develop between 24 and 48 hours after the meal; nausea and diarrhoea follow, and there is a rapid rise in pulse and temperature. As trichinosis progresses, *oedema* develops in the face and eyes, with a pain in the chest, a cough and breathlessness. In severe cases trichinosis can be fatal, but treatment usually ensures a complete recovery. This consists of anti-helminthic drugs to destroy the worms, and *corticosteroid* drugs to control the inflammation.

Toxocariasis is caused by Toxocara canis, a roundworm that lives in the intestines of infected dogs. Children pick up the eggs when they play on surfaces and soil contaminated by dog faeces, then transmit them to the mouth by sucking the fingers. The larvae hatch in the stomach, and spread through the body, sometimes causing *asthma*, *splenomegaly*, and an increase in certain types of white blood cell *(p21)*. Occasionally, a growth forms around dead larvae that have become trapped in the eyes, and causes permanent blindness. Usually, however, toxicariasis is a very mild illness, and may not even be noticed by the child. Again, hygiene *(p334)* is important in the prevention of the disease. Children should be encouraged to wash their hands frequently, and discouraged from sucking dirty fingers. Dogs should be not exercised in areas in which children play.

Hookworms are found throughout the world. There are a number of different species, but all thrive in conditions where sanitation is poor, hygiene is lax and drinking water has been inadequately purified. Hookworm larvae live in the soil, and usually enter the body by penetrating the skin. They travel to the lungs in the blood, then move up the airways into the mouth, where they are swallowed, reaching the small intestine.

The worms attach themselves to the intestinal wall in large numbers, causing severe bleeding, diarrhoea and *anaemia*. Diagnosis of the infestation, known as ancylostomiasis, is by examination of the faeces, in which eggs can be seen. Hookworm disease is treated by regular dosages of special drugs, and iron is given to treat the anaemia. If the condition is not treated, sufferers become dangerously weakened, and may eventually die.

The filarial worms are confined to South East Asia and Africa. One type of worm, onchocerca, is believed to affect more than 20 million people, and causes serious eye disease—*see blindness*. Another filarial worm, Wuchereria bancrofti, is transmitted to humans by the bite of an infected mosquito. This worm lives in the lymph system *(p21)*, causing elephantiasis, a condition in which the area drained by the affected lymph vessels—usually the scrotum or leg—becomes grotesquely swollen around ten years after the initial infestation.

In general, an infestation of worms is difficult to diagnose, unless the eggs or worms are visible on the skin, in the *faeces* or on an X-ray. This is because many worms produce no symptoms, and some cause symptoms that mimic those of other diseases. Suspected cases may be confirmed by blood tests—*see Special Tests. p84*—and by examining the faeces for eggs. Once the worm has been identified, however, modern anti-helminthic drugs, formulated to eliminate specific parasites, work quickly and have few side-effects. Sometimes, however, worms cause damage to the tissues before the diagnosis is made and treatment can begin. Such damage is often irreversible.

For this reason, personal hygiene, household cleanliness and adequate cooking of food are of vital importance—*see Hygiene, p334*.

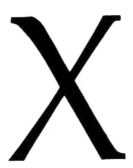

XANTHELASMA—see Xanthoma

XANTHOMA

Deposits of fatty substances, such as cholesterol, in the skin, that appear as soft yellow spots.

Three types of xanthoma— xanthoma multiplex, disseminatum and tuberosum—are hereditary, and in these the fat deposits can form anywhere on the body. The most common form of the condition, however, is xanthoma palpebrarum, also known as xanthelasma palpebrarum, in which the fat deposits are found on the eyelids, or in the creases of the palm.

The condition most often affects middle-aged and elderly people, and is more common in women than men. In itself it is usually of no consequence, but it may be a symptom of poor fat metabolism *(p44)*, or simply a sign of an excess of fats in the blood. In this case the presence of fat deposits may be an early warning of a vascular problem, such as *atherosclerosis*. Xanthomata may also be associated with diseases such as *myxoedema*, *diabetes mellitus*, or primary biliary *cirrhosis*.

As the formation of xanthomata is sometimes an indication of serious disease, a doctor should be consulted when soft yellow spots are noticed on the skin; he or she may advise a reduction of the amount of fat in the diet.

XANTHOPSIA

A condition in which the vision has a yellow tint (it is sometimes called 'yellow vision'). It is a side effect of an overdose of, or sensitivity to, the drug *digitalis*, which is used to increase the efficiency of a weak heart. The drug is effective, but the condition of those taking it must be monitored carefully, because the body breaks down digitalis slowly, so it may build up in the blood.

XEROPHTHALMIA

A disease caused by a deficiency of vitamin A *(p322)*, which is associated with *malnutrition* and diseases affecting the digestion, such as *coeliac disease*.

When the epithelial cells, which form the outer layer of the skin and line the cavities and hollow organs of the body, are deprived of vitamin A, they flatten and form a layer of horny tissue. As a result, the sebaceous glands and hair follicles in the skin and the tear glands of the eyes become blocked.

The eyes gradually become dry, and if the condition is not treated *keratomalacia* may develop. In this disease, the cornea *(p32)*, the front part of the eyeball, softens. It becomes thickened and opaque, and eventually ulcerates and perforates, causing blindness.

If xerophthalmia is diagnosed in its early stages, however, this problem can easily be avoided. It is treated successfully by dealing with the vitamin A deficiency—*see Diet, p322*. The immediate discomfort caused by the dryness of the eyes can be relieved by bathing them with a saline solution or a proprietary eye lotion. Repeated and prolonged exposure to dust and glare may produce symptoms similar to those of xerophthalmia, but these soon disappear if the eyes are rested.

XEROSTOMIA

A condition known as 'dry mouth' that is caused by a reduction in the secretion of saliva. People who habitually breathe through the mouth, or sleep with the mouth open, commonly experience this problem. Sometimes, however, xerostomia is the result of

dehydration, or a reduction in the level of body fluids, that may be caused by *fever, diarrhoea*, states of intoxication with alcohol and narcotic drugs, or *diabetes mellitus*. In these cases xerostomia is relieved when the root cause is treated.

XYY MAN—see Chromosomes

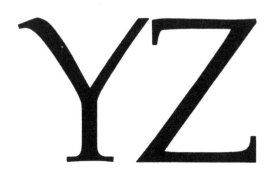

YAWS

A contagious diseases, occurring mainly in the tropics, similar to *syphilis*. Unlike syphilis, however, it is not necessarily transmitted by sexual contact. Yaws is a major problem in South America, the West Indies, parts of Africa and the Far East. Between 1950 and 1960, the World Health Organization treated more than 60,000,000 people for yaws.

Yaws is caused by the micro-organism Treponema pertenue, one of a group of *bacteria* called treponemes. A similar organism, Treponema pallidum, causes Syphilis.

The disease is transmitted by close bodily contact, and so is a particular hazard in poor countries where whole families sleep together on one mattress. The bacterium is thought to enter the body through minute cuts and bruises in the skin.

The first sign of yaws is a skin rash that usually appears about a month after contact. The rash most commonly affects the buttocks or legs and eventually ulcerates. A few weeks later it spreads over the whole body, affecting particularly the moist folds of the skin in the groin and armpit. The long bones of the body and the bones of the nose may swell and become painful. At this stage the disease is very infectious, although the sufferer does not feel ill.

After a few months, the outward signs of yaws may disappear, though sometimes they persist in a less serious form. However, if the disease has not been treated, from five to ten years later, more serious symptoms will appear. *Lesions* develop on the skin, and grow to form deep ulcers. The long bones

and the bones of the skull, nose and palate swell and become distorted, causing gross deformities.

Yaws is treated either by penicillin or tetracycline. Both these drugs are *antibiotics*, and are extremely effective against the disease. As a result, the gross deformities of the second stage of yaws are rarely seen nowadays.

YELLOW FEVER

A *viral* disease transmitted to humans by the bite of an infected mosquito. The insect acquires the virus by biting an infected person or animal, and remains infective for the rest of its life. Yellow fever occurs throughout the tropics, with the exception of the northernmost parts of Africa and some parts of Central and South America.

A mild attack of yellow fever may cause *fever, proteinuria*, or protein in the urine, and mild *jaundice* because of the effect of the virus on the liver and kidneys. In more severe attacks, which may occur in people with little or no *immunity*, the fever may be very high, with *rigors*, a headache, backache and a coated tongue. The patient feels extremely ill and usually vomits copiously. There is also photophobia, or pain in the eyes on exposure to bright light.

Usually, the fever subsides within about four days, and recovery begins. Occasionally the illness progresses, however, and causes serious, and sometimes fatal damage to the liver and kidneys. There is no specific treatment for the disease, other than careful nursing and supportive measures, such as administering fluids directly into a vein, by means of a *drip*, when there is severe vomiting.

Yellow fever can be prevented by

immunization with a live strain of a similar virus. This confers a degree of protection for about ten years. Unlike most other immunizations, the yellow fever vaccination is carried out only at special vaccination centres and is not available at a family doctor's surgery.

ZINC

Small quantities of zinc in the diet are essential for good health, since the metal activates a number of enzymes (p32) that are vital to metabolism. Normally, sufficient quantities of zinc are absorbed, mainly from meat and vegetables. As a result, zinc deficiency is fairly rare, though when it does occur it may cause *anaemia* and, in children, a general failure to thrive.

However, zinc is also used in medical preparations, mainly in those used to treat skin complaints. Zinc and castor oil cream is a well-known remedy for nappy rash and zinc oxide is the basis of a number of soothing ointments. It is one of the constituents of calamine lotion, used to treat mild sunburn and itchy rashes caused by *allergies*. Cotton bandages impregnated with zinc oxide paste are used to treat varicose eczema.

Zinc undecanote, another zinc compound, is a fungicide—that is, it destroys fungi—and is sometimes used in the treatment of athlete's foot, or *tinea pedis*; zinc sulphate, taken by mouth, is thought to speed up the healing of leg ulcers.

ZOLLINGER ELLISON SYNDROME

A rare condition in which there is excessive secretion of the hormone gastrin and consequent peptic ulceration. It is caused by a tumour, or tumours, of the gastrin-producing cells of the islets of Langerhans in the pancreas—*see islet tumours of the pancreas*. The excess gastrin produced stimulates the production by cells in the lining of the stomach of hydrochloric acid. This, in turn, makes the the stomach extremely acidic and causes ulceration, both in the stomach and in the rest of the digestive tract *(p40)*, such as the oesophagus and the small intestine.

The acidity of the stomach also inactivates some of the pancreatic enzymes *(p44)*, reducing the efficiency of digestion, and causing changes in the bile *(p40)*, leading to malabsorption of fats. These two problems cause *diarrhoea* and *steatorrhoea*, in which the stools are pale and fatty.

Zollinger Éllison syndrome is suspected in any patient who has multiple ulcers. The diagnosis is confirmed by an X-ray in conjunction with a barium meal, and by measuring the amount of gastrin secreted—*see Special Tests,p84*. If the tumour responsible can be located, it is removed by surgery. This is not always possible, however, and as the level of gastrin cannot be controlled by drugs, the most effective treatment in such cases is a total *gastrectomy*, the removal of the stomach and thus of the cells that produce the excess acid.

ZOONOSIS
Any diseases that usually affect animals, but can also be contracted by man. *Rabies* and *brucellosis* are two examples of zoonoses. People who are closely involved with animals, such as vets and those who work on farms or in abattoirs are the most at risk.

ALTERNATIVE MEDICINE

MANY PEOPLE believe that the therapies and practices of alternative medicine can supplement — and sometimes even supplant — the orthodox treatments and remedies prescribed by conventional doctors. At the very least, they cannot be ignored. This section examines alternative medicine's key principles and beliefs, assesses insofar as possible their effectiveness and finally provides an A-Z guide to the subject's therapies and practices.

Alternative medicine

Alternative, or complementary, medicine comprises all those forms of treatment that are not taught in ordinary medical schools. This exclusion from the orthodox curriculum, however, is the only thing that many of the alternative treatments have in common; alternative medicine is not a unified discipline but includes a great variety of often very disparate therapies.

Unorthodox forms of therapy have always existed, but they have attracted increasing attention in the last ten or 15 years. This may seem surprising in view of the remarkable successes of modern medicine, but there are a number of reasons why patients still seek alternative treatment. Sometimes orthodox doctors are perceived as rigid and authoritarian, or as uninterested in the environmental and emotional causes of disease, whereas alternative medicine is said to treat the whole person. Some patients are afraid of the side effects of conventional treatment, while others have diseases for which there is at present no satisfactory orthodox treatment, or symptoms for which no conventional diagnosis has been found. There is therefore plenty of scope for methods of treatment that are claimed to be safe, effective, and holistic.

How far are these claims justified? On the whole, it is true that alternative treatments are safe. However, this safety is only relative. Acupuncture, for example, carries certain definite risks and should only be performed by properly-trained practitioners. Osteopathy, likewise, can be dangerous if performed inexpertly, while herbal medicines are not necessarily free from side effects; in general, the only kinds of treatment that are entirely safe are the ineffective ones. A more subtle form of risk arises from the possibility that the practitioner, if not trained in orthodox medicine, may fail to diagnose a serious disease, such as cancer. Fortunately, however, problems of this kind are fairly rare.

The effectiveness of alternative medicine is hard to judge. There is no doubt that many patients feel better for various kinds of alternative treatment, but critics usually say that this is owing to the placebo effect—in other words, it is merely suggestion. Few alternative treatments have been subjected to the kind of critical scientific evaluation that has been applied within the orthodox branch. However, scientific studies have been carried out to a limited extent in the case of certain kinds of alternative therapy (mainly acupuncture, osteopathy, and homoeopathy), and they have given a fair amount of support to claims for their efficacy. In any case, so far as the individual is concerned, what mainly matters is whether he or she feels better.

Choosing a therapist

Normally the first step should be to consult your general practitioner. He or she may perhaps be trained in one or more forms of alternative therapy, and, even if this is not the case, he may well be sympathetic to the idea and be willing to refer patients for this kind of treatment. Sometimes a family doctor will have a good reason for not wishing a patient to have alternative treatment, in which case his opinion should be respected, but, unfortunately, there are still a few doctors who still resist such therapies.

Some forms of alternative treatment are available within the NHS; this is true of acupuncture, homoeopathy, and osteopathy, for example, though in some cases it is necessary to travel quite long distances to obtain treatment. Most alternative medicine, however, is practised privately, and the majority of practitioners do not have an orthodox medical qualification. Non-medical therapists sometimes claim that they are better suited to practise holistic medicine because they have not been subjected to the mechanistic indoctrination they think an orthodox training entails, but this is a doubtful argument.

Patients who decide to seek help from a non-medical practitioner should remember that, in Britain, there is at present no statutory control of alternative medicine, and anyone can set up as a practitioner, with or without training. However, the longer-established therapies mostly possess organizations for training and the maintenance of professional standards, and prospective patients would be well advised to make sure that any non-medical therapist belongs to such an organization.

ACUPUNCTURE

Acupuncture is part of the vast and complex system of traditional Chinese medicine. It is ancient—some people believe it was practised in prehistoric times—but the traditional system as it exists today was largely developed in the Middle Ages and later.

Traditional acupuncture is based on the idea that there is a subtle fluid, called *chi*, which flows through the body in the arteries and veins and also in special channels (the so-called meridians). Disease is thought to result from imbalance in the flow of *chi*, leading to disturbance in the functioning of the various internal organs, and the acupuncture treatment is intended to restore the flow to normal. The traditional acupuncturist makes use of a complicated system of pulse diagnosis, which is supposed to reveal the way the *chi* is flowing through the internal organs, and he inserts needles into the "acupuncture points" in order to correct imbalances in this flow. Usually large numbers of needles (20 or more) are inserted and left in place for up to half an hour, and electrical stimulation may be used. There are a number of practitioners of traditional acupuncture in the west; most are not medically qualified.

The theory of traditional acupuncture sounds strange to people with a modern scientific training. Attempts to prove the existence of *chi*, acupuncture points and channels, the phenomena of pulse diagnosis, and so on have largely been unconvincing, and in the past this led many doctors to dismiss the whole thing as mumbo-jumbo. However, there has long been a small minority who have been convinced that, for whatever reasons, acupuncture does work, and in the last few years modern research has begun to suggest ways in which it might do so.

Acupuncture has been known in the west since the 17th century, and interest in it has periodically fallen off and revived ever since. The modern phase began with President Nixon's visit to China in 1972, since when it has been practised and studied by a small, but enthusiastic,

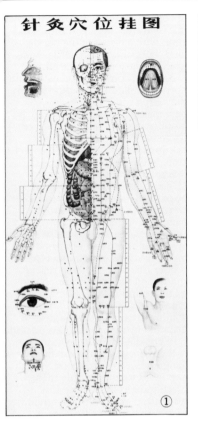

Acupuncturists believe there are 12 main groups of acupuncture points spread over the body, which join to form 12 meridians. Through these, 'chi', the body's vital energy, runs. By examination, including checking the six meridian pulses in each wrist, which meridians need their 'chi' balances restored is determined and the balance of the opposing Yin (negative) and Yang (positive) forces in the body. Once diagnosis has been established, the acupuncturist selects the appropriate points and inserts his needles.

number of western doctors. As a result there has grown up what might be called a scientific form of acupuncture. In this, the traditional explanations of how acupuncture works are largely discarded in favour of ideas based on modern notions of anatomy and physiology. This makes the theory of the subject easier to accept for western doctors, although in practice the difference between the two approaches is not always that great.

It has been recognized for a long time in the west that patients may develop zones in their muscles that hurt when they are pressed and from which pain may radiate to other areas, giving rise to patterns of what is called referred pain. Various names have been applied to these zones; today they are most often called trigger points. It has been found that there is a considerable resemblance between the distribution of these trigger points, as recorded in western medical texts, and classic Chinese acupuncture

points, and many researchers have concluded that they are really the same thing.

Needling these trigger points often seems to relieve or abolish various kinds of symptoms, sometimes permanently but more often for a variable time, and much of modern scientific acupuncture is based on this, though other methods are used as well. As a rule, doctors practising this type of acupuncture find they need to insert fewer needles and for a shorter time than traditional acupuncture practitioners, although it is interesting that in the ancient texts the ideal is said to be to use the fewest possible number of points, or even just one.

Whichever approach is used, traditional or scientific, acupuncture is a relatively safe technique, with two provisos: the acupuncturist must know anatomy thoroughly and he must avoid transmitting infection. Deaths have resulted from accidental insertion of needles into various organs, especially the lungs, and there have been many cases of transmission of hepatitis; recently, there have been a few cases of transmission of AIDS. Because of the risk of spreading infection, pre-sterilized needles should be used and should be disposed of after use; if these rules are adhered to, no infection can be transmitted.

Acupuncture is an effective form of treatment for many disorders, including various kinds of arthritis, certain kinds of neuralgia, headaches, allergies, and period pains. However, it does not work for everything by any means, and about thirty per cent of people appear not to respond to it at all. Moreover, acupuncture seldom seems to cure disease; rather, it alleviates symptoms to a greater or lesser extent for a time—weeks or months as a rule. It therefore usually has to be repeated at intervals.

The main advantages of acupuncture are that—if competently performed—it is relatively safe, and it is effective in some disorders for which there is little effective orthodox treatment. Its main disadvantages are the need in most cases to repeat it and the fact that—contrary to what is sometimes claimed by enthusiasts—it can hurt. However, the degree of pain is not very great, being comparable to that of a blood test.

ALEXANDER TECHNIQUE
Advocates of this technique believe that both physical and mental ill health are partly caused by the incorrect use of the body over many years—often since childhood. They

believe that if people habitually adopt an incorrect posture—with tensed muscles, humped backs, crossed legs and jutting chins—the nervous system and the muscles cannot function properly, and there is a lack of co-ordination and of balance.

Most people, according to the theory, constantly abuse their bodies without being aware of it. They have been doing this for so long that their incorrect posture has become a normal and natural one. By adulthood, most people have developed habits of muscular attitude and tension that are harmful, because such habits cause physiological, emotional, behavioural and structural changes. They do not realize that they tend to stand with their weight on one hip, so twisting the spine and putting the back out of line; or that the habitual tension in their shoulders affects breathing and eyesight.

These habits can be corrected through a painstaking and meticulous process of re-education—the Alexander Technique. Teachers retrain the patient in the correct use of the body, so that a conscious awareness of correct posture and body alignment is developed. The process involves relearning many things that are taken for granted, such as, sitting, standing, lying down, getting up and walking. One of the main aims is to 'free the neck', through an awareness of the tension in the neck and shoulders and the use of special techniques to release this tension.

The Alexander Technique demands considerable commitment from the patient. Usually, about three sessions are needed a week for the first few weeks of treatment, though this reduces as the treatment progresses. An individual session can also last for some time, depending on the special problems of each patient.

The technique has proved particularly helpful to actors and musicians, who often find that incorrect posture has an adverse effect on their performance. In fact it was invented by an actor, Frederick Matthias Alexander, who found that the quality of his voice improved greatly after the posture of his head and neck had been corrected. The treatment is also said to be of benefit in helping people with a number of conditions. These include neck pain, depression, sexual problems, muscle spasms, rheumatism and psychological problems.

AUTOGENIC TRAINING, BIOFEEDBACK and

VISUALIZATION

These three alternative therapies are listed together because, in each, the patient is taught to use conscious thought to exercise a degree of control over some functions of the body, such as pulse rate, blood pressure and brain rhythms. This was once thought to be impossible, because of the way the nervous system is constructed. Recent investigations, however, many of which have been concerned with the control of chronic pain, have shown that, with training, the conscious brain can control some of the functions of the autonomic system—see The Nervous System, p32.

In autogenic training, invented in the 1920s, the patient is taught how to 'talk' the mind and body into a state of deep relaxation. The patient lies on his or her back on a bed, or sits in a chair, with the arms to the sides and legs slightly apart, and runs through the following formula: 'My right arm is heavy and warm; my left arm is heavy and warm ....' This is continued for each part of the body, with each phrase being repeated three times; the whole exercise is performed twice each day. Usually, the body responds by feeling heavier and warmer—the rise in temperature can be measured. The deep state of relaxation that results is said to help resolve many of the conditions that are caused by stress and emotional disturbances.

Biofeedback uses similar techniques to those taught in autogenic training. In this case, however, the various body functions which the patient is attempting to influence are monitored. The patient can then see the effect of his efforts on pulse rate, perspiration on the skin, brain rhythms, blood pressure and tension in the muscles. By the use of an electroencephalograph, or EEG machine, for example, a patient can be taught to change the rhythm of the brain from a Beta wave, seen during consciousness, to an Alpha wave, indicating relaxation. Once the patient has learned exactly what has to be done to alter his body functions, the monitoring equipment becomes unnecessary.

This technique has been used successfully to reduce blood pressure, to decrease the level of cholesterol and to reduce the frequency of epileptic fits. It has also been shown that biofeedback helps in the treatment of asthma, headaches and muscular problems.

Visualization is another technique that utilizes the principle of 'mind over body'. It can be applied to almost any medical problem, and has been used with some success in orthodox as well as alternative medicine. Carl Simonton, a Texan doctor who specializes in the study and treatment of cancer, has been in the forefront of the use of this technique.

Simonton uses visualization therapy alongside the more conventional treatments of the disease. He urges his patients to conjure up pictures of their cancer cells, and then to imagine them under attack from the drugs that he prescribes and from the body's own defence systems. The patients imagine, and sometimes draw, their white blood cells as knights on white chargers, or as vicious white sharks which gobble up the cancer cells.

The technique does not work with every patient. Much depends on the patient's self-image, on his will to live and his belief in his own ability to affect the progress of the disease. Some of Simonton's results, however, have been astonishingly successful.

Other techniques, such as 'Silva Mind Control', also use the principle of visualization for healing, but their success is less well attested. In these techniques patients are urged to concentrate on an image of the way they would like to be, and to erase any image of their unhealthy bodies.

CHIROPRACTIC and OSTEOPATHY

Both chiropractic and osteopathy involve manipulation of the spine and joints of the body. Manipulative techniques are used to some extent by physiotherapists and by an increasing number of doctors as part of the treatment of conditions in which the skeleton and musculature is affected. However, chiropractors and osteopaths rarely have medical qualifications, and rely solely on manipulation.

Chiropractors believe that nearly all disorders of the body are the result of a disruption of nervous and muscular activity. This is itself caused by a misalignment of bones at the joints, most frequently of the intervertebral joints of the spine. Chiropractors attempt to correct such a misalignment, and relieve symptoms, by vigorous and often violent manipulation of the joints.

Osteopaths have similar beliefs, but use a more indirect form of treatment. First they may use a combination of massage and gentle manipulation of the joints, tendons and muscles, and then apply stronger pressure. They move the body so that the areas above and below a misaligned joint are tensed in opposition to each other, and then release the tension, and the locked joint, with a thrust of the hands. A loud, but painless, 'crack' is often heard as the joint is released.

Both chiropractors and osteopaths normally take a full medical history; they often use X-rays to help make a diagnosis and to monitor the progress of treatment. Sometimes only one session of manipulation is necessary to effect a cure, but more often a course of treatment is required.

Manipulation has been shown to be particularly effective in the treatment of back and neck pain, where the record of chiropractors and osteopaths is more impressive than that of orthodox medicine. Some practitioners also believe that they can help relieve conditions such as asthma, migraine and disorders of the digestive system by manipulation, but this claim is disputed by many orthodox doctors.

In unskilled hands, manipulation of the spine and joints can be very dangerous. For this reason, it is important to consult only those practitioners who belong to a recognized association—in the case of chiropractors the British Chiropractors Association (BCO); for osteopaths, the Register of Osteopaths, the Society of Osteopaths or the British Naturopathy and Osteopathy Association.

HEALING

Of all the alternative therapies, the art of healing has probably the most practitioners, and the most followers. There are faith healers, psychic healers, spiritual healers and natural healers, but all share a common principle—the belief in their ability to channel a healing force.

Different types of healers attribute their powers to different sources. Faith healers claim to work through their patients' religious convictions, while psychic healers work through what they call their 'spirit guides'. Other healers talk of a divine, universal healing power which they can channel to people in need. Healers do not think of themselves as the source of healing power but as the conduit for it; through this power, the patient cures himself. Only a few people have the special gift which enables them to lay on hands and channel this power to the patient.

There is some dispute as to whether it is necessary for the patient to have either religious faith or belief in this method of healing for the technique to work. Some healers regard this as essential; others believe all that is necessary is a rapport between patient and healer, as scepticism or mistrust can 'block off' the healing energy.

Usually, the healer lays his or her hands on the patient's body, either on the head or on the affected area. Some healers, however, place their hands at some distance from the body. The resulting sensation is often intense; it can vary between a feeling of hotness, coldness or tingling. A feeling of great calm is said to follow a successful healing.

Nobody knows exactly how healing works. Practitioners claim, variously, that healing energy flows through their hands into the patient's body; that they change the pattern of the patient's brain waves; and that healing is achieved through the metaphysical powers of the healer's own personality. All agree that their effect on the patient's state of mind is of the utmost importance. Healers believe that negative thoughts and emotions, such as anger, hostility and guilt, can all lead to illness, and that by healing the mind they can cure illness.

Healers have been consulted about the whole range of medical conditions, and some notable successes have been reported. But as with many other alternative therapies, it is almost impossible to submit healing to controlled scientific analysis, and, therefore, to explain the phenomenon. This area of alternative medicine is particularly susceptible to false claims and confidence trickery, but, on the other hand, there is some evidence to support some of its practitioner's claims. In one study, healers were shown to change the brain rhythms of their patients—both were producing Alpha and Theta waves, those found while daydreaming and during deep sleep respectively.

HERBALISM

This is one of the oldest and most widespread forms of medical treatment in the world. Until a century ago, nearly all medicines were chemicals derived from plants—digitalis from the foxglove, for example, and reserpine, a medicine used to treat high blood pressure, from rauwolfia, or snakeroot. It is only in recent years that herbalism has become an 'alternative' therapy.

Practitioners of herbalism believe that the effect of the chemical, called the active ingredient, is reduced if, as with modern drugs, it is separated from the other substances contained in the plant. Some herbalists claim that the natural substances other than the active

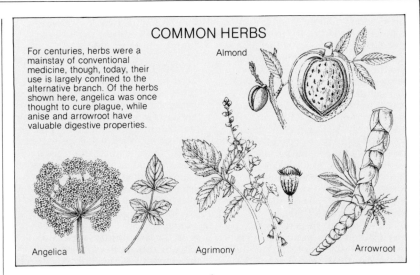

COMMON HERBS

For centuries, herbs were a mainstay of conventional medicine, though, today, their use is largely confined to the alternative branch. Of the herbs shown here, angelica was once thought to cure plague, while anise and arrowroot have valuable digestive properties.

Angelica

Almond

Agrimony

Arrowroot

ingredient control and enhance the activity of that ingredient. Because of this belief, they combine various herbs and plants into one mixture, usually either a liquid extract, a tincture diluted with distilled water, a powder, or in tablet form. As yet, there is insufficient scientific evidence to prove or disprove this claim.

Herbalists use many of the techniques of orthodox medicine to make a diagnosis. They may, for example, use a stethoscope and a sphygmomanometer—*see The Doctor, the Patient and the Disease, p70.* As well as herbal remedies, treatment is also likely to involve a change in the patient's lifestyle, and sometimes a change of diet. Like other alternative therapies, herbalism is concerned with the health of the whole body, not just with curing a specific disease or symptom. Treatments work slowly, but are thought to be cumulative in effect.

Herbalists treat a wide range of disorders, but claim to be particularly successful in their management of chronic complaints. These include arthritis, rheumatism, hypertension (high blood pressure), eczema, ulcers, allergies, and disorders of the digestive system.

Herbalism has its dangers, however. Plants and herbs are not necessarily safe because they are 'natural'. An incorrect dosage can turn a powerful herbal medicine into a harmful poison, or cause side-effects. For this reason, many herbal remedies are now subjected to rigorous scientific testing, in the same way as orthodox drugs. Unlike the latter, however, herbal remedies are rarely standardized, or subject to quality control. Imported herbal preparations have occasionally been found to contain dangerous substances, such as lead.

These dangers can be reduced if the patient ensures he or she consults a member of the National Institute of Medical Herbalists. This body provides training in the basics of medical science and medical law, as well as in herbalism.

HOMOEOPATHY

Homoeopathy is a system of medicine that arose in Germany thanks to the work of one man, Samuel Christian Hahnemann (1755-1843). Hahnemann was an orthodox doctor who became disillusioned with the medical treatments of his day, which depended on massive blood-letting and the administration of large and often toxic doses of complex drug mixtures. An experiment which he carried out himself led him to believe that the right way to treat disease was by what he called the simillia principle: namely, that drugs should be chosen on the basis of their ability to reproduce the symptoms of the disease.

In addition to the simillia principle, Hahnemann introduced some other ideas which in their day were thought to be revolutionary. He said that medicines should be given as single substances, not mixtures, and doses should be repeated only until the symptoms improved and thereafter only if they returned. He also introduced the idea that the effects of medicines should be ascertained by testing them on healthy people, a procedure which he called proving.

Probably Hahnemann's most contentious idea, however, and the one that has most strongly captured public imagination, was to dilute medicines literally to vanishing point. He started doing this at quite a late stage in his career, and not all his followers, either then or now, have been happy about it. However, the method is widely used by homoeopaths today; the usual procedure is to take an extract of the active medicine (the mother tincture) and then to dilute it progressively, using either 1:10 or 1:100 steps, with each dilution forming the starting point for the next one. Such dilution may be repeated six, 12, 30, or 200 or more times, yielding preparations in which it would be expected that no molecule of the original substance would be found. At each step of dilution the mixture is shaken hard—this is called succussion— and is thought to be essential if the treatment is to be effective.

Homoeopathic prescribing is based largely on symptoms, and is as far as possible tailored to suit the physical and mental characteristics of the individual patient. Thus, especially in a case of longstanding disease, the homoeopath may inquire exhaustively into the patient's reaction to weather, sleeping pattern, food likes and dislikes, and so on. However, this is not necessary in every case, and moreover individual prescribers vary considerably in their methods. There is no single right way to practise homoeopathy.

Having decided on a medicine to try, the prescriber may give it either as a single dose in the form of a liquid, a powder, or a tablet (all these are mutually equivalent), or else as a dose to be repeated once or twice a day for a longer period; again, there are many variations from one prescriber to another. The patient is seen again after a week or two (in the case of a chronic disorder) and then the medicine may be continued, changed, or stopped, depending on what has happened after the first dose.

Some homoeopaths believe that patients will often feel worse before they feel better; this was Hahnemann's teaching, although he also said that the "aggravation" might be very slight and transient. Not all homoeopaths have been convinced about the inevitability of aggravations, and some find that they rarely occur.

Because homoeopathy is largely prescribed on the basis of symptoms, in principle it can be applied to the treatment of most diseases; but clearly medicine has moved on a great deal since Hahnemann's day and it would no longer be appropriate to treat everything homoeopathically, ignoring modern medicine completely. Homoeopathic doctors today, therefore, use homoeopathy in conjunction with conventional treatment, selecting one or other as appropriate and, if necessary,

combining the two. In this way patients can receive the benefit of both forms of treatment.

HYDROTHERAPY

Hydrotherapy—the treatment of illness by the use of water—has been practised since the time of the ancient Greeks and Romans. Today, it is considered to promote general well-being, but not to cure disease. Hydrotherapy still has a place in many hospitals however, for water is an ideal medium for remedial exercise, as part of a programme of physiotherapy following muscle damage, paralysis, or a stroke.

In the last century, water was often drunk for its curative properties. Continental spas claimed that their water helped to cure a wide range of diseases.

The type of water therapy still found at spas, especially in Germany, is rigorous and invigorating, but unlikely to be curative. In the Priessnitz Method, patients are sponged down with cold mountain water, wrapped in wet sheets and then immersed in ice cold baths or drenched with cold showers. A fellow German, Kneipp, recommended walking barefoot through cold water, on dew-laden grass or on snow first thing in the morning. Another form of treatment found in Europe is called 'thalassotherapy'—the patient is deluged by jets and showers of hot and cold salt water.

The popularity of spas has been on the wane for many years, but hydrotherapy is still practised at the health farms which have replaced them. Sitz baths, found at many modern health farms and *naturopathic* clinics, are invigorating and stimulate the circulation. The patient sits in a small bath, up to the waist in hot water, for a few minutes, and then transfers to a cold water bath.

HYPNOTHERAPY

In hypnotherapy, the techniques of hypnosis are used to lead the mind into a state of great suggestibility. The hypnotist puts the subject into a hypnotic trance by means of a process called 'induction'. There are several methods, but, most commonly, the hypnotist asks his subject to stare at something, such as a flower, and then, using a deep, monotonous voice, suggests that the subject's eyes are becoming heavier and heavier. Around five per cent of all subjects go into a deep trance very easily on the first attempt; the majority may require several sessions to be able to pass into a trance state with ease.

Not everyone can be hypnotized, however. To some extent, the process depends on the subject's willingness to surrender control of his or her 'self', and on the degree of trust placed in the hypnotist. Many people worry that they will be forced to say or do something embarrassing or harmful under hypnosis. This is almost impossible, because a part of the mind seems to stay alert and monitor what is happening.

During a hypnotic trance, the subject normally experiences a feeling of well-being and deep relaxation. The hypnotist can then explore doubts and feelings that are normally excluded from the subject's conscious mind. He can lay bare traumatic incidents that may have occurred during childhood, and implant suggestions that will help to adjust behavioural patterns.

As a result, the technique can be of great help in the treatment of emotional illnesses, phobias and bad habits; some people have been helped to give up smoking, alcohol, or other drugs by hypnosis.

Hypnotism has also been used to help boost self-confidence, and to treat insomnia. bed-wetting, and hypertension.

Hypnotism has also been used to give relief from pain. A patient who has been hypnotized can often block off sensations of pain during childbirth, for example, or a dental operation—the technique has been strikingly successful in the field of children's dentistry.

Orthodox doctors and dentists who practise hypnotism belong to the British Society of Medical and Dental Hypnosis. Alternative practitioners, who have not qualified as doctors or dentists, belong to either the British Hypnotherapy Association or the British Society of Hypnotherapists. It is inadvisable to consult any hypnotist who is not a member of one of these three organizations.

NATUROPATHY

Practitioners of naturopathy, called naturopaths, attribute many diseases to an 'unnatural' lifestyle. They believe that illness is caused by a build up of toxins, or poisons, in the body—the inevitable consequence, they say, of a bad diet, inadequate exercise and stress. Naturopathic treatment, therefore, involves a change of diet and an exercise programme, as well as massage and *hydrotherapy*.

Naturopaths first attempt to rid the patient of poisons in order to allow the body's own healing systems to function. This is done by fasting, ideally at a health farm or residential clinic. Individual techniques vary, but, generally, only water and fruit or vegetable juices are allowed. At home, the fast might last for up to three days; under supervision, in a residential clinic, it could last for anything up to ten days.

Hunger pangs normally disappear after the first two days of a fast, but during this time there may be a feeling of general illness, with nausea, a furry tongue and bad breath. Naturopaths believe that these symptoms are proof that the toxins are being eliminated.

After the fast, the patient's diet is closely controlled. Fresh, natural, unprocessed foods are recommended: whole grain foods, such as brown rice and wholemeal bread, and large raw-vegetable salads. Stimulants such as tea or coffee are banned, as are refined products, such as white flour and sugar. Some naturopaths insist on a strict vegetarian diet, while others allow small quantities of white meat.

Naturopaths recommend exercise, to help strengthen the body so that it can make its own recovery, and massage, to tone up the muscles, stimulate the circulation and speed up the disposal of toxic wastes. They may also suggest a change of lifestyle to help reduce stress. But, because they disapprove of some forms of orthodox treatment—for example, the use of antibiotics to reduce inflammation—saying that these disturb the natural order of the body, and because they sometimes recommend extremes, such as fasting, any proposed naturopathic treatment should be discussed with your doctor.

OSTEOPATHY—see Chiropractic and Osteopathy

RADIESTHESIA and RADIONICS
In both these therapies, the practitioner aims to heal the patient at a distance. The methods used, which defy scientific explanation or confirmation, rely on concepts such as telepathy and extra-sensory perception (ESP).

Radiesthetists use a pendulum and slide rule as diagnostic and healing tools, while radionic practitioners use a 'black box'. Neither type of practitioner needs to see or examine a patient, but works on a 'witness'—something that has been taken from the patient, such as a drop of blood on a piece of blotting paper, or clippings of hair or nails.

Unlikely as it may seem, radiesthetists claim that they can 'dowse' a patient's illness, and

prescribes the appropriate alternative treatment for it, by placing a specially made pendulum over the 'witness'. A number of different techniques are used, but, usually, the diagnosis is indicated by the degree and angle of the pendulum's swing. This is judged against a calibrated slide rule placed on the east-west axis.

Practitioners of radionics place the 'witness' inside a 'black box' that contains magnets and resistors, but is not operated electronically. A series of up to 24 dials are then calibrated until the practitioner thinks that he or she feels some resistance—the machine is now claimed to be 'tuned in' to the patient. The dials are then reset to correct the imbalances found while tuning in, and the machine 'switched on'—though no electric current is used—to 'broadcast' healing vibrations to the patient.

Both sets of practitioners claim that they can treat almost every disease. They say that the machinery used is merely an aid—the effectiveness of the therapies lies in the sensitivity of the practitioner. Such claims seem highly unlikely, but there is one piece of evidence to support them. The Royal Society of Medicine found, in a series of controlled tests on the effectiveness of radionics, that diagnoses made by the technique were correct slightly more often than could be accounted for by chance.

REFLEXOLOGY
At the turn of the century, this therapy was known as 'zone therapy'. Now 'reflexology' is the more popular term. Reflexologists believe that the organs of the body can be treated by stimulation of specific points on the feet, and, in some cases, on the hands.

According to this theory, the feet make up a map on which every part of the body is marked—the left and the right foot have a different topography, though some areas are identical. The main areas of the map are the soles of the feet, though some information is displayed on the sides and upper parts.

The reflexologist massages the feet by pressing gently with the edge of the thumb or forefinger and rotating it clockwise. When making a diagnosis, he or she feels for tiny nodules of a gritty substance which feel painful when touched. This pain is sometimes felt not only in the foot, but in the organ which corresponds with the particular area of the foot. When the diagnosis is made, the reflexologist applies deep massage to the area that has been located. This can hurt considerably, but the

pain lessens as the treatment progresses, and the organ—so it is claimed—returns to health. A typical treatment session lasts about 45 minutes.

Reflexologists claim a considerable degree of success for their treatment of disorders, such as constipation, bladder, kidney and gall stones, sinusitis, asthma, migraine and stress. Some practiioners also claim to have successfully treated disorders of the endocrine and digestive systems, sexual disorders, sciatica and muscular tension.

There is no scientific confirmation for these claims, nor any explanation of how the treatment works. The gritty nodules used in diagnosis have never been discovered at a post mortem examination, and there is no scientific evidence of a connection between the feet and all areas of the body.

SHIATSU
A therapy derived from *acupuncture*, which has been developed over the last 45 years. The word 'shiatsu' means 'finger pressure' in Japanese; in the therapy pressure is applied to more than 600 acupuncture points by finger, thumb or palm. The degree of pressure, and the point at which it is directed, depends on the patient's state of health.

Originally, shiatsu was devised as a preventive therapy that would relieve fatigue, stimulate the body and promote health. Nowadays, it is often used as a diagnostic and healing therapy. To make a diagnosis, the practitioner massages the body lightly, detecting irregularities solely by touch. The principle of treatment is similar to that of acupuncture. The practitioner massages the appropriate points of the body to promote the flow of healing energy that, it is claimed, runs through the acupuncture meridians towards the affected organ. Shiatsu therapists claim that their technique is painless, but some patients have found that this is not always the case.

Like some other practitioners of alternative medicine, shiatsu masseurs believe that other therapies must be combined with their own if the best results are to be achieved. Japanese practitioners, for example, prescribe a macrobiotic diet, consisting only of pure vegetables, and a stress-free lifestyle.

VISUALIZATION—see Autogenic training, Biofeeback and Visualization

ZONE THERAPY—see Reflexology

YOU
AND YOUR
HEALTH

FROM BIRTH TO DEATH, the risk of illness and disease is always present. This section of the book is a guide to the all-important topic of preventive medicine, showing you what steps you can take to keep yourself healthy and what you can do to cope with some of the problems that can arise to affect your well-being and so put you — and others — at risk. As well as offering simple, down-to-earth advice on topics such as exercise, diet and hygiene, it also gives invaluable information on subjects of concern to every reader, such as contraception and the danger areas of bodily abuse, such as alcoholism and drug addiction.

Connections

Cross-connections Refer back to the A-Z sections for full information about the entries listed here.

Exercise *p315*
Arteriosclerosis
Arthritis
Back pain
Blood pressure — *see*
Hypertension
Heart attack — *see*
Myocardial infarction
Heart failure
Hernia
Hypertension
Obesity

Ante & post natal *p319*
exercises
Back pain
Diverticular disease
Heart disease

Diet *p321*
Anaemia
Cancer
Cold
Colitis
Constipation
Diabetes
Diverticular disease
Fissure
Haemorrhoids
Heart disease
Hypertension
Irritable bowel syndrome
Menorrhagia
Obesity
Rickets
Stroke — *see*
Cerebrovascular accident
Tumour

Abuses of the body *p328*
Alcoholism
Anaemia
Arteriosclerosis
Benzodiazepine
Bronchitis
Buerger's disease
Cancer
Cardiomyopathy
Cirrhosis
Coma
Depression
Epilepsy
Hallucination
Heart failure
Lung cancer
Narcolepsy
Neuropathy
Pancreatitis
Stroke — *see*
Cerebrovascular accident

Tuberculosis
Ulcer
Virus

Stress *p332*
Anxiety
Blood pressure — *see*
Hypertension
Depression
Dysmenorrhoea
Hypertension
Indigestion — *see*
Dyspepsia
Influenza
Phobia
Pre-menstrual tension
Psychosis
Tranquillizers
Virus

Hygiene *p334*
Acne
Bacteria
Carrier
Cholera
Colds
Diarrhoea
Epidemic
Faeces
Food poisoning
Gingivitis
Gonorrhoea
Hepatitis
Herpes
Influenza
Lead poisoning
Lice — *see Pediculosis*
Peridontal disease
Plaque
Ringworm — *see Tinea*
Roundworm — *see Worms*
Salmonella
Scabies
Smallpox
Syphilis
Tinea

Sex & contraception *p338*
Anaemia
Arthritis
Blood pressure — *see*
Hypertension
Breast lumps
Chromosomes
Cystitis
Diabetes
Dysmenorrhagia
Dyspareunia
Ectopic pregnancy
Embolism
Episiotomy
Gingivitis
Gonorrhoea
Herpes
Infertility

Impotence
Liver disorders
Menarche
Menopause
Menorrhagia
Migraine
Pre-menstrual tension
Psychotherapy
Sexually transmitted
diseases
Smegma
Sterilization — *see Tubal
ligation; Vasectomy*
Syphilis
Thrombosis
Tubal ligation
Urethritis
Vaginismus
Vaginitis
Vasectomy

Routine checks *p346*
Breast lumps
Cataract
Diphtheria
Eye tests — *see Specials
tests, p84*
German measles — *see
Rubella*
Glaucoma
Gonorrhoea
Hypochondria
Immunization
Penile discharge
Poliomyelitis
Rubella
Sexually transmitted
diseases
Tetanus
Tuberculosis
Uterine cancer
Vaginal discharge
Venereal disease — *see
Sexually transmitted disease*
Whooping cough

Home nursing *p352*
Aspirin
Constipation
Dehydration
Depression
Diarrhoea
Faeces
Headache
Incontinence
Nausea
Virus
Vomiting

**Looking after disabled
people** *p358*
Arthritis
Depression
Down's syndrome
Meningitis

Mental subnormality
Multiple sclerosis
Occupational therapy
Parkinson's disease
Phenylketonuria
Physiotherapy
Poliomyelitis
Rubella
Speech therapy
Spina bifida
Strokes — *see*
Cerebrovascular accident

Looking after old people
p363
Arteriosclerosis
Arthritis
Bronchitis
Dementia
Depression
Heart disease
Hypothermia
Incontinence
Insomnia
Multiple sclerosis
Occupational therapy
Prostrate disorders
Prolapse
Pneumonia
Stroke — *see*
Cerebrovascular accident

Death
Anti-depressants
Anxiety
Constipation
Depression
Insomnia
Opiates
Tranquillizers
Vomiting

Exercise

It is estimated by the Health Education Council that around 90 per cent of the population of Britain is unfit; 200,000 people die each year from heart attacks. It is very likely that these two facts are related. Yet by exercising for a total of only one hour each week, you can improve the function of your heart, add tone to your muscles, and increase the suppleness, stamina and strength of your body. By following a simple exercise programme, you will be more alert, sleep better, feel better, and look better.

How fit are you?

There is no need to go through a complicated series of physical tests to determine whether you are fit. You will benefit from exercise if:
* Running for a bus or climbing a couple of stairs leaves you puffing and panting
* You have difficulty in getting to sleep and you feel tired the next day
* Your joints feel stiff
* You have difficulty in walking briskly on the flat and talking at the same time
* You have a continual feeling of pessimism or depression
* Your clothes, the scales and the mirror all tell you that you are overweight and out of shape.

What exercise does for you

Exercise can greatly improve the performance and efficiency of your cardiovascular system, and your muscle tone. The heart, the most important muscle in the body, will pump blood more efficiently, ensuring that oxygen reaches the tissues quickly and that waste products are eliminated before they have time to accumulate.

If you are unfit, the heart has to work harder and beat faster to pump the necessary amount of blood through the system, and waste products—*see Metabolism, p44*—stay in the body for a longer time. This accumulation of waste products may lead to arteriosclerosis, the formation of deposits in the arteries, which can increase the resistance to the flow of blood. Because the heart has to work harder to overcome this resistance as a result, the blood pressure is raised, and a continual strain is put on the system. During stress or exercise, this strain is increased; the cells of the body require more oxygen in order to produce more energy, but the lungs, heart and blood vessels of a person who is unfit cannot cope with the

To limber up, spend two or three minutes on some simple stretching exercises designed to increase mobility. Do them slowly, ten times each and breathe normally.

1 Feet apart and hands on hips, tip your head back and look at the ceiling. Roll your head slowly round to the right, then towards the floor, then to the left and finally back towards the ceiling again. Repeat the same sequence but in the opposite direction.

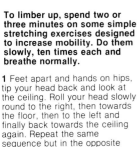

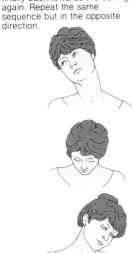

4 With feet apart, stretch your arms in front of you. Keep your eyes on your right hand, swing your right arm to the right as far as possible, while keeping it straight. Return it to the front and repeat with the left arm.

2 Feet apart and hands at sides, lean to the right, sliding your right hand down your leg. Come back up again, then lean to the left, sliding the left hand down.

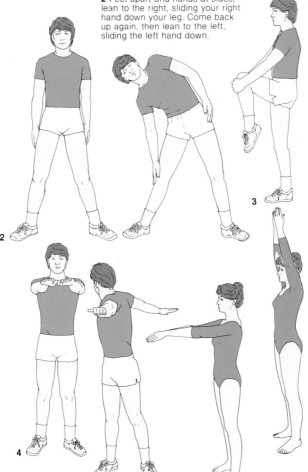

3 Feet together, bring one knee up to your chest, using your hands if necessary. Bend down so that your forehead touches your knee. Repeat with the other knee.

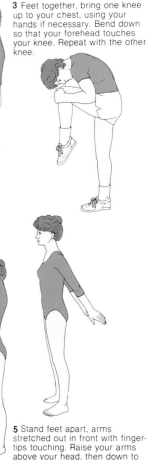

5 Stand feet apart, arms stretched out in front with finger-tips touching. Raise your arms above your head, then down to the sides of the body, pushing each arm backwards at the same time.

extra demand. The result is a racing heart, puffing and panting.

Why you need to be fit
You may think that your body, and in particular your heart, will not suffer if you are not fit, provided that you are not subjected to any undue exertion. It is true that increased mechanization and the use of the car can mean less of the kind of exercise that would have been common for our great-grand-parents. However, the lifestyles of today tend to involve more stress and that, too, can take its toll.

The term 'stress' does not just mean hard work. Stress involves excessive demands on mental energy and emotions. You can be under stress if you are thwarted in some way—if, for example, you are stuck in a traffic jam, or, more seriously, if your career is not progressing as you think it should—see Stress, p332.

During times of stress, the hormone adrenaline is pumped into the bloodstream to prepare the body for extra effort. It releases glycogen from the liver and muscles to provide fuel for the cells; it also makes the heart beat faster, thus raising the blood pressure,

so that food and oxygen circulate more quickly.

The other hormone released at times of stress is noradrenaline. It is produced in response to anger, aggression and frustration. It helps to release fat from the body's food-stores, widens the blood vessels that supply the muscles, and shuts down those supplying the stomach, so that the fat can be diverted to the muscles alone. Noradrenaline, too, raises the blood pressure.

The action of both these hormones, released as a response to stress, causes extra work for the heart and cardiovascular system. If this is working efficiently, the extra demands do not cause any problems; if that is not the case, the heart can be put under strain, causing hypertension and the possibility of a heart attack or heart failure. The fact that exercise improves the cardiovascular system and expands the lungs is the most important reason for keeping fit. The heart can be trained, through physical exercise, to cope with the extra demands of stress and physical exertion: this will not rule out the possibility of heart problems, but it will significantly reduce the chances

of such a problem developing.

Part of your exercise programme should include periods of deep, regular breathing for relaxation. Try to breathe slowly and deeply while relaxing every muscle in your body, and divert your mind by counting slowly up to 10. Other relaxation techniques are shown on p333. They can reduce stress generally: in fact, once learnt, the techniques can be used to lower tension in most stressful situations. The first thing that cardiac patients are taught after a heart attack is how to reduce stress by relaxation—they are also urged to stop smoking and to lose weight if necessary.

Will you lose weight?
Obesity is a medical condition, and causes problems over and above those of a lack of fitness. The only sure way to lose weight is to reduce your intake of food and fattening drinks, observing a sensible, well-balanced diet—see p321. Exercise alone will not take the kilos off, but, in combination with a sensible diet, exercise can help to quicken the process by which stored body fat is burned up—recent studies have shown that exercise may help to increase the metabolic

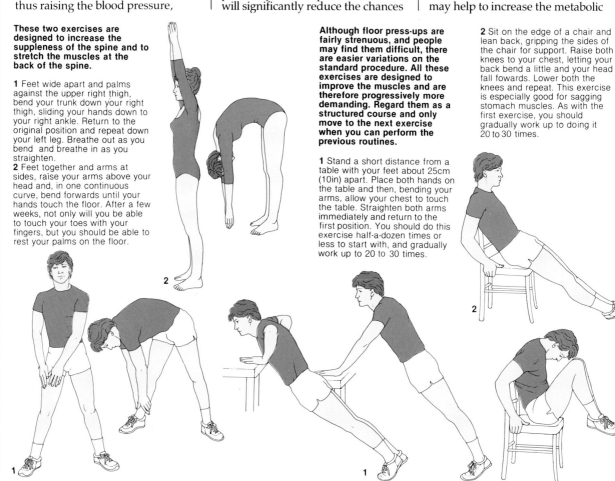

These two exercises are designed to increase the suppleness of the spine and to stretch the muscles at the back of the spine.

1 Feet wide apart and palms against the upper right thigh, bend your trunk down your right thigh, sliding your hands down to your right ankle. Return to the original position and repeat down your left leg. Breathe out as you bend and breathe in as you straighten.
2 Feet together and arms at sides, raise your arms above your head and, in one continuous curve, bend forwards until your hands touch the floor. After a few weeks, not only will you be able to touch your toes with your fingers, but you should be able to rest your palms on the floor.

Although floor press-ups are fairly strenuous, and people may find them difficult, there are easier variations on the standard procedure. All these exercises are designed to improve the muscles and are therefore progressively more demanding. Regard them as a structured course and only move to the next exercise when you can perform the previous routines.

1 Stand a short distance from a table with your feet about 25cm (10in) apart. Place both hands on the table and then, bending your arms, allow your chest to touch the table. Straighten both arms immediately and return to the first position. You should do this exercise half-a-dozen times or less to start with, and gradually work up to 20 to 30 times.

2 Sit on the edge of a chair and lean back, gripping the sides of the chair for support. Raise both knees to your chest, letting your back bend a little and your head fall forwards. Lower both the knees and repeat. This exercise is especially good for sagging stomach muscles. As with the first exercise, you should gradually work up to doing it 20 to 30 times.

rate, the speed at which food is used by the body. Exercise also tightens muscles so that you appear to be less fat; floppy abdominal muscles, for example, make the stomach look larger, and if these are toned up the stomach appears flatter.

A note of caution

To get fit and keep fit, you need to exercise for only one hour each week, preferably in three 20-minute or two 30-minute spells. It is very unwise to embark suddenly on prolonged bouts of exercise if you have been taking little exercise beforehand. Your progress should be gradual, attempting a little more each week. Over-exertion will not make you more fit, and it may be dangerous.

If you are in any doubt about your ability to take any form of exercise, seek professional medical advice. (If you are overweight, over 40, have or have had a heart or lung condition, may be pregnant, or have not taken exercise for many years, you should ask the advice of your doctor in any case). You should not take exercise if:
* You have eaten a meal less than two hours earlier

* You are tired
* You are ill—even if you only have a cold
* It is too cold. Keep warm during and after exercises. If you exercise at home, do so in a warm, ventilated room with the minimum of clothing.

You should stop exercising immediately, and consult your doctor if you experience:
*Excessive tiredness
*Excessive, unnatural breathlessness
*A pain or a feeling of tightness in the chest, arm, back, or joints
*Dizziness
*Headache.

Some types of exercises should be avoided. Women should remember that, because of their anatomy, press-ups may be difficult. The double-leg exercise, in which you lie on the floor on your back and raise both legs very slowly off the floor, is not recommended—it can strain the muscles of the abdomen and may cause a hernia. Jumping exercises should be avoided if you are very unfit or overweight.

Above all, remember not to overdo your exercises. When your body tells you to stop, do so.

What type of exercise?

Once you have allocated a number of short periods each week for exercise—adding up to no more than one hour—you can decide whether to exercise indoors or outdoors. Whichever you choose, it is the overall effect that matters: there is little point in performing only one type of exercise as it will only tone one set of muscles—and will also be extremely boring. Choose a variety of different exercises, to spread the beneficial effects over the whole of your body, and to maintain your interest.

Outdoor exercises

Most people feel that outdoor exercises must be healthier than indoor ones, mainly because of the fresh air. If you live in a town which has high levels of air pollution, this is not necessarily true. Outdoor exercise, however, is beneficial, because it often involves several sets of muscles at the same time.

Jogging, swimming, bicycling, squash and tennis are all good forms of exercise, since all involve deep breathing and many repetitive pumping movements of the arms and legs. These forms of exercise are called 'aerobic', because they

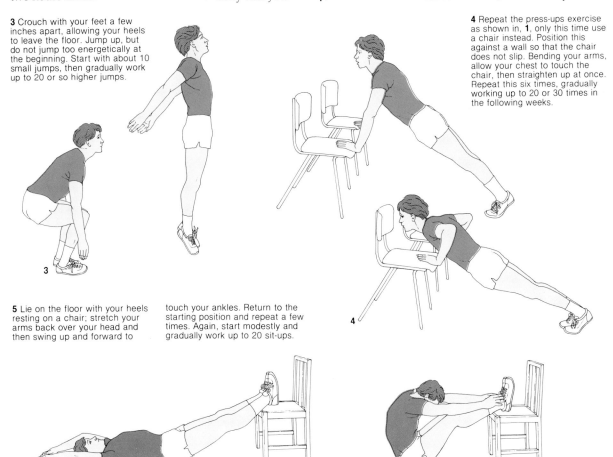

3 Crouch with your feet a few inches apart, allowing your heels to leave the floor. Jump up, but do not jump too energetically at the beginning. Start with about 10 small jumps, then gradually work up to 20 or so higher jumps.

4 Repeat the press-ups exercise as shown in, **1**, only this time use a chair instead. Position this against a wall so that the chair does not slip. Bending your arms, allow your chest to touch the chair, then straighten up at once. Repeat this six times, gradually working up to 20 or 30 times in the following weeks.

5 Lie on the floor with your heels resting on a chair; stretch your arms back over your head and then swing up and forward to touch your ankles. Return to the starting position and repeat a few times. Again, start modestly and gradually work up to 20 sit-ups.

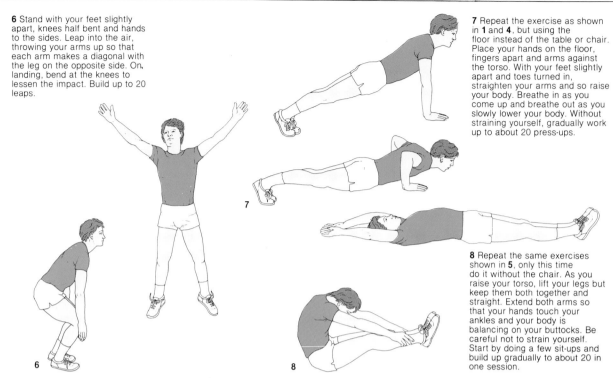

6 Stand with your feet slightly apart, knees half bent and hands to the sides. Leap into the air, throwing your arms up so that each arm makes a diagonal with the leg on the opposite side. On landing, bend at the knees to lessen the impact. Build up to 20 leaps.

7 Repeat the exercise as shown in **1** and **4**, but using the floor instead of the table or chair. Place your hands on the floor, fingers apart and arms against the torso. With your feet slightly apart and toes turned in, straighten your arms and so raise your body. Breathe in as you come up and breathe out as you slowly lower your body. Without straining yourself, gradually work up to about 20 press-ups.

8 Repeat the same exercises shown in **5**, only this time do it without the chair. As you raise your torso, lift your legs but keep them both together and straight. Extend both arms so that your hands touch your ankles and your body is balancing on your buttocks. Be careful not to strain yourself. Start by doing a few sit-ups and build up gradually to about 20 in one session.

increase the efficiency with which air is breathed and oxygen transported around the body. However, for full effectiveness, aerobic exercises should be performed for at least 12 minutes, without a rest. Many team sports do not fulfil this criterion, and are less effective than individual exercises. This is because they often involve long periods of inactivity, interspersed between short, intense bouts of exertion.

Swimming is an excellent aerobic exercise, especially if a variety of strokes are used, because all the muscles are exercised equally. Sufferers from arthritis or back problems, and the overweight, find swimming a convenient form of exercise because the water supports their weight. Walking is also a good form of exercise, provided that you walk briskly: a leisurely amble, or even a walk at normal pace does not constitute exercise.

Exercise at home

There are an infinite number of exercises that you can perform at home. If you are prepared to spend money on your fitness programme, a static bicycle or a rowing-machine will be particularly effective in giving tone to your legs and heart. But without such aids, simple exercises such as running on the spot, repeatedly sitting down in a chair and then standing up, or dancing energetically, will still help to improve your fitness.

The number of exercises given in this section may seem daunting at

first, but as the weeks go by, you will find that you are able to perform more and more of them in your weekly hour; soon you will come to welcome the variety of exercises available. It does not matter which exercises you choose as long as there is a good mix of activities: all parts of the body should be exercised with the aim of achieving suppleness, strength and stamina. To monitor your progress, keep a log of the exercises that you perform at each session, and record how many times you were able to repeat them. You will be surprised how quickly you improve.

Stamina

Running on the spot can be done anywhere, and is one of the best exercises for developing your physical endurance, particularly for improving the function of the heart and lungs. Start by running for around 30 seconds, and after a few months build up to five minutes. Britain's Health Education Council also rate brisk bicycling, jogging, and energetic swimming as excellent for developing stamina.

As with all exercise, do not overdo any of these activities at the start of your fitness programme. It is all too easy to overstrain the heart if you are unaccustomed to exercise, and the results can be tragic. If you have any doubts about your fitness, you should consult a doctor. In any case, it is advisable to prepare for such activities by walking as much as you can, and by doing the limbering-up

exercises described earlier on a regular basis. Make sure that you wear suitable shoes: they should fit snugly, but not too tightly, and be designed specifically to absorb the constant jarring on the skeleton. When you start stamina exercises, be sure to take plenty of rest periods. When jogging, for example, walk first, jog for a minute or two, walk, then jog a little more. Finish by walking for five minutes. As the weeks go by, you can gradually increase the time you spend jogging.

Quality of life

Exercise taken on a long-term basis increases your suppleness, strength and stamina. It can reduce high blood-pressure, and studies have shown that the pulse rate is lower at all times in those who exercise than in those who do not. Clearly, if you are fit you can cope more efficiently with the physical and mental demands of everyday life in the 20th century. Carrying heavy loads, such as shopping, presents less of a problem when the muscles are strong and the heart is pumping efficiently. Moreover, the effects of stress will be reduced, you will feel more alert and will sleep better. Exercise is not guaranteed to make you live longer, but it will improve the quality of your life. But remember, to enjoy all the benefits of fitness you must continue your exercise programme—one hour of exertion each week is not much to pay for such benefits.

Ante-natal and post-natal exercises

Birth is one of the most exciting and challenging events of a woman's life. Not only is it a profound emotional experience, but it is also a time when the body undergoes major changes, readying it for labour, birth and feeding. The demands made on the body during pregnancy and labour make physical preparations—exercises and posture correction—invaluable.

You should exercise to improve your physical condition, to prepare for the special stresses that will be encountered by your muscles, joints and tissues, to ensure maximum suppleness during birth, to achieve a quicker return to fitness after birth, and to make pregnancy itself more comfortable. However, any exercise programme should be gradual—over-exertion will not make you more fit and may harm your baby. Professional medical advice should always be sought before embarking on any course of exercise. Remember, above all, not to attempt anything that you would have found strenuous before pregnancy.

Walking and swimming are the best forms of exercise outside the home. It is perfectly safe to go swimming right up to the last day of pregnancy, so make use of your local pool or the sea, if it is nearby and warm enough. Walk and swim after the birth too, and remember that babies take to the water quickly,

so it will not be long before you can swim together.

Posture
The benefits of regular exercise during pregnancy are greatly reduced if your posture is not good. Backache is common when carrying a child, so remember to stand up straight, and do not succumb to the temptation of slumping forward. Wear flat shoes whenever you can: high heels always strain the back, and the problem becomes worse when the line of gravity moves during pregnancy.

When you sit down, choose a chair that gives good support, and do not slump. If you are tired, try and rest while lying on your side. Too much lying or sleeping on the back is not recommended, as it impedes the circulation. When you get up from the floor or the bed, do so slowly to prevent dizziness. Get up from the floor by first going on all fours, and from the bed by first swinging the legs over the side, then sitting for a few minutes before rising.

Ante-natal exercise
These exercises are designed for pregnant women, but many of them can usefully be performed after birth as well. You should do each exercise twice at first, gradually increasing to five times. Alternate the different

exercises so that various parts of your body are involved. Exercise for as long as you feel comfortable: stop before you get tired, begin to shake or are unable to control the movement. Always rest and relax between exercises. The exercises should ideally be performed on the floor, but you can use a bed if you find it more comfortable.

Invisible exercises
It is important to perform the exercises outlined here during pregnancy, and to keep generally fit. But you will probably not feel like taking formal exercise every day. Some exercises, however, can be performed while you are ironing, standing on a station platform, or watching television. You should be aware of your breathing rate all the time, and you should try to take regular, even breaths. Practise the backward and forward movements of the pelvis whenever you can.

When you are watching television, or chatting, choose a chair that gives good back-support, put your feet up and exercise your calves and feet. Bring your toes towards you so that you feel the muscles at the back of the legs stretch. Circle your feet around and around, forwards and backwards. This will aid the circulation in your feet and legs, which have to take a

Your body has to work harder during pregnancy than at any other time in your life. An increasing and often uncomfortable pressure in the abdomen impedes breathing, for instance, yet efficient breathing is essential to provide the developing baby with an adequate supply of oxygen. For this reason, both pregnancy and the eventual birth will be much easier if you have learned to control your breathing in advance. The following exercises will help you to achieve this. They should be practised during pregnancy but they are also an essential part of labour.

1 Lie on the floor with a pillow beneath your head and relax. Place your hands on each side of your lower ribs and breathe in and out, feeling your ribs rise and fall as you do so. Remember to breathe moderately and slowly to avoid becoming dizzy.

2 Try to breathe in through your nose when you inhale and, at the same time, feel your abdomen rise. When you exhale, concentrate on your abdominal muscles: pull them inwards and force the air out through your mouth, blowing softly as you do so.

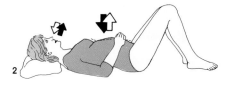

During labour During the first stage of labour, the neck of the womb dilates to allow birth to take place. At this time, efficient breathing will ensure a regular supply of oxygen to both mother and baby. It also enables the mother to concentrate on the physical effort involved.

Breathe in and out as shown in the second pre-natal exercise and continue to do so during the contractions of the uterus. It helps to establish a rhythm by emphasizing the exhalations.

During the second stage of labour, the baby moves out of the uterus, through the dilated cervix and into the vagina. Good control of breathing is required and this, too, can be practised in advance.

Co-ordinate your breathing with the tensing and relaxing of your abdominal muscles, as in the second exercise. During the delivery you will be asked to push as you exhale, but do not practise this during pregnancy, for obvious reasons.

At the moment of delivery, you will feel an almost uncontrollable urge to push, but you will have to blow, breathe out or pant instead. This is when the midwife checks that your cervix is fully dilated and the umbilical cord is in the right place. Practise controlling this urge to push by blowing out through the mouth while your abdominal muscles are relaxed.

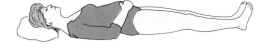

The gradually increasing weight at the front of the body during pregnancy alters the body's centre of gravity, and, as a result, more and more strain is placed on the back and abdominal muscles. You can counter this by doing reaching, stretching and bending exercises to increase the mobility and suppleness of your back. When you are bending or lifting, make sure that your knees and not your back take the strain.

1 Lie on your back on the floor with your arms at your sides, the palms of your hands palm up, and your legs straight out. Bend your feet upwards, pulling the toes forward and pressing the backs of the knees down so that the calf muscles are stretched. Try to flatten the small of your back against the floor by pulling in your abdominal muscles. Do the same with the back of your neck by pulling the shoulder blades together. Hold the muscles in this position for a few seconds and then relax.

2 Lie on the floor with your knees bent and your lower back flattened so that your pelvis is tilted back. Incline your head forwards and breathe in slowly. As you breathe out, raise the upper part of your body but keep your waist on the floor. Return slowly to a lying position and relax. To begin with, and in the later weeks of pregnancy, you will find it easier to lie with your arms outstretched.

2a, 2b As you progress through the middle months of pregnancy, try holding your arms in front of you, and then, a couple of weeks later, clasping your hands behind your head. This exercise increases the mobility of your back and, at the same time, tones up the muscles in your abdomen.

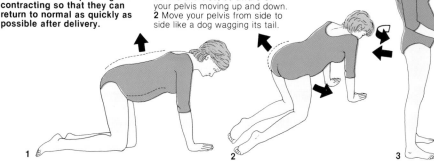

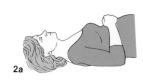

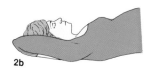

The muscles on the floor of the pelvis are vitally important during pregnancy for they need to be as supple as possible when the moment of birth arrives. They should also be accustomed to expanding and contracting so that they can return to normal as quickly as possible after delivery.

1 Get down on your hands and knees and push your back up like an angry cat. Then let your back return slowly to the normal position, but do not allow your back to dip downwards. As you do this exercise, be aware of your pelvis moving up and down.
2 Move your pelvis from side to side like a dog wagging its tail.

3 Stand up straight with your feet several inches apart and your knees slightly bent. Move your pelvis gently from side to side, rotate it one way and then the other, and finally move it slowly from front to back.

You should also try to practise contracting and relaxing the muscles of the vagina, urethra and anus while doing each of the exercises described here. These particular muscles need to be strong so that you can have more control during delivery and an enjoyable sex life after the birth. Strong urethral muscles can provide some insurance against the incontinence that sometimes occurs before and after labour.

Muscles, known as adductors, lie on the inside of the thighs and control the movement of the hip and the pelvis. They need to be as flexible as possible for labour, so these exercises should be practised whenever you can.

1 Sit on the floor with your back straight and draw in your feet so that the soles touch. Hold one knee with each hand and press down slightly on the knees. You will feel the muscles stretch inside the upper thigh. Relax and repeat the exercise.

2 Cultivate the habit of sitting on the floor tailor-fashion, with legs apart, knees bent and ankles crossed. This is a good stretching exercise for the adductor muscles in both thighs and relaxes the floor of the pelvis.

good deal of the physical strain of pregnancy.

Post-natal exercise
After the birth of your baby, you should continue with the exercises that you performed during pregnancy. This is important, firstly because your muscles will have been greatly stretched and therefore will be in need of toning; and, secondly, because exercise helps to eliminate the waste products that have accumulated in the muscles and tissue during labour. Exercises for regular breathing, and for the back, pelvis, legs and feet are recommended.

Take medical advice before you start on an exercise programme after, as well as before, the birth. If you have had a Caesarean delivery, there will be some exercises that you should not do, and it is wise in any case to seek the advice of your doctor. In some cases, depending on your condition, different exercises may be suggested.

The exercises should not be thought of as a chore. Listen to music while you do them and relax. Remember that they are good for you, and good for your growing baby—and after the birth, your breast-milk will be better if you are in good shape.

Diet

A sensible and well-balanced diet is essential for a healthy and vigorous life. We eat to provide fuel, vitamins and minerals for our bodies. But when we eat to excess, or eat the wrong foods, we run the risk of disease. The right balance of foods, in the right quantities, can not only make us thin and keep us thin; it can also help to protect us against common medical conditions, such as heart disease and diverticular disease.

Basic energy requirements

About half of the energy needed by the body is required to power the muscles used in daily life. The rest is used up in the maintenance of the body—see Metabolism, p44.

Individual energy requirements vary widely. Some people use over three times more energy each day than others. Most of these differences are due to the varying amounts of energy needed for different physical activities. Other factors are body weight, age and, to a lesser extent, climate. The speed with which energy is used by the body, the metabolic rate, also varies from person to person.

All these factors are interrelated in a complex way. Without a lengthy series of tests, it is impossible to predict exactly how much energy a person needs over an average day, or even for a specific activity.

The average energy expended in a number of routine activities is given in the diagram on p323. From this table, it is possible to calculate that an 'average' middle-aged man, weighing 65kg (10 stone) uses about 2380 calories a day: 524 during eight hours of sleep; 856 while at work in a sedentary, office job for eight hours; and 1000 in a variety of activities, such as household chores, hobbies and television watching. Men who weigh more than 65kg, or who have more active jobs, use more energy. The equivalent figure for an average woman who weighs 55kg (8.5 stone) is 1900 calories per day.

Energy in food

The amount of energy in foods varies tremendously. Some foods, such as vegetables, have practically no energy value; others, such as cooking oil, margarine and butter, have a value as high as 950 calories per 100g (3.5 oz). The energy value of a food depends on the amount of water that it contains, and the chemical form in which the energy is held.

Fats head the list of high-energy foods, followed by carbohydrates, such as sugar and starch, then protein. Starchy foods, such as bread, potatoes, pasta and rice, contain so much water that up to ten times more starch than fat has to be eaten to produce the same amount of energy. However, if fat is added to starches when they are cooked, the energy content increases markedly. Chips fried in fat or oil have four times the energy value as the same quantity of boiled potatoes; weight for weight, biscuits have twice the energy value of bread.

Most of an individual's energy input should be from starches. In fact, 40 per cent of the energy in the average British diet is derived from fat.

Energy balance and weight

If the input of energy from food exceeds the use of energy through physical activity, the balance is stored as fat. Many people accept that they will put on weight as they grow older. This is not a natural or inevitable process, however, and, ideally, a person's weight should remain constant after he is fully grown. There is only one way to achieve this—to adjust the number of calories eaten to the number of calories used.

About 20 tons of food are eaten during an average lifetime, and only a small energy imbalance can have an extraordinary cumulative effect. An extra 50 calories each day, from an extra knob of butter at breakfast, or from driving to the shops instead of walking for ten minutes, can result in a weight gain of 20kg (3.25 stone) in ten years.

To lose weight, most people will need to eat at least 1000 calories less than their average daily expenditure of energy. If this is done, the body has to mobilize its stores of fat to make up the deficit. A diet that

THE RULES OF HEALTHY EATING

Many doctors believe that high-fibre diets make a positive contribution to health. As well as aiding weight loss as part of a calorie controlled diet, fibre helps prevent constipation by softening the faeces, so that they are easy to pass. By increasing the bulk of the food residue in the intestine and softening it by retaining fluid, it gives the bowel more soft matter to push through, and so lessens the strain on it. This is an important feature in relieving the symptoms of diverticular disease. It increases the bacterial content of the bowel; a high-fibre diet encourages the growth of protective bacteria.

Increasing the fibre content in your food helps you slim in two ways. Firstly, high-fibre food generally contains fewer calories, but more bulk, than the same amount of low-fibre food and needs more chewing. This helps you feel fuller and so reduces your appetite. Secondly, high-fibre food reduces the energy absorbed from food, while also ensuring that the energy that is absorbed is absorbed more slowly.

Food	g	Food	g
Wheat bran	44.0	Srping greens (boiled)	3.8
Haricot beans (uncooked	25.4	Lentils (boiled)	3.7
Butter beans (uncooked)	21.6	Bananas	3.4
Puffed wheat	15.4	Carrots (boiled)	3.1
Almonds	14.3	White flour	3.0
Coconut (fresh)	13.6	Cabbage (boiled)	2.5
Crispbread	11.7	Apples (peeled)	2.0
Cornflakes	11.0	Oranges	2.0
Wholemeal flour	9.6	Tomatoes (fresh)	1.5
Peanuts	8.1	Lettuce	1.5
Peas (uncooked frozen)	7.8	Potatoes (boiled)	1.0
Brown flour (85%)	7.5	White rice (boiled)	0.8
Muesli	7.4	Porridge (cooked)	0.8
Raisins (dried)	6.8		
Spinach	6.3		
Sweetcorn (canned)	5.7		
Brown rice	5.5		
Brown bread	5.1		

Which foods contain fibre? The chart (above) shows the fibre content of some popular foods, the figures showing the weight of fibre per 100g of the food. Use it as a guide to the high-fibre foods that are good for you and cut down on others.

contains 1200 calories should cause a gradual weight loss of 1kg (2.2lb) each week for the average person. Although many gimmicky diets are devised to sugar the pill, there are no easy ways to slim. The only method that is consistently effective is to eat less than you require to fulfil your body's energy demands

Over the last 20 years, low-carbohydrate diets (restricted in sugar, sweets, cakes, biscuits, bread and potatoes) have often been recommended. Nowadays, most nutritionists suggest a different approach, because of the risks of a high intake of fat in such a diet. They allow small portions of low-energy foods, such as lean meat, bread and potatoes, but cut out entirely all high-energy foods. Food cooked in fat is prohibited,and a low-fat spread is substituted for butter. Allowing 120 calories for such a spread, a flexible 1200 calories diet, made up from low-energy foods, would consist of:
Breakfast—100g (3.5 oz) or two-and-a-half medium slices of wholemeal bread, low-fat spread, grilled tomato
Lunch—50g (1.75 oz) of grilled lamb chop (with the fat removed), 200g (7 oz) jacket potato, any vegetable or salad without dressing, two pieces of fresh fruit
Dinner—50g (1.75 oz) of minced lean stewing steak, tomato, mushroom, onion and fresh tomato sauce (no fat), 200g (7 oz) cooked wholewheat spaghetti, two pieces of fresh fruit
To drink—300g (0.5 pint) of skimmed milk plus water. No alcoholic drinks are allowed.

Staying thin
The ideal body weights for men and women, according to their heights and their builds, are shown in the diagram on p324. Once these ideal weights have been achieved, more high-energy foods, such as butter, chocolates, cheese and fatty meats, can be gradually added to the diet, but it is important to keep a close, regular check on your weight for at least a year. Even then, you must eat sensible, well-balanced foods to stay slim.

Protein
Protein is part of the structure of each of the millions of cells of our body. It is needed to replace old tissues, and to build new tissues—see Metabolism, p44. Some protein is discarded when old tissues are broken down, and between 50g and 70g (1.75-2.5 oz) must be provided each day in the diet to replace it.

The average diet in the Western world supplies at least this much, partly because foods rich in protein,

such as meat, fish, cheese, eggs and milk, are readily available. Bread and other foods made from cereals are important sources of protein, and make up a quarter of the total protein intake. Peas, beans and nuts are also rich sources.

Vitamins and minerals
Vitamins and minerals are also part of the structure of every cell in the body, and are of fundamental importance in the maintenance of body functions. Many have a specific role: the B vitamins are needed for the release of energy from food; iron and folic acid (a B vitamin) are necessary for the formation of blood; vitamin A is a part of the chemical structure of the light-sensitive areas of the eyes. Calcium is a vital component of bone, and zinc is needed for the sense of taste and flavour—See The Digestive System, p40.

Vitamins and minerals are found in nearly all foods except 'empty calorie' or 'junk' foods. In the West, vitamin and mineral deficiencies are rare among those who eat a normal, balanced diet. Sometimes, however, they may be caused by problems other than those of inadequate nutrition. People from tropical countries who now live in northern Europe may not be exposed to enough sunshine for their needs: too little vitamin D is manufactured, calcium cannot be absorbed from the intestine, and a condition of the bones called rickets may be the result. Menorrhagia, or heavy menstrual bleeding, may lead to anaemia, and iron deficiency in women. These conditions may be remedied by supplements of vitamin D and iron.

Vitamin pills and tonics.
Serious diseases that threaten life can develop in the absence of some vitamins and minerals, but only tiny quantities are needed to prevent the onset of these conditions. Claims for the curative or protective powers of large doses of vitamins rarely have any human experimental basis; such

WHAT CALORIES ARE
Protein, carbohydrate and fat have different amounts of energy locked up inside them. When you use up a specific quantity of fat, for example, a specific amount of energy is released. This energy is measured in calories. Scientifically speaking, one Calorie (with a large 'c') is the equivalent of 1000 calories (with a small 'c') or one kilocalorie.

claims are particularly common for those vitamins for which there are no dramatic deficiency symptoms. Vitamin E is a good example of this—it has been said, variously, to prevent wrinkles, prolong life and revitalize sexual powers. Where such claims for vitamins have been investigated, they have usually been found to be misleading.

More recently, it has been suggested by the American scientist Linus Pauling that huge doses of Vitamin C both prevent and cure the common cold and other viral infections. These theories are as yet unproven. At the very least, however, they are good reasons for choosing a diet that contains plenty of the fruit and vegetables with these vitamins.

If a sensible diet is observed, it is debatable whether the expense of vitamin pills and tonics can be justified. If you do use vitamin supplements, take care. While vitamin C is harmless in any quantity, Vitamins A and D are fatal poisons in large doses.

Special needs
Children, pregnant women and nursing mothers need more protein, vitamins and minerals than normal to allow for growth. These can be obtained from a vitamin pill prescribed by the family doctor, which contains iron and folic acid, and extra milk.

The elderly need less energy, because they are less active on the whole, but the same amounts of protein, vitamins and minerals as younger people. Foods that are high in energy but are poor sources of essential nutrients—fried foods, cakes, pastries, and biscuits—are best avoided. Tinned meats, fish, vegetables and eggs can easily be prepared, stored and chewed, and are a good source of nutrients. At least 300g (0.5 pint) of milk should be taken each day, together with extra vitamin D, if an elderly person cannot spend much time in the sunshine.

Diet and disease
In the earlier part of this century, the main nutritional problems were poor health and stunted growth, caused by diets lacking in iron, vitamins and sometimes protein. Over the past 30 years, the pattern of disease has been changing. Now the major nutritional problem is obesity, or fatness.

The use of new technology has reduced the expenditure of energy in physical work and in daily life. At the same time there has been a steady increase in the availability of high-energy foods. The result has

The energy used in various activities by a man of 65kg (10 stone) and a woman of 55kg (8.5 stone)

Activities	cals 0.5	1	1.5	2	2.5	3	3.5	4	4.5	5	5.5	6	6.5	7	7.5	8
Asleep in bed																
Sitting quietly																
Standing quietly																
Cooking																
Light cleaning																
Moderate cleaning (polishing)																
Walking at 5kmph (3mph)																
Sedentary work																
office																
driving																
Light industry																
garage repairs, laundry work																
electrical work																
Recreations																
seated (knitting)																
light (golf, sailing)																
moderate (dancing, riding)																
heavy (athletics, football)																

Men ▮ Women ▯   Approximate amount of energy used on average each minute

been an increase in the incidence of heart disease—it now accounts for 25 per cent of all deaths in Britain—hypertension, or high blood pressure, strokes, cancers of the large intestine, and other disorders of the bowels.

Evidence of the importance of diet in these diseases has come from two lines of research. Scientists have examined the foods eaten in parts of the world in which these diseases are rare, such as Africa, and have compared them with the foods eaten in industrialized countries. They have also carried out careful experiments to see how the body reacts to changes in the diet.

Neither of these two approaches has given any definite proof of a clear relationship between the type of diet an individual eats and the pattern of disease that may develop ten or 20 years later. It is extremely difficult to measure a person's daily diet accurately; furthermore, the extent to which the body copes with the components of the diet varies tremendously from one person to another. Without expensive mass-screening tests, the relationship is not easy to establish.

In the absence of proof, and because if such theories were proven, there would be significant economic repercussions for the agricultural, food-manufacturing and catering industries, the role of diet in disease is subject to much debate and controversy. This centres primarily around five components of the diet: fat, cholesterol, dietary fibre, salt and sugar.

Fat
On average, we eat about 100g (3.5 oz) of fat each day—this is around 40 per cent of our total energy intake. There is substantial evidence that a more sensible amount would be around 75g (2.5 oz), or 30 per cent.

In experiments in a number of countries, the number of people dying from heart disease and from cancers of the intestines has been closely linked with the amount of fat and animal products that they have consumed, the main sources being meat, milk, butter and cheese. The incidence of such diseases is much higher where these foods are eaten in large quantities. A high-fat diet is thought to increase the amount of bile secreted by the liver and alter the level of hormones circulating in the bloodstream. In so doing, fat encourages the growth of cancerous tumours in the large intestine. Most of the evidence that a lower fat intake would be beneficial, however, is based on research into the cause of heart disease.

Cholesterol
Some studies have shown that people who have high levels of cholesterol in the blood run an increased risk of suffering from heart disease in later life. However, the link has yet to be proven conclusively.

Cholesterol is manufactured in the body, and also taken in as food. The main sources are eggs, meat, cheese, butter, milk, cream and animal fats in general. Plant foods contain no cholesterol, while the quantities in margarine vary, depending on whether plant or animal oil is used in its manufacture.

Both the type of fat in food and its quantity can affect the amount of cholesterol in the blood. The level can be lowered if less fat is eaten, or if polyunsaturated margarine, or corn, sunflower or safflower oil is used for frying and cooking, instead of animal fats, such as butter and lard. Most margarines and vegetable oils, as well as olive oil, are unsuitable because they do not contain enough polyunsaturated fats. For those people who have a tendency to be overweight, it is more sensible to eat less fat overall.

Although many people can eat foods containing a high level of cholesterol without it affecting the cholesterol level in their blood, experiments have shown that others are more sensitive. People with a relative who already suffers from heart disease are advised to eat no more than two or three eggs a week, and to restrict their intake of other foods rich in cholesterol. This is because there is an hereditary factor in heart disease.

Dietary fibre
The cell walls of virtually all plants contain a greater or lesser amount of dietary fibre, or roughage. Dietary fibre cannot be digested by the body. It passes through the digestive tract and stimulates the intestine to pass on food; it also provides the bulk that makes stools solid.

Wholemeal bread, wholegrain cereals such as wholemeal pasta and oats, peas, beans, nuts and products with added bran are the best sources of dietary fibre. White flour, rice, vegetables and fruits contain rather less. Wholemeal bread is preferable to bran as a source of fibre, because it contains less phytic acid, a substance that interferes with the absorption of minerals such as iron, calcium, magnesium and zinc.

A diet that is low in fibre causes constipation, though most people would need to double their

intake of fibre before its effect was noticeable. Large amounts of fibre are given in the treatment of diverticular disease, in which small pockets develop in the wall of the large intestine and tend to become infected in diverticulitis. A sensible diet contains 40g (1.4 oz) of fibre each day, twice the present average intake.

Fibre also alters the way in which bacteria use or break down many substances in the large intestine, some of which can cause cancer. It may reduce the contact of these substances with the intestinal wall as well. There is some evidence that people who eat a high-fibre diet are at less risk from cancer of the intestine.

A high-fibre diet is also thought to be useful in the treatment of conditions such as haemorrhoids, anal fissures, colitis and irritable bowel syndrome, but insufficient research has been carried out to assess its value in these problems properly. There is little evidence that dietary fibre actually protects the body against these conditions.

Such a diet may, however, be of some help in the treatment of diabetes. Several studies have shown a marked improvement in diabetics after treatment with a low-fat, very high-fibre and high-starch diet. There is a significant reduction in the amount of insulin needed and a reduction in the blood level of cholesterol. In the long term, this diet may reduce the risk of

complications in diabetes, such as heart disease.

Salt
The body requires very little salt to maintain its body chemistry, but most people eat considerable amounts of it—both in cooking and at the table. It is also added to a variety of foods by manufacturers. Sometimes it is used as a preservative, but more often for taste. It is present in bread, butter and margarine, while monosodium glutamate, a form of salt, is added to virtually all 'convenience foods'. Unprocessed food, however, contains very little salt.

Hypertension, or high blood pressure, can be a symptom of a number of medical conditions, or a disease itself. In many people its cause is uncertain, but in those with a family history of hypertension there seems to be a relationship between a high level of salt in the diet and high blood pressure. A proportion of people seem to be particularly sensitive to this.

Since hypertension markedly increases the possibility of a stroke and is a major risk factor in heart disease, some family doctors now screen their patients for the problem—especially when there is a family history of heart disease. Part of the treatment for those with high blood pressure is a reduction in the intake of salt. Table salt should not be used, and it should be omitted entirely in cooking. Salt substitutes should be used instead.

Desirable weights for adults of medium frame, aged 25 and over

Height (no shoes)		Weight (indoor clothes)				
		Women		Men	
Metres	Feet	Kilograms	Stones	Kilograms	Stones
1.42m	4ft 8in	44-49kg	6st 12lb- 7st 9lb		
1.45	4 9	45-50	7 0 - 7 12		
1.47	4 10	46-51	7 3 - 8 1		
1.49	4 11	47-53	7 6 - 8 4		
1.52	5 0	49-54	7 9 - 8 7		
1.55	5 1	50-55	7 12 - 8 10	54-59kg	8st 6lb- 9st 3lb
1.58	5 2	51-57	8 1 - 9 0	55-60	8 9 - 9 3
1.60	5 3	53-59	8 4 - 9 4	56-62	8 12 - 9 10
1.63	5 4	54-61	8 8 - 9 9	58-63	9 1 - 9 13
1.65	5 5	56-63	8 12 - 9 13	59-65	9 4 -10 3
1.67	5 6	58-65	9 2 -10 3	61-67	9 8 -10 7
1.70	5 7	60-67	9 6 -10 7	63-69	9 12 -10 12
1.73	5 8	62-69	9 10 -10 11	64-71	10 2 -11 2
1.75	5 9	64-70	10 0 -11 1	66-73	10 6 -11 6
1.78	5 10	65-72	10 4 -11 5	68-75	10 10 -11 11
1.80	5 11			70-77	11 0 -12 2
1.83	6 0			72-79	11 4 -12 7
1.85	6 1			74-82	11 8 -12 12
1.91	6 2			76-84	11 13 -13 3
1.93	6 3			78-86	12 4 -13 8

NB – If of light frame, subtract 3kg (7lb) from the lowest weight and 5kg (11lb) from the highest weight
– If of heavy frame, add 4kg (9lb) to the lowest weight and 6kg (13lb) to the highest weight
– Allow 2kg (4.5lb) for clothes if female; 4kg (8lb) if male

A sensible diet

	Energy (cals)	Protein (g)	Fat (g)	Starch (g)	Sugar (g)	Fibre (g)	Cholesterol (mg)	Calcium (mg)	Magnesium (mg)	Iron (mg)	Zinc (mg)	Vitamin B1 (mg)	Vitamin B2 (mg)	Vitamin C (mg)	Vitamin A (µg)
Breakfast															
Wheatflakes 35gm (1.4oz)	121	4.0	1.2	23.3	2.1	4.4		11	42	2.6	0.7	0.09	0.02		
Sugar 5gm (0.2oz)	15				5.0										
5 slices wholemeal bread[1]	452	18.4	5.7	83.3	4.4	17.8		48	195	5.2	4.2	0.55	0.13		
Thinly spread butter, or polyunsaturated margarine, for 5 slices			145	0.1			16.4	46[2]	3						166
Marmalade 20gm (0.8oz)	52				14.4	0.1		7		0.1				2	2
Milk, for cereal and drinks during the day, 450gm (0.75 pint)	290	14.8	17.1		63		540	54	02	1.6	0.18	0.86	7	173	
Lunch															
1 small slice of chicken 30gm (1.2oz)	42	7.4	1.6				22	3	7	0.2	0.5	0.02	0.06		
1 small slice of cheese 30gm (1.2oz)	119	7.8	10.0				21	240	75	0.1	1.2	0.01	0.15		103
Lettuce, tomato 100gm (4oz)	14	0.9			2.8	1.5		13	11	0.4	0.2	0.06	0.04	20	
Small piece fruit cake 40gm (1.6oz)	143	2.0	5.2	6.0	17.2	1.2	16	24	10	0.6	0.2	0.04	0.02		
Fresh orange 120gm (4.8oz)	42	1.0			10.2	1.8		49	16	0.4	0.2	0.08	0.02	46	7
Dinner															
Lentil soup, no fat, 200gm (8oz)	93	7.1	0.3	15.2	0.7	3.5		12	23	2.3	0.9	0.15	0.06		3
2 thin pork escalopes, 50gm (2oz)	111	16.1	5.3				55	4	15	0.6	1.7	0.44	0.13		
Mushroom sauce 100gm (4oz)	52	1.1	3.8	0.8	3.1			30	4	0.3	0.3		0.05		
Large jacket potato, 250gm (10oz)	204	3.5	0.2	61.0	1.5	6.0		6	37	0.7	0.5	0.25	0.10	15	
Peas (2oz)	21	2.5	0.2	0.5	1.7	2.5		15	11	0.7	0.3	0.12	0.03	7	50
Carrots 100gm (4oz)	19	0.6			4.2	3.1		37	6	0.4	0.3	0.05	0.04	4	2000
Stewed apple 150gm (6oz)	90	0.4			23.4	2.4		21	30	0.3	0.1	0.03	0.03	16	4
Natural yoghurt 100gm (4oz)	52	5.0	1.0		6.2		7	180	17	0.1	0.6	0.05	0.26		6
Nut topping 10gm (0.4oz)	52	1.1	5.2	0.2	0.3	0.5		6	13	0.2	0.3	0.03	0.01		
Total (rounded up)	2129	94	73	190	114	45	230	1249	566	15	14	2	2	117	2624

[1] These values are given under breakfast for convenience, but the slices of wholemeal bread may be eaten at other times of the day. Butter or margarine should be thinly spread - only 20gm (0.8oz) is allowed per day.
[2] This value is for butter only.

Processed foods with a high level of salt should be avoided—salt and sodium-containing additives are declared on the labels.

Because nationwide screening for sensitivity to salt would be impractical, it has been suggested that food manufacturers should voluntarily reduce the level of salt and sodium additives in their products. Baby-food manufacturers have already done this, but a wider response seems unlikely in the near future.

Sugar
Sugar, whether white or brown, is an ingredient of confectionery, cakes, biscuits and soft drinks. It is an 'empty calorie' food, providing energy but no other nutrients; it also causes dental decay. As this has been realized it has become less popular as a food. The annual consumption of sugar has been falling steadily since the mid-1950s, and continues to fall today.

Sensible and healthy eating
The basic principle of sensible eating is to halve the amount of high-energy, fatty or sugary, foods. Low-energy foods can be eaten freely.

A sensible diet should contain all the most important sources of each nutrient. Bread, milk, cheese and meat contain the most protein; oranges the most vitamin C; and carrots the most vitamin A. Normally dairy fats supply the majority of vitamin A, so it is important that dark green vegetables or carrots are eaten regularly to make up for the reduced intake of cheese, butter, eggs and cream. Similarly, wholegrain cereals, nuts and pulses should be eaten to make up for reduced amounts of meat protein, as well as for their fibre content.

The risks inherent in our present eating habits are large, especially for those who are susceptible to particular diseases, or have a family history of them. Shopping habits, and even life-style, will have to be changed if these risks are to be reduced. Foods that in the past were thought to be luxuries, but are now commonplace, such as cream, pastries and lavish helpings of meat, should be once more limited to special occasions. The level of risk that any individual runs cannot yet be forecast accurately. But it is sensible to make these sacrifices, and to follow the example of most nutritionists and doctors by eating less high-energy food and more dietary fibre. As a result, you will be less likely to contract diseases, look better, and feel better.

Vitamins (Summary of vitamins significant in human diet)

	Chief functions	Results of deficiency	Characteristics	Good sources	Daily allowances recommended
VITAMIN A Provitamin, carotene	Essential for maintaining the integrity of epithelial membranes. Helps maintain resistance to infections. Necessary for the formation of rhodopsin and prevention of night blindness.	*Mild:* Retarded growth. Increased susceptibility to infection. Abnormal function of gastrointestinal, genitourinary and respiratory tracts due to altered epithelial membranes. Skin dries, shrivels, thickens, sometimes pustule formation. Night blindness. *Severe:* Xerophthalmia, a characteristic eye disease, and other local infections.	Fat soluble. Not destroyed by ordinary cooking temperatures. Is destroyed by high temperatures when oxygen is present. Marked capacity for storage in the liver. Excessive intake of carotene from which vitamin A is formed may produce yellow discoloration of the skin (carotenaemia).	Animal fats butter cheese cream egg yolk whole milk. Fish liver oil. Liver. Vegetable 1. green leafy, esp. escarole, kale, parsley 2. yellow, esp. carrots. *Artificial:* Concentrates in several forms. Irradiated fish oils.	*Males (Ages 10-75+ yrs):* 4500 to 5000 I.U. *Females (Ages 10-75+ yrs):* 4500 to 5000 I.U. *In pregnancy:* 6000 I.U. *In lactation:* 8000 I.U. *Children:* 2000 to 3500 I.U. *Infants:* 1500 I.U.
THIAMINE Vitamin B$_1$	Important role in carbohydrate metabolism. Essential for maintenance of normal digestion and appetite. Essential for normal functioning of nervous tissue.	*Mild:* Loss of appetite. Impaired digestion of starches and sugars. Colitis, constipation, or diarrhea. Emaciation. *Severe:* Nervous disorders of various types. Loss of coordinating power of muscles. Beriberi. Paralysis in man.	Water soluble. Not readily destroyed by ordinary cooking temperature. Destroyed by exposure to heat, alkali, or sulphites. Is not stored in body.	Widely distributed in plant and animal tissues but seldom occurs in high concentration, exception in brewer's yeast. Other good sources are: Whole grain cereals Peas, Beans Peanuts Oranges Glandular—heart, liver, kidney Many vegetables and fruits Nuts. *Artificial:* Concentrates from yeast. Rice polishings. Wheat germ.	*Males (10-75+ yrs.):* 1.3 to 1.5 mg. *Females (10-75+ yrs.):* 1.0 to 1.1 mg. *In pregnancy:* 1.1 to 1.2 mg. *In lactation:* 1.5 to 1.6 mg. *Children:* 0.6 to 1.2 mg. *Infants:* 0.2 to 0.5 mg.
RIBOFLAVIN Vitamin B$_2$	Important in formation of certain enzymes and in cellular oxidation. Normal growth. Prevention of cheilosis and glossitis. Participates in light adaption.	Impaired growth. Lassitude and weakness. Cheilosis. Glossitis. Atrophy of skin. Anaemia. Photophobia. Cataracts.	Water soluble. Alcohol soluble. Not destroyed by heat in cooking unless with alkali. Unstable in light, esp. in presence of alkali.	Eggs Green vegetables Liver Kidney Lean meat Milk Wheat germ Yeast, dried Enriched foods.	*Males (10-75+ yrs.):* 1.3-1.7 mg. *Females (10-75+ yrs.):* 1.3-1.5 mg. *In pregnancy:* 1.8 mg. *In lactation:* 2.0 mg. *Children:* 0.6 to 1.2 mg. *Infants:* 0.4 to 0.6 mg.
NIACIN Nicotinic acid Nicotinamide Antipellagra vitamin	As the component of two important enzymes, it is important in glycolysis, tissue respiration, and fat synthesis. Nicotinic acid but not nicotinamide causes vasodilation and flushing. Prevents pellagra.	Pellagra. Gastrointestinal disturbances. Mental disturbances.	Soluble in hot water and alcohol. Not destroyed by heat, light, air or alkali. Not destroyed in ordinary cooking.	Yeast Lean meat Fish Legumes Whole grain cereals and peanuts Enriched foods.	*Males (10-75+ yrs.):* 14 to 20 mg. *Females (10-75+ yrs.):* 12 to 16 mg. *In pregnancy:* 15 mg. *In lactation:* 20 mg. *Children:* 8 to 15 mg. *Infants:* 5 to 8 mg.
VITAMIN B$_1$2 Cyanocobalamin	Produces remission in pernicious anaemia. Essential for normal development of red blood cells.	Pernicious anaemia.	Soluble in water or alcohol. Unstable in hot alkaline or acid solutions.	Liver Kidney Dairy products. Most of vitamin required by humans is synthesized by intestinal bacteria.	*Males and Females (10-75+ yrs.):* 5 to 6 mcg. *In pregnancy:* 8 mcg. *In lactation:* 6 mcg. *Children:* 2 to 5 mcg. *Infants:* 1 to 2 mcg.

What vitamins do The chart here shows what vitamins the body needs, what they do, what foods contain them and the results of vitamin deficiency. I.U. is an international unit, a common form of medical measurement.

	Chief functions	Results of deficiency	Characteristics	Good sources	Daily allowances recommended
VITAMIN C Ascorbic acid	Essential to formation of intracellular cement substances in a variety of tissues including skin, dentine, cartilage and bone matrix. Important in healing of wounds and fractures of bones. Prevents scurvy. Facilitates absorption of iron.	*Mild:* Lowered resistance to infections. Joint tenderness. Susceptibility to dental caries, pydrrhoea, and bleeding gums. *Severe:* Haemorrhage. Anaemia. Scurvy.	Soluble in water. Easily destroyed by oxidation; heat hastens the process. Lost in cooking, particularly if water in which food was cooked is discarded. Also loss is greater if if cooked in iron or copper utensils. Quick frozen foods lose little of their vitamin C. Stored in the body to a limited extent.	Abundant in most fresh fruits and vegetables, esp. citrus fruit and juices, tomato and orange. *Artificial:* Ascorbic acid. Cevitamic acid.	*Males* *(10-75⁺ yrs.):* 40 to 60 mg. *Females* *(10-75⁺ yrs.):* 40 to 55 mg. *In pregnancy:* 60 mg. *In lactation:* 60 mg. *Children:* 40 mg. *Infants:* 35 mg. The infant diet is likely to be deficient in vitamin C unless orange or tomato juice or other form is added.
VITAMIN D	Regulates absorption of calcium and phosphorus from the intestinal tract. Antirachitic.	*Mild:* Interferes with utilization of calcium and phosphorus in bone and teeth formation. Irritability. Weakness. *Severe:* Rickets, may be common in young children. Osteomalacia in adults.	Soluble in fats and organic solvents. Relatively stable under refrigeration. Stored in liver. Often associated with vitamin A.	Butter Egg yolk Fish liver oils Fish having fat distributed through the flesh, salmon, tuna fish, herring, sardines Liver Oysters Yeast and foods irradiated with ultraviolet light. Formed in the skin by exposure to sunlight. Artificially prepared forms.	*Males and Females* *(10-22 yrs.):* 400 I.U. After age 22, none except during pregnancy or lactation. *In pregnancy:* 400 I.U. *In lactation:* 400 I.U. *Children:* 400 I.U. *Infants:* 400 I.U.
VITAMIN E Alpha tocopherol	Normal reproduction in rats. Prevention of muscular dystrophy in rats.	Red blood cell resistance to rupture is decreased.	Fat soluble. Stable to heat in absence of oxygen.	Lettuce and other green, leafy vegetables. Wheat germ oil Margarine Rice.	*Males* *(10-75⁺ yrs.):* 20 to 30 I.U. *Females* *(10-75⁺ yrs.):* 20 to 25 I.U. *In pregnancy:* 30 I.U. *In lactation:* 30 I.U. *Children:* 10 to 15 I.U. *Infants:* 5 I.U.
VITAMIN B₆ Pyridoxine	Essential for metabolism of tryptophan. Needed for utilization of certain other amino acids.	Dermatitis around eyes and mouth. Neuritis. Anorexia, nausea, and vomiting.	Soluble in water and alcohol. Rapidly inactivated in presence of heat, sunlight, or air.	Blackstrap molasses Meat Cereal grains Wheat germ.	*Males and Females* *(10-75⁺ yrs.):* 1.4 to 2.0 mg. *In pregnancy:* 2.5 mg. *In lactation:* 2.5 mg. *Children:* 0.5 to 1.2 mg. *Infants:* 0.2 to 0.4 mg.
FOLIC ACID Folacin	Essential for normal functioning of haematopoietic system.	Anaemia.	Slightly soluble in water. Easily destroyed by heat in presence of acid. Decreases when food is stored at room temperature. NOTE: A large dose may prevent appearance of anaemia in a case of pernicious anaemia but still permit neurological symptoms to develop.	Glandular meats Yeast Green, leafy vegetables.	*Males and Females* *(10-75⁺ yrs.):* 0.4 mg. *In pregnancy:* 0.8 mg. *In lactation:* 0.5 mg. *Children:* 0.1 to 0.3 mg. *Infants:* 0.05 to 0.1 mg.

Abuses of the body

Many people do not realize that the human body is a delicate machine that can easily be abused. It consists of chemicals, and is controlled by a complex series of chemical reactions. As our understanding of these has developed, other chemicals, drugs that can adjust the chemistry of the body to deal with disease, have been discovered and brought into use by man. The process takes many years. Drugs are tested thoroughly before use, and even then are only prescribed in controlled quantities and in known situations. Yet every day, enormous numbers of people either eat, drink, smoke or inject drugs whose effect can be deadly.

Smoking.
One of the main reasons that people smoke is that cigarettes contain nicotine, an addictive drug that increases the level of adrenaline in the bloodstream. This chemical causes the small blood vessels to contract, increases the blood pressure and raises the pulse rate—see Blood and lymph, p21. It also increases the likelihood of plaque formation, a build-up of cholesterol and fats on the walls of blood vessels, causing arteriosclerosis, and frequently heart disease or a stroke.

If you inhale tobacco smoke, a number of toxic substances enter the body. These irritate the lining of the bronchi and bronchioles, the air passages of the lungs. As a result, the bronchi become inflamed and the cells of their linings secrete large quantities of mucus, which may become infected. The amount of mucus present also reduces the surface area of lung tissue available for the absorption of oxygen—see The Respiratory System, p28—causing breathlessness. Habitual smokers nearly always suffer from this condition, which is called chronic bronchitis.

One of these substances is a gas called carbon monoxide, which combines with the haemoglobin contained in red blood cells to reduce the amount of oxygen that the blood can carry. If a woman smokes while she is pregnant, carbon monoxide can cross the placenta, and infiltrate the blood of the developing baby. This stunts foetal growth and increases the likelihood of a

The relationship between smoking cigarettes and lung cancer, first realized early in the 1960s, is summarized in the graph (above). It charts the correlation in England and Wales between the increasing number of cigarettes smoked and the increasing deaths from lung cancer. throughout the course of this century. The average number of cigarettes smoked by a man each day rose steadily from about 1900 until after World War 2, when they became much more expensive. Since then the number has oscillated up and down: the downward trends following the publication of reports on the subject and rises in tobacco tax. Deaths from lung cancer in men have paralleled the rise in smoking, reaching a maximum around 1960 and falling off gradually ever since. The story for women is different. The average number of cigarettes smoked by a woman each day rose sharply in World War 2 and has roughly doubled since. The death rate from lung cancer among women was originally much lower than in men, but has recently started to rise quite sharply and is continuing to do so.

miscarriage.
Tobacco smoke also contains carcinogens—substances that cause cancer. Though it is impossible to prove that smoking actually causes cancer—people who smoke may have a predisposition towards the disease—the link between cigarette smoking and cancer of the lungs, mouth and throat has been proved beyond any reasonable doubt.

The incidence of a number of other kinds of cancer is increased in smokers. These include cancer of the cervix, of the uterus, cancer of the bladder, and cancer of the pancreas.

If you smoke cigarettes
* The risk of contracting lung cancer is increased by up to 25 times, depending on how much you smoke and for how long you have smoked.
* You are ten times more likely to contract cancer of the mouth or throat.
* You are twice as likely to die of heart disease —the risk is even higher if you are a woman who is taking the contraceptive pill.
* You will almost certainly develop chronic bronchitis,
  *If you have a duodenal ulcer, smoking will probably delay its healing.
* You will suffer from a higher incidence of colds, coughs and sore throats.
* You are shortening your life by ten to 15 years—by five and a half minutes for each cigarette.
  *You are being antisocial: the smoke you exhale is not only unpleasant for other people, it can do them actual harm. In families where one or more people smoke, children have an increased liability to coughs and colds. The non-smoking wives or husbands of smokers have a greater incidence of lung cancer than the spouses of non-smokers.
  *If you are pregnant, you are certainly likely to have a smaller baby than normal. The baby may be less intelligent, and its lung function may be somewhat reduced, both at birth and later, even into adult life. There is an increased likelihood of your baby dying either in the late stages of pregnancy or soon after birth; indeed, in countries where cigarette smoking is common, it may be the most important preventable risk factor for death of the baby in

Alcohol in small doses is a stimulant and may well be good for you. But in large doses it is a depressant and a poison which the body takes up to 24 hours to remove from the time you stop drinking it. Eating food before or as you drink will slow down the alcohol absorption from your intestine. Once in the blood, alcohol is broken down by the liver, excreted in the urine and breathed out through the lungs. It is also broken down far more quickly in the evening than in the morning or the middle of the night. The illustration *(right)* correlates the volumes of different drinks the level of alcohol they will produce in the blood and the effects they are likely to have upon an average person weighing about 70 kilograms (11 stone). They are the results of medical research involving blood tests and observations of the behaviour of a wide sample of people. Small people are likely to be affected quickly, while some people break down alcohol more easily than others. In addition, the speed with which you consume a drink will alter the level of alcohol in your blood: sipping a pint of beer raises your blood alcohol level more slowly than gulping down a glass of whisky. The volume of alcohol varies from drink to drink. Most beers and lagers have 5% alcohol by volume; real ales may be as much as 9%; table wines between 9 and 13%; fortified wines, such as port and sherry, about 20%; and spirits about 40%.

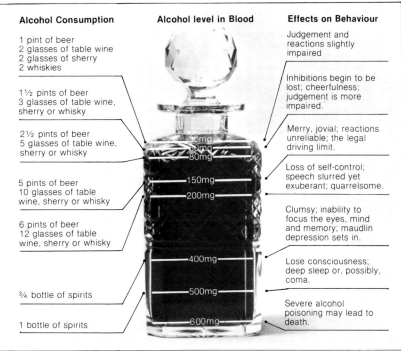

Alcohol Consumption

1 pint of beer
2 glasses of table wine
2 glasses of sherry
2 whiskies

1½ pints of beer
3 glasses of table wine, sherry or whisky

2½ pints of beer
5 glasses of table wine, sherry or whisky

5 pints of beer
10 glasses of table wine, sherry or whisky

6 pints of beer
12 glasses of table wine, sherry or whisky

¾ bottle of spirits

1 bottle of spirits

Alcohol level in Blood

50mg
60mg
80mg
150mg
200mg
400mg
500mg
600mg

Effects on Behaviour

Judgement and reactions slightly impaired

Inhibitions begin to be lost; cheerfulness; judgement is more impaired.

Merry, jovial; reactions unreliable; the legal driving limit.

Loss of self-control; speech slurred yet exuberant; quarrelsome.

Clumsy; inability to focus the eyes, mind and memory; maudlin depression sets in.

Lose consciousness; deep sleep or, possibly, coma.

Severe alcohol poisoning may lead to death.

late pregnancy.
* You increase the risk of contracting thrombo-angiitis obliterans or Buerger's Disease, a progressive degeneration of tissue which may necessitate amputation of the feet.

Stopping smoking
It is important to realize that, for many people, smoking is addictive, and that giving up any such drug can be extremely difficult and traumatic. But more than eight million people in Britain have given up, while in the USA in 1980, nearly one million stopped smoking, following a campaign by the American Cancer Society.

First of all, decide on a day on which you will definitely stop smoking, and stick to your decision. Throw away all your cigarettes, lighters and ashtrays. Identify the times when you are most likely to want a cigarette—after meals, on the telephone or in times of stress—and try to reorganize your life to avoid moments of temptation. Often, it is easier to stop smoking in company rather than in isolation, so look for advertisements for 'smoking-withdrawal' groups in your local newspaper.

There is no point in changing to cigars or a pipe. The risk of lung cancer decreases slightly, but the risk of mouth and throat cancer increases, nicotine still enters the blood, and you will still be shortening your life substantially. Low-tar cigarettes still kill too, so the only sensible course of action is to stop smoking tobacco completely. When you have finished your last cigarette, think of yourself as a non-smoker. Avoid smoking-sections of a train or bus, and try to frequent places in which you would not be allowed to smoke, even if you wanted to. Gentle forms of exercise, such as walking or jogging—*see Exercise, p316*—will keep you busy and help you to feel better, but it may be sensible to seek medical advice first if you have been living a sedentary life.

You will often feel the need to have something in your mouth. Chew gum (preferably sugar-free gum to reduce the risks of tooth decay), or, better still, nibble on fruit or raw vegetables. Make sure, however, that you do not eat more than usual, or you will put on weight—*see Diet, p322*. Reformed smokers often find that they do not know what to do with their hands. Play with a key ring, fiddle with worry-beads or doodle with a pencil, but, above all, do not reach for a cigarette, whatever the temptation.

Heavy smokers, or those who have smoked for many years, often find that they suffer from a variety of physical and mental side-effects when they give up tobacco. These are 'withdrawal' symptoms, caused by the body's adjustment to the withdrawal of a drug on which it has become dependent. As the lungs clean themselves of mucus and tar, the result may be a bad cough, an upset stomach and extra susceptibility to colds and virus infections. There are often mental effects: a person who has given up smoking may become irritable, tense and find it difficult to concentrate, while their mood may fluctuate between depression and elation. Usually, these problems only last for three to four weeks, but sometimes they can persist for several months. Eventually, however, the symptoms subside.

During this trying period, there are a number of things which can help the reformed smoker to persevere. Alternative medicine techniques, such as acupuncture and hypnosis — *see Alternative Medicine, p305*—have often been used to good effect, while some smokers have found that proprietary medicines that make cigarettes taste foul are helpful. Recently, a chewing gum containing nicotine has proved effective—it can be prescribed by your family doctor, but only on a private prescription. However, this gum still costs less than a packet of cigarettes.

Alcohol

Like nicotine, alcohol is a toxic and addictive drug. But while cigarette smoking is now widely recognized as anti-social, and is on the decline as a result, the consumption of alcohol increases each year. Changing social conventions have made it acceptable for women and young people to drink; many people, in all sections of society, drink far more than is good for their physical and mental health. Even though definitions of alcoholism, an addiction to alcohol, have been modified many times, the number of men in Britain diagnosed as alcoholics doubled between 1966 and 1975, while the number of women trebled. Of the 33 million people who are estimated to drink alcohol in Britain today, over 300,000 are thought to be alcoholics.

In moderation, alcohol is pleasant and relaxing. It may even, according to some researchers, be beneficial—one small glass of whisky taken each day may help to control arteriosclerosis, but the benefits are lost if more is drunk. Alcohol acts on the nervous system and the brain, first as a stimulant, then, as more is drunk, as a depressant. It is a poison, and excessive consumption causes stupor, unconsciousness, coma and death. Often, people who have drunk enough to become unconscious die through inhalation of their own vomit.

Inside the body, alcohol is detoxified, or broken down into harmless compounds by the liver. In the process, liver cells are destroyed. Normally, the liver replaces these cells quickly, but if an excessive amount of alcohol is drunk every day, the liver is unable to repair the damage. The result is a progressive, and finally fatal, condition called cirrhosis of the liver.

The amount of alcohol the liver can tolerate naturally varies from person to person, but you probably suffer from some degree of cirrhosis if you have drunk around four and a half pints of beer, or one bottle of wine, on most days for between five and 15 years. For women, these quantities are much smaller. Unless cirrhosis is advanced, men normally recover full liver function if they stop drinking; women, however, only recover liver function in around a

third of cases.

Alcohol has many other effects on the body. It can cause a fatal disease of the pancreas called pancreatitis, which may occur suddenly, or develop gradually. Through its action on the nervous system, alcohol may cause neuropathy, a progressive and debilitating disease of the nerves. It may also cause cardiomyopathy, or damage to the muscles of the heart, leading to heart failure. Alcohol also increases the risk of peptic ulcers and cancers of the digestive tract.

Despite considerable publicity and stiff penalties, drunken drivers are still responsible for a horrific number of deaths on the roads. Incapacity caused by the drug is also a frequent cause of accidents in the home.

Heavy drinking may also lead to vitamin deficiencies, especially of folic acid and Vitamin B, and so cause anaemia, though it is not known for certain whether this is caused by the action of alcohol, or by the nutritional deficiencies that are common among heavy drinkers. Similarly, the excessive use of alcohol lowers resistance to conditions such as tuberculosis, though it is not known whether this is an effect of the alcohol itself, or of the squalid conditions in which many alcoholics live.

Alcohol also has an effect on the mind and personality. This is fully described in an earlier section—*See The A-Z of Medicine*. It may cause difficulties in personal relationships; the loss of friends; poor performance at work, and possibly job loss; neglect of children; financial problems; and violence within marriage, separation and divorce. Tragically, alcoholics are often unaware of their own deterioration, and become angry and resentful if the possibility that they are suffering from the disease is even suggested to them. Turn to the instant checklist—if you think that you may be an alcoholic, or that a friend or relative is addicted to alcohol, you must seek help, or persuade the victim to do so.

Where to get help

First, you should contact your family doctor, health visitor, or a social worker. He or she is trained to assess the extent of the problem and will be able to advise the best course of action for you to take. In addition, there are many organizations specializing in this problem, which offer the victim both understanding and practical help. Probably the best known of these is Alcoholics Anonymous.

Around 100 years ago, the only drugs in daily use were alcohol and nicotine. The great strides made by medicine and science since then have made a whole range of new drugs available. Many of these are extremely dangerous, and illegal; others are frequently prescribed by doctors—in some cases too frequently—and are equally dangerous when misused.

The abuse of any drug can be dangerous. It may cause physical damage, which may be fatal if the drug is taken regularly or in large dosages; it may be physically addictive—the body comes to be dependent on a constant supply of the drug; it may be psychologically addictive—the mind and personality come to depend on the drug. The body develops a tolerance to some drugs, and in order to feed the addiction, larger and larger doses may be necessary, increasing the danger of irreversible damage.

The image of a drug-taker as disreputable, unconventional and young is totally obsolete. It is thought that millions of people in Britain, in particular women, are addicted to one of three types of drug that are prescribed by doctors —amphetamines, barbiturates and tranquillizers. Many of these people do not realize that they are addicted until it is too late, and never think of themselves as drug addicts. All these drugs are also abused by so-called 'recreational users'—people who take drugs purely for pleasure.

'Recreational' drugs

Amphetamines, barbiturates and tranquillizers are drugs used primarily for a medical purpose, though they are sometimes purchased illegally and taken for amusement. A number of other drugs are also purchased and used in this way for 'recreational' purposes. Many false claims are made for the harmlessness of these drugs. In fact, their effects are not fully known, and will not be established without years of experiment—after all, it took several hundred years for the dangers of smoking to be realized. It is clear, however, that many recreational drugs are highly addictive, cause untold misery and deprivation, and are eventually fatal.

Drug takers are often secretive, resourceful and sly. As a result, it is often extremely difficult to know if a friend or relative is abusing drugs. There are, however, some clues.

Look for changes in the person's personality, routine and health.

DRUGS AND DRUG ABUSE

There are specific physical symptoms of drug abuse *(right)*, as well as changes in behaviour which indicate the existence of the problem. Common drugs which can be abused or addictive are outlined *(below)*. As well as looking for the physical signs, ask yourself such questions whether the person is losing weight, dreamy or disinterested in the world at large? Does he or she speak incoherently or show a lack of concern for his or her appearance? Is he or she unusually moody, elated or lethargic? Look also for tell-tale signs of heroin addiction, such as syringes, teaspoons with burn marks, small envelopes and needle-marks on the arms or legs. If you feel that someone close to you is abusing drugs, try to persuade them to seek help. Consult your family doctor as well, for a GP is bound by an oath of confidentially and will know where to find specialist advice.

The eyes may be sore or red; the pupils may be dilated or constricted.

Breathing may be fitful or irregular.

The hands may be shaky or trembling.

The nose may be irritated or runny. The person may constantly sniff or rub and scratch the nostrils.

The person may feel nauseous.

Needle-marks like punctures in the veins of the arm.

Medical drugs

Amphetamines. Also called 'speed', or 'uppers'. amphetamines speed up the metabolism, increase energy and lift depression. They may be prescribed by doctors in the treatment of narcolepsy and, at one time, were given in the form of 'diet pills'. The use of amphetamines to lose weight is, in the long-term, ineffective and is now strongly condemned by many doctors. Amphetamines are psychologically addictive, and their use over a long period can lead to disastrous psychological problems.

Barbiturates. Also called 'downers', or 'sleepers', barbiturates were once the most widely prescribed from of 'sleeping pill'. They are psychologically addictive and can be fatal if an overdose is taken; nowadays, most doctors prescribe benzodiazepine drugs, such as Valium, instead. These are less dangerous in large doses. A form of barbiturate called phenobarbitone is still used in the treatment of epilepsy, however, while barbiturates are given by injection in some forms of anaesthesia.

Tranquillizers. Tranquillizers are prescribed by doctors to relieve anxiety, restlessness and agitation. They are commonly given in the treatment of depression and in other mental disorders. Though, unlike barbiturates, they are rarely fatal in large doses, tranquillizers have been proved to be physically and psychologically addictive in recent years. Withdrawal symptoms, for instance, have been observed in patients who have ceased to take tranquillizers but the drugs, particularly Valium and Librium, are still very widely prescribed.

Recreational drugs

Cocaine. A white, crystalline powder that is produced from cocoa leaves and usually sniffed. In recent years, cocaine has become a 'fashionable' drug: it causes an intense feeling of exhilaration and energy, and increases concentration. Cocaine can be fatal in large doses, and frequent use can lead to a psychological addiction. It causes serious damage to the membranes and central partition of the nose, which may rot away in a heavy user, and leads to circulatory problems. The possession of cocaine is against the law.

Glue and Dry-Cleaning Fluid. The abuse of these substances has become a considerable problem in recent years. They are inhaled to give a feeling of exhilaration and intoxication—the result, however, is not predictable, and some users experience mental confusion and hallucinations. The act of glue-sniffing is dangerous, and sometimes causes suffocation; the practice can be psychologically addictive, and can cause serious, and sometimes fatal, damage to the heart, brain and liver.

LSD (Lysergic Acid Diethylamide) Also called 'acid', LSD can be taken either in liquid or tablet form. It causes extraordinary hallucinations, called 'trips', which can be horrific. The drug is not physically addictive, but can cause distorted perceptions that lead to dangerous behaviour—the conviction that one can fly, for example. The long-term effects of LSD are strongly debated, but the drug sometimes has a serious effect on the stability of the mind—in fact LSD is occasionally used in the treatment of severe mental disorders. Unauthorized possession of LSD is a criminal offence.

Cannabis. Also called 'marijuana', 'dope', 'grass' or 'hash', cannabis is made from the Indian Hemp plant, and either smoked or eaten to produce mild intoxication and lethargy. There is considerable debate about the addictive properties of cannabis, and its long-term effects on the body and mind. Some researchers, however, have reported that the drug is considerably more likely to cause cancer than the tobacco with which it is often smoked. Even though the possession of cannibis is illegal, it is estimated that millions of people use the drug regularly.

Heroin. A derivative of opium in powdered form that is either inhaled or injected into the body. Heroin causes a feeling of intense intoxication and elation, which changes to drowsiness and nausea. It is extremely addictive, both physically and psychologically, and is especially dangerous because the addict develops a tolerance to the drug. More and more heroin is needed to feed the user's craving, until a fatal dosage level is reached. Giving up the drug is a difficult and extremely unpleasant experience for an addict. The possession of heroin is an offence in Britain and America, but in Britain heroin addiction is treated as a medical, rather than criminal, problem.

The problem of stress

Stress is a problem that is becoming increasingly common, given the strains of life in the highly technological society of today. Though it is not something that can be counted, weighed or measured, the condition is known to be the result of excessive demands on physical or mental energy. It can cause fatigue, unhappiness, emotional problems, and, in the long-term, illness.

How stress develops
Everyone has a different level of tolerance to demands on their mental energy. As a result, it is difficult to forecast when stress will occur, what sort of people it will affect and to what degree. Some people can cope with high levels of mental pressure and with extreme physical demands; others quickly become aware that they have reached their limits of tolerance. When this happens, they often show signs of emotional disturbance and a lack of energy, both of which may indicate a vulnerable state of health. Most people find that constant efforts to solve a problem or to ward one off cause stress, which may lead to illness.

Each individual reacts in a different way to any situation that may cause stress. Some people, for example, may find the prospect of a party delightful, while for others it may be a worrying thought and so the cause of considerable stress. People also have moods—a person who normally feels capable may, at other times, feel emotionally vulnerable and unable to cope with a difficult situation. Such changes in mood are the result of a complex interaction between social contentment and physical well being. They may expose an individual to stress, and so to illness.

How stress leads to disease is not completely understood. What is known, however, is that the hormone adrenaline is manufactured during times of stress, and that its continual presence may lead to an increase in blood pressure, or hypertension. Stress also reduces the body's general resistance to infection. Again, however, it is impossible to be specific. Just as different situations cause stress in different people, so individuals react to the problem in varying ways. There are a number of 'stress illnesses', but it is not known why, for instance, stress may cause headaches in one person, but depression or indigestion in another. It is possible that a predisposition, or an inherited trait, influences the type of illness caused by stress in an individual.

Symptoms and signs of stress
The reasons why it is important to recognize signs of stress are clear cut and obvious. If allowed to increase unchecked, they can lead to disease. As such symptoms vary from person to person, it is sensible to make a note of the warning signs that are specific to you.

In the case of serious worry, or if something happens to make you tense or upset, one of the obvious signs of stress is often a disturbance in normal eating and sleeping habits. Lack of sleep causes fatigue and a consequent inability to make decisions, while inadequate nourishment results in both a lack of energy and indigestion. Both problems adversely affect the general state of health, and lower resistance to disease.

Some common indications of stress, such as aches in the muscles and feelings of extreme tiredness, are also early symptoms of influenza, or other viral infections. Scientists have different views about the cause of these symptoms. Some think that such aches and pains may, in fact, be caused by stress, and not by the virus. They believe that stress reduces the resistance to disease so that the virus can take hold. Perhaps the most common consequences of stress are anxiety and depression.

Anxiety can make a person agitated, vacillating and confused; the problem is associated with feelings of mental tension and with headaches. Depression, in contrast, may cause a person to become withdrawn and inactive. It is associated with fits of crying, early-morning wakening and loss of weight. These problems are recognizable medical conditions, and very different from normal, shortlived, changes of mood.

Once you have taken stock of your individual symptoms and signs of stress, it is important to identify the problems that are causing them.

Write down all the major worries that you have, and any minor causes of irritation as well, and think of the practical steps you could take to overcome them. Sometimes, the major stresses cause the minor stresses and irritations, but often it is an accumulation of minor stresses that contribute to eventual disease.

Stress and illness
Stress is rarely the single cause of an illness. More frequently, it tends to emphasise existing bodily weaknesses. A minor problem may hardly be noticed in normal circumstances, but during times of stress it may grow worse, as part of a general deterioration of health. This is often the case in PMT, or premenstrual tension, and in dysmenorrhoea, or painful menstruation.

If stress is extreme or prolonged, it can lead to exhaustion, a state in which physical and psychological deterioration leads to illness. Such illnesses can take the form of an imbalance of hormones, the chemical controllers of the body and particularly to an increase in the level of adrenaline. The result of this is high blood pressure. They can also be apparent in a loss of weight through an excessive expenditure of energy, and in mental disorders.

Certain conditions are known to have definite links with stress, and are called 'stress-related diseases'. Hypertension, an increase in blood pressure which may lead to heart disease, is among these. Perhaps the most obvious stress-related diseases, however, are mental and emotional disturbances. Extreme stress may cause such serious anxiety, tension, aggression, depression or even a phobia, a concentrated and focused form of anxiety, that psychiatric help is necessary.

Not all psychiatric problems, however, are caused by stress. Some forms of depression, and psychoses, in which an individual loses touch with reality, have internal causes, and are not reactions to stress. Even so, these often become worse at times of stress.

Such extremes of normal emotions are regarded as medical conditions, reactions to stress that can be treated and cured. Your family doctor will be able to give

RELAXING NATURALLY

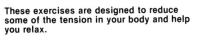

These exercises are designed to reduce some of the tension in your body and help you relax.

1 Reach up and out with your arms and have a good stretch and a yawn if you feel like it. Stretch out and contract the muscles in one leg and then the other.

2 Raise your arms in front of you to the level of your shoulders and then let them drop loosely so that they 'swish' past your hips. Bring your arms back to the starting position and repeat the exercise several times.

3 Stand upright with your arms almost touching above your head and your feet turned outwards. Let your arms drop loosely so that they cross in front of you. Raise up your arms sideways and repeat the exercise. Remember to relax your arms and try to establish a rhythm that captures a sensation of flight.

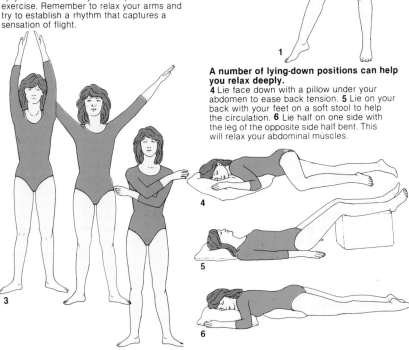

A number of lying-down positions can help you relax deeply.
4 Lie face down with a pillow under your abdomen to ease back tension. **5** Lie on your back with your feet on a soft stool to help the circulation. **6** Lie half on one side with the leg of the opposite side half bent. This will relax your abdominal muscles.

STRESS AND ULCERS

Contrary to popular belief, stress, worry and anxiety do not mean that you will inevitably develop ulcers. These are, however, what doctors term contributory factors. So, too, are excessive smoking, drinking and irregular, rushed meals. What seems likely is that many people are predisposed to ulcers. If you are related to someone with an ulcer, or if your blood group is O, you are three times more likely to develop one yourself. It is also thought by some doctors that factors such as stress can trigger the ulcer to which that person is already predisposed.

Stomach and duodenal ulcers are commoner among certain professions than among others. People particularly at risk include journalists and business executives. Statistics show that 15 per cent of males will suffer from an ulcer before the age of 40; the age group most at risk is between 45 and 55. Women are four times less likely than men to have a duodenal ulcer, but are just as likely to suffer from stomach ulcers.

advice and treatment in the first instance. If additional help is needed to give further counselling or specific treatments, the family doctor may refer you to a specialist.

How to cope
The best way to relieve stress is to deal with the problems and worries which are responsible for the condition. Unfortunately, stress seems to inhibit the skills of decisiveness and clear thinking that are needed for this. The answer is to seek help and support from a friend, a relative, or from your family doctor. You will be able to talk through your problems—in itself, this often clarifies the problems and reduces the stress as a result.

Nowadays, many family doctors see this type of support as an essential part of medicine. It is unlikely that your problems are unique, so the doctor may well be able to suggest a solution to them, or

give you sound practical advice.
Sometimes problems, especially those involving personal relationships or financial worries, cannot be solved easily. Even if you cannot solve a problem without difficulty, you can take steps to reduce the stress that it causes, and so limit its harmful effects on the mind and body. One way to achieve this is to practise specific relaxation techniques.

Stress can also be reduced by the enjoyment that comes from following a hobby or pastime. The choice of activity is governed by personal taste—as long as it does not overtax a person physically or emotionally. Some people find relaxation and mental diversion in music, chess or a good book; others prefer a holiday, a change of scenery or a pleasant walk. Even demanding sports can help to release tension.

Sometimes, however, people find a relief from stress in drugs, such as

the nicotine in tobacco or alcohol. These are undeniably relaxing, but expose the body and mind to considerable dangers—*see Abuses of the Body, p328*. Eventually, cigarettes or alcohol may become a harmful addiction.

Doctors often prescribe tranquillizers, such as Valium, to reduce stress. In the short term, these drugs often perform their function well—if the full course is taken—giving a temporary relief from stress during which problems can be solved. In the long term, however, they do not cure stress, but only disguise it. People taking such drugs run the risk of becoming psychologically and physically dependent upon them. If possible, it is far better to reduce stress by the use of relaxation techniques, and to avoid it by making a determined effort, with the help of doctors and friends, to solve the problems that are causing it.

Health and hygiene

Personal cleanliness and hygiene are not merely conventional social graces—they are a vital part of preventive medicine. How clean we keep ourselves and our surroundings, and the steps we take to ensure that what we eat and drink is as fresh and pure as possible, provide some of the keys to good health.

How infections are spread

Infections are caused when the body is invaded by microscopic alien particles commonly called 'germs', viruses or bacteria. Most of them are spread by people who are suffering from a particular ailment or by 'carriers'—that is, those who carry the germs in their bodies, but do not show any symptoms of infection. Depending on the type of germ, a person may be infectious for some weeks before symptoms develop, and for some days after they have disappeared.

Germs may be spread from person to person in several different ways. Infections of the respiratory tract, such as colds and influenza, are characteristically transmitted by droplet infection, or airborne spread. When someone sneezes or coughs, a fine spray of saliva and germ-carrying secretions is released to be carried in the air. The droplets in this spray may be inhaled by others, who thus pick up the germs of the disease.

The greatest risks of this occurring are in overcrowded and poorly ventilated places, but you can take steps to lessen them, both for yourself and for others. If you are suffering from a respiratory infection, cover both your mouth and nose with a clean handkerchief before coughing or sneezing, and try to keep your distance from other people; if you do not have an infection, make sure that rooms are well aired and that you avoid those who have a cold or sniffle.

Some diseases are transmitted by direct physical contact of one body with another—smallpox can be passed by the touch of skin on skin; serum hepatitis by the contact of body fluids, such as blood, saliva, semen or mucus secretions. This form of transmission is especially common in the venereal, or sexually transmitted diseases, such as syphilis, gonorrhoea and herpes genitalis— *see 'Sex and Contraception', p338.*

Depending on the life-span of disease organisms outside the human body, infection may also be carried by objects that have been contaminated by a sufferer, such as an unsterile thermometer, or crockery. Contrary to popular belief, however, syphilis and gonorrhoea cannot be caught from towels or lavatory seats—the organisms that cause them can only live outside the human body for about 20 seconds. The virus that causes herpes genitalis, however, is now thought to have the ability to survive away from the human body for up to 72 hours. This condition, which can even be transmitted through the print of a hand on a wash-basin, is now a serious health problem in America.

Germs are excreted in the faeces of both sufferers and carriers in the case of many diseases—salmonella and infective hepatitis among them. These germs may infect another pers n by the oral-faecal route. As a result of inadequate hygiene, germs in the faeces are transferred to the hands, or to flies, and so contaminate food, toys and crockery; they are passed to the eventual sufferer when anything so contaminated is placed in the mouth. Drinking water may also become contaminated by faeces—

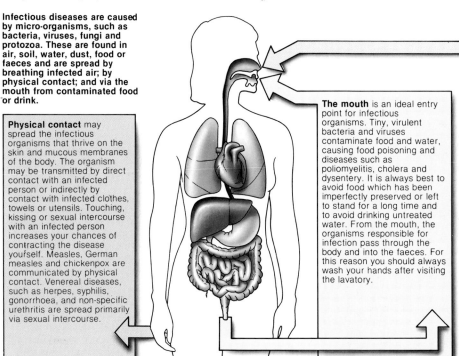

Infectious diseases are caused by micro-organisms, such as bacteria, viruses, fungi and protozoa. These are found in air, soil, water, dust, food or faeces and are spread by breathing infected air; by physical contact; and via the mouth from contaminated food or drink.

Physical contact may spread the infectious organisms that thrive on the skin and mucous membranes of the body. The organism may be transmitted by direct contact with an infected person or indirectly by contact with infected clothes, towels or utensils. Touching, kissing or sexual intercourse with an infected person increases your chances of contracting the disease yourself. Measles, German measles and chickenpox are communicated by physical contact. Venereal diseases, such as herpes, syphilis, gonorrhoea, and non-specific urethritis are spread primarily via sexual intercourse.

The mouth is an ideal entry point for infectious organisms. Tiny, virulent bacteria and viruses contaminate food and water, causing food poisoning and diseases such as poliomyelitis, cholera and dysentery. It is always best to avoid food which has been imperfectly preserved or left to stand for a long time and to avoid drinking untreated water. From the mouth, the organisms responsible for infection pass through the body and into the faeces. For this reason you should always wash your hands after visiting the lavatory.

The air is the primary medium for spreading some diseases of the respiratory tract, such as colds, influenza, tuberculosis and diphtheria. The old rhyme 'coughs and sneezes spread diseases' is true, because the offending viruses or bacteria are rapidly expelled from the body in tiny droplets. A cough, for instance, expels the air at speeds up to 300m/sec (990ft/sec), spraying the droplets over people, clothes, surfaces or food. Many types of organisms will die as soon as the droplets dry out, but some remain virulent for a long time. Sneezes shower droplets over a three- to four-metre area. Apart from spreading the germs that cause respiratory diseases, they can release Staphylococcus aurens into the air. This bacterium, which is found in the pus of boils and septic wounds, forms colonies in the noses of a third of the population. When these people sneeze, the bacterium fills the air and infects any wound in the vicinity.

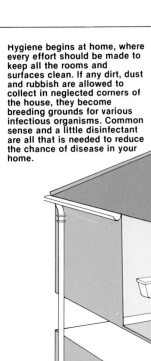

Hygiene begins at home, where every effort should be made to keep all the rooms and surfaces clean. If any dirt, dust and rubbish are allowed to collect in neglected corners of the house, they become breeding grounds for various infectious organisms. Common sense and a little disinfectant are all that is needed to reduce the chance of disease in your home.

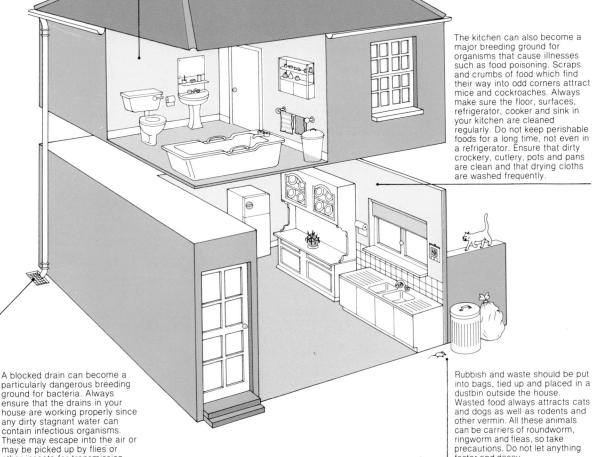

The bathroom and lavatory can become major sources of infection if they are not kept clean. Any infectious organisms, excreted in the faeces or shed from the skin and mucous membranes while washing, will readily multiply if given half a chance. It is important to wash regularly; to have clean towels; to scrub the bath, basin and lavatory with disinfectant on a weekly basis; to put your dirty clothes in a linen basket; to wash your hands after using the lavatory; the clean the floor, skirting boards and door handles regularly; to empty kitchen rubbish every day.

The kitchen can also become a major breeding ground for organisms that cause illnesses such as food poisoning. Scraps and crumbs of food which find their way into odd corners attract mice and cockroaches. Always make sure the floor, surfaces, refrigerator, cooker and sink in your kitchen are cleaned regularly. Do not keep perishable foods for a long time, not even in a refrigerator. Ensure that dirty crockery, cutlery, pots and pans are clean and that drying cloths are washed frequently.

A blocked drain can become a particularly dangerous breeding ground for bacteria. Always ensure that the drains in your house are working properly since any dirty stagnant water can contain infectious organisms. These may escape into the air or may be picked up by flies or other insects for transmission.

Rubbish and waste should be put into bags, tied up and placed in a dustbin outside the house. Wasted food always attracts cats and dogs as well as rodents and other vermin. All these animals can be carriers of roundworm, ringworm and fleas, so take precautions. Do not let anything fester and decay.

this is the main cause of epidemics of cholera—though the problem is sometimes the result of poor sanitation rather than inadequate hygiene.

There are therefore three main routes for the spread of infection—droplet infection, physical contact and the oral-faecal route. It is not realistic to expect to eliminate the possibility of contracting an infectious disease, but the chances can be dramatically reduced by the application of common sense and the simple rules of hygiene. Common sense dictates that you should keep away from sources of droplet infection, and avoid physical contact with those suffering from disease, but the rules of hygiene in the home, and personal hygiene, are the best weapon against infection by the oral-faecal route.

Food hygiene
When shopping, you should always select fresh goods, especially in the case of fish or meat. Check the 'sell by' date on any packages, and avoid any shop in which food is left uncovered, working surfaces are dirty or animals and flies are tolerated.

You should be scrupulous in the preparation of food. Cuts or abrasions on the hands should be covered with waterproof dressings, fingernails clean and trimmed, long hair tied back and aprons clean. All these may be sources of contamination. Before cooking, it is advisable to wash and examine all food carefully—especially fresh fruit—handling it as little as possible. Other members of the family should also be discouraged from handling food, unless you are sure that they are scrupulously clean too. Make sure that surfaces in the kitchen are clean, and soak dishclothes and mops in disinfectant once a week.

Food should never be stored for too long, even in a refrigerator. Bacon, for example, should not be kept for more than seven days; check the 'eat by' date if it is given on the package. Dishes cooked at home should not be left in the refrigerator for longer than two days, and if reused, should be thoroughly reheated. Generally, however, you should not reheat any

DENTAL HYGIENE

Recent statistics show that an alarming number of adults have lost all their teeth. This reflects the fact that standards of dental hygiene are very low even though this has developed into a science of its own over the last 20 years.

Tooth decay is caused by the continuous deposition of plaque — a sticky and colourless film of saliva, bacteria and food debris — on the teeth. Everyone suffers from this, as a simple test shows. if you buy some 'disclosing' tablets from a chemist and use one before cleaning your teeth, you will see a dramatic pink film on them. However, by paying attention to dental hygiene (far right), you will prevent the formation of much of this plaque, and help to avoid any damage the plaque might cause if left to its own devices. Proper hygiene will also prevent bad breath and, if you are a smoker, will help to keep your teeth free from the yellow stains of nicotine.

The process of tooth decay starts when sugar comes into contact with the bacteria in the plaque. An acid is formed, which dissolves the enamel on teeth so exposing their structure to decay. An excess of plaque will also spread to the gums, causing inflammation and damage to their tissues. Occasionally, only the gums themselves are affected. This causes gingivitis, in which the gums becomes red and swollen, and bleed when they are brushed. When plaque is very severe, it affects both the jawbone around the teeth and the tissues deep within them. The result is peridontal disease, in which the gums recede and the teeth become loose, sometimes even falling out.

The acid formed by the bacteria and the sugar will attack your teeth for up to an hour after eating something sweet. However, if you end your meals with cheese, this will neutralize the acid. Fruit and raw vegetables such as celery are less effective, but they do massage the gums and help to keep your teeth clean.

Dental hygiene poses special problems for children and pregnant women. A baby's milk teeth should be cleaned twice a day from the moment they first appear. At first, use a piece of gauze dipped in toothpaste and then progress to a brush as the child grows older. A child's diet, like an adult's, should contain as little sugar as possible in order to reduce the chance of tooth decay as well as for dietary reasons. Take your child to the dentist as soon as he or she can walk. If you are confident and treat the visit as a matter of routine, the child is more likely to feel reassured. Children should have a check-up every four months (right).

Pregnant women often suffer from gum problems or tooth decay. They should be particularly careful about dental hygiene, visiting the dentist frequently for a check-up.

Dentures or false teeth are often a trap for bacteria and particles of food. They should be removed every night, cleaned and kept moist. A number of proprietary preparations can be used to clean dentures. Many of them will also remove unsightly stains. In addition, be careful when biting and chewing your food, since this puts pressure on the ridges of the gums. The result may be inflammation of the gums which may lead to a mouth ulcer. Dentures should be checked regularly by a dentist, who should be consulted immediately if they cause any discomfort.

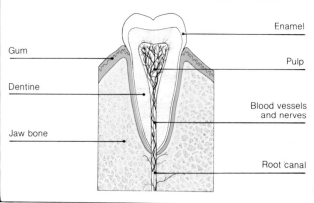

Gum

Dentine

Jaw bone

Enamel

Pulp

Blood vessels and nerves

Root canal

Milk teeth appear at around six months, are fully formed by the age of six and are replaced by 32 adult teeth in adolescence (right). Each jaw has four incisors, **1**, for cutting, two canines, **2**, for tearing, four premolars, **3**, and six molars, **4**, for grinding. The wisdom teeth are the two back molars on each jaw and appear after adolescence. Each tooth (left) is rooted to the jaw. This soft root, supplied by blood and nerves, is protected by a hard but sensitive layer of bone called dentine. The tooth above the gum is covered in enamel, the hardest substance in the body.

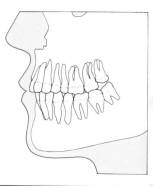

meat or meat products, nor should you keep meat for more than a few hours at room temperature. Canned foods should be eaten as soon as they are opened, or stored for no longer than two days in a refrigerator, while frozen poultry should be completely defrosted before cooking. If you have a freezer, check the manufacturer's recommendations to see how long food can be left frozen—it varies between three and six months—but, in any event, never refreeze any food once it has been defrosted.

Ignoring such simple precautions may lead to stomach upsets, and, in some cases, to food poisoning.

Hygiene in the home
The cleanliness of the food you buy is a day-to-day concern, but the importance of pure drinking-water is often forgotten. It is vital that the water supply to your home is safe and free from contamination. If you suspect that there is any problem with the water supply, call a plumber. If there is a fault in the main drainage or the sewage system, you should also inform the public health department of your local authority. Many older houses contain lead piping. If this is the case with your house, you may be risking lead poisoning. The only course is to replace the original lead pipes with new ones. A grant to help with this work may be available from the local authority.

However, the particles that cause disease are not just carried by contaminated food and water. They are nearly always found wherever there is dirt. In order to reduce the chances of contracting a disease, you should keep your home as clean as possible. Wrap up all rubbish well, and make sure that your dustbin or refuse sack is tightly sealed and regularly emptied or removed. Keep all crockery and kitchen utensils clean, and throw away any that are cracked—food particles can become trapped in the cracks, and attract germs. Defrost and clean the refrigerator regularly.

Particular attention should be paid to the bathroom and lavatory—the easiest places for contamination by faeces to occur. It is essential to clean the lavatory, wash-basin, taps and bath, or shower, at least once a week with a powerful domestic disinfectant. If a member of the family has a stomach upset or diarrhoea, this should be done once a day. Make sure that each person has his own flannel and towel, and that they are washed regularly.

Pests and parasites
Some old houses, and, on occasions, modern blocks of flats, can easily become infested with pests, such as mice or cockroaches. If you find evidence of pests in your own home, contact the public health department of your local authority immediately. Pests can carry disease. It is not only mice and cockroaches that may be sources of infection, however. Your own family pets can transmit diseases, such as ringworm, a fungal infection of the skin, and roundworm, a parasite that lives in the intestines. If your pet has fleas, they may sometimes affect you as well. You should ensure that family pets are kept

Cleaning your teeth When you clean your teeth, use a flat-headed brush which has bristles that are neither too hard nor too soft. Your dentist will advise you on this. If you use your toothbrush properly, you will almost certainly have to replace it every few months; after this, it will be too worn and dirty to be of use. Brush down on your upper teeth and brush up on your lower ones, **1**, from the gums to the edges of the teeth. Brush the backs of both your upper and lower set of teeth, **2**, and then clean the surfaces with a scrubbing action, **3**. It usually takes around three minutes to remove all the plaque. Until you have become accustomed to this routine, check that the plaque has been removed by using a 'disclosing' tablet.

Dental floss is also very useful for removing debris from underneath the gums. The floss is a thin, strong thread which you can buy either waxed or unwaxed from a chemist. By passing the thread backwards and forwards through the spaces between your teeth, **4**, you can remove food debris and plaque from areas which are hard to reach. It also massages your gums.

Many dentists *(left)* recommend a fluoride toothpaste, because this chemical strengthens the teeth and makes them more resistant to decay. You should, if possible, clean your teeth after every meal; if this is impossible, then you should clean them after breakfast and last thing at night at the very least.

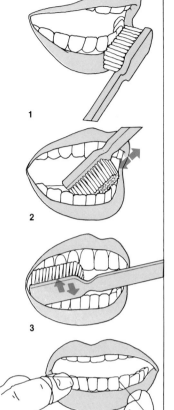

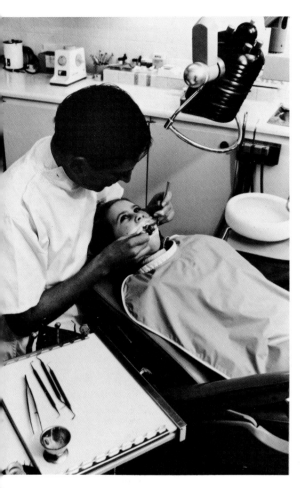

---

clean and healthy, and that children, especially, do not come into contact with animal faeces.

Personal hygiene

Personal cleanliness is not just a social matter. It is vital if you are to ensure, as far as possible, that the environment of your body and clothes you wear, is not one that encourages the breeding of bacteria and parasites.

Waste products are excreted through the skin in the form of sweat, a large part of which is grease and salt. This is an ideal environment for bacteria to breed, and to cause infection. The unpleasant aroma of body odour is caused by the combination of sweat and bacterial activity. Parasites, such as nits or crabs, the various forms of lice , or scabies , tiny mites that burrow beneath the skin, also thrive on dirt—though they may be caught by a clean person after physical contact with someone who is dirty. Simple, old-fashioned, washing is the answer.

How often you need to wash depends on how dirty you become during your day, but most people wash thoroughly, bath, or shower at least once a day. Particular areas of the body need special attention, particularly those that contain sweat glands. The armpits and the groin should be washed frequently, especially in hot weather. The use of a deodorant is no substitute, as few brands stop sweat secretion completely, while perfume disguises, but does not prevent, the presence of bacteria. Men who have not been circumcised should pull back their foreskins and wash the tips of their penises regularly, while both sexes should wash the whole genital area frequently. Adolescents who suffer from acne and greasy skin should pay particular attention to the face and shoulders.

Particular attention should also be paid to the feet, which tend to perspire freely; after washing them, the area between each toe should be dried thoroughly. This helps to prevent infection by tinea pedis, or athlete's foot, a fungal infection that is often contracted through use of communal changing rooms or towels.

Most important of all, however, is that hands should be washed after using the lavatory. Microscopic particles of faeces, and the disease-producing particles that they contain, can easily pass through the thickness of a sheet of lavatory paper to contaminate the hands. If these are not washed, infection can spread through the oral-faecal route, described above, with ease.

Clothes also form a part of the body's environment, and may harbour or encourage the presence of disease-producing organisms. When the skin cannot breathe, sweating and bacterial action is encouraged, so socks and tights should be changed every day. Shoes made of synthetic materials contain no pores to allow the feet to breathe, so, ideally, shoes with leather uppers should be worn. All clothes, and all bed-linen, should be regularly washed or dry-cleaned to kill any bacteria or parasites that may be present, and to destroy the environment on which they thrive.

Sex and contraception

Sex and sexual awareness are both integral parts of life from birth to death. Sexual and emotional awareness starts in babyhood and continues through puberty and adolescence until it becomes a healthy, rewarding and fulfilling part of adult life. This section of the book charts and explains this development. It also covers contraception and the physical and mental problems that can affect sexual feelings and relationships at any stage of life.

Sexuality in the early years
Until about the age of six months, all babies are emotionally selfish. They will normally show love or affection to anyone who provides them with food, warmth and comfort. Now, however, babies become aware of the individual identity of the person who spends the most time with them and actively strive to win that person's affection. This is part of what psychologists term the bonding process, which is believed to influence how stable a child's future relationships will be. Usually, though not always, this takes place between mother and baby.

At about this time, too, infant sexuality first becomes noticeable. For a baby, suckling at the breast is not only a means of obtaining food—it is also pleasurable in itself. The baby may also derive pleasure from sucking its thumb and its toys. This stage of development is called 'mouthing'.

Breast feeding is therefore desirable in emotional terms for both mother and baby. Bottle feeding can be an adequate substitute where breast feeding is impossible. The person feeding the baby should ensure that there is as much involvement and bodily contact during bottle feeding as there would be during breast feeding. This can be reinforced by feeding the baby while naked, so that the baby is aware of the warmth and smell of the person feeding it.

The toddler
As babies grow up they develop physical and social skills through play. At first this play is mainly imitative—toddlers copy the activities of the adult with whom they spend the most time. Young children quickly learn that particular parts of the body produce a pleasant feeling when touched. A boy will discover that rubbing his penis is pleasant. Little girls enjoy massaging their clitoris or fingering their vagina.

All children go through this stage of genital play. Though this may sometimes cause embarrassment to adults, it is quite normal, and it is wrong to scold or punish children for doing it. Such attitudes can only create feelings of shame and guilt, and can have long-lasting effects on children's future sexuality.

The same need for adult patience and understanding applies to toilet training. This is the first bodily function over which the infant gains total control, but the age at which this happens may vary widely. Generally toddlers can stop wearing nappies during the day by the age of about two and a half. It is important for adults not to become over-anxious during this period, especially if a child is slow to respond. Worry can escalate into a conflict between adult and child, in which both will be the losers. Pressure on a child to conform is always counter-productive. Not only will the whole process take far longer; the child may also become burdened by repressed feelings of guilt, which can be emotionally damaging.

Growing up
As toddlers, boys and girls play together, seemingly unaware of the sex difference between them. As they grow older, however, chromosomal and hormonal differences start to affect their behaviour patterns. The physical differences between the sexes become apparent first of all—the presence or lack of a penis is a fact which sometimes worries young girls, for instance. The child's natural response is to ask questions and, rather than avoiding them, this may be the time to explain the facts of life, at least in basic terms. It is important for the adult not to be embarrassed and to be as clear and as straightforward as possible. Failure to tackle the subject means that the child may well become dependent on piecemeal, superficial and inadequate information he or she may pick up from other children television and newspapers This may confuse and frighten the child.

As children grow up, they naturally segregate themselves into single-sex groups and often tend to denigrate the other sex.

Puberty and adolescence
Adolescence is often a difficult stage for both parents and children. For teenagers, it is a time of great mental and physical change and adjustment, when they suddenly find that they are no longer children—yet neither are they adults.

Most of the changes are caused by the adult sex hormones, which the body starts manufacturing at the beginning of adolescence. Girls usually become aware of such changes a year or so earlier than boys, when they start to develop breasts and grow pubic and axillary hair—that is, hair in the armpits. They generally start their first periods around the age of 11 or 12 years, though menstruation may begin as early as eight or as late as 18. A boy grows facial and body hair; his voice breaks and his penis and scrotum grow larger and more conspicuous from the age of 12 or 13 years. He also starts to have involuntary night-time emissions of semen—often called 'wet dreams'. Both sexes may feel emotionally confused by the many changes that are taking place. Adolescence is also a time for gaining independence from parents, and this involves questioning most of the ideas and rules that have been taken for granted in childhood. Teenagers' own relationships are changing as well, as their sexual feelings awaken. Instead of spending the majority of their time with groups of their own sex, they gradually start to form attachments to members of the opposite sex.

Masturbation is common in both sexes. Boys manipulate their penises to achieve erection and ejaculation. Girls masturbate by massaging the clitoris with their fingers to achieve a climax, though, as opposed to boys, this result may be produced involuntarily as well. The clitoris can be stimulated by other means—by the friction produced by tight clothing, for example.

Adolescence is also the time for 'pashes' or 'crushes'—that is, hero worship, often of an older person of the same sex. Such feelings are often intense and passionate although they are rarely completely consummated physically. They should not be confused with homosexuality, but seen as a perfectly normal stage of heterosexual development.

Some teenagers, however, do form homosexual attachments, either as a phase or as a permanent development. This raises two problems, one moral and the other legal. In Britain, for instance, homosexuality is illegal between men under the age of 21. If you find that a daughter or son is having a gay relationship, it is important to examine your own attitudes to homosexuality and to try your best to come to terms with any preconceptions you may have about the issue. Your teenager may feel very apprehensive about your reaction and be terrified of rejection.

The first sexual relationships with the opposite sex are usually innocent and involve relatively little physical contact. As confidence increases, however, the behaviour of each couple becomes more openly sexual as they progress from holding hands and a peck on the cheek to more intimate caresses—so-called 'heavy petting'. This may culminate in sexual intercourse, although such behaviour is modified by the prevailing moral climate and by social or religious customs.

The first experience of sexual intercourse is likely to be memorable for a variety of reasons, both good and bad. Some teenagers expect it to be purely pleasurable and are disappointed; others will remember it as a positive experience. Girls in particular face a particular physical fact; if the hymen, the membrane which covers the entrance to the vagina is intact, the loss of their virginity will cause some bleeding and soreness as the result of its rupture. Foreknowledge of this can help stop making love for the first time from becoming a traumatic experience.

Whenever the possibility of a relationship progressing to full sexual intercourse exists, contraception should be considered. This raises both ethical and practical problems. The legal age of consent—below which sexual intercourse between heterosexuals is a criminal offence—is still 16, and some doctors feel strongly that to prescribe any form of contraception for girls below this age is wrong. Others believe that this view is old-fashioned and short-sighted, since any girl who feels mature enough to have sexual intercourse will probably do so. Modern opinion is that it is more sensible to encourage contraception than deal with an unwanted pregnancy. If getting advice is a problem, it is best to turn to one of the special advisory centres that have been set up to advise teenagers on sex and contraception, such as the Brook Advisory Centres.

The adult

Human sexual behaviour is immensely varied. There is no 'right way' to make love; sexual variations are really only limited by the imagination of the partners and their individual sex drives.

In Western society today, heterosexuality is still the norm, though it is now widely accepted that homosexuality is not a perversion, and that two people of the same sex have as much chance of establishing a loving, satisfying relationship as heterosexuals.

Sexual myths

How the sexual act itself is performed and its frequency may be affected by a number of factors, including the mood, age, physical and mental health of the partners as well as their basic sexual drives.

The frequency of intercourse may vary enormously from once or twice a year at one end of the scale to once or twice a day at the other. In an established relationship, it usually averages once or more a week.

HYGIENE AND SEX

Anyone who is sexually active should be aware of the dangers of contracting a sexually transmitted diseases. These range from well-known diseases, such as syphilis and gonorrhoea, to problems that have been recognized more recently, such as non-specific urethritis (NSU) and herpes genitalis. All the sexually transmitted diseases are described in the A-Z section of this book.

The likelihood of contracting a sexually transmitted disease, or STD, increases with the number of sexual partners. There is also a direct relationship between the incidence of cervical cancer in women and the number of sexual partners they have enjoyed. Though barrier methods of contraception—such as the use of condoms—give some protection against venereal disease, the decline in their use, due to the popularity of the contraceptive pill has been linked to the general increase in the incidence of venereal disease. The only sure way to avoid contracting a sexually transmitted disease is to make love with partners in a relationship which is stable enough to minimize the risk of infection. By the same token, it is vitally important that anyone who has a sexually transmitted disease should avoid all sexual activity until free from infection, and that he or she should co-operate fully with doctors to enable them to trace, and then treat, any partners who may be unwittingly transmitting the disease to others.

A number of other, less serious, conditions can affect the sexual organs. Some of these are transmitted sexually, and some are not, but all can be avoided to a large extent if the simple rules of hygiene are observed by both partners.

Cystitis is a common problem in women, probably because the openings of the urethra, vagina and rectum are so close together. Daily washing of the genital area, together with careful cleansing after defaecation, helps to avoid the possibility of cystitis. It is important to wipe the rectum from front to back so that germs are not spread from it into the urethra.

Cystitis can sometimes be caused by intercourse—the condition known as 'honeymoon cystitis'. It is thought to occur because germs are forced into the lower part of the urethra by the friction of the penis during intercourse. A change in the position used for lovemaking, urination before and after intercourse, and washing the vulva after intercourse all help to prevent the problem.

While it is sensible to wash the vulva and vagina gently with warm water, the old-fashioned practice of douching the inside of the vagina with a stream of water and antiseptic is positively dangerous. It destroys the bacteria normally living in the vagina, which are an essential part of the region's defences against disease.

Even if such precautions are observed, infections may set in on occasions. Any persistent, offensive vaginal discharge should be reported to the doctor, as should any bleeding between the periods, during pregnancy or after the menopause, unless hormone therapy has been prescribed.

Hygiene is just as important for men as for women. Old skin cells and debris tend to accumulate under the foreskin of the penis; this smegma, as it is called, should be removed by pulling back the foreskin and washing underneath it every day.

In all partnerships, a full understanding of the physical mechanics of intercourse and orgasm is important—*see Sex and Reproduction, p54.* However, the sexual act has always been surrounded by a large number of myths and misconceptions, which have led to tensions and misunderstandings in many relationships.

It is a myth, for instance, that there is only one way in which a woman can experience a satisfactory orgasm. This was exploded by the Hite report, in which Shirley Hite, an American researcher, asked 3,000 women (heterosexual, bisexual and homosexual) how they experienced orgasm. About one-third of the sample replied that they climaxed through the sensations produced by the penis in the vagina alone. Many others said that they enjoyed intercourse accompanied by direct clitoral stimulation, while others preferred clitoral stimulation alone. They also indicated that there is no clear-cut difference between a vaginal and a clitoral orgasm, and that where a difference exists, one is in no way superior to the other. The male orgasm, for its part, actually consists of two stages, although it is impossible to have the first—the 'point of no return' when the sperm meets the semen—without it being followed immediately by the second—the urethral contractions that force the sperm and seminal fluid out of the penis.

Modern research shows, too, that the belief that the male sex drive is greater than the female has no foundation.

Parenthood
In some instances, the birth of a baby can make it difficult for couples to sustain their sexual relationship. This may be due to physical problems after the birth, such as those caused by a painful episiotomy and stitches. A woman may feel very tired through coping with the baby's constant needs. For his part, the father may feel excluded from the relationship between mother and child and may even be jealous of the new arrival. Both parents may feel overwhelmed by the idea of their new responsibilities. On top of this, living conditions may be cramped. Discussing problems like these openly can help matters; if the couple can maintain their own relationship with one another as well as the baby, then all three can only benefit.

Growing older
Like adolescence, middle age is a time of uncertainty and change.

Children have usually grown up, left home and are starting families of their own. Retirement often means a drastic change in life style—indeed, many people see it as a threat—while waistlines frequently thicken, hair recedes or turns grey and the skin wrinkles. All these factors can sap confidence and sometimes combine to convince people, wrongly, that they can no longer enjoy sex or make love adequately. Some people respond to these fears by simply putting an end to their sex lives; other respond by trying to make new sexual conquests as a form of reassurance.

Women also have to face the inevitable fact of the menopause. This is when their periods cease and the level of female hormones in their bodies gradually drops. To some, the end of the ability to reproduce means the end of their interest in sex, though, for many, the menopause relieves the worry of accidental pregnancy. To others, the menopause is an excuse to escape from a boring or unsatisfying sexual relationship. In fact, there is no evidence that the sexual drive diminishes after the menopause. Nor is there any physical reason why older people should abandon sex. Men and women who are secure in their relationships and have many years of satisfying and confident sexuality behind them can continue to enjoy making love.

As old age approaches, physical facts may inevitably alter love-making techniques. After the menopause, the vagina and vulva become a little thinner and drier, due to the lowered hormone levels in the body. This condition, called senile vaginitis, can be treated by local application of oestrogen creams and the use of lubricants.

Arthritis of the hips may make it impossible for a woman to open her legs wide enough for penetration. A man suffering from shortness of breath or a heart condition may worry about the physical effort involved if his usual position is on top of his partner. Both these problems can be solved by finding new, more comfortable, less stressful ways of making love and by oral and manual stimulation of the genitals. Two physically and emotionally mature people should be able to satisfy each other, whatever their ages. This applies even if one or both are disabled

Sexual problems
Both men and women often face sexual problems, though it has only recently become acceptable to admit that they exist. Following the lead of William Masters and Virginia

Johnson in the USA, a branch of psychiatry—psychosexual therapy—has been established to deal with many of these problems, and its success rate is high.

Womens' problems
Women face two main sexual problems, which may be linked. The first is vaginismus, in which the muscles at the entrance of the vagina contract to become so tense that penetration is impossible—even manual penetration by a doctor in the course of a physical examination. The vagina is tight and dry, while the woman herself feels tense and anxious. The condition tends to occur in women who have not come to terms with their own sexual desires. They fear sex and the loss of control it entails.

Vaginismus may also occur after years of unsatisfying sex which eventually have the effect of putting the woman off making love altogether. Supportive discussions with a psychosexual therapist can greatly help women with this problem. The first step may be to help the patient to overcome her distaste for the sight and feel of her own genitals and then to teach her to masturbate, perhaps with the help of a vibrator. The aim is to encourage her to learn about her body and its responses in private and in her own time. Later, she can communicate what she has learned to her partner. The process can be slow, but, eventually, full, satisfying intercourse is possible.

The other main female sexual problem is called orgasmic dysfunction. A woman with this problem apparently enjoys sex but is unable to climax, or achieve orgasm. The psychological reasons for this are complex, but often, as with vaginismus, a fear of losing control is involved. Women with this problem often do not understand the physiological aspects of the so-called orgasmic cycle, and therefore do not ask their partners for the extra stimulation that may be necessary. Instead, they remain on the 'plateau phase' preceeding orgasm. Sometimes, too, ignorance on the part of both partners can be a factor; the woman may not realize that she needs help from her partner, or she may lack understanding of her problems. Eventually she may become so frustrated that she loses interest in sex altogether.

Psychosexual therapy for orgasmic dysfunction is aimed at helping both the woman and her partner to overcome any barriers which have built up between them because of frustration and

THE RHYTHM METHOD: MONITORING TEMPERATURE

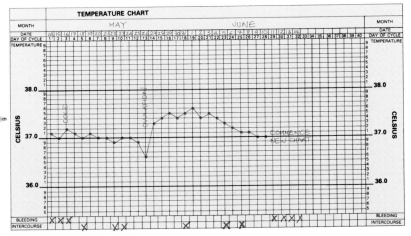

Monitoring the body temperature orally, or via the rectum or vagina, is one way of establishing a safe period. On ovulation, the temperature rises and remains higher than normal until the next menstrual cycle begins. Before using this contraceptive method, the temperature changes should be carefully monitored for a minimum of six months.

resentment. They are taught to give pleasure to each other—first by kissing and caressing, but stopping short of intercourse. By removing intercourse as a goal to be achieved at all costs, the couple learn to please each other without worrying about the sexual act itself. By taking the pressure out of sex, they are both able to relax and enjoy it more. As therapy progresses, their understanding of each other's physical and emotional needs increases, and eventually full sexual intercourse can be resumed.

Men's problems
Men have two main sexual problems—impotence and premature ejaculation. Most men occasionally experience impotence, the inability to have successful intercourse. There are various reasons for this. Excessive drinking, for instance, often makes it impossible to sustain an erection, while certain drugs, illnesses, pressure at work or fear of failure may also cause impotence. If this problem happens repeatedly, a vicious circle of worry impairs performance still further.

Psycho-sexual therapy has a very high success rate in such cases. The object, again, is first to minimize anxiety and fear of failure, so enabling both partners to regain their confidence in their ability to give and receive pleasure. Intercourse is avoided at first; instead the couple learn to give each other sensual pleasure by caressing their bodies. The next stage is genital caressing by hand or mouth. In this way confidence builds up. Both partners begin to enjoy sex more and can eventually progress to

successful, satisfying intercourse.

In premature ejaculation, the man ejaculates almost immediately on achieving an erection, or on penetration of his partner. A specific technique which can help with this problem is the squeeze technique. When the man feels that he is about to ejaculate, he withdraws his penis and his partner places thumb and forefinger around the penis, just below the glans, or head, and squeezes gently for a few seconds. This can be repeated a number of times until both partners feel satisfied.

Loss of libido
In the majority of cases, sexual problems have a psychological basis. However, loss of sexual drive can have physical causes as well. Women can be affected by the contraceptive pill, pregnancy or menopause, or by plain physical tiredness. There may be a specific gynaecological problem—especially in cases of painful intercourse, called dyspareunia—so a physical examination is always advisable. Men, too, can suffer from physical conditions that lead to sexual problems, and these must be treated before psychosexual therapy begins.

In general, though, reducing pressure to perform sexually, understanding and rest are all that is required, plus psychosexual therapy to help with any underlying sexual problem.

Contraception
Today there are a number of different methods of contraception, or family planning, as it is sometimes termed, and each has its advantages and disadvantages. No

single method is 100 per cent reliable, completely safe and available to both sexes.

The choice of contraceptive method depends on a number of factors, including the age, preference, specific physical problems and religious beliefs of both partners. Many doctors are now well-trained in this field, and can give advice based on their personal knowledge of the patient. Less personal but sometimes more up-to-date information is available from the various specialist family planning clinics.

The five methods of contraception are discussed in order in this section. The term 'failure rate' is used frequently. A failure rate of 10% means that out of every 100 women who use the method for one year, on average ten will become pregnant during that year.

Natural methods
The two natural methods of contraception are coitus interruptus and the rhythm method. The latter is the only contraceptive technique considered acceptable by the Roman Catholic Church—and then only between married couples.

Coitus interruptus, or withdrawal, is based on the idea that, if a man withdraws his penis from the vagina before ejaculation, then no sperm pass into the vagina.

Advantages:
* A natural method,
* Needs no prescription, preparation or equipment
* Has no medical risks.

Disadvantages:
* Not very effective. The method has a failure rate of about 20% to 25%, because it is difficult to judge the exact moment of withdrawal accurately. In any case, some sperm may seep out in the seminal fluid during arousal, before ejaculation
* Withdrawal detracts from the sexual satisfaction of both partners, especially the woman's.

The rhythm method is based on avoiding intercourse during the fertile time in the menstrual cycle. There are three ways in which this can be calculated—through the calendar, by temperature and examination of cervical mucus. All three methods aim to establish the date of ovulation.

Women ovulate, or produce eggs, 14 days before each menstrual period. If they have a regular 28 day cycle—that is, a period starts on day one, and the next period starts on day 29—then the date of ovulation is easy to calculate, as it comes midway between two periods. However, many women have variable menstrual cycles, and must make a calculation based on the length of both the shortest and longest cycles to decide when to avoid intercourse. The length of the cycle should be measured for a minimum of six consecutive months, so that the number of days in both the shortest and longest cycles can be established, before these calculations can be used as a basis for contraception.

Intercourse must be avoided for four days before ovulation as sperm can live for up to three days in the womb—and for four days after ovulation Using these rules, the first and last unsafe days according to each length of cycle have been calculated and listed in the table below.

THE CALENDAR METHOD

Length of cycle	First unsafe day	Ovulate on day	Last Unsafe day
20	2	6	10
21	3	7	11
22	4	8	12
23	5	9	13
24	6	10	14
25	7	11	15
26	8	12	16
27	9	13	17
28	10	14	18
29	11	15	19
30	12	16	20
31	13	17	21
32	14	18	22
33	15	19	23
34	16	20	24

Monitoring is essential to establish the length of longest and shortest period.

If, for example, the shortest cycle is 24 days, then the first unsafe day is day six, which is probably immediately after the period. If the longest cycle is 30 days then the last unsafe day is 20—so the couple must not have sex between days 6 and 20. This is called the calendar method of determining the date of ovulation.

Another method of calculating the time of ovulation is by temperature. A woman's temperature dips slightly before ovulation, rises again by about half a degree Centigrade (3.13°F) within 24 hours of ovulation, and stays elevated until the next period. This is due to the effect of the hormone progesterone.

There are two ways of taking the temperature. It can be either taken by mouth first thing in the morning on getting up, or by inserting a thermometer into the rectum or vagina. Both methods are accurate,

but the second is more so than the first. In the strictest version of this method, intercourse is not allowed from the end of a period until a temperature 0.2°C (0.4°F) higher than the average for the previous week has been recorded for three consecutive days. This may mean that intercourse is only safe between day 18 and day 28. A less strict version of the temperature method allows intercourse during the first few days of a cycle after the end of a period.

The date of ovulation can also be calculated by another technique, known as the Billings method, or the mucus method. This is based on the fact that a woman's cervical mucus changes in quantity and consistency throughout her menstrual cycle. At ovulation, the mucus is copious and stringy, while the opening of the cervical canal is wider than at any other time in the cycle. The Billings method is the most reliable way of calculating the date of ovulation—its failure rate is around 15% as against 47% for the calendar method—but many women find it difficult to learn. No women should attempt to use this technique unless they have received training in it. This may be available from the family doctor, but is also given by Family Planning Clinic and the Catholic Marriage Advice Council.

Many women use two of these three methods of determining the date of ovulation at the same time. This is extremely advisable, since the extra safeguard reduces the failure rate significantly.

Advantages:
* A natural method, approved by the Roman Catholic Church
* No prescription or equipment is necessary
* Has no medical risks.

Disadvantages:
* Fairly difficult to calculate the safe period accurately. The temperature method may be upset by illness, for example, and so be unreliable; the calendar method relies on the average length of cycle worked out over six months; the Billings method is difficult to learn
* Can only be used with confidence by women who have a regular menstrual cycle; one study showed that only 8% of women had perfectly regular cycles
* May mean up to 14 days of sexual abstinence during the cycle, which, together with the period itself, leaves only about ten days available for unprotected intercourse.
* Not very effective. Estimates for the failure rate vary: for the 'strict' temperature method around 7%; for

the less strict version around 19%; for the calendar method between 20% and 47%; Billings method around 15%.

Barrier methods
In all barrier methods, sperm is prevented from reaching the womb, and, therefore, the egg, by a barrier made of rubber. There are two types: the sheath, worn by men, and the diaphragm, or Dutch cap, worn by women.

The sheath is known by a variety of names, including prophylactic, condom, French letter, johnny, and Durex—a trade name that has passed into common usage. It consists of a very thin tube of latex rubber, similar to the finger of a rubber glove, but much finer. This is slipped on to the erect penis before penetration of the vagina. The sheath ends in a teat, which catches the sperm as they are ejaculated and prevents them from reaching the womb. It is important that the sheath is properly put on and kept in place until after the penis is withdrawn, so that no sperm escape. In case this happens, and as an additional precaution, spermicidal pessaries should be inserted high up in the vagina.

Over 150 million sheaths are purchased in Britain each year, and it is estimated that they are used by about 25% of men.

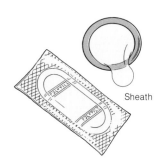

Sheath

Advantages:
* Cheap and easily available. May be bought without a prescription at chemists and other shops, or obtained free of charge at Family Planning Clinics
* The woman is not only protected from unwanted pregnancy, but from the medical risks of other methods
* Some degree of protection against sexually transmitted diseases; also thought by doctors to give some protection against cervical cancer.

Disadvantages:
* May decrease the pleasure felt by the man
* Has to be put on after an erection, but before penetration,

thus interrupting love-making.
* Failure rate of between 10% and 15%

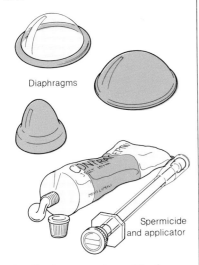

Diaphragms

Spermicide and applicator

The diaphragm and cap. The four types of device defined as diaphragm and cap are the cervical cap and vimule which fit over the cervix; the vault cap, which fits in the vault of the vagina; and the vaginal diaphragm, which fits over the cervix and the vault of the vagina. The most commonly used of these is the vaginal diaphragm. This is a thin sheet of rubber stretched over a circular spring; it is covered with spermicidal jelly and inserted into the vagina not more than two hours before intercourse. If a longer time elapses before intercourse, or if intercourse occurs repeatedly, spermicidal pessaries or more jelly must be placed in the vagina without dislodging the cap. It is left in place for eight hours after intercourse, then removed, washed and dried to be used again.

Various sizes of vaginal diaphragm are available, and it is essential that the correct one is fitted by a doctor, or a specially qualified nurse. A diaphragm is not difficult to insert, but there is a knack to doing this, which can be quickly taught. After the initial fitting, most doctors recommend that the woman practises inserting the diaphragm for a week, while using other methods of contraception, and returns to the surgery for a check-up to see that she is inserting it correctly before relying on the method. They also advise her to check the diaphragm for tears and holes at routine intervals and to have a new one prescribed after a year.

Advantages:
* Quite reliable. When it is used conscientiously, the failure rate is as low as 2%

* Has no serious medical risks.

Disadvantages:
* Has to be fitted by a trained person and refitted after childbirth or after much weight has been gained or lost
* Occasionally women who are prone to urinary tract infections, contract cystitis after using the diaphragm, probably because it presses on the urethra, the tube which passes from the bladder to the outside
* A minority of women are allergic to spermicides.
* Unless the diaphragm is put in place before intercourse is expected, its use can interrupt the spontaneity of love-making.

Hormonal methods
Hormonal methods of contraception work by disrupting the natural balance of female hormones, with the result that an egg is not released at ovulation. There are two hormonal methods—the oral contraceptive pill and the controversial drug Depo-Provera.

The oral contraceptive pill
This consists of a course of tablets containing either one or both of the female hormones oestrogen and progesterone. Two main types of contraceptive pill are available: the combined pill and the progesterone-only pill. Both are among the most reliable of all contraceptives.

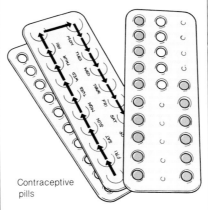

Contraceptive pills

The combined pill is a combination of two synthetic hormones, oestrogen and progesterone, that act together to prevent ovulation by mimicking the way in which ovulation is suppressed during pregnancy. One pill is taken every day for 21 days (or 22, depending on the type of pill), after which there are seven (or six) pill-free days. During this week, withdrawal bleeding occurs, so-called because it is triggered by the withdrawal of the hormones. It is similar to a period. Some manufacturers make packs of 28 pills, of which the extra seven are

in fact sugar covered placebos, containing no hormones. This is to help women who prefer to stick to a routine of taking a pill each day.

Two more types of combined contraceptive pill have recently been introduced. These are the triphasic and biphasic pills. A course of triphasic pills contains three different combinations of oestrogen and progesterone, so that the amount of hormone taken during different times of the menstrual cycle varies as it does in nature. This is thought to make the contraceptive effect even more reliable, and to reduce the incidence of possible harmful side-effects. The biphasic pill works on a similar principle, but there are only two different combinations of hormones in each monthly packet. With both types of pill, it is important to take them in exactly the order indicated on the packet.

If a woman forgets to take a combined pill, and if she is less than 12 hours late in taking it, she should take the pill she has forgotten as soon as she remembers, and continue as normal. This short delay should not leave her unprotected. The next pill should be taken at the normal time. If she is more than 12 hours late protection cannot be guaranteed, since ovulation may have occurred; she should use additional precautions, such as a sheath, or diaphragm and spermicide, for the rest of the cycle. If a woman misses more than one pill she will probably have a withdrawal bleed, similar to that expected at the end of the packet. In this case, she should continue taking the pill as usual, but also take other contraceptive precautions until things return to normal.

Advantages:
* Highly effective if taken correctly—the failure rate is around 0.7%
* Easy to take
* Has a beneficial effect on dysmenorrhoea (period pains) and PMT (pre-menstrual tension)
* Reduces incidence of pelvic infections and benign breast lumps
* Improves menorrhagia (heavy periods), making periods light and reducing risks of anaemia
* Makes timing of periods predictable and controllable
* Does not interfere with the spontaneity of love-making.

Disadvantages:
* Not suitable for women with medical or family histories of high blood pressure, thrombo-embolic disorders such as DVT (deep vein thrombosis) and pulmonary embolism, liver diseases or diabetes

* Increases the risk of thrombo-embolic disorders—circulatory diseases are four times more' common in combined pill users. Not recommended for women over 35 who are heavy smokers
* There may be amenorrhoea, or a lack of periods, for a few months after stopping the pill
* Slightly increases risk of congenital abnormalities in children conceived immediately after stopping the pill. (For this reason, and in order to re-establish a regular menstrual cycle so that the date of conception can be calculated, women are advised to stop taking the pill and rely on other methods for around three months before they wish to become pregnant).
* Requires a prescription and regular checks of blood pressure, weight and urine
* Side-effects are common. These may include nausea, headaches, migraine, cramps in the legs, gingivitis, breast enlargement, weight gain due to fluid retention, a tendency to cystitis, urinary tract infections or loss of libido. Some or all of these may disappear after the first few packets of pills, or after a change to another brand containing slightly different ingredients
* May reduce quantity of breast milk when taken by breast-feeding mothers
* May interact with other drugs. The efficacy of the pill is not usually reduced, except in the case of barbiturates and a drug called Rifampicin, used to treat tuberculosis
* Diarrhoea and vomiting may interfere with the absorption of the pill, and other precautions should be used after an attack.

The progesterone-only pill is also called the mini-pill, and contains no oestrogen. It is taken on every day of the menstrual cycle, exactly at the same time each day. It works by changing the characteristics of the cervical mucus so that sperm find it impossible to penetrate the womb. It is also thought to change the lining of the womb in a way that makes it impossible for a fertilized egg to implant, and, in high dosages, inhibits ovulation.

It is vital that the progesterone-only pill is taken at the same regular time, preferably a few hours before love-making. If the pill is taken more than three hours late, the woman should consider herself unprotected and use additional precautions, such as a diaphragm and spermicide, or her partner should wear a sheath. These precautions must be continued for the next fortnight. However, she should continue to take the remainder of the course of pills to avoid a withdrawal bleed. If two consecutive pills are missed, then the dosage should be doubled for the next two days and additional precautions taken for the same reasons.

Advantages of the progesterone-only pill:
* Highly effective, though not so reliable as the combined pill. Has a failure rate between 2% and 3%
* May be used by women over 35 who smoke, and cannot take the combined pill because of the risk of thrombo-embolic complications
* May be used by diabetics and women with mild hypertension
* Easier to remember than the combined pill because taken at the same time every day, though some women find this a disadvantage.
* Can be taken while breast-feeding as it does not diminish the supply of milk
* No increase in incidence of birth defects in children conceived immediately after stopping the pill
* Does not interfere with the spontaneity of love-making.

Disadvantages of the progesterone-only pill:
* Has to be taken at the same time every day.
* Causes an irregular pattern of bleeding: the frequency of periods may vary.
* Incidence of ectopic pregnancies increases slightly
* There may be side-effects, though these are generally less severe, and less common, than those caused by the combined pill. They include: weight gain, nausea, headache, decreased breast size and decreased libido. Some or all of these may disappear after the first few packets have been taken, or after a change to a brand with slightly different ingredients
* There may be amenorrhoea, or a lack of periods, for a few months after stopping the pill.

Depo-Provera is the trade name for a drug called medroxyprogesterone acetate. Depo-Provera is a long-acting progesterone. It is injected into a muscle, and gradually released into the blood-stream over a period of up to three months. This is a highly effective method of contraception, with a failure rate of less than 0.5%.

Unfortunately, Depo-Provera is a highly controversial drug. It has similar drawbacks to the progesterone-only contraceptive pill, though menstrual irregularities are more frequent and more severe, as well as a number of other disadvantages. Few statistics cover long-term use of the drug, but it appears that, in some cases of frequent use, there may be a permanent loss of periods and permanent infertility. In addition, Depo-Provera is unsuitable for diabetics, and may, in rare cases, cause diabetes.

For these reasons, the drug is only licensed for short-term use in Britain, though it is widely used in a number of other countries, including America.

Depo-Provera has one distinct advantage, however: it is a reliable method of contraception for women who cannot remember to take a pill each day, and who find other methods unsuitable. These are sometimes given to women who have just been immunized against German measles, who must not become pregnant for three months, and to women who are waiting for their partner's sperm count to become negative after a vasectomy.

Controversially, Depo-Provera is also given to psychiatric patients who cannot be relied on to use other methods of contraception. While recognizing that the use of this drug is sometimes the only way of avoiding unwanted pregnancies, many doctors believe that Depo-Provera should be prescribed only if the person who is taking it fully understands and appreciates its risks.

Interception methods
Two methods of contraception prevent a fertilized egg from implanting in the womb: an intra-uterine device and post-coital contraception. These are known as interception methods, because they intercept the fertilized egg. They are both effective, but some people have a moral objection to them, believing that life begins at the moment of conception.

An Intra Uterine Device (IUD) is a small plastic shape that is placed in the uterus. The presence of any foreign object in the uterus is thought to prevent implantation of the fertilized egg. There is a variety of designs, some containing copper, which has an additional spermicidal action, and others containing progesterone. While the main effect of an IUD is to intercept a fertilized egg, the use of spermicide or progesterone in a device enhances its contraceptive effect, and may in itself help to prevent fertilization.

The IUD is inserted into the womb under sterile conditions by a doctor trained in family planning in the surgery or Family Planning clinic. No anaesthetic is required, although the procedure may be

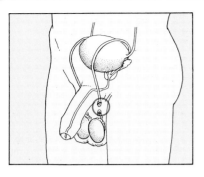

Male sterilization is carried out by surgically sealing the vas deferens, the tubes which carry sperm to the urethra, in an operation called a vasectomy under a local anaesthetic. Because some sperm may be stored in the testicles, contraception must continue until tests show the semen is sperm-free.

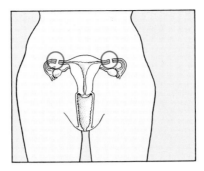

Female sterilization is carried out by surgically sealing the Fallopian tubes to block the passage of the ovum. The operation, called a tubal ligation, is done under general anaesthetic. An instrument called a laparoscope is inserted through two small cuts made just beneath the navel and used to seal off the tubes.

positive pregnancy test and then seek a legal abortion
* Can be used to help victims of rape.

Disadvantages:
* Nausea may be a side effect of pill
* May be unnecessary. Doctors believe that the risk of pregnancy after one unprotected intercourse during ovulation is around 25%.

Sterilization

In both men and women, sterilization must be considered as a permanent method of birth control. The method involves tying off the tubes—in men the vas deferens and in women the Fallopian tubes—through which the sex cells travel. As a result, no sperm can be ejaculated—though there is still seminal fluid—and no eggs can reach the womb to be fertilized. In neither case does sterilization have any effect on sexual activity.

In women, the operation is called a tubal ligation. It is usually performed with a laparoscope under general anaesthetic—*see Special Tests, p.84.* Occasionally it is performed at the same time as a Caesarian section for the delivery of a final baby. In men, the operation is called a vasectomy, and does not require a general anaesthetic.

Since sterilization is irreversible in all but a few cases, it should not be undertaken lightly. Most doctors insist on a period of counselling and discussion, involving both partners, before they are prepared to recommend anyone for an operation. Sterilization is rarely carried out immediately after the birth of a child, for example, but delayed for around six weeks, so that both partners can discuss the implications of the operation. Especially in the cases of single people, doctors are reluctant to perform a sterilization unless they are sure that the request has been extremely carefully considered. The only time it may be actively recommended is for strong medical reasons, as in the case of someone who has strong moral objections to contraception, but who realizes that a further pregnancy could be fatal for her and her child.

Advantages:
* A permanent, safe method of birth control, especially for women who cannot use the pill or IUD, with no serious medical risks

Disadvantages:
* Permanent—can rarely be reversed successfully
* Women may experience heavier, more painful periods after tubal ligation.

uncomfortable. The device has a plastic string hanging from it into the vaginal canal, so that the woman can check to see that it remains in position.

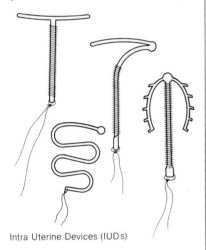

Intra Uterine Devices (IUDs)

Advantages:
* Highly effective—the failure rate is between 2% and 5%
* Can stay in position—depending on type—for up to five years
* The woman does not have to remember to take a pill, or to lose the spontaneity of love-making by inserting a diaphragm
* Generally works well for mature women who already have a family
* Can be used for post-coital contraception.

Disadvantages:
* A high proportion of pregnancies that occur are ectopic or tubal; sometimes this results in infertility later
* Some evidence of increased incidence of intra-uterine infections
* May cause painful, heavier periods
* Sometimes the device is expelled naturally

* The risks and disadvantages are greater for young women who have never had babies, and who may have more than one sexual partner
* Requires expert insertion under sterile conditions. Insertion may occasionally be rather painful, especially in women who have not had babies, and there is a slight danger that the uterus may be perforated during insertion.

Post-coital contraception is a form of contraception that can be used after a woman has had unprotected intercourse. Two methods are commonly used, the pill and the IUD. For reasons of conscience, not all family doctors are prepared to give post-coital contraception, which has only recently become available. In cases of difficulty, a Family Planning Centre should be contacted.

A woman who fears that she may have become pregnant should consult her doctor or attend a family planning clinic within 72 hours of unprotected intercourse.

There are two possible forms of treatment. In the first, she isprescribed a large dosage of oestrogen in the form of two combined oral contraceptive pills, each containing 50 micrograms of a chemical called ethinyl oestradiol. Two more pills are taken exactly 12 hours later, and, as a result, the woman usually has a period at the expected time. Alternatively, she can be fitted with an intra-uterine device up to five days after unprotected intercourse, with the same result.

Advantages:
* Highly effective
* Immediate help for a woman who fears unwanted pregnancy. She does not have to wait until two weeks after a missed period for a

Routine health checks

'Preventive medicine' means just what the term implies. Modern medicine lays great stress on suggesting to people they should eat, exercise and live in order to reduce the chance of disease. But the early detection and recognition of disease is also an important part of preventive medicine. Many diseases can be cured relatively easily if only they are diagnosed at an early stage. In this section, all the simple, but vital, routine checks that you can perform on your own are discussed, plus the check-ups which you can, and on certain occasions should, ask your doctor to perform.

If you are worried about your health, go and see your family doctor. If the doctor thinks your worries are soundly based, he may send you to hospital for special tests—these are free. If the doctor cannot find any cause for concern, but you would still like to have a complete check-up, he or she will arrange a private check-up. Full check-ups are also available through most private medical insurance schemes.

Examination of the breasts

A woman's breasts are made up of fat, connective tissue and milk-producing glands, so, quite naturally, they are a little lumpy when pressed. However, if a lump suddenly appears, the skin of the breast seems to have thickened, or there is a bloody, green or brown discharge from the nipple, you should consult your doctor immediately.

Harmless lumps in the breasts may be caused by cysts, blocked milk ducts, benign, or non-cancerous, tumours, or by scar tissue. Sometimes, however, a lump may be caused by cancer. Breast cancer is one of the largest causes of death in women—there is a one in 16 chance of contracting the disease. You are more at risk than others if:

* Anyone in your family has suffered from breast cancer, especially after the age of 40
* You have never been pregnant, or had your first child after the age of 30
* You started your periods early (before 12), or had a late menopause (after 50)
* You have been exposed to high

EXAMINING THE BREASTS

Examine your breasts once a month and compare their shape and size, paying particular attention to your nipples. If you follow this procedure, you are much more likely to notice any changes in them.

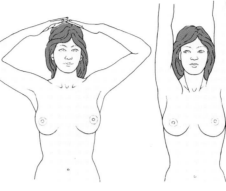

Stand naked in front of a mirror with your hands on your head. Look for any differences between your breasts and see if your nipples turn in, out or up. Look for any lumps, rashes, swellings or discolorations

Stretch your arms above your head for a few moments. This position will give you another opportunity to compare your breasts, to examine your nipples and to detect any differences between them.

Place your hands on your hips and push inwards. This will tighten the muscles on the top of your chest and will emphasize any dimple in the skin of your breasts, or an abnormality of your nipples.

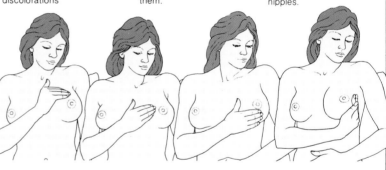

Lie down on the floor with a folded towel under your left shoulder. Examine the tissue of your left breast with the first three fingers of your right hand. Press firmly but gently towards your chest wall, rotating your fingers in small circular movements. Start at a point above the nipple and work outwards around your breast. Pay attention to your nipple and familiarize yourself with the normal consistency of your breast. Sometimes the tissue underneath makes them naturally lumpy. Feel every part of your breast at least three times. After several examinations you will be able to tell if there is any unusual lump or swelling forming in the tissue.

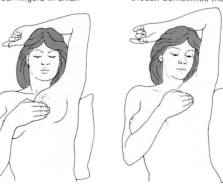

Bend your arm at the elbow and raise it above your head. Examine your left breast again, especially the outermost part which can now be felt with more certainty. Finally, feel the 'tail' of the breast as it extends towards your armpit. After examining your left breast, move the towel to your right shoulder and repeat the examination on your right breast.

An internal examination of a woman's womb *(right)* is often performed by her family doctor at the same time as a cervical smear. This is known as a 'bimanual examination' because the doctor uses both hands to explore the vagina, cervix and womb. The doctor places two fingers of one hand into the vagina and presses down on the abdomen with his other hand *(below)*. In this way doctors check the womb's size, shape and position. They look for abnormalities, such as cysts or lumps, check the tone of the internal muscles and examine the ovaries and vulva.

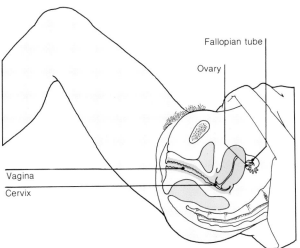

Fallopian tube

Ovary

Speculum

Wooden spatula and slide

Vagina

Cervix

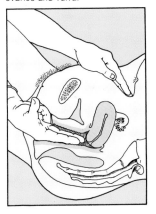

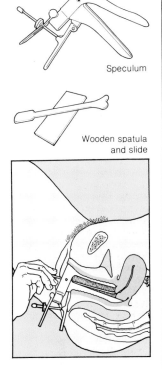

A cervical smear, or 'Pap' test, can detect cancer of the cervix at an early stage. The test is painless and simple; it cannot be carried out during menstruation. The doctor first widens a woman's vagina with an instrument called a speculum *(above right)* and examines the cervix. With a wooden and disposable spatula *(above right)*, the doctor scrapes a sample

from the cervical lining *(right)* and smears it on to a slide. The doctor also makes two further smears by scraping the walls of the vagina and cervical canal. The three slides are then stained with a chemical dye and examined under a microscope. The doctor looks for certain abnormal cells which are an indication that cervical cancer is developing.

dosages of radiation
* You have had cancer of the colon or of the endometrium, the lining of the womb

All women should examine their breasts at least once a month. Follow the steps shown in the illustrations here, and, if you discover a lump, see your doctor as soon as possible. Around 80 per cent of lumps are not malignant, or cancerous, but it is vital to rule out even the smallest possibility of the disease. He will probably send you to hospital for a tissue biopsy—*see Special Tests, p84*—when a small sample of the suspected tissue will be removed from the lump under local anaesthetic and examined under a microscope for any sign of malignancy.

Cervical smears
Cancer of the cervix, or neck, of the womb, affects around 5,000 women in Britain annually. This condition, called cervical cancer, is thought by scientists to be linked to sexual activity—women are more at risk if they started to have sex at an early age, if they became pregnant when young, or if they have had a number of sexual partners.

Fortunately, it is possible to detect cervical cancer at an early stage by a simple test called a 'cervical smear', or a 'Pap Test', after its Greek inventor, Dr Papanicolau. The procedure is simple, usually

painless, and takes only a few minutes. Your doctor will widen, or dilate, the vagina with an instrument called a 'speculum', and then scrape a few cells from the lining of the cervix with a spatula. The cells are examined microscopically to detect any cancerous changes. Out of every 1,000 smears, only about 20 will show any serious abnormalities, and, of these, only around three will require treatment.

Doctors recommend that women should have a smear test every three to five years, up to the age of 35, and then every two to three years thereafter. Many doctors, however, perform a smear test as a matter of routine in the course of a consultation about contraception. As a result of early diagnosis, and advances in treatment, more than 90 per cent of those women found to have cervical cancer can be completely cured.

Your family doctor will usually perform an internal examination at the same time as a cervical smear. He may place two fingers inside your vagina, and press the outside of your abdomen with his other hand—this is called a 'bimanual' examination, because both hands are used and enables the doctor to check the position, size and shape of your womb. The doctor will also examine the vulva, and sometimes check the tone of the internal muscles. Often, the condition of the

cervix and vagina will be examined visually by shining a light through the speculum.

Children
Children pass through many stages between birth and adolescence, continually acquiring new skills and new patterns of behaviour. The ages at which such skills are acquired varies widely from child to child, so you should not worry if your child walks, say, a little earlier or a little later than the child next door. But it is important that the development of your child is carefully monitored, so that any abnormalities can be detected and treated.

Most family doctors run 'well-baby clinics', at which regular developmental checks are performed on children, usually at intervals of six weeks, six months, ten months, 18 months and two years. Your baby will be checked to see what progress has been made since the last visit—the doctor will ask questions about the baby's activities, and observe the baby's play. In this way, any problems in your child's development can be spotted quickly, and worries dealt with effectively and put to rest. The development chart here gives the standard schedule for these.

Your child should also be immunized, or vaccinated, against a number of diseases—*see Natural Defences Against Disease, p52.*

Growth and development

Every child spends the first years of life learning social skills, first through play and imitating others, and later at school. Gradually, he or she learns how to move about, talk and relate to other people.

Each step forward is a milestone of development, forming the basis for checks carried out by your doctor in the practice Baby Clinic; substantial deviations from the norm may indicate the existence of a problem which must be solved. This chart outlines the main features of childhood development, the dates shown being those at which the average baby performs specific tasks. Remember, though, that children develop at different rates and some may be faster or slower to learn some skills than others. Some babies miss out whole stages of development, for instance, perhaps progressing straight from shuffling around on their bottoms to walking, without going through the crawling stage, so small deviations from the dates given here are no cause for alarm. However, if you are worried that there is something wrong, then consult your family doctor and health visitor, who are there to check and advise.

IMMUNIZATIONS

Age	Immunization against
Three months	First Diptheria, Tetanus and Whooping cough injection (Pertussis)
Five months	Second Diptheria, Tetanus and Whooping cough injection Oral Polio
Nine months	Third Diphtheria, Tetanus and Whooping Cough injection
Fifteen months	Measles injection
Pre-School	Diptheria and Tetanus injection Oral Polio
Ten to fourteen years	BCG vaccination if necessary by injection Rubella injection for girls
School leaving	Tetanus injection Oral Polio

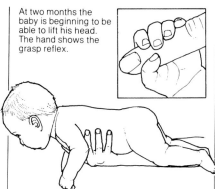

At two months the baby is beginning to be able to lift his head. The hand shows the grasp reflex.

Six weeks to two months By about six weeks, the baby can hold his head in line with his body for a few minutes. He cries if he is hungry or has wet himself. He spends a good deal of time asleep. He can see things close-up, but distant objects are blurred. When the palm of the hand is stroked with a finger, he grasps the finger firmly. This is called the grasp reflex; it disappears during the second month after birth.

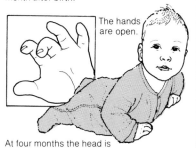

The hands are open.

At four months the head is held high and the baby is kicking.

Three months By about three months, the baby can hold his head up when held horizontally. When lying on his tummy, he supports himself on his forearm and so is able to lift his head and upper chest off the floor. He starts to play with his fingers and watches people moving around him. He gurgles with pleasure when happy and may turn his head in the direction of a noise. When held standing, he sags at the knees.

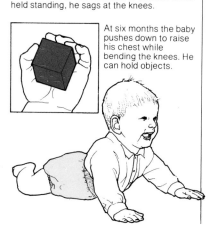

At six months the baby pushes down to raise his chest while bending the knees. He can hold objects.

Six months By now, the baby can usually hold his head up and his back straight when held in a sitting position. He can usually roll over from front to back and turns his head and eyes from side to side to look around. When held standing, he puts his weight on his feet and bounces up and down. He is more alert, following people's movements with head and eyes and turning towards sound. He is interested in toys and can hold small objects, such as a building brick, in the palm of the hand. He can also pass toys from one hand to the other, but loses interest quickly if he drops them.

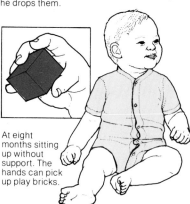

At eight months sitting up without support. The hands can pick up play bricks.

Eight to ten months The baby can sit unsupported on the floor for about ten minutes. He may attempt to crawl and reaches forward for toys out of his reach. He climbs to a standing position, using furniture to support himself. He points and pokes at objects with his forefinger, but he cannot put toys down voluntarily, so drops them. He babbles loudly, usually words like 'Da-Da', and is able to understand one or two simple words, such as 'No' or 'Bye'. He is able to hold and chew a rusk and may have a few teeth. He holds his feeding cup while being fed. He is able to distinguish between family and strangers and may be shy with the latter.

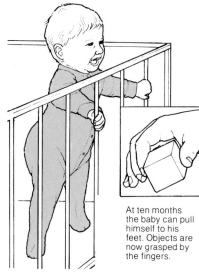

At ten months the baby can pull himself to his feet. Objects are now grasped by the fingers.

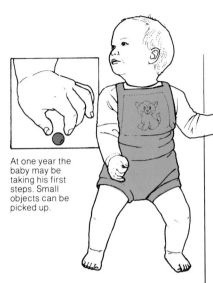

At one year the baby may be taking his first steps. Small objects can be picked up.

One year He will sit alone on the floor for a long time and can reach a sitting position from a lying one. He can walk with someone holding his hand or alone by holding on to furniture (some babies can walk alone or crawl up a few stairs). He can pick up small objects by grasping them, between thumb and index finger, and can put toys down deliberately. He is very interested in everything that is happening around him and likes pictures. He can hold two cubes at the same time, one in each hand. He talks incessantly in his own language — some of which is recognizable to adults — can understand some words and often will obey very simple commands. He can drink from a cup on his own and likes to be allowed to help with dressing and feeding.

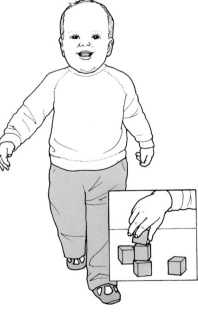

At about 18 months old the toddler's walking has become steady. At this stage the child will be keen to explore and may attempt to walk upstairs. He will also bend down and pick things up and will enjoy building things such as towers of bricks.

15 to 18 months By now he is walking independently, though his legs will be wide apart and his steps uneven. He can crawl up stairs, but finds coming down them more difficult. He can pick up small objects easily and can build a tower of two and later three cubes after being shown how . He likes books with pictures and will try to scribble with crayons. He can say a few words but manages to get most of what he wants by pointing and making noises.

He drinks from a cup, can hold a spoon and tries to feed himself. He also helps with dressing and realizes when he is wet and needs changing.

By eighteen months, he is much more assured when walking and climbing stairs and can run a few steps though he frequently bumps into things. He is beginning to show a preference for either the right or the left hand.

He talks more and can say up to 20 words, though he can understand many more. He begins to learn the names of various parts of his body and will point to them if he is asked to do so. He probably knows the names of a few animals and some household objects.

At about three years old the child will be able to build a higher tower and construct a bridge with bricks. Many children of this age enjoy helping in the house with washing dishes, dusting and cleaning.

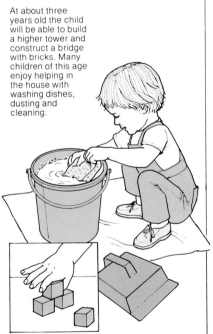

Two to three years As he grows older, he learns to go up and downstairs safely, play with a ball and ride a small tricycle or pedal car.

He can build progressively taller towers of cubes, draw a line and later a circle. He enjoys looking at books, having stories read to him and joins in songs and nursery rhymes.

His vocabulary is continuously increasing and he can understand and obey more complex commands. He clamours for attention and often physically clings to his parent s He likes to get his own way and has an occasional tantrum when thwarted. In particular, he is not used to sharing his toys or his parents and so may be very jealous of a new baby.

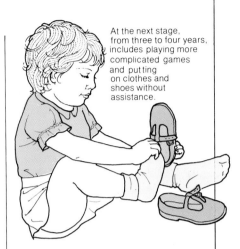

At the next stage, from three to four years, includes playing more complicated games and putting on clothes and shoes without assistance.

Four to five years The young child is now much more sure of himself physically and emotionally. He can go up and downstairs without holding on to bannisters and can climb trees, hop, skip, and jump.

He can throw, kick and catch a large ball and can manipulate small objects easily. He enjoys drawing and painting, can copy letters, and draw a stick man. He knows what several colours are, and his full name and address and can count up to 20. He eats with a knife and fork and can dress himself fully, apart from tying his shoelaces.

He is very sociable, playing happily with other children, and looks forward to going to school, though he may be upset at first.

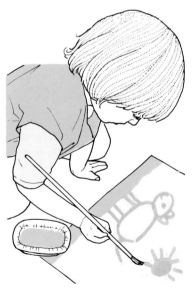

Developmental checks Routine checks are performed at specific intervals to check the baby's development. The actual age at which these tests are carried out may vary from clinic to clinic. Your health visitor or family doctor will advise you when to bring your baby for a developmental check.

Checks are usually carried out at six weeks, eight months, eighteen months, three years and before the child starts school.

Most vaccinations are straightforward, but one in particular causes parents some concern. This is the immunization for pertussis, or 'whooping-cough'. The vaccine causes serious side effects in a small proportion of cases—around one in 100,000 vaccinations.

Unfortunately, the publicity given to these side-effects has deterred many parents from agreeing to vaccination—in 1974, 78 per cent of British babies were vaccinated against pertussis; by 1978, the figure had fallen to 31 per cent. As a result, there have been a major succession of whooping-cough epidemics. In the last major epidemic, 105,000 children caught the disease, 27 children died, and there were 17 cases of serious brain damage.

Talk things over thoroughly with your family doctor, who will advise if there are any potential problems, and make your own decision. Remember, though, that the risk of a child dying from pertussis is significantly higher than the risk of side-effects from the vaccine.

Eye examinations

Problems with vision can be caused by a disease of the eyes, or by purely optical difficulties in focusing. In the first case, a doctor should treat the problem; in the second an optician can prescribe glasses or contact lenses to deal with the problem.

Opticians are trained to notice eye defects caused by disease, and will recommend that you see your doctor in such cases. Normally, your eyes will be tested with an eye chart that contains letters of decreasing size. The optician will examine the retina of the eye with an ophthalmoscope, and, if necessary, specify the lenses you need to correct your vision. This service, and a range of glasses, is available from the National Health Service free of charge; however, this only applies to a restricted variety of standard frames and lenses and there is a substantial charge for other ones.

Babies should have their eyes tested regularly from the age of six months, and children should be checked frequently during the school years—children suffering from conditions like short-sightedness, called myopia, or long-sightedness, called hypermetropia, often fall seriously behind in their education.

The older you are, the more common optical problems become. This is because the tissue of the lens of the eye becomes less and less elastic. As a result, many old people experience difficulty in focusing on

EYE EXAMINATION

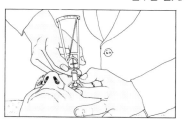

The aqueous humour is constantly drained away and replaced. When the drainage is blocked, as in glaucoma, fluid accumulates and the pressure in the eye increases. A tonometer *(above)* presses down on the cornea and measures resistance. The more it resists, the higher the pressure.

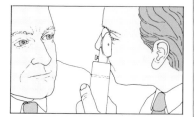

The ophthalmoscope *(above)* shines a fine beam of light on to the back of the eye. It allows an optician to see where the light falls and so discover if the retina has become detached. It also determines the opacity, the cloudiness, of the lens, which, in a cataract, is high.

close objects. The problem can be rectified by the use of glasses that magnify, or of bi-focal glasses, in which only one part of the lens magnifies.

In addition, there are two serious medical problems that can affect the eyes in old age. Glaucoma is a common cause of blindness that affects one in every 50 people over the age of 40. It is a gradual and progressive disease, caused by an increase in the pressure of fluid within the eye, but it can be treated, either by special eye-drops, or, more rarely, by surgery. All people over the age of 40 should have their eyes checked regularly by the family doctor. Otherwise the disease may not be detected and treated until it becomes obvious at a late stage. A cataract, an opaque film that forms over the lens of the eye, can also cause blindness. Cataracts often develop so slowly that they can be left untreated, but sometimes it becomes necessary to remove them surgically, so early detection is vital.

Venereal disease

If you are sexually active and have a number of partners, you run the risk of contracting a form of venereal disease, or VD. This holds true for both homosexuals and heterosexuals, and for people of all classes and cultures.

The incidence of venereal disease has risen considerably in the last decade. This is partly due to a change in sexual attitudes and partly caused by a decline in the use of condoms, which give protection against infection. If you think that you may have contracted a venereal disease—there may be a discharge from the penis in men, or the vagina in women, sores on the genitals, or pain on urination—you should see your doctor immediately. If this embarrasses you—though there is no reason for this—attend a VD clinic at your local hospital. This is

sometimes called a 'special' clinic, or an STD (for 'sexually transmitted diseases') clinic. No appointment is necessary.

Only around 50 per cent of people attending VD clinics are found, after tests, to have a venereal infection. If the diagnosis is positive, treatment will be prescribed, and the staff will insist that you contact anybody with whom you have had sex in the recent past. This is vitally important, both for the health of your sexual partners, and to prevent the spread of venereal diseases. If you are unwilling to contact such partners yourself, a social worker will do it for you.

Unfortunately, women are often unaware that they have a venereal disease—80 per cent of women who have gonorrhoea, for example, show no symptoms. As a result, many doctors recommend that women who are sexually active have routine tests for venereal disease, as part of their programme to achieve and maintain good health.

CHEST X-RAYS

Mass miniature radiography (MMR) was at one time widely practised in the UK. Vans containing X-ray equipment were a familiar site in town centres and university campuses. People were encouraged to have a chest X-ray once a year in order to detect pulmonary tuberculosis or lung cancer in their early stages.

This practice has been discontinued for two reasons. Firstly, pulmonary tuberculosis is very rare, except in some immigrant communities where MMR is still practised. Secondly, annual chest X-rays were found to expose people to harmful levels of radiation, especially women who were not aware that they were pregnant.

Nowadays, the commonest reason for having a chest X-ray is if your doctor suspects a serious bronchial complaint or if you run a special risk of contracting a lung disease. People exposed to fine dust, such as miners and workers in the asbestos industry, are at special risk because they are likely to suffer from pneumoconiosis.

COPING
WITH
SICKNESS

SICKNESS IN THE FAMILY is a problem everyone has to face at some time or other. Coping with sickness shows you what you can do — either as patient or nurse — to deal with the problem of illness in the home. It looks at the special problems that can face the disabled and elderly, and ends with practical, yet compassionate, advice on coming to terms with death.

Home nursing

At some time or other, it is almost inevitable that most people will have to nurse a sick relative or child. Sensitive, careful nursing is a vital factor in speeding recovery; it also makes a great difference to the comfort of anyone confined to bed for more than a short time. Fortunately, most home nursing is far from complicated. It requires a basic knowledge of the simple nursing techniques, described in this section, and common sense.

The sick room

The first rules of home nursing govern the effective organization of the sick room. It is extremely important that this is organized and arranged with care. A hygienic, controlled and cheerful environment can make a great difference to how the person who is ill feels, and so help to speed recovery.

The room should be warm and well-aired. As far as possible, you should exclude draughts, because the sick, especially the elderly, are very susceptible to chills. The room temperature should be kept at around 20-23 C (68-74°F), and the air kept moist. Place a bowl of water on a table, or, if you have a central-heating system with humidity controls, set the humidity at 30-60 per cent. (It may be a good idea to buy a small, single-room humidifier, if a sick person is confined to bed for a long period). Make sure that the air is always fresh—a stale atmosphere is unhygienic and depressing. Something as simple as a bowl of flowers will brighten up the room, and raise morale.

One particular point worth remembering is that sick people often cannot tolerate bright lights. This is particularly true for someone with a fever or headaches. You may have to draw the curtains or lower the blinds during the day, depending on the patient's wishes. Sick children, on the other hand, often feel frightened and lonely in the dark, and a dim light by the bed can help to comfort them. A night-light is also useful for the elderly, who sometimes can wake up during the night in a confused state.

Make sure that everything your patient may need is close at hand—tissues, soft drinks, books, magazines and a radio or television. A bell can be very useful for the times when the patient needs to attract attention.

Remember that continual noise can be very irritating, so you should try to create a peaceful, quiet atmosphere. If the patient wants to be left alone, respect his wishes, but if he feels like company, be ready to draw him into activities.

The bed

A sick person's bed should be comfortable and accessible. There

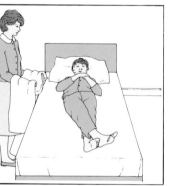

1 Changing the bed Linen should be changed frequently, so it is important that both sides of the bed are accessible.

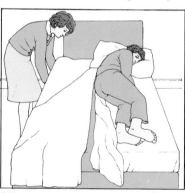

4 Place a clean sheet on the side of the bed away from the patient and tuck it in, leaving the rest of the clean sheet in the middle.

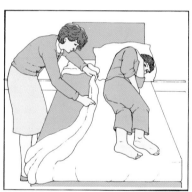

2 Remove the duvet or the top sheets and blankets and gently but firmly roll the patient over to one side of the bed.

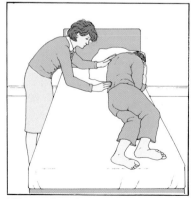

5 Roll the patient carefully over the old and new sheets in the middle of the bed and on to the freshly-made half.

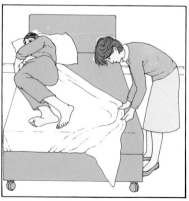

3 Detach the bottom sheet, roll it as far as you c   towards the centre of the bed and tuck it underneath the patient's body.

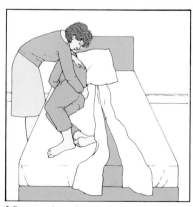

6 Remove the soiled sheet completely. Pull the clean sheet through and tuck it in tightly. Make the top of the bed as usual.

THE SICK ROOM

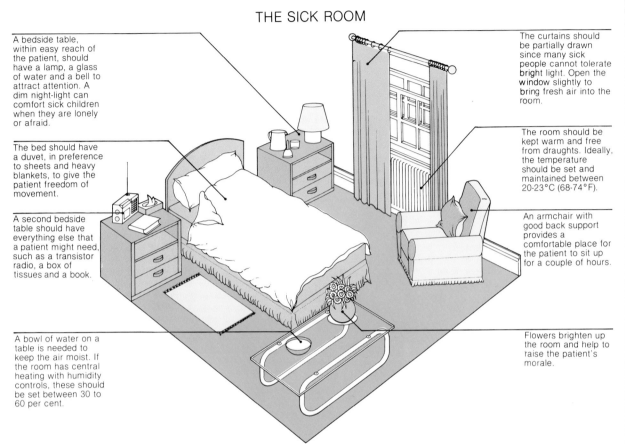

A bedside table, within easy reach of the patient, should have a lamp, a glass of water and a bell to attract attention. A dim night-light can comfort sick children when they are lonely or afraid.

The bed should have a duvet, in preference to sheets and heavy blankets, to give the patient freedom of movement.

A second bedside table should have everything else that a patient might need, such as a transistor radio, a box of tissues and a book.

A bowl of water on a table is needed to keep the air moist. If the room has central heating with humidity controls, these should be set between 30 to 60 per cent.

The curtains should be partially drawn since many sick people cannot tolerate bright light. Open the window slightly to bring fresh air into the room.

The room should be kept warm and free from draughts. Ideally, the temperature should be set and maintained between 20-23°C (68-74°F).

An armchair with good back support provides a comfortable place for the patient to sit up for a couple of hours.

Flowers brighten up the room and help to raise the patient's morale.

should be enough space for someone to stand on either side of the bed—this is especially important when the sheets of a bed-ridden patient are being changed.

If the patient is elderly or disabled, the bed should be near to the ground—this will make it much easier for him to get in and out of it. A light duvet is the best bed covering since it gives the patient freedom of movement, but, if sheets and heavy blankets are used, a bed cradle—a framework underneath the bedclothes—can help to take the weight off the legs. The district nurse, contactable through the family doctor, may be able to supply this—see *Looking After the Disabled.*

The mattress should be firm enough to support the patient properly. If you have a soft mattress, try placing boards beneath it. Special 'fracture' boards can sometimes be hired—your district nurse will be able to advise you about this.

Bed-linen should be changed as often as necessary. Frequent

changes will be needed if the patient is restless or feverish; if he is incontinent, plastic mattress-covers and special 'incontinence pads' can be used. If the patient can move, ask him to sit in a chair while you change the sheets. When a patient is bed-ridden, however, use the step-by-step technique shown in the diagram on page 352 to change the sheets while he lies in bed. This seems complicated, but becomes easy with a little practice.

Personal hygiene

For reasons of morale, comfort and hygiene, it is important that a sick person washes regularly. A patient with a fever, or one who is incontinent, may need to wash several times each day. Normally, he or she will be able to use the bathroom, but, if he is too weak, or confined to bed, you may have to give a 'bed-bath'. The way to do this is shown in the diagram on page 354; the same method can be used if the patient is able to sit in a chair.

If you are ill, this will often be reflected in the condition of your mouth. A high temperature and a reduced appetite may lead to the tongue becoming furred. This results in an unpleasant taste in the mouth, which may further reduce the appetite. The problem can be avoided if the patient cleans

DAILY ROUTINE

To organize a patient's day is just as important as organizing the sick room. Work out a daily routine with the patient, trying to combine his or her needs with the necessary nursing routines. Serve meals, give the medication, take the temperature, change the dressings, wash the patient and make the bed at set times of the day. For the sake of a patient's spirits and morale, try to fulfil any reasonable request at the time it is most required. However, do not allow the patient to abuse your role as nurse by indulging him or her unduly.

GIVING A BED BATH

It is important, for reasons of morale, comfort and hygiene, that a sick person washes regularly. A patient suffering from a fever or incontinence may need to wash several times a day. Normally, the patient will be able to wash in the bathroom, but if he or she is confined to bed then a bed-bath must be substituted. The bed-bath procedure *(below)* can be modified and still used if the patient is able to sit in a chair. After you have washed the body, allow the patient to rinse the hands in a bowl of fresh water rather than wiping them.

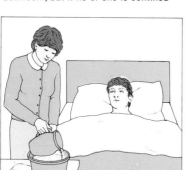

1 Before giving the patient a bed-bath, make sure the room is warm. You will need hot water, a bowl, two flannels, two towels, soap, talcum powder and clean night-clothes.

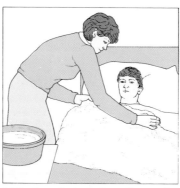

2 Offer the patient a bed-pan. Remove the top covers from the bed and cover the patient's chest with a towel to prevent him from getting wet and cold.

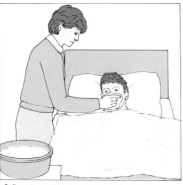

3 Starting with the face, neck and ears, wash and dry each part of the body separately. Only expose the part of the body you are washing. When you dry, pat the skin with the towel.

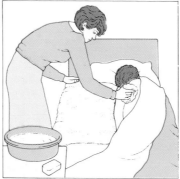

4 Roll the patient on to the side and place the towel on the bed. After washing the back, wash the armpits, groin and, if the patient is a woman, the underpart of each breast.

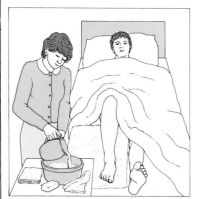

5 Change the water after washing the groin and buttocks. Bend one leg and place the towel under it. Wash the leg, foot and between the toes. Repeat this for the other leg.

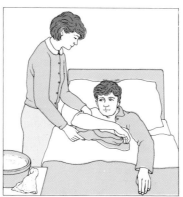

6 After all the parts of the body have been washed and thoroughly dried, dust the patient with talcum powder and help put on clean night-clothes.

his teeth regularly, and drinks frequently. A mouthwash, such as a glycerine and thymol mixture, should also be used each day.

In order to clean a coated tongue, mix two teaspoonfuls of bicarbonate of soda with a little water. Soak a small piece of gauze, from the First Aid Box, in the solution, wrap it round your finger and gently wipe the tongue, or ask the patient to do this himself.

Posture and exercise
Sick people should be encouraged to sit up in bed whenever possible. This helps the patient to breathe properly, and also makes him feel less of an invalid. Use a backrest, or a number of pillows, to make the shape of an armchair—this will make the patient comfortable, and give him firm support.

You may have to help the patient into a sitting position. It is easy to slide a small child up the bed, or to lift him bodily, but in order to move a heavier patient, you will need help. If the patient is able to push with his own feet, you and your helper should stand one on either side of the bed. Each of you should crook one of your arms through one of the patient's arms, and then move slowly towards the top of the bed, pulling the patient up.

If the sick person is helpless, a different technique must be used. The two of you should stand opposite each other, one on each side of the bed, and join your hands under the widest parts of the patient's hips and shoulder. Simultaneously bend the knees, and lift the patient together. It is vital that both of you lift properly, both for your own safety and that of the patient. When lifting:
*Always lift by bending the knees and then straightening the legs. Never lift with your back
* Keep your legs apart and lean close to the patient
* Always lift in unison with the other helper
* Never attempt to lift a patient who is too heavy for you—send for extra help.
A patient can be lifted out of bed in exactly the same way. This is important, because continual bed-rest can cause constipation, muscle weakness, circulatory problems and bedsores.
To avoid such problems, a sick person should be encouraged to take as much light exercise as his physical condition permits. Patients who are confined to bed should flex their arms and legs, while those who can get out of bed should be encouraged to take short walks

LIFTING A PATIENT OUT OF BED

Unless they are completely bed-ridden, sick people should be encouraged to spend as much time out of bed as possible. Sitting up in an armchair in the sunlight for a couple of hours, say, does wonders for many invalids in helping to keep their spirits up; more importantly still, there are also sound medical reasons for getting a patient out of bed for at least a brief period during the day. Continual bed-rest can lead to problems such as constipation, muscle weakness, circulatory difficulties and bedsores — all of which are both unpleasant and can affect the patient's spirits.

Lifting a patient out of bed is not a complex procedure, provided that a few simple commonsense rules are followed. It is important to remember, for instance, that two people will be needed to take the weight; otherwise you will risk damaging yourself, as well as dropping the patient.

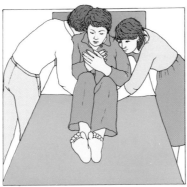

1 Two helpers, standing on each side of the bed, link hands beneath the patient's thighs. With their other hands, they firmly hold the patient's back above the hip.

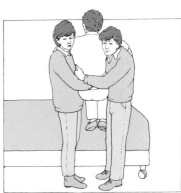

2 Sitting on the edge of the bed, the patient rests the armpits on the shoulders of the helpers who, with their knees bent, lift the patient by straightening their legs.

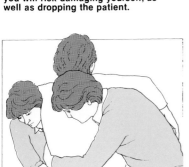

3 Viewed from behind, the helpers' arms can be seen crossing the lower back, their shoulders tucked under the armpits and their hands linked beneath the thighs.

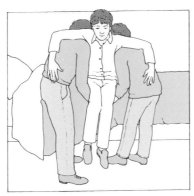

4 On standing up, the helpers walk slowly towards a chair, with the bulk of the patient's weight taken by their shoulders and their hands clasped under the thighs.

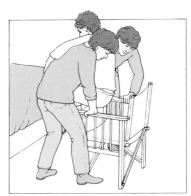

5 Releasing their hold on the patient's back, the helpers steady themselves on the chair. They bend their legs to take the strain of lowering the patient into the chair.

around the sick room. Walking frames and sticks will give confidence and support—*see Looking After Disabled People, p358.*

The lavatory

The use of the lavatory can be a source of great embarrassment to a sick person if he or she is dependent on others for the performance of this most personal of bodily functions. The problem should obviously be approached with considerable sensitivity and tact.

Bedridden patients may use a bedpan, a urinal, a glass or plastic bottle. Though many people find it physically difficult to use a bedpan, the district nurse will be able to help overcome any problems—she can also give information on the various different types of bedpan available for those with special needs. Make sure that the bedpan is warm, clean and dry before giving it to the patient.

Urinals can be obtained from most chemists. They are convenient to use, though less so for women than men, portable and discreet. Care should be taken when they are removed from the bed, however, because they tend to spill easily. Both urinals and bedpans should be kept scrupulously clean with disinfectant.

Patients who can move from the bed but cannot reach the lavatory usually prefer to use a commode—a chair with a lavatory seat and a container—which can be kept covered in the sick room. Most people find a commode easier to use, and less inhibiting, than a bedpan or a urinal.

Diet

Illness often reduces the appetite. This is not necessarily a cause for alarm, because the human body can survive for a considerable time without any solid food. It is important, however, that a sufficiently high intake of liquids is maintained—especially if an excessive amount of fluid is lost

HOME NURSING

District nurses are employees of the local health authority and care for patients in their own home. As reliable mobile nurses, they visit the home of anyone who is sick and look after any patient recently discharged from hospital with a long-term or a terminal illness. They provide reassurance and, as a source of medical advice, are an important link between the hospital and the patient's GP. They change dressings, administer drugs and medication, organize meals, home help and any special service the patient needs.

TAKING A TEMPERATURE

A clinical thermometer is graded and marked in degrees according to one of two temperature scales, Centigrade, or Fahrenheit. The chart (*top right*) helps you to convert degrees Centigrade to Fahrenheit and vice versa. Before taking a patient's temperature, shake the mercury towards the bulb at the end with a few downward flicks of the wrist (*below*). Make sure the mercury level is below the point indicating the normal temperature of 37°C (98.6°F). Depending on a patient's age, there are three ways that can be used to take the temperature (*right*).

Bulb of mercury

| 95°F | 96.8 | 98.6 | 100.4 | 102.2 | 104 | 105.8 | 107.6 | 109.4 |
| 35°C | 36 | 37 | 38 | 39 | 40 | 41 | 42 | 43 |

Armpit temperatures are 0.5°C (1°F) lower than mouth temperatures.

Normal mouth temperature 36-37°C (98.6-99.5°F)

Rectal temperatures are 0.5°C (1°F) higher than mouth temperatures.

Temperatures of 41°C (105.8°F) and over may cause body convulsions in children under five.

Always clean the thermometer before and after use.

For patients over the age of seven, put the thermometer's bulb under the tongue, close the mouth and leave it there for a minute.

For a child under seven, put the thermometer into the armpit and leave it there for three minutes with the arm folded across the chest.

To take a baby's rectal temperature, insert the thermometer about an inch and hold it in place by keeping the buttocks together.

through sweating, diarrhoea or vomiting. The danger signs of dehydration, a dangerous reduction of body fluids, are—a dry tongue, sunken eyes and a reduced, concentrated output of urine.

Water is the easiest thing for the body to retain. By adding sugar or a fruit flavouring to it you will provide extra calories, as well as making the drink more appetizing. Fruit juices or proprietary fruit squashes are also useful, as long as they do not cause nausea, but they should be 'still'; carbonated, or gaseous, drinks tend to distend the stomach, and reduce the appetite still further.

If the sick person is not hungry, he should not be forced to eat vast amounts, but tempted with small, frequent, tempting and nourishing meals. A suitable diet includes boiled fish, lightly boiled or scrambled eggs, vegetable or fruit purées, jellies and yoghurts. Fatty foods may cause nausea, while, apart from providing calories, they have little nutritional value—*see Diet, p321.*

Problems: bedsores
Bedsores are reddened, painful areas of skin which may break down into open sores if left untreated. They are caused by the continual pressure of the bed against the skin, and are especially likely to develop if the patient is wet or dirty. Nutritional deficiencies, such as an ill-balanced diet or a lack of vitamins and iron, exacerbate the problem.

Some people are more likely to develop bedsores than others. Likely sufferers include those who lie in bed or sit in a chair in the same position for long periods; the overweight or those who are very thin, when they are seriously ill or elderly; and those whose condition makes it impossible for them to move. The buttocks, heels, hip bones, elbows, spine and shoulders are the areas most at risk, as the greatest pressure is felt at these points.

The danger signs that indicate a sore is developing are: discoloration of the skin, soreness at the site, or a small break in the skin. If you notice any of these, try to encourage the patient not to lie on the affected area. Cover the sore with a sterile dressing from the First Aid Box in order to prevent infection, and consult your family doctor or district nurse.

Bedsores can, however, be prevented. Encourage the patient to take up a new position in bed at least every two hours—if he is unable to move, you should turn him over yourself. Keep the skin clean and dry by frequent washing especially if the patient is incontinent. Barrier creams, such as zinc and castor oil, may help to reduce soreness—they are available from your local chemist—while gentle massage of the skin in danger areas with soap and water is often helpful.

Special equipment designed to reduce the pressure between the patient and the bed is available from the district nurse or the welfare agencies. These aids include: 'sorbo' rings, sheepskin covers, and, in extreme cases, 'ripple' mattresses and water beds — *see Looking After Disabled People, p358.*

Problems: incontinence
Incontinence—the unintentional release of urine or faeces—can cause great distress, both to the sick person and the home nurse. A person who cannot control urination should be encouraged to empty his bladder by using a bedpan, urinal or commode regularly—about every two hours. This procedure will help to avoid accidents and can be especially important for the elderly, who generally have a reduced capacity for the storage of urine in the bladder. People suffering from

incontinence can learn to control the release of urine, but the process takes time and commitment on the part of both the patient and the nurse.

Even if the patient is too ill to eat properly, it is important that he opens his bowels regularly if he is constipated because there is often a slight leakage of faeces in constipation. The problem can be avoided if a balanced diet is followed and exercise taken. If the patient does become constipated, the addition of high-fibre foods, such as bran, to the diet will help to restore regular bowel movements—*see Diet, p321.*

Incontinence pads and mattress covers are available from the district nurse, and in some areas an 'incontinence laundry service' is provided by the local authority.

Problems: fevers

In many illnesses, particularly those caused by viral infections, the temperature of the body rises. This causes a number of symptoms which make up the condition generally termed 'fever'.

Establishing what the body

temperature is with a clinical thermometer is an important guide to the progress of the illness. You must remember, however, that the temperature is only one indication of the state of health. A high temperature in children, for example, may be caused by overactivity or crying; often people can be seriously ill with a normal temperature. The significance of various temperatures is shown in the diagram.

A person with a fever should be made as comfortable as possible.

Because the skin plays an important part in the regulation of the body temperature allowing the direct loss of heat, all excessive clothing should be removed, leaving just loose-fitting night-clothes. This will help reduce the temperature, while the aspirin or paracetamol from the First Aid Box — junior aspirin or a weak solution of paracetmol in the case of children—will effectively reduce it still further.

A high fever can cause serious dehydration, so the sufferer will need plenty of extra fluids. Lack of appetite is an associated symptom, but when the patient feels hungry again you should only give him small quantities of easily digestible foods, gradually increasing the amounts as he recovers.

If the temperature reaches high levels—over 39.7°C (103.5°F)—it can be very useful to sponge the patient down, especially if he is a child. Remove all the patient's clothes, and sponge him liberally with tepid, not cold, water. Do not dry the patient off, but allow the water to evaporate—it is the process of evaporation that reduces the temperature.

Patients who are confined to bed for long periods of time are likely to develop bedsores on some part of their bodies. The patient's weight on the bed is carried by particular areas or pressure points *(right)*. Bedsores will develop at one or more of these points unless preventive measures are taken. Always keep the sheets dry, clean and free from wrinkles. If necessary, purchase a synthetic, washable sheepskin to use as an undersheet as this will provide an extra cushion between the patient and the mattress. Encourage the patient to change positions at least once every two hours and to do some simple exercises to improve the circulation to the limbs. Sheepskin boots can protect the ankles and heels. Inflatable or foam-rubber rings, bed-cradles, ripple or water beds, and a number of other aids can also be obtained with the help of your district nurse or health visitors.

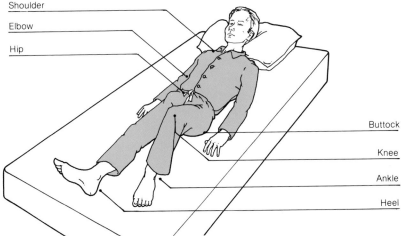

Shoulder
Elbow
Hip
Buttock
Knee
Ankle
Heel

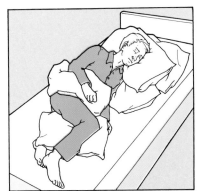

Place an inflatable or foam-rubber ring inside a pillow case and carefully position it under the buttocks of the patient.

Separate the legs and support the arms with pillows to protect the elbow and the knees of a patient lying permanently on one side.

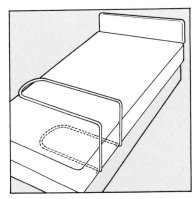

Position a bed-cradle in such as way as to keep the weight of the bedclothes away from the patient's legs and feet.

Looking after disabled people

Disabled people face an enormous range of problems. Their physical powers are restricted, yet they have to live in a world designed almost exclusively for those who have normal functions. They may be dependent on other people, and have no sense of control over their own lives. Relatives and friends, too, will have to come to terms with the presence of a disabled person in their lives, and adjust their attitudes accordingly. But with help, understanding, and the support of the community, many disabled people can overcome their problems, and lead a full and satisfying life.

There is no formal definition or classification of disability, so it is difficult to say how many people are affected by the problem. It is thought that around three million people in Britain suffer from a significant disorder of a limb, sight, hearing, balance or mobility. About a quarter of these suffer from a severe disability. Between 120,000 and 300,000 people use a wheelchair, and, of these, almost half are confined to it.

Though some people are disabled from birth, as a result of a congenital abnormality, such as severe spina bifida, the main causes of disability are the diseases associated with old age: arthritis, strokes, Parkinson's Disease and conditions of the cardiovascular and respiratory systems. Conditions that may affect people at any age, such as multiple sclerosis, accidents and diseases that necessitate amputation of a limb and polio, account for only a small percentage of the disabilities, so that the average age of the disabled is high—around 50.

Problems of disability
Disabled people do not just have physical disabilities: they are normally handicapped in many areas of life. They may be confined to a wheelchair and so find it difficult to move around the house. Outside the house, they may not be able to use public transport, or enter the majority of buildings, without considerable difficulty. Often, a disabled person becomes dependent on others for shopping or cleaning, or for the basic chores of looking after himself or herself, dressing, bathing and using the lavatory.

Many disabled people are isolated and lonely—it has been estimated that around 25 per cent live alone—and the majority have a weekly income that is about half the national average. They are unlikely to be able to overcome the financial handicap, because it is extremely difficult for a disabled person to find a job. Studies have shown that it is four times easier for an able-bodied school-leaver to find work than his disabled counterpart.

It is important to realize that, for these reasons, a disabled person has not only lost the use of a part of his body. He has also lost the ability to control his own life and to enjoy the activities that the able-bodied take for granted. However, through rehabilitation, medical care and support from the family, community and voluntary organizations, a disabled person can regain some of his independence, and enjoy a rewarding life. To achieve this, a family should not be overprotective, or he will become increasingly dependent on them, and fail to realize his full potential.

Help for the disabled
Because there is no effective medical treatment for many disabilities, disabled people must be helped to overcome their handicaps. One way of doing this is to adapt a disabled person's environment so that he can regain some of his independence.

Adaptations in the home may make a tremendous difference to the disabled person's morale—a number of these are shown in the illustrations in this section. Many can be supplied by the social services office of the local authority. The Disabled Living Foundation can also give advice on a wide range of aids and gadgets that help with cooking, cleaning, eating, washing and even gardening.

About 50 per cent of disabled people are thought to live in substandard housing conditions that cannot be adapted adequately. For such people, local authorities, housing associations and voluntary organizations provide purpose-built housing. Unfortunately, however, the demand for such housing far outstrips the supply.

Other aids, such as a wheelchair, artificial limbs or 'POSSUM' equipment are supplied by the Department of Health and Social Security on the recommendation of a family doctor. 'POSSUM' stands for 'patient operated selector mechanism', and this equipment can be used to control electrical devices, such as televisions, typewriters and doorlocks. The DHSS also pay a monthly 'mobility allowance' to those who are unable to walk, or virtually unable to walk, and to those for whom exertion would be a danger to life. Some voluntary organizations help disabled people who receive a mobility allowance to buy or lease a car.

A disabled person, or his relatives, may be entitled to a number of special benefits, which are paid by the DHSS. There is no charge for medical prescriptions for those 'with a continuing physical disability which prevents someone from leaving home without help'. An 'attendance allowance' is available for a severely handicapped person over the age of two who needs constant attention; an 'invalid care allowance' is for people who cannot work because they are caring for a person who is receiving an attendance allowance.

One of the most important functions of the DHSS is to help disabled people to find a job. Disablement Resettlement Officers (DROs) at the local Employment Office can advise disabled people about jobs, and liaise with employers. Large firms are now expected to employ at least 3 per cent of their staff from the pool of the disabled. Before a job is arranged, the DRO may arrange for a disabled person to attend an employment rehabilitation course.

A number of services are also designed to help in the social integration of disabled people. Local authorities have a statutory duty (the Chronically Sick and Disabled Persons' Act 1970) to provide services that improve the quality of life for the disabled. For this purpose, the Act defines a disabled person as someone who is blind, deaf or dumb, or who is 'substantially and permanently handicapped by illness, injury or congenital deformity'. These services include: day centres, holidays, a mobile library and the provision of a television, radio and telephone.

A large number of voluntary agencies provide similar services, and also run clubs, meetings, functions and holidays.

The aftermath of a stroke

A stroke, a cerebrovascular accident or CVA, is the third most common cause of death in Britain, after heart disease and cancer. After a major stroke, 30 per cent of victims die within one week, and about 50 per cent within one year. Around 15 per cent recover completely, while the remainder suffer varying degrees of disability. So the aftermath of a stroke does not necessarily mean severe disability. Through remedial techniques and support and encouragement from the family, a victim can recover many of his former powers.

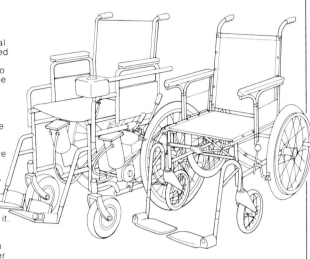

A wheelchair is essential for any physically disabled person who cannot walk and yet is not confined to bed. Once they overcome an initial reluctance, people who depend on wheelchairs consider them to be an extension of themselves. They save themselves energy and, as scientists invent new aids and gadgets, acquire more and more independence. The standard wheelchair *(far right)* is manually operated and needs much muscle power to move and stop it. Modern wheelchairs are battery-powered with a hydraulic braking system *(near right)* and a number of optional attachments.

POSSUM SYSTEMS

The Possum Selector Unit (PSU 3) gives a severely disabled person control over the immediate environment. By gently puffing or sucking on a tube, a disabled person can turn a pneumatic switch on or off. This allows him to operate an electronic unit which gives an on/off control of some electrical appliances. These are shown on an indicator panel *(below)*, which lights up when the appropriate appliance is selected. There is also a microswitch which, when attached to a finger for example, is so sensitive it can operate the PSU 3 whenever the finger moves. The Possum-Link system *(below right)*, with six switches and a door interlock unit, is designed for those who can move slightly but lack mobility and control.

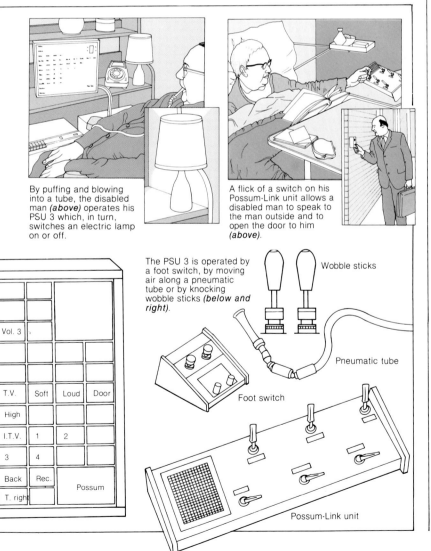

By puffing and blowing into a tube, the disabled man *(above)* operates his PSU 3 which, in turn, switches an electric lamp on or off.

A flick of a switch on his Possum-Link unit allows a disabled man to speak to the man outside and to open the door to him *(above)*.

The PSU 3 is operated by a foot switch, by moving air along a pneumatic tube or by knocking wobble sticks *(below and right)*.

Wobble sticks

Pneumatic tube

Foot switch

Possum-Link unit

Start	Reset							
Alarm	Hold.		Off					
Call	Reset	Buzz	Vol. 1	Vol. 2	Vol. 3			
Phone	Reset	Off						
I-com	Reset	Off						
Misc	Reset	Off	Light	Book	T.V.	Soft	Loud	Door
Heat	Reset	Off	Low	Med	High			
T.V.	Reset	B.B.C.	1	2	I.T.V.	1	2	
Radio		Off	1	2	3	4		
Tape	Reset	Off	Play	Fwd.	Back	Rec.	Possum	
Bed		Up		T. left	T. right			

Doctors often disagree about whether a victim of a stroke should stay at home or go to hospital. Often the decision is easy, because there is no one at home who can give the considerable amount of care that is needed in the early stages. There are a number of advantages to hospital admission, however. The type, size and site of the stroke can be evaluated, and a clear idea of the likely outcome obtained. After the crisis of the first week has passed, a full assessment can be made of the damage—a stroke may affect any or all of the faculties and senses: movement, speech, vision, sensation, calculation, understanding, writing, personality and mood. On the basis of this assessment, the remedial team—doctors, nurses, the physiotherapist, speech therapist, occupational therapist and psychologist—will develop a scheme of therapies aimed at rehabilitating the patient and improving his mobility.

After about four weeks, the patient is usually ready to return home, or, if he is lucky, to one of the small number of rehabilitation units that are available. At home, relatives should gradually take over the role of the remedial workers, with the aim of helping the victim to live as independently as possible.

A victim often feels a great sense of loss. He may have lost his job, his control over his own life and his financial security, as well as some of his physical abilities. He may also experience a sense of isolation, because sometimes he has difficulty in understanding what people are saying, or in communicating with them. This often causes severe depression. The relatives must react with great sensitivity, and help him by their support and understanding. The victim should be encouraged to feel that he has a part to play in his recovery, but should not be told that the problem will pass quickly—he will soon discover that this is not the case, and lose heart.

Mental handicap

There are thought to be around 160,000 people in Britain who suffer from severe mental handicap. The problem may be caused by inherited or congenital disorders, such as Down's syndrome, also called mongolism, which accounts for about a third of mentally handicapped people, phenylketoneuria, or PKU, and hydrocephalus; by injuries during birth or illnesses before birth, such as rubella and meningitis. Milder forms of handicap, such as educational subnormality, or ESN, can even be caused by a lack of

stimulation in the environment—the problem is much more common among low-income groups.

It is difficult to define mental handicap precisely. The Mental Health Act of 1959 defined subnormality as 'arrested or incomplete development of mind which includes subnormality of intelligence'. The dividing line between mild and severe subnormality is usually drawn at the IQ of 50. This is a purely medical and legal definition. Recently there has been a trend towards the definition of mental handicap through the way in which a person responds to and follows the conventions and demands of society. As a result, the emphasis of care has moved from the hospital towards community care at home, in a foster-home, or in a home run by the local authority or a voluntary organization. Here mentally handicapped people can be educated and trained from an early age to cope with modern society and to make full use of their potential.

It is essential that mental handicap is detected as early as possible in children, and that parents are told frankly what the problem is, and what the outcome will be. The parents will often feel angry and bitter, and may look on their child with repulsion. Sometimes they feel guilty, as if they are in some way responsible for the child's disability. They will often be helped if they express these feelings, and talk them over with other people—especially those who have been through the same situation.

However, it is important that parents do not become over-indulgent with the child, because this can cause behavioural problems. Mentally handicapped children have much the same social and emotional needs as other children, so rules must be set, and adhered to. This is better for the child in the long term.

The continuous care of a mentally handicapped member of the family is often extremely draining, both physically and emotionally. To help ease this strain, parents should take advantage of the wide range of facilities and services available for the handicapped child who lives at home. These include: special day nurseries, special playgroups, special school nurseries, special schools and Gateway Clubs. Short-term care, to give the parents a break, is sometimes available in specialist hospitals, or in homes run by the local authority, or by voluntary organizations. These organizations, as well as the Family Fund , may also help with holidays.

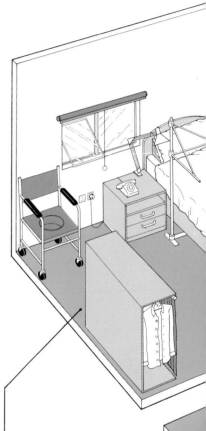

The routines of day-to-day living which the majority of people take for granted can present major problems to the physically disabled. However, with a little ingenuity and expense, a house or flat can be easily adapted (below) to make living safer, more comfortable and more convenient for a physically disabled person.

In the bedroom, the bed is raised on special blocks to make it easier to reach from a wheelchair. It is covered with a lightweight duvet instead of heavy blankets to make sleeping more comfortable. Beside the bed is a tall, sturdy frame with a triangular fixture at the top; gripping this allows a disabled person to rise to a sitting position. The bedside table has sliding drawers, an adjustable lamp and a telephone. The window, which is hung in the middle to make it easier to open and close, has a roller-blind with a long ring-pull instead of curtains. On the wall, there are raised electrical sockets in which plugs with easy-grip handles can be inserted. In the corner, there is a commode. The small wardrobe is as high as a chest of drawers and has a curtain hanging over the front instead of doors. It provides easy access to, and ample space for, a variety of clothes.

The bathroom has a door at least 32in (80cm) wide and space enough to turn a wheelchair round. The toilet has grab rails at either side. The wash basin is shallow to make room for a wheelchair and the mirror is hung low. The taps on the basin and bath are single-lever operated. To make it easier to get in and out, the sloping bath is higher at one end and has bars either side and on the wall. On the bottom there is a non-slip pad and beside the bath is a non-slip bath mat. The light switch cord is long with a ring at the end for easy grip.

The kitchen has a work surface equipped with a microwave oven to make cooking easier and a bread bin with a sliding door. The surface has two drawers: one has room underneath for a wheelchair and is adapted into a chopping board and mixing bowl; the other is divided vertically for the easy storage and removal of pots and pans. Adjacent to this surface is a cooker with space underneath and, for easy grip, cross-shaped knobs and pans with large handles. For easy access, an electrical socket is placed beside the control knobs on the cooker instead of on the wall. A cupboard is hung fairly low on the wall and has round shelves which swivel about, bringing items stored at the back within easy reach. Bar handles on the cupboard are attached diagonally for ease of grip and opening. Underneath the shallow sink there is space for a wheelchair and a pedal rubbish bin. The tap is operated by a single lever: a slight push of the lever one way produces hot water while the other way gives cold water. Beside the sink there is a cupboard with sliding trays and racks for storing vegetables and fruit.

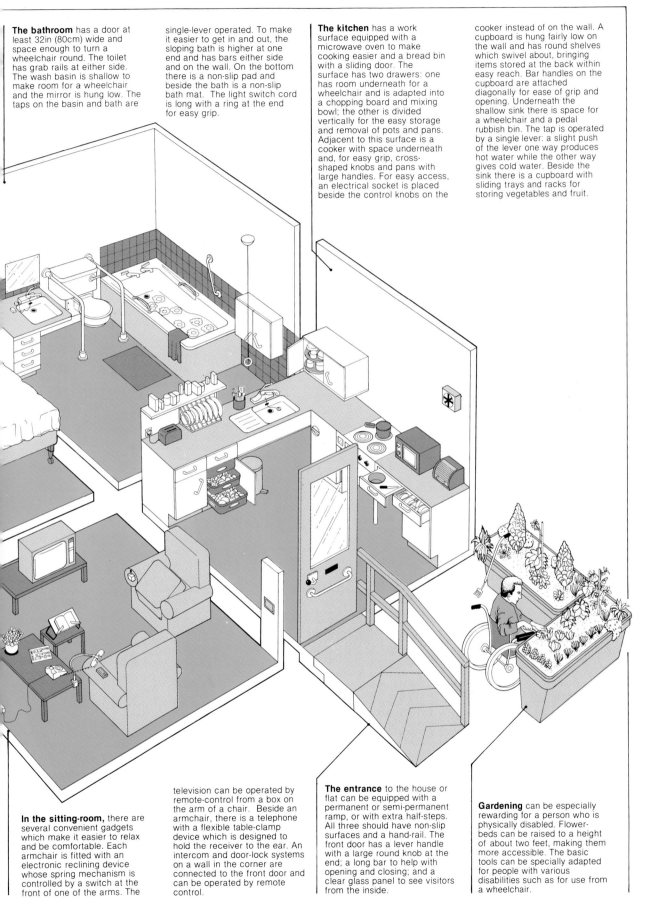

In the sitting-room, there are several convenient gadgets which make it easier to relax and be comfortable. Each armchair is fitted with an electronic reclining device whose spring mechanism is controlled by a switch at the front of one of the arms. The television can be operated by remote-control from a box on the arm of a chair. Beside an armchair, there is a telephone with a flexible table-clamp device which is designed to hold the receiver to the ear. An intercom and door-lock systems on a wall in the corner are connected to the front door and can be operated by remote control.

The entrance to the house or flat can be equipped with a permanent or semi-permanent ramp, or with extra half-steps. All three should have non-slip surfaces and a hand-rail. The front door has a lever handle with a large round knob at the end; a long bar to help with opening and closing; and a clear glass panel to see visitors from the inside.

Gardening can be especially rewarding for a person who is physically disabled. Flower-beds can be raised to a height of about two feet, making them more accessible. The basic tools can be specially adapted for people with various disabilities such as for use from a wheelchair.

AIDS FOR THE ELDERLY AND THE DISABLED

A wide range of domestic aids are available for people who are either elderly and frail, physically disabled or both. Such aids and special appliances are vital when grip is weakened, muscular co-ordination impaired or mobility curtailed. Everyday routine activities such as eating, drinking, cooking, moving about the house, cleaning, dressing and so on, are made far easier and safer, while the quality of life is greatly improved.

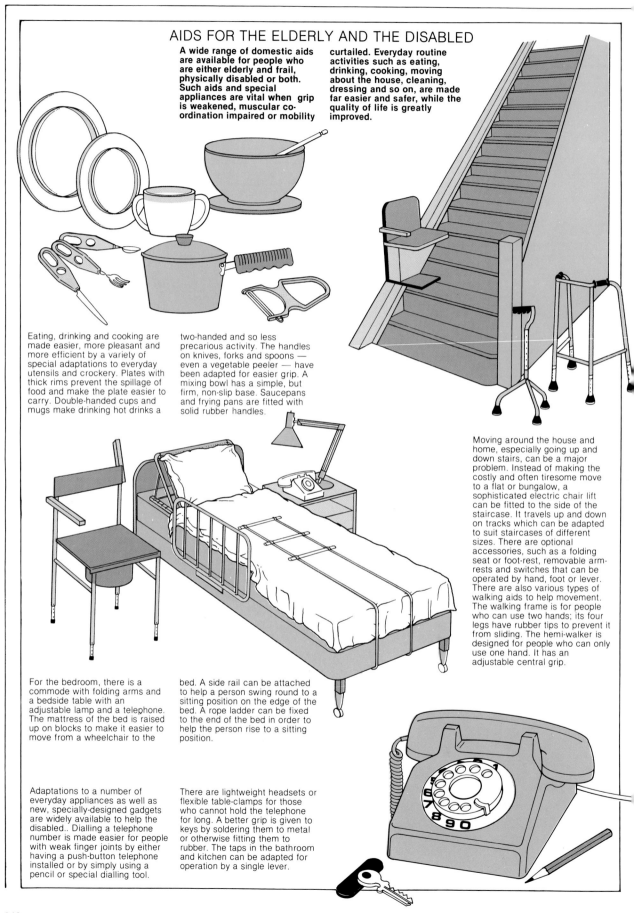

Eating, drinking and cooking are made easier, more pleasant and more efficient by a variety of special adaptations to everyday utensils and crockery. Plates with thick rims prevent the spillage of food and make the plate easier to carry. Double-handed cups and mugs make drinking hot drinks a two-handed and so less precarious activity. The handles on knives, forks and spoons — even a vegetable peeler — have been adapted for easier grip. A mixing bowl has a simple, but firm, non-slip base. Saucepans and frying pans are fitted with solid rubber handles.

Moving around the house and home, especially going up and down stairs, can be a major problem. Instead of making the costly and often tiresome move to a flat or bungalow, a sophisticated electric chair lift can be fitted to the side of the staircase. It travels up and down on tracks which can be adapted to suit staircases of different sizes. There are optional accessories, such as a folding seat or foot-rest, removable arm-rests and switches that can be operated by hand, foot or lever. There are also various types of walking aids to help movement. The walking frame is for people who can use two hands; its four legs have rubber tips to prevent it from sliding. The hemi-walker is designed for people who can only use one hand. It has an adjustable central grip.

For the bedroom, there is a commode with folding arms and a bedside table with an adjustable lamp and a telephone. The mattress of the bed is raised up on blocks to make it easier to move from a wheelchair to the bed. A side rail can be attached to help a person swing round to a sitting position on the edge of the bed. A rope ladder can be fixed to the end of the bed in order to help the person rise to a sitting position.

Adaptations to a number of everyday appliances as well as new, specially-designed gadgets are widely available to help the disabled.. Dialling a telephone number is made easier for people with weak finger joints by either having a push-button telephone installed or by simply using a pencil or special dialling tool.

There are lightweight headsets or flexible table-clamps for those who cannot hold the telephone for long. A better grip is given to keys by soldering them to metal or otherwise fitting them to rubber. The taps in the bathroom and kitchen can be adapted for operation by a single lever.

Looking after old people

Today, largely due to the success of modern medicine, more people than ever before are living into old age. In Britain alone, there are now around nine million people, or 17 per cent of the population, over the age of retirement; three million over the age of 75, and 500,000 over 85. These numbers are on the increase.

Many old people live full, independent and contented lives, adjusting fully to the problems old age can bring. Like any machine, the body deteriorates with age and will inevitably slow down to a greater or lesser degree. This section of the book is not intended for them; it is intended to help people who find it difficult to come to terms mentally with the effects of the ageing processes, or are so affected by them physically that they cannot survive unaided.

A loss of value

Old people often feel, wrongly, that they no longer have any value or status in society. While many still feel valuable as grandparents, members of a church or voluntary workers, others begin to feel that they have no part to play in the community. This often leads to depression. It also encourages the growth of a feeling of isolation, which many old people feel is their greatest problem.

Old age can also be a time of growing dependence on others. An old person may have to rely on an outsider's help to perform tasks that have been second nature for decades—shopping, cleaning, getting dressed, and even using the lavatory, for instance. Roles and relationships may change as a result: a daughter, for example, may act as a parent to her ailing mother or father, whose needs are like those of a child. This reversal of roles can be both unsettling and stressful. To treat an elderly person like a child causes many problems, and may even encourage child-like behaviour, such as incontinence. As well as losing the feeling that they are valued by the family and society, old people may gradually lose the ability to control what is going on in their lives. They will often appear bloody-minded, angry or even aggressive as a defence against these changes, and ungrateful for what others try to do on their behalf. Some old people may respond by withdrawing and becoming depressed, and may need medical help as a result.

Confusion

Another common problem of old age is that of confusion: an old person may not know the day of the week, or even the year. This may be caused by dementia but is often the result of being cut off from the mainstream of life—if he or she has no regular visitors, has lost interest in the television and radio and no longer reads the newspapers, every day seems very much the same. As the normal activities and interests of life become more remote, some old people also begin to pay less attention to their diet and personal appearance.

The psychological problems caused by age and the loss of a worthwhile role in life may be exacerbated by poverty and poor housing conditions. A great number of old people live in flats and houses that lack essential amenities, such as hot water, inside lavatories and proper heating. Those on fixed incomes and inadequate state pensions are usually unable to cope with the financial problems that substandard housing brings. Their answer is often to cut down on the food and fuel that is essential for good health—this in part accounts for the large numbers of deaths from hypothermia—the gradual and finally fatal reduction of the body temperature.

All these problems, together with the physical ones described below, can usually be solved given time and patience. In the main, the people who shoulder the burden are relatives, friends and neighbours. If they can come to understand the physical and mental problems that old people sometimes face, relatives and friends can help enormously, merely by providing sensitive care, support and practical help. However, they represent only one segment of a complex network of organizations and individuals who care for and support the elderly. A wide range of statutory services is provided as a legal requirement by local authorities and the National Health Service: there are also numerous voluntary agencies, charities, pressure groups and advice centres, all of which can offer practical advice and help if required.

Medical problems

Old people are prone to many disabling diseases, such as heart problems, bronchitis, arthritis and strokes—but some conditions are due to old age itself, and can cause problems that may be very distressing to the sufferer and relatives alike.

Perhaps the most distressing of these conditions is generally known as chronic organic brain disease. There are two types of brain disease: senile dementia, in which the brain shrinks gradually and deteriorates, and arteriosclerotic dementia, in which small areas of the brain die. In the first condition, mental deterioration is constant, but gradual; in the second an old person may suddenly become mentally confused as the immediate result of the attack.

Both conditions cause dementia, a problem that affects every aspect of an old person's intellect, memory, emotions and behaviour. The most noticeable symptom is the failure of short-term memory. This may be accompanied by an impairment of judgement and reasoning, and by insomnia. As the problem develops, a sufferer may become, in medical jargon, 'disoriented in time and space'—he will be unaware of where he is, or what day or time it is. Sometimes an old person may lose control of his sexual impulses and expose himself or make sexual advances.

There may also be delusions: often the sufferer becomes convinced that people are stealing from his house, or interfering with the water-pipes. As his personality disintegrates, the old person may become incontinent and may fail to feed and warm himself. Often such old people become careless with fires and wander from the house at any time of day and in all weathers; moods may also change quickly from elation to depression.

Though they can sometimes be controlled, both forms of dementia are incurable. Unfortunately chronic organic brain disease is common: it affects one in ten of those over 65, and one in five over 80. It puts a tremendous strain on the supportive network and on those who have to watch the personality of a loved one disintegrate.

Sometimes old people are affected by a problem that can easily be confused with senile dementia. It is sometimes called 'acute brain syndrome'. In this condition an old person may suddenly become confused, have hallucinations and appear agitated. The problem may be caused by pneumonia, circulatory problems and even drugs that have been prescribed for another condition. Fortunately, once the underlying cause has been detected, the symptoms usually clear up.

There are two other problems that often affect old people—hypothermia and incontinence. Hypothermia is extremely common and has a social cause: old people who do not have sufficient money for their needs tend to economise on fuel and heating. As a result their body temperature slowly falls, until, when it is below 35°C (95°F), the face and hands may appear warm and flushed, but the sufferer feels drowsy. Unless First Aid is given promptly—see p369—the sufferer will eventually die; in fact hypothermia accounts for a considerable number of fatalities in this age group.

Incontinence, on the other hand, usually has a physical cause. In men it may be a disease of the prostate gland and, in women, a prolapse of the bladder. In both sexes incontinence may also be caused by an infection of the urinary tract or by damage to the central nervous system, such as acute or chronic brain disease, or to the spinal cord in conditions such as multiple sclerosis. Faecal incontinence, however, is more rare than urinary incontinence. It may be caused by constipation if watery faeces escape round the obstruction, or be a result of depression or schizophrenia. Both types of incontinence can cause great distress to the sufferer and to the people who are responsible for his care and support. Again, patience and understanding is the key to the problem, plus adequate home nursing —see p352.

Helping the old

The problems of age can rarely be cured, although symptoms can be relieved, but practical help and support often improve an old person's condition beyond recognition. When looking after an old person, the most valuable form of support is understanding. The relative, friend, neighbour and voluntary worker must be able to appreciate the old person's psychological problems, as described above, and draw on all their reserves of patience, kindness and understanding. It is important that an old person is not treated like a child, however much he may act like one; that his wishes and preferences are respected; and, above all, that he is encouraged to retain an interest in the world and a sense of value and usefulness to society. Apart from these psychological considerations, the life, and health, of an old person may be considerably improved by recourse to the many supportive organizations that are available.

The majority of services for old people are obtainable through the Social Services Department of your local authority: ring and ask to speak to a social worker. The problems of old age are daunting, but it is surprising how much improvement can be made if they are tackled one by one. The golden rule is to concentrate on what the old person sees as a problem. It will usually be covered by one of the following services:

Adaptations—many minor adaptations to the household environment can be carried out by the local authority under the terms of the Health Services and Public Health Act, 1968. They include handrails, ramps, sliding-doors and small water heaters.

Aids—aids to daily living are provided by local authorities under the same legislation as above. They include bathseats, raised toilet-seats, fireguards, commodes and many other items that can substantially improve the quality of an old person's life and prevent serious accidents.

Day Centres—these provide company and activities for elderly people who might otherwise be alone. Transport to and from the day centre is often provided.

Holidays—most authorities provide short holidays for the elderly in special centres, or grants towards a holiday, provided that the candidates meet certain criteria.

Home Help—some old people qualify for a home help, who will assist with shopping, cleaning and household duties. Many old people find this service invaluable.

Homes—some authorities allow old people who are disabled to spend one or two weeks in a residential home—the intention is to give the relatives who look after such old people a holiday themselves. Some authorities also allow old people to spend the day at a home, and so give an old person the opportunity to keep his own home.

Laundry—in many areas a laundry service collects and delivers linen and clothes for old people who are incontinent.

Luncheon Clubs—places where a small charge is made for a hot meal, but also where an old person can meet other people of his own age.

Meals-on-Wheels—a most useful service for those who are housebound or unable to cook for themselves and also for those who have lost interest in preparing meals.

Occupational Therapist—a paramedical worker who is skilled at assessing the need for the aids and adaptations discussed above, and who can also suggest physical and psychological therapies that help an old person retain an interest in life and a capability for activity.

Rent/Rate Rebates — old people who live on small incomes are often entitled to rebates, but rarely apply for them.

Sheltered Housing — specially adapted flats or bed-sits that usually have a resident warden. This type of housing is invaluable for old people, but, unfortunately, there is often a waiting list.

Social Worker — the person who monitors and advises on the services in this list. Approach a social worker about any problems you may have in caring for an elderly relative.

Telephone—a local authority may pay for the installation and rental of a telephone if an old person is vulnerable or isolated.

The services listed above are provided by local authorities, though not all authorities provide all of the services. Another range of services is also provided by the National Health Service. To obtain these, contact the family doctor.

Aids and Adaptations—Area Health Authorities provide various aids and adaptations for home nursing under the provisions of the National Health Service Acts. These include bed-hoists, special beds and mattresses and incontinence pads.

Bath Attendants—may be provided to help disabled or frail elderly people with bathing.

Day Hospitals—an old person may attend a day hospital on one or more days a week, so that professional

WHERE TO GO FOR HELP

Local Authorities
Social services are provided by the local authority and, to find out what these are and what you are entitled to claim, you should telephone or write to your local Social Services Department. Local authorities may provide grants for minor household adaptations, such as handrails and ramps for the disabled, as well as bath seats, raised toilet seats, fireguards and commodes. They run day centres for the elderly, and often provide transport to and from them. They may offer grants for short holidays, provide a home help to assist with shopping and cleaning, and run short-stay or long-stay residential homes. In many areas, local authorities provide laundry services in cases of incontinence. They run luncheon clubs, where hot meals are provided at a nominal charge. The meals-on-wheels service provides meals in the home for the housebound or bedridden. Social workers will advise on the possibility of rent or rates rebates, while the authority may provide sheltered housing — specially adapted flats, usually with a qualified resident warden — and may even pay for a telephone to be installed.

Social workers and occupational therapists have individual functions, though they work closely together. The former advise on the availability and monitor the effectiveness of the various social services. The latter assess which of the services are suited to particular cases; they also advise on psychological and physical therapies.

Both your doctor and your local welfare services can provide practical help to help you care for an elderly relative. If you are faced with this responsibility, always find out what both can do to help you in your task.

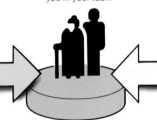

National Health Service
To obtain the range of services provided by the National Health service, first contact your doctor. These services include the provision of bed-hoists, special beds and mattresses, and incontinence pads, if required. Your doctor can also arrange attendance at special clinics, together with transport to and from them. In the home, bath attendants can be provided to help the disabled or frail with bathing; in addition, many services normally found in hospital, such as those of an optician or chiropodist, can also be provided at home.

District nurses and health visitors will also visit. The former help with home nursing, while the latter monitor general health and well-being and will organize the services listed here.

---

treatment, such as physiotherapy, and support can be given while the old person retains his own home. Transport to and from the day hospital can usually be provided.

District Nurses—visit on the recommendation of the family doctor. They help with every aspect of nursing in the home and may order nursing aids.

Domiciliary Services—many services available in hospital can also be provided at an old person's home, including those of a chiropodist, optician and occupational therapist. Sometimes a geriatrician or psychogeriatrician, specialists in the diseases that affect old people, will make a home visit to a housebound person at the request of the family doctor.

Health Visitors—are concerned with the general health and well-being of an old person. They will visit frail and vulnerable old people in their area, and give advice on diet, budgeting, and any of the services mentioned here. Health visitors are usually attached to a family doctor's practice or a health centre.

It is also worthwhile to make contact with the local office of the Department of Health and Social Security to check whether an old person is entitled to supplementary benefit. If this is the case, the old person may also be entitled to single discretionary payments to provide essential equipment for the home—a heater or a bed, for example. These payments may also be provided for emergency repairs and decoration. Some old people may qualify for a heating allowance, while those who need to be attended for all or part of the day may be entitled to an attendance allowance.

So far the services that have been discussed are all provided by government or local government agencies. However, many of these professional resources are under-financed and over-stretched, and it may also be wise to contact one of the many voluntary organizations that help to care for the elderly. Some are mainly pressure groups, but others can be approached for grants, advice or volunteer visitors; several organizations provide specially adapted housing that is in great demand. Among the best known of these organizations are 'Help The Aged', 'Age Concern', 'Task Force' and the WRVS (addresses are given on p408), but there are many others, some of which, as part of a growing trend, are self-help groups run by the elderly themselves.

The last resort
Sometimes the network of community care breaks down, and relatives, friends, the professional services and voluntary organizations can no longer cope. At this time the question of institutional care arises. Often the old person has become so frail physically or mentally that falls in the house, wandering or self-neglect have put his health at risk.

It is always difficult to say when this risk becomes unacceptable—especially because the old person is usually prepared to accept a higher level of risk than those caring for him, as he wants to stay in his own home. The wishes of an old person must always be respected, but if nursing care or treatment that cannot be given at home is required, then admission to hospital may be necessary. Usually the move is temporary, but occasionally it is permanent.

If an old person is able to walk, dress and feed himself, perhaps with help, admission to an old people's home might be considered. Some homes are run by local authorities, others by voluntary organizations and private enterprise. Admission should always be with the consent of the old person, and in the case of local authority homes an assessment of the case by a social worker is necessary. In fact it would be sensible to consult a social worker and make use of his specialist knowledge and advice before arranging for the admission of an old person to any type of home. In certain exceptional circumstances, covered by Section 47 of the National Assistance Act, an old person may be compulsorily removed from his home, but this is very rare.

It is important to remember that the majority of confused and bed-ridden people remain in their own homes—not in hospital or an old people's home. Institutional care should only be considered as a last resort, when an old person can no longer receive the necessary care and attention at home from friends, relatives and neighbours, or from the numerous other sources of help that are available.

Coming to terms with death

Most people find it difficult to talk about death, yet it is something that all of us must face, sooner or later. Death is not a subject that can be ignored—nor should it be, for a dying person can be greatly comforted by the support of his friends and loved ones, and by modern nursing techniques. This section also deals with the problems bereaved relatives face after death, when they have to cope not only with their own grief but the practical details of registration and the funeral.

Preparations for death

Often, relatives will know that a patient is dying, but the patient will not have been told. This can put a great burden on them, because they have to reassure the patient that all is well, but at the same time prepare themselves for his or her death. It is always difficult to know whether a dying patient should be told about his condition. Usually doctors, who have considerable experience of this dilemma, try to work out wheher the patient wants to know and respect his decision.

Some patients do not want to know that they are dying, and their wishes should be respected. Sometimes, patients think that they may be dying, but do not want to have their suspicions confirmed. This situation may be upsetting for the relatives: they are unable to say their farewells properly, and a feeling that they have been deceitful may cause some guilt after the death.

Often, however, a patient feels relief, rather than distress, when the fact that he is dying is brought out into the open. He is able to share his fears and worries with the people closest to him, while the relatives can prepare themselves emotionally for what is to happen.

It is very important that someone who is dying is allowed to talk as freely as he wants about his feelings and his fears. He should not, however, be forced to do so if this is not his wish. Often, he will experience anxiety, grief, loneliness and a sense of failure. The most helpful response is to listen carefully, and to allow him to bring these feelings out into the open. They will not then be so overpowering, and he may be able to face death with a less troubled mind. It is also important that the patient is allowed to control his own life as much as possible, to look after his own affairs and take part in family decisions.

All people react differently to death, but in general a patient who has been told that he is dying goes through the following stages. First, he may refuse to accept that the doctor's diagnosis is correct. This is a defence against something that is too painful to contemplate. Gradually, he becomes more dependent on others, and as a reaction to this may become demanding or aggressive. Finally he may become extremely depressed, as he realizes that he is losing his independence and control over his own life. This may grow worse if the patient is in severe pain.

Relatives can help by visiting regularly and often, by listening with understanding and sympathy, and by reassuring the patient that he will not be alone at the end.

Medical care

About 20 years ago, doctors began to realize that a patient who died at home or in a general hospital could suffer much unnecessary pain and distress. As a result the hospice movement, which developed in Dublin in the middle of the nineteenth century, gathered momentum. Hospices are medical institutions that are devoted to the care of the terminally ill and their families. The expertise that hospice staff have developed in this field, since the pioneering work at two world-famous London hospices, St Joseph's and St Christopher's, has had a great influence on the care of the dying throughout medical practice.

Hospices attempt to eliminate pain, and other distressing problems, so that the dying patient can prepare himself, and his affairs, for death. Since severe pain is disabling and exhausting, every effort is made to control it before it becomes severe. This is achieved by the delicately gauged use of high dosages of opiates, such as morphine—the risk that the patient will develop a tolerance or addiction to these drugs is minimal.

Great care is taken to treat other common symptoms of terminal disease, such as constipation, vomiting and breathlessness, as these can lower the patient's morale and reduce his resistance to pain. Through their skill and experience, the doctors and nurses make sure that the hospice is a happy place, where death is almost always peaceful.

There are now more than 30 hospices in Britain, most of them under the control of the National Health Service. In order to discuss the possibility of treatment in a hospice for someone who is terminally ill, you should consult your family doctor.

Community support

The majority of the services available to old people—*see Looking After Old People, p362*—are also available to a person who is dying at home. The key figure in the network of community support is the District Nurse. As well as helping to nurse the patient, by guarding against bed-sores, applying dressings and giving injections, she can advise on many aspects of home care, such as getting in and out of bed, using a bedpan and lifting. The Health Visitor will assist her, the activity of both being co-ordinated by the doctor—*see also Home Nursing, p352.*

The District Nurse can also provide a number of aids which will make the patient more comfortable, and so increase his morale. These include bed cradles, hoists, commodes and special mattresses. Either the District Nurse, or a bathing attendant, will also help to bath the patient.

A number of aids, such as a television or telephone, can be provided by the local authority under the terms of the Chronically Sick and Disabled Persons Act, 1970. Anyone who is terminally ill is covered by this Act, and every effort should be made to use it, and any other services, to make a patient more comfortable in his last illness—no matter how short a time he or she has to live.

Ask at your local Department of Health and Social Security office about an 'attendance allowance' and an 'invalid care allowance'; if you are entitled to Supplementary Benefit, you may also claim allowances for a special diet for the patient, laundry and heating. In exceptional circumstances, the DHSS may pay for a permanent helper to live in your house.

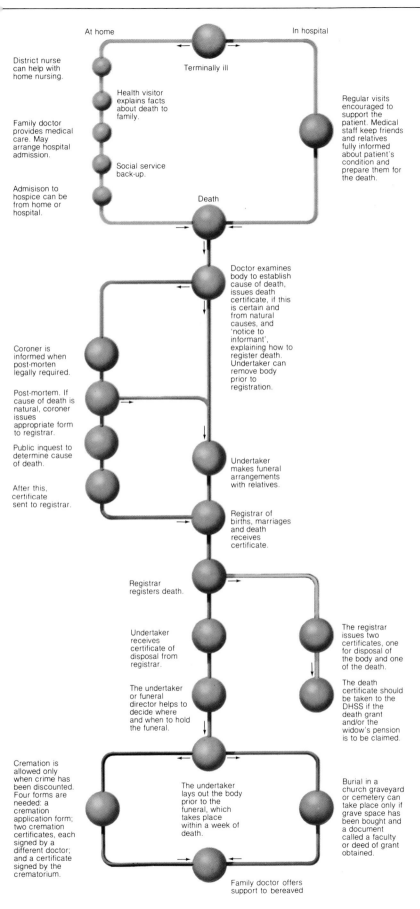

At home

In hospital

Terminally ill

District nurse can help with home nursing.

Health visitor explains facts about death to family.

Regular visits encouraged to support the patient. Medical staff keep friends and relatives fully informed about patient's condition and prepare them for the death.

Family doctor provides medical care. May arrange hospital admission.

Social service back-up.

Admission to hospice can be from home or hospital.

Death

Doctor examines body to establish cause of death, issues death certificate, if this is certain and from natural causes, and 'notice to informant', explaining how to register death. Undertaker can remove body prior to registration.

Coroner is informed when post-morten legally required.

Post-mortem. If cause of death is natural, coroner issues appropriate form to registrar.

Public inquest to determine cause of death.

After this, certificate sent to registrar.

Undertaker makes funeral arrangements with relatives.

Registrar of births, marriages and death receives certificate.

Registrar registers death.

The registrar issues two certificates, one for disposal of the body and one of the death.

Undertaker receives certificate of disposal from registrar.

The death certificate should be taken to the DHSS if the death grant and/or the widow's pension is to be claimed.

The undertaker or funeral director helps to decide where and when to hold the funeral.

Cremation is allowed only when crime has been discounted. Four forms are needed: a cremation application form; two cremation certificates, each signed by a different doctor; and a certificate signed by the crematorium.

The undertaker lays out the body prior to the funeral, which takes place within a week of death.

Burial in a church graveyard or cemetery can take place only if grave space has been bought and a document called a faculty or deed of grant obtained.

Family doctor offers support to bereaved

Coping with death. Only one person in four dies a quick death. For the majority of people, death can be a drawn-out process, involving a slow decline over weeks or even months, either at home or in hospital. This decline can be the result of a terminal illness, such as cancer. Equally, what can happen is that the body's resistance is so weakened it cannot resist effectively when, eventually, the final disease attacks.

The aim of modern medicine is to make the process of death as peaceful and as painless as possible for the person who is dying, relatives and friends. When someone is dying at home, the local doctor and the practice support team will do all they can to relieve any pain and distress. In hospital, care, sympathy and reassurance are the three watchwords for medical and nursing staff alike.

Doctors also recognize that their responsibilities do not end with the death itself. The support and care they can offer the bereaved is of equal importance.

A number of voluntary organizations also help with the care of the dying. The Marie Curie Foundation has a number of homes for the terminally ill, and provides night-nursing and help for patients in their own homes. The National Society for Cancer Relief provides financial help for those who suffer from cancer. This can be for nursing fees, fuel bills, visitors' fares and holidays. This organization is at present developing the Macmillan Home Care Service, which will help the terminal patient to remain in his own home for as long as possible.

After death
When a relative or friend dies, especially if the death is unexpected, the response is one of overwhelming grief. 'In the midst of grief, there is life' is a cliche, but, nonetheless, it is true. Before the healing process of grief can run its course, the relatives have to attend to the practical details of registration of the death and the funeral.

The first step is to call the family doctor, so that he or she can examine the body and certify the death. He will also be able to advise on the correct procedure to be followed. Every death that occurs in Britain must be registered by the Registrar of Births and Deaths. The Registrar's office is normally at the Town Hall. He or she will want to see the doctor's certificate, usually within five days of the death. On the certificate, the doctor states the place and date of death, and, 'to the best of his knowledge and belief', the cause of death. On the certificate is a 'Notice to Informant'—the informant is the nearest relative who was present at the death, or who was in attendance at the last illness.

A doctor may not sign the medical certificate unless he has attended the dead person in the 14 days before the death, or unless he has seen the body. Even if he has done this, he may not sign the the certificate if the cause of death is unknown or in doubt; if the death was sudden or the result of an accident; if the death was unnatural or suspicious. These cases, as well as those in which the death occurred during an operation, or was due to industrial disease or poisoning, are referred to the doctor or lawyer who holds the office of Coroner (or Procurator Fiscal in Scotland).

The coroner will usually order a post mortem examination—a detailed inspection and analysis of the organs and tissues—in order to determine the cause of death. If the post mortem shows that the death had a natural cause, he will send a pink form, a substitute for the medical certificate, direct to the Registrar and take no further action.

The coroner will hold an inquest if the cause of death was violent or unnatural, if it was an accident or an industrial disease, or if it is still not known. An inquest is a legal proceeding, held in public. Relatives may attend, and may be represented by a lawyer—indeed, this is advisable if there is an insurance claim. After the inquest has decided the cause of death, the coroner will send a medical certificate to the Registrar.

On presentation of the medical certificate, the Registrar will ask for details of the dead person's life and the circumstances of his death. After formally registering the death, he will give the 'informant' two certificates—a 'certificate of disposal' and a 'certificate of registration of death'. There is no cost for these certificates, but there is a small charge for copies of them—which may be necessary for insurance, probate, or when the dead person is to be cremated.

On the back of the certificate of registration of death is a form that should be completed and presented at the local office of the DHSS. A small 'death grant', depending on the age of the deceased, is available to offset the expenses of the funeral. If a close relative of the deceased receives Supplementary Benefit, he may be eligible for a larger grant from the DHSS towards basic funeral expenses. In cases where no relative, friend or executor is able to make the arrangements for the funeral, the local authority, or the hospital authority, if the person died in hospital, has a statutory duty to do so, under the National Assistance Act, 1948.

The certificate of disposal should be given to the undertaker, sometimes called a funeral director.

DONATION OF THE BODY AND ORGANS

The deceased, or the relatives of the deceased, may decide to donate an organ for transplant or the whole body to a medical school. If an organ is to be donated for transplant, it must be removed almost immediately. A kidney must be removed within half an hour and the eyes, to be used in a corneal transplant, within six hours.

It is sensible to obtain at least two detailed estimates before choosing an undertaker, because funeral costs can be high. The funeral director will help and advise on all the arrangements for the funeral, and his calm, reassuring presence can be a great comfort at a difficult time. He will 'lay the body out'—a process in which the body is washed, the orifices closed with cotton wool, the eyelids closed and the mouth propped shut. If the deceased died in hospital, this will have been done by the nursing staff. Unless children are frightened by the idea, it may be a good idea to allow them to see the body at this time, so that they can say goodbye, and come to terms with the death.

The funeral will normally take place within a week. If the body is to be cremated, extra certificates will be required: one from the doctor at the crematorium, and two more signed by different doctors. Your family doctor will be able to arrange this, but most doctors make a charge for the service .

Bereavement and grief

Grief is a long process, which starts as soon as a family is told that one of its members is dying. Nevertheless, the experience and the expression of the intense sadness of grief is a healing process. It gives physical and emotional outlets to the pain of bereavement.

Individual responses to bereavement vary, but, in general, they form a pattern. An understanding of this pattern can help people to cope with their sorrow.

At first, the bereaved person feels numb. He or she is in a state of shock. Often the family will talk about inconsequential things, and appear unaware of what has happened. This is usual, and should not cause guilt. After a few days, a bereaved person will begin to experience pangs of grief: he may be in great distress, which may manifest itself in physical symptoms, such as shortness of

breath and a feeling of choking. He may also suffer from insomnia, restlessness, anger and an inability to concentrate. He is likely to be preoccupied with thoughts of the dead person and, probably in a subconscious attempt to bring the dead person back to life, to have vivid illusions of the presence of the deceased.

The funeral is a ritual focus and expression for grief. After it, the pangs of grief are often replaced by severe depression, and sometimes an unjustifiable feeling of guilt. These feelings may continue for some considerable time.

The bereaved should be allowed, and even encouraged, to express their grief. They may need to talk at length about the person they have lost, to go over the events of the weeks before death and even the death itself. This may be painful for others, but it is an important part of the way in which grief runs its course. After some months they may need reassurance that it is reasonable for them to stop grieving and start to remodel their lives.

Sometimes, bereaved people become suicidal, or suffer from serious and prolonged depression. In these cases psychiatric help may be necessary. In the normal grief of bereavement, however, anti-depressants and tranquillizers should be avoided, unless, of course, they are prescribed by the family doctor. Drugs such as these merely subdue and repress the natural expression of grief, and delay the acceptance of a new life. If grief continues for too long, however—the normal period varies with the individual, but is, on average, around six weeks—then treatment with anti-depressants or tranquillizers may be necessary.

The expression of grief is especially important for children. It is thought that children suppress grief more than adults, and sometimes even feel responsible for the death. This may cause depression in later life. Children should be encouraged to grieve, and allowed to see others grieve openly. Their feelings about the death should be discussed, and they should be reassured that they are not to blame.

Bereaved people may be helped by talking to others who have suffered a similar loss. A number of organizations fulfil this need and specialize in counselling the bereaved. Among them are: Age Concern, The Society of Compassionate Friends (for bereaved parents), Cruse (for widows), The Stillbirth Association and The Samaritans.

FIRST AID

WHEREVER YOU MAY BE,
you may be faced with a
medical emergency. While the
scale of such emergencies
obviously varies, taking the
appropriate action is still vital.
This section of the book
helps you to do this.
For ease of access, emergency
life-saving techniques, such as
artificial respiration, are given
first, followed by an A-Z
of First Aid.
In addition, there is a guide to
what should be included in the
home First Aid box and
medicine cupboard, while the
section ends with instant check
lists to danger spots in and
around the home.

Emergency techniques/ Mouth-to-mouth ventilation

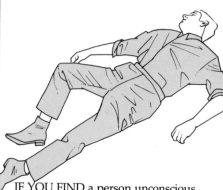

IF YOU FIND a person unconscious, go through the *action checklist*. If there is more than one person, someone should get an ambulance immediately. Do not move the casualty except to save his life. Do not leave an unconscious person alone.

IF THE AIRWAY is clear but the casualty is not breathing, start mouth-to-mouth ventilation immediately (see box for dealing with babies and small children). If this is not possible, because of facial injuries or if the casualty is pinned face down, use one of the following methods of ventilation:

Mouth-to-nose ventilation. If you cannot seal the casualty's mouth with your mouth, follow the method on this page but substitute the nose for the mouth. Close off the mouth. Blow air into the nose.

ACTION CHECKLIST
1. Stay calm and call for help
2. Check consciousness and breathing
3. If casualty is not breathing, open airway
4. If he or she is still not breathing, give mouth-to-mouth ventilation | **(1)**
5. Check pulse **(4)**
6. If heart has stopped, there is no circulation. Start heart massage at once *(p372)*
7. If there is a wound, control serious bleeding
8. Place casualty in the correct recovery position *(p375)*
9. Prevent shock *(p374)*

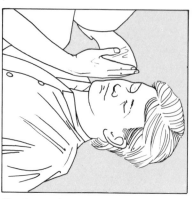

Check consciousness. Loosen any tight clothing around the neck. Then check consciousness. Quickly and gently tap the face and talk to the casualty. If you get a response you know he is conscious.

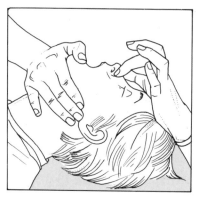

1. Keeping the neck arched, hold the chin forward with one hand and pinch the nostrils closed with the other. It is vital that the lungs are inflated as soon as possible.

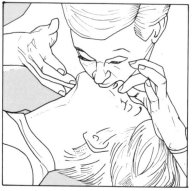

2. Take a deep breath and place your mouth over the casualty's, making sure the seal is tight. Blow five good breaths into the mouth. Watch to see the chest rise and fall.

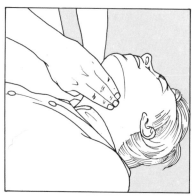

4. If the chest has risen, check the pulse on the neck before continuing ventilation. Check carefully, the pulse may be very faint. If there is no pulse turn to *heart massage (see p372).*

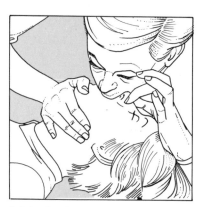

5. If the chest has risen and a pulse is present, blow another good breath into the mouth. Watch for the chest to rise as you do this.

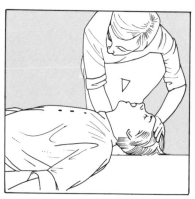

6. Watch the chest go down. Give another good breath into the mouth. Continue giving a breath every five seconds, until the casualty starts to breathe.

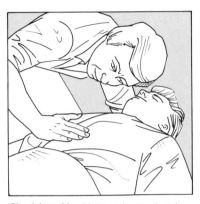

Check breathing Listen at the mouth and check chest and abdomen for movement. If breathing has ceased, open airway; if not, check pulse. If no pulse, start *heart massage (see p370)*. If pulse present, put casualty in *recovery position (see p375)*.

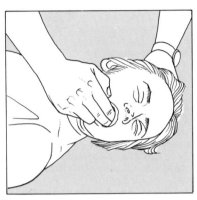

Clear the mouth With your finger, remove any possible obstructions from the airway. Remove dentures, if worn.

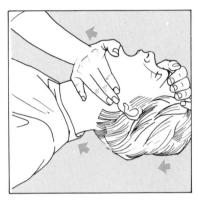

Open airway With one hand on forehead and the other behind neck, tilt head back. Then push jaw forward to lift tongue. If breathing starts, place casualty in the *recovery position (see p375)*.

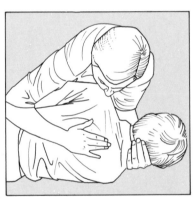

3. If the chest does not rise, clear the airway by pulling the casualty on to the side towards you. Give two sharp slaps between the shoulder blades.

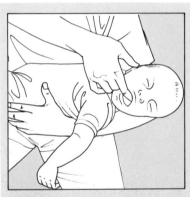

Babies and infants
1. Cradle the baby on your knee, supporting trunk and head. Tilt the head back slightly, then clear out the mouth.

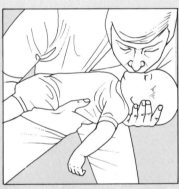

2. A tight mouth-to-mouth seal may be difficult, so place your mouth over the baby's nose and mouth. Give a gentle breath into the baby's lungs and watch for the chest to rise.

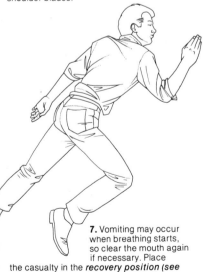

7. Vomiting may occur when breathing starts, so clear the mouth again if necessary. Place the casualty in the *recovery position (see p375)*. Do not leave him, especially if unconscious.

3. If the chest does not rise, turn the baby over and give a gentle tap between the shoulder blades. Return to mouth-to-mouth ventilation.

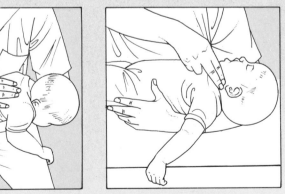

4. Check pulse on the neck. If no pulse turn to *heart massage (see p372)*. Otherwise continue with one breath every two seconds until breathing starts.

Emergency techniques/Heart massage

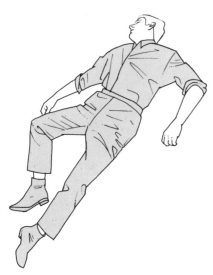

HEART MASSAGE can be dangerous if the casualty's heart has not stopped beating. Do not proceed unless the heart has stopped.
If the heart has stopped, the casualty will show the following signs:

1. Unconsciousness
2. No pulse. Check the carotid pulse on the neck, not the wrist pulse
3. Breathing will usually have stopped, but casualty will be gasping for breath
4. The pupils of the eyes gradually dilate
5. Skin becomes ashen and the body limp.

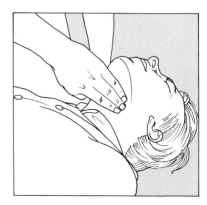

1. Check carefully for a pulse. The carotid pulse in the neck is the most accurate and reliable. The pulse may be very faint, so check the neck thoroughly. If any pulse is present, do not start heart massage.

SPECIAL CASES

Heart massage for two people
Heart massage can be given more effectively if there are two of you to carry it out. One should compress the chest, the other should give mouth-to-mouth ventilation. Start by giving four breaths and check the heartbeat. If the heart is still not beating, give five compressions. Then alternate a good breath and live compressions until the heart restarts. The person giving ventilation should check the pulse and eyes regularly. If the heart starts, stop the massage immediately, but continue ventilation until breathing is restored.

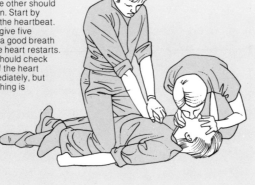

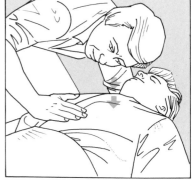

5. Listen for the heart beat by placing your ear on to the chest. If you are satisfied that the heart has stopped, start heart massage.

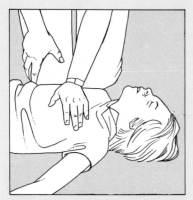

Young children If giving heart massage to young children, follow the steps on this page, but use only one hand for compressions and press gently.

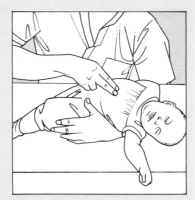

Babies If giving heart massage to a baby, use only two fingers on the chest. Give two compressions every second and press gently.

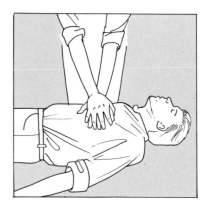

9. Repeat the compressions a further five times at the same rate *(see step 7)*.

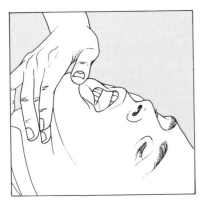

2. The complexion will be pale and ashen if the heart has stopped. The lips may turn bluish and the arms and legs become limp.

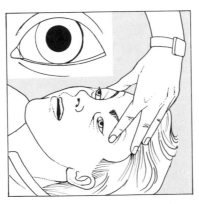

3. Another characteristic sign of heart failure is dilation of the pupils of the eyes. If they are dilated, the black centres of the eyes will be enlarged to cover almost the whole eye.

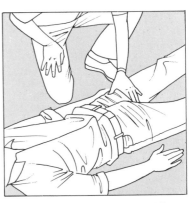

4. The femoral pulse in the groin should be checked, if the carotid pulse cannot be detected but a heart beat is still suspected. The femoral pulse is located in the groin.

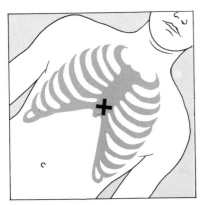

6. Quickly locate the heart area by running your fingers up the inside of the rib cage until you feel the tip of the breast bone. Just above this is the heart area and massage point.

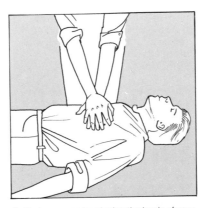

7. Start massage by placing the heels of your hands on top of each other on the chest and, with arms straight, press down firmly five times at one second intervals.

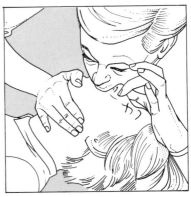

8. After the first five compressions, give a good breath by mouth-to-mouth ventilation.

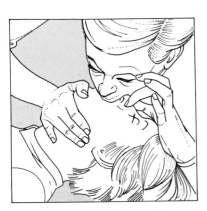

10. After these five compressions, give a further breath of mouth-to-mouth ventilation. Check the heart by seeing if the carotid pulse has restarted and if the eyes and lips are returning to normal. If not, continue with the cycles of compressions to breaths.

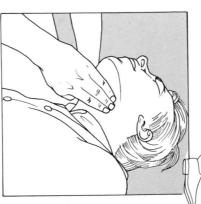

11. Continue to check the pulse regularly as you give a breath. Also check the eyes to ensure the pupils are still dilated. Stop heart massage as soon as the heart starts beating.

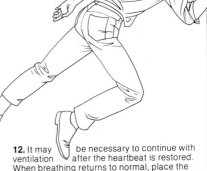

12. It may be necessary to continue with ventilation after the heartbeat is restored. When breathing returns to normal, place the casualty in the *Recovery Position (see p375)* but do not leave alone.

Emergency techniques/ Recovery position/Shock

THE ABC OF EMERGENCY RESUSCITATION

In any emergency, where life is obviously at imminent risk, it is vital to take prompt action, but, at the same time, to ensure that all such actions are calm and logical. Resist the pressure to do anything without first thinking about what you are doing and the consequences of the steps you are taking.

Remember, too, that witnessing a medical emergency can and will have its effects upon you. Your pulse rate may well increase and your hands may well tremble. Panic is infectious, so try at all times to remain clear-headed and collected. Always follow the three basic principles given here in any emergency; they may well be life-saving.

A-AIRWAY

Ensure the airway is clear and keep it clear. The airway can be blocked by the tongue, dentures, or by the posture of the casualty. Take the appropriate steps to deal with the problem.

B-BREATHING

If breathing ceases for longer than a few moments, brain damage starts and, unless respiration is restored, the casualty will die. The only effective methods of artificial respiration are mouth-to-mouth and mouth-to-nose ventilation; the Holger-Nielsen method of resuscitation is now considered ineffective by medical authorities.

C-CIRCULATION

If the heart stops beating, blood cannot be pumped around the body, with brain damage and death as the results. Always check the pulse — ideally the carotid pulse in the neck, not the wrist or groin pulses — to see whether the heart is beating or not. The carotid pulse is the best one to check because it is close to the heart and easy to detect. The only way to re-establish the circulation, if the pulse has ceased, is by external chest massage. When faced with any emergency, you must assess the position carefully before proceeding. Ensuring that the airway is clear is the first and most important step; if it is blocked, no other treatment can be effective. Remember, too, that blockage can occur during resuscitation, primarily through changes in head and neck positions, so it is important to re-check the airway frequently.

Clearing the airway can be the only form of emergency treatment required; if so, the casualty's breathing will recover spontaneously. If this does not happen, artificial ventilation must be started immediately and continued until breating is re-established. It is equally important to check the pulse and listen for a heart beat; if there is no pulse and a heart beat cannot be detected, external chest massage must be performed.

SHOCK

SHOCK IS a state caused by a sudden drop in the supply of oxygenated blood to the body. It can be caused by loss of breathing, heart stoppage, severe injury, loss of blood and other serious conditions.

If a casualty is in a state of shock, some of the following features will be present:
1. Extremely pale complexion
2. Clammy skin and sweating
3. The pulse will be shallow
4. Breathing will be irregular
5. The pupils will be enlarged
6. Casualty may complain of thirst
7. Casualty may feel nauseous
8. Unconsciousness may occur.

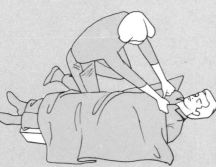

Loosen clothing Place casualty on his back with the legs raised if possible. Cover if necessary. Get help quickly.

To treat shock:
1. Loosen casualty's clothing
2. Lay the casualty down
3. Raise legs if possible
4. Keep casualty warm. Cover if necessary, but do not use hot water bottles or a heater
5. Moisten lips with water, but do not give an actual drink
6. Never give alcohol
7. Keep a constant check on breathing and pulse
8. Talk to casualty, reassure and make comfortable
9. Do not move unnecessarily
10. If you think it is safe to leave casualty, go for help as soon as possible.

THE RECOVERY POSITION is used when a casualty is unconscious, but is breathing. Do not move the casualty, however, if there is a back injury. The recovery position ensures that the airway remains open and allows ventilation. By widening the air passage, it also ensures that the airway cannot become blocked – by, say, the tongue curling up at the back of the throat – and that vomit in the mouth can drain off easily. If a casualty's breathing seems to be difficult or noisy, he or she must be placed in the position at once. Do not leave an unconscious person alone. Check regularly to ensure he or she is breathing and the heart is beating.

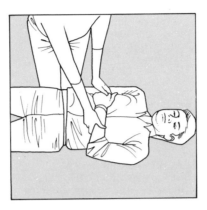

1. Kneel beside the casualty (if he or she is already face down go to step **5**). Ruck the near hand under his hip.

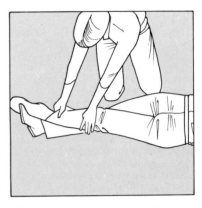

2. Bring the far arm over the chest. Cross the legs by bringing the far leg across towards you.

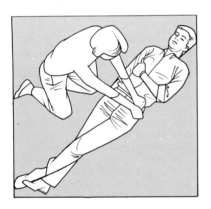

3. Grasp clothing at the far hip and pull on to the side towards you until resting on your knees.

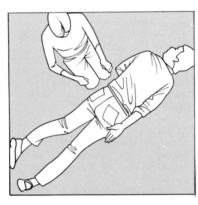

4. Place on front with care. The head should be on to one side and facing towards you.

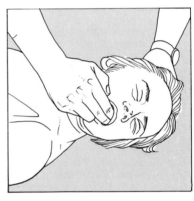

5. Tilt head upwards to ensure that the airway remains open and in case the casualty vomits.

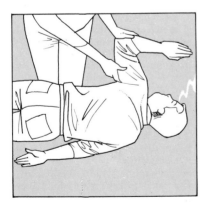

6. Pull the far arm clear of the body. Bend the near arm up, so that the hand is close to his face.

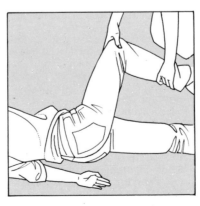

7. Keeping the far leg straight, bend the near leg at the hip and knee. Do not leave an unconscious casualty alone.

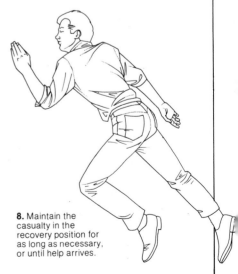

8. Maintain the casualty in the recovery position for as long as necessary, or until help arrives.

The A-Z of first aid

ABDOMINAL PAIN
There are many causes of abdominal pain, including constipation, indigestion, period pains, cramp, colic or wind. If the pain is not accompanied by headache, vomiting, fever or diarrhoea, it is probably not serious and will not last for long. If any pain in the abdomen persists, or is severe, seek the advice of a doctor. If the pain is at the top of the abdomen consult a doctor immediately – pains in this area may be caused by heart problems. If the pain follows an accident or a heavy blow, or if there is swelling and tenderness, seek medical help – it may be the result of an internal injury. Otherwise, abdominal pain may be caused by constipation, food poisoning, menstruation, wind or a pulled muscle.
See also Wounds & serious bleeding, Internal bleeding, Muscle strain, Food poisoning.

ABRASIONS *See Cuts & scratches.*

ACCIDENT *See Road traffic accident.*

ACID *See Poisoning.*

ALCOHOL
The effects of alcohol depend on the amount in the bloodstream. Initially alcohol acts as a stimulant, but as more is drunk it causes consecutively depression, confusion, stupor, unconsciousness, coma and finally death through poisoning. At any stage after confusion, a person who is intoxicated also risks death through the inhalation of vomit while unconscious.
The effects of alcohol may be dramatically worsened as a result of interaction with another drug or medicine. If a person appears to be considerably more intoxicated than is warranted by the amount of alcohol consumed, try and find out if he has taken any drugs, if so what they were, and seek medical help.
Remember never to give alcohol to an injured person, or to a casualty suffering from shock – you will make his condition worse

ACTION
In cases of paralytic drunkenness, take immediate action:
1. Place him in the recovery position, *see p375.*
2. Clear the airway, *see p371.*

3. Keep checking breathing and pulse – you may have to give artificial respiration and/or heart massage, *see pp370-374.*
4. Send for medical help.

ARTIFICIAL RESPIRATION *See Emergency Techniques, pp370-375.*

ASPHYXIATION
See Emergency Techniques, pp370-375.

BACK INJURIES
Back injuries fall into two main categories – fractures of the spine and back strains. The latter are common, particularly in sports, and occur when the back muscles are overstretched – and, in extreme cases, torn – by over-exertion. Follow the procedures below, but, if there is any doubt, treat the injury as a potential fracture.
A violent injury to the spine may involve both splintering of the spinal vertebrae and damage to the spinal cord. Such a fracture is extremely dangerous. Any victim of a road accident or serious fall may well suffer spinal damage.

ACTION
1. Do not attempt to move the casualty if you have the slightest suspicion that the back may be fractured
2. Summon medical help.
3. If the casualty is conscious, ask him to wiggle his fingers and toes, but prevent him from moving any other part of the body. If fingers or toes cannot be moved, this suggests a serious back injury. Tell the doctor or ambulanceman what you have done
4. If help is on the way, steady the head and support the feet. If this is delayed, bandage ankles, feet, thighs and knees together, placing padding between the legs. Do not move the casualty
5. Give artificial respiration and/or heart massage if necessary (*see Emergency Techniques, pp370-375*).

Slipped discs occur when a person bends, or attempts to lift a heavy object and the discs in the spine are affected. As a result of these abnormal stresses, a section of the disc between the bones in the spine become displaced, so that it puts pressure on a nerve.
A slipped disc may be frightening for the victim. The effects vary, but

the onset is usually sudden and there is considerable pain; sometimes feeling in the legs and lower abdomen is lost.

ACTION
1. Reassure the casualty
2. Though pain and immobility make it difficult, try to make the casualty comfortable, laying him on a flat surface
3. Call for medical help.

Pulled back muscles should be treated by keeping still, painkillers, rest and, if necessary, medical help. Immediately after the injury, the application of ice may help to relieve the pain; later on, heat will be comforting.

BANDAGING *See facing page.*

BIRTH *See Childbirth.*

BITES AND STINGS
In Britain, bites and stings are rarely dangerous. They may cause pain and discomfort, but this usually passes reasonably quickly. If, inflammation and swelling develop, you should consult your doctor, since infection may have set in.
In other countries, the situation is much more complicated. Rabies is not uncommon in Europe, America and parts of the Far East, and anybody who has been bitten by a dog, cat or another small mammal should be taken to a hospital immediately. In the case of other bites or stings, seek medical attention whenever you are in any doubt.
Remember, therefore, in Europe, America and the Far East, always to seek immediate medical help after a bite from a dog or cat. In Britain seek immediate medical help if the animal appears rabid – wild-eyed and frothing at mouth

ACTION – ANIMAL BITES
1. Calm and reassure the casualty
2 Wash the wound and apply a clean, dry dressing – *see Wounds & serious bleeding.*
3. Seek medical help. Bites carry the risk of infection and your doctor may recommend an antibiotic or an anti-tetanus injection, especially if the wound is dirty.

Bee and wasp stings are painful, but not normally dangerous. In some
continued p379

BANDAGES AND DRESSINGS

Bandages and dressings are protective coverings which are normally applied directly to wounds to help control bleeding, absorb any discharge and lessen the risk of infection.

Bandages are used to keep dressings in place. In addition, they are used to provide support and prevent movement in the case of a fracture, so giving the damaged bones the opportunity to heal.

It is not difficult, in theory, to tie a bandage, or apply a dressing, but the stress of coping with an emergency often makes it more difficult. The first priority is always to stop serious bleeding.

Points to remember
Whenever possible, wash your hands and, if bleeding is under control, clean a wound prior to bandaging it. Always apply a dressing directly on to the wound; never slide it into position.

Always keep a variety of bandages and dressings in a First Aid Box. In an emergency, however, use anything that comes to hand as a bandage, as long as it is clean. Never use fluffy dressings over open wounds, as they will stick to the injury.

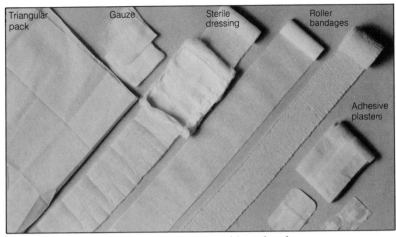

Triangular pack — Gauze — Sterile dressing — Roller bandages — Adhesive plasters

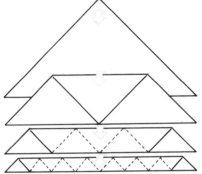

Making a bandage
There are many different types of bandage available, each suited to various purposes (*above*). Some you can make yourself. A triangular bandage for use as a sling can be cut from a linen or calico square. Once made (*left*), the bandage can be converted into a broad or narrow one in a series of simple steps. Fold the point of the triangle towards its base, having first created a narrow hem along it. Then, fold the bandage in half and, to narrow it still further, fold in half once more.

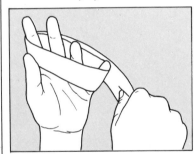

Making a ring bandage
1. Fold a clean bandage into a narrow strip, position it across your fingers and wind one end round to make a loop.

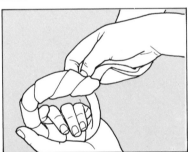

2. Pass the other end of the bandage through the loop. Wind it around the loop and pull tight.

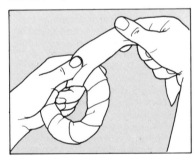

3. Continue building up the thickness of the loop until the bandage has been used up and a solid ring formed. Tuck the end in.

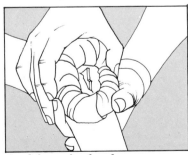

Applying a ring bandage
1. Place the ring bandage in position over a dressing. Put the loose end of the securing bandage under the ring and wrap it around twice.

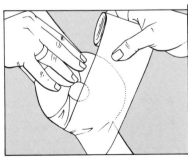

2. Work the bandage around the ring diagonally, passing the bandage under the limb and over the ring as shown until the ring is secured.

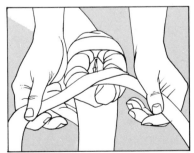

Improvisation In emergencies, use any suitable clean material. Here, a tie is being used to secure the ring.

BANDAGES AND DRESSINGS

Roller bandages can be used to keep dressings in place, support strains and sprains and to apply pressure to control bleeding. After applying a roller – or any other – bandage, always check the circulation to make sure the bandage is not tight enough to impede it. Normally, roller bandages are made of linen, cotton or gauze. Though they have standard lengths, they are available in various different widths to suit particular parts of the body. Check you have the correct width bandage before you start and also that the bandage is rolled tightly.

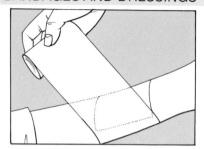

Applying a roller bandage
1. Place the free end of the bandage around the injury and wrap it around the limb once to secure the end.

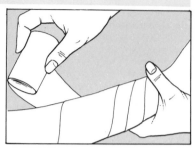

2. Work up the limb in a series of spirals, allowing each one to overlap the previous one by two-thirds. Finish with a straight turn. Secure the end.

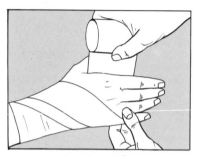

Bandaging hands and feet
1. Make a straight turn across the wrist and continue down. At the hand, pass between thumb and forefinger.

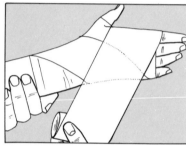

2. Criss-cross the bandage over the palm and back again, up to the root of the nail of the little finger. Bandage back to the wrist. Secure the end.

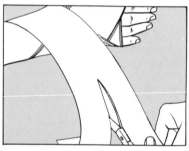

Securing the bandage Cut down the centre of the bandage to form two ribbons. Tie these off at the bottom and secure the ends with a reef knot.

Sterile unmedicated dressings are recommended by doctors as the best possible protection for large wounds and are available in a variety of shapes and sizes to suit various injuries. The dressings themselves consist of a cotton wool pad and layers of soft gauze, mounted on a roller bandage. As the name implies, they are factory sealed in protective wrappings; such a dressing should not be used if the seal is found to be damaged or broken. In an emergency, however, use any clean, dry, absorbent material as long as it is not fluffy, as strands can become embedded and cause infection.

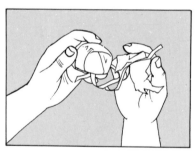

Applying a sterile dressing
1. Always wash your hands if possible. Release the dressing from the pack carefully, checking for damage.

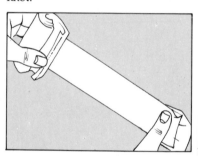

2. Hold the end of the bandage and the dressing in one hand and unwind a suitable length of the bandage with the other.

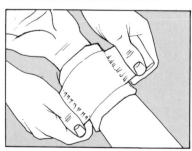

3. Place the dressing on the wound, gauze side down. Control its positioning by placing your thumbs on the edges; it should be central.

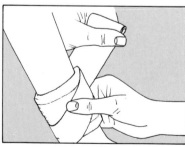

4. Wind the bandage around dressing and limb to secure the dressing. Continue bandaging until the dressing is covered as in the normal roller procedure.

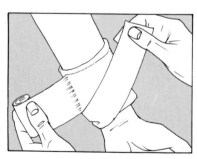

5. Secure the bandage by tying a reef knot. Check the circulation to make sure the bandage is not too tight.

continued from p376
people, however, they can cause an allergic response that requires immediate treatment. If this is the case, use the appropriate emergency technique (see pp370-375) and send for medical help. Otherwise:

ACTION – INSECT STINGS
1. If the sting is visible, remove it with a pair of tweezers
2. Apply anti-histamine cream to the sting or vinegar to a wasp or bee sting and soda solution to ant stings.
3. Try to prevent the casualty from scratching the sting – this only causes the poison to spread.

Snake bites demand prompt treatment. The American Rattlesnake and the European Adder, the only poisonous snake found in the wild in Britain, are both members of the 'Viper' family. Snakes of this type are shy and rarely bite unless in self-defence – when somebody has trodden on them, for example. The bite is painful, but the quantity of venom transferred by the bite is rarely large enough to make the injury fatal. The state of shock that normally results from a snake bite is often more dangerous than the venom.

Never attempt to suck poison from a bite or sting.

ACTION – SNAKE BITE
1. If possible, kill the snake. Preserve the body for later identification, so that the appropriate serum can be given
2. Lay the casualty on the ground
3. Calm and reassure the casualty, who will almost certainly be in a state of shock
4. Wash the wound and apply a dry dressing
5. Keep the casualty still – do not allow the casualty to walk
6. Treat for shock (see Emergency Techniques, p374)
7. Send for medical help.

BLEEDING See Cuts & scratches and Wounds & serious bleeding.

BLISTERS
A blister is a fluid-filled bubble that develops between two layers of the skin. It may be caused by a burn, sunburn, or by friction. Although a blister is a result of damage to the skin, it also has an important part to play in the healing process, protecting the underlying tissue and allowing regeneration to take place.

ACTION
1. Do not prick the blister or try to peel it off – in due course it will dry out and flake off
2. If the blistered area is likely to be

exposed to further damage, it should be covered with a dry dressing
See also Burns & Scalds.

BONES See next page

BREATHING FAILURE
See Emergency Techniques, pp370-375.

BRUISES
A bruise is the outward sign of bleeding beneath the skin as a result of pressure or a blow. Blood from damaged vessels seeps into the tissues, causing swelling, discoloration and soreness. The characteristic changes of skin colour at the site of a bruise are the result of the gradual degeneration of the components of blood.

ACTION
1. The flow of blood to the area of the bruise may be reduced by raising the injured part
2. Apply a cold compress – a clean cloth or towel soaked in cold water – or fill a plastic bag with ice cubes, wrap it in a towel and hold gently over the bruised area. Unless it is deep-frozen, steak will have no effect – cold water or ice is more economical
3. If there is a tendency to bruise very easily, or without discernible cause, consult a doctor

Black eye A bruise around the eye. The eye is extremely delicate, and a blow hard enough to have created a black eye may have caused more serious damage. In severe cases, or if there is any disturbance to vision, consult a doctor. Otherwise treat as above.

BURNS, SCALDS AND SUNBURN
Burns can be among the most serious of common accidents. They carry an associated risk of shock and infection for adults and children, but the dangers for babies and children are especially serious because of the proportionally larger area of skin affected by even a minor burn, and the increased severity of shock (see Emergency Techniques, p374. In all cases, other than for a small burn in an adult, medical attention is necessary. If burning is extensive, send for an ambulance immediately.

Burns, scalds and sunburn produce essentially the same effects. Burns may be caused by the sun, by heat, chemicals, electricity or friction, while scalds are, by definition, caused by hot liquids, such as cooking oil or steam.

Before treating electrical burns, ensure that the current has been turned off. The casualty is likely to be in a state of shock and may have

lost consciousness – immediate treatment of both of these problems (see Emergency Techniques) is the priority. Medical help is essential.

ACTION
1. Cool the area of the burn by placing it under a cold-water tap, or by immersing it in water. If this is not possible, as in the case of a chest burn, pour cold water over the area. Keep the burn in water for at least 10 minutes, or until the pain subsides
2. If the skin has been scalded and clothing over the scald is still warm, remove it – the heat the clothing retains may do further damage
3. If the clothing has been burnt, do not remove it. It will be sticking to the burn, and should only be removed by trained medical personnel
4. If the burn has been caused by chemicals, remove the clothing – chemicals that have soaked into the clothes may cause further damage. Remember to protect your own hands before touching the clothes
5. If the burn is large or deep, send for medical help, especially if the casualty is a baby or small child – while waiting for medical help, treat for shock (see Emergency Techniques, p374)
6. If the burn is not serious, apply a sterilized dressing. Do not use an adhesive dressing or plaster, which may stick to the affected area
7. Do not apply grease or ointment to a burn. It does not help; it will need to be cleaned off later and may increase the damage
8. Do not touch a burn or apply fluffy material such as cotton-wool to it: this will stick and increase the problem
9. Do not let the casualty move
10. Do not give alcohol, or hot tea. You may, however, give small sips of cold water – unless the casualty is unconscious, in which case give nothing
11. Do not prick blisters.

CAR ACCIDENT See Road Traffic Accident.

CHEMICAL BURNS See Burns & Scalds.

CHILDBIRTH See p.388.

CHOKING
The most common cause of choking is a physical obstruction to breathing – a particle of food or gulp of liquid that has 'gone down the wrong way'. In other words, the piece of food has been taken into the airway rather than the oesophagus, the tube that leads to the stomach.
continued p382

BONES—FRACTURES AND DISLOCATIONS

In an injury, bones may fracture or break, or they may become dislocated at the point where they meet in a joint. Of the two conditions, a fracture is potentially more serious, so, if there is any doubt, always treat the injury as a fracture.

There are four main types of fracture. The most serious is when the damaged bone has broken through the skin. In this type of injury, called an open, or compound, fracture, the risk of subsequent infection is high. If the skin is not broken, the fracture is said to be closed. If the bone is only partially broken, the injury is called a greenstick fracture. This type of fracture is usually seen only in teenagers and younger children, whose bones have a degree of flexibility that adult bones do not possess.

A joint is said to be dislocated when the bones articulating at the joint are displaced. There are two possible causes. A strong force, either direct or indirect, can wrench the bone involved out of its normal position into an abnormal one. Alternatively, the same result can be produced by a sudden muscular contraction.

Remember that broken bones and dislocations both require medical attention as soon as possible. If you can, seek medical help at once. Remember, too, that a casualty should not be moved more than necessary – ideally, not at all – until medical help arrives. Break this rule only if the casualty's life is at risk, if there is a danger of further injury – especially if the initial injury involves the back or neck – or if the casualty is in the open and exposed to severe weather.

ACTION
1. It is likely that a casualty has a fractured bone or joint if there is pain and swelling at the site of the injury, with discoloration of the skin. It will prove impossible to move or control the affected joint or limb without causing the casualty considerable pain, while there will be much tenderness at the site of the fracture, especially if gentle pressure is applied to the area involved. The casualty may be in a state of shock, or unconscious
2. Assess the situation. Deal with any breathing problems (*see Emergency Techniques, pp370-375*), severe bleeding (*see Wounds and serious bleeding*) and unconsciousness as the first priority
3. If the facture is open, protect the wound

4. Immobilize the injured part by securing it to a sound part of the body with bandages and padding. In some cases, particularly leg injuries, extra bandages and splints may be needed. Try to move an injured limb as little as possible during the process of immobilization. If this is unavoidable, grip either the hand or foot, depending on which is appropriate, and move the limb gently, but firmly, away from the body. Take care not to release the limb suddenly
5. If possible, raise the injured part slightly. This will reduce the flow of blood to it and so lessen pain and swelling
6. Loosen any constricting clothing and keep the casualty warm. Treat for shock if necessary (*see Emergency Techniques, p374*)
7 Do not offer the casualty anything to drink or eat. Medical treatment of the injury may necessitate a general anaesthetic
8. In the case of a dislocation, never try to put bones back into their normal positions
9. Seek medical help.

Lower arm injuries often involve the wrist, with considerable pain at the site of the fracture.

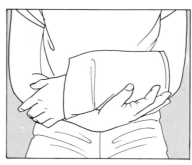

1. Support the injured limb by placing it across the casualty's chest. If forearm or wrist are involved, place some soft padding around them, plus padding between them and the chest.

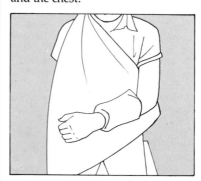

2. To fit a sling, support the injured arm, making sure that the wrist and

hand are slightly higher than the elbow. Take a triangular bandage and slide it between chest and forearm via the hollow between chest and elbow, so that one end lies over the shoulder of the sound arm. Take the bandage round the back of the neck to the front of the body on the injured side.

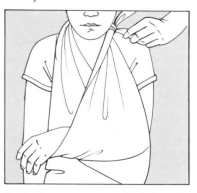

3. Continue to support the injured forearm and carry the bandage up over the affected area. Tie it off above the collar bone with a reef knot.

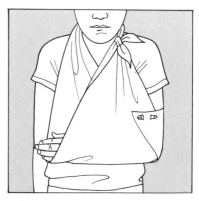

4. Secure the loose point at the elbow by pinning it to the front of the bandage with a safety pin. Check position and tightness.

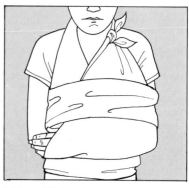

5. For additional support, secure the arm by placing a broad bandage over the sling and around the chest. Tie this on the uninjured side.

Elevation slings are necessary when it is important to raise and support the forearm and hand. Such slings should be used if the chest or shoulder is injured, or if the hand is wounded and bleeding.

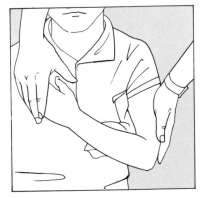

1. Get the casualty to support the injured limb and position the forearm across the chest, so that the fingertips are just below the opposite shoulder. Cradle the arm in a triangular bandage, easing the base of the bandage under the arm and carrying one end over the back to meet the other at the front of the uninjured shoulder.

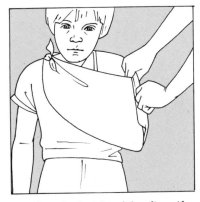

2. Adjust the height of the sling, if necessary, and tie the ends with a reef knot above the collar bone. Tuck the point in and secure it.

If the elbow is damaged and the arm is extended, never bend the arm, as you would to make a normal sling. This will not only cause the casualty further pain, but will also damage the tissue. Ask the casualty to lie down and place the injured arm by the side. Put padding between arm and side, then strap the former to the latter, using three broad bandages – one around the upper arm and trunk, one around the forearm and one around the wrist and thighs. The casualty should be moved only by stretcher.

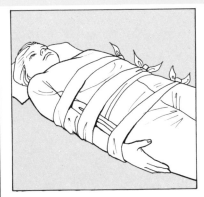

Leg injuries can involve both the tibia and fibula. Tibia fractures are often open, because the bone is covered only by a thin layer of skin and tissue. Fibula fractures often occur as the result of an ankle wrench and can be easily mistaken initially for a severely sprained ankle.

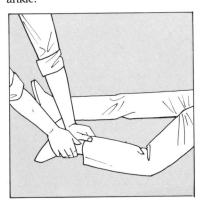

1. Support the limb and gently move it to alongside the undamaged one.

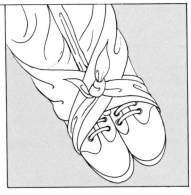

2. Place padding between knees and ankles and bandage the legs together, using a figure-of-eight bandage for the ankles and a broad bandage for the knees. Increase the number of bandages if necessary – one around the thighs, one around the lower legs and one below the fracture. Do not bandage over the fracture site.

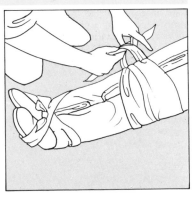

3. If a splint is to hand, place it alongside the injured leg. The splint should reach from crutch to foot. Use the padding and the five bandages, as described above, to secure legs and splint. Unless the leg swells around the ankles, keep the shoes on, as they help to support the injury.

Injuries to the thigh bone should be treated in the same way as other leg injuries, but require extra support. The injured thigh will probably be turned outwards; place the leg in its natural position by gripping the foot and moving the limb firmly, but gently. Place a splint alongside the inside of the injured leg and another, longer, one along the outside. This second splint should reach from the armpit to the foot. Secure this with two extra broad bandages, one around the pelvis in line with the hips and the other across the chest below the armpits. Bandage the legs as before, finishing off with a figure-of-eight bandage around the feet.

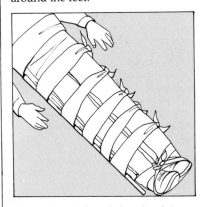

A casualty with an injured pelvis should not be moved, as there may be damage to the internal organs or to the spine. Ask the casualty not to urinate, then immobilize by placing padding between the legs and securing them as you would do for a leg injury. If possible, place two wide bandages around the hips.

BONES—FRACTURES AND DISLOCATIONS

With an ankle or foot injury, do not remove footwear, which gives support to the injured part, unless there is swelling. Keep weight off the damaged limb and support the foot from the knees down with cushions and pillows.

Knee-cap fractures occur when the small bone in the front of the knee breaks as a result of a blow or muscle strain.

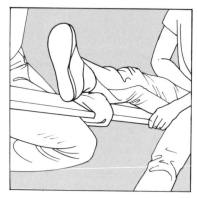

1. If the knee is bent, and cannot be straightened by the casualty, do not attempt to straighten it yourself. If the casualty can straighten his knee, raise and support the injured leg.

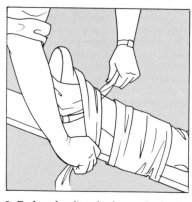

2. Pad and splint the leg at the back from thigh to ankle. Secure the splint with bandages above and below the knee, and with a figure-of-eight bandage around the feet as with a leg injury.

With a broken or dislocated jaw, remove any teeth or dentures that have been dislodged. If there are no other injuries, place the casualty in a sitting position with the head well forward; if the casualty has severe injuries (other than to the back or hip, in which case do not move), or is unconscious, place him in the recovery position (*see Emergency Techniques, p375*).

Support the jaw by means of a pad underneath the chin (*right*).

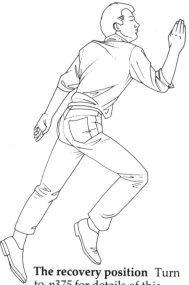

The recovery position Turn to *p375* for details of this technique.

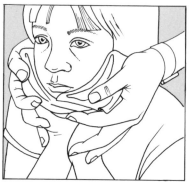

Either hold it in place by hand, or by means of a bandage tied on top of the head.

Dislocated shoulders and hips are Shoulders and hips are both 'ball and socket' joints and either may become dislocated when strong pressure forces the ball out of socket. Do not attempt to force the joint back into place. Support a dislocated shoulder in a sling and secure a dislocated hip joint in the same manner as a fractured pelvis. In both cases treat for shock (*see Emergency Techniques, p374*) and send for medical help.

Dislocated fingers are a common injury. The most frequent joint at which a finger dislocates is that nearest the palm of the hand. It is possible to reposition the joint yourself – pull the finger straight, apply a gentle but firm pressure away from the hand and slide the finger sideways until it clicks back into place. Do not use force. If the procedure is difficult or painful, stop immediately and seek medical advice.

continued from p379

If the airway is completely blocked, the casualty will be unable to breathe or to cough and will slowly turn blue. Loss of consciousness may follow. If the airway is partially blocked, the casualty will cough in spasms, in an attempt to dislodge the obstruction.

An attack of asthma may also cause the victim to choke, but the cause is not an obstruction. Muscles of the small bronchioles of the lungs go into spasm, so that no air can reach the point of gas exchange. A sufferer from asthma will normally carry an inhaler, or tablets, to relieve such an attack.

ACTION

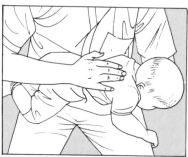

1. Babies Support chest and abdomen and smack gently between the shoulder blades

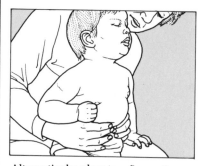

Alternatively, place two finger-tips together just above the navel as shown and press gently upwards

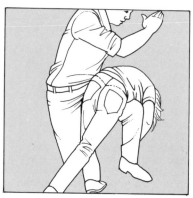

2. Children Lay face downwards across your knee and slap hard between the shoulder blades

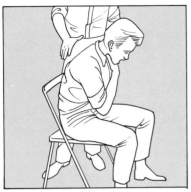

3. Adults Treat adults by leaning them forward and striking between shoulder blades.

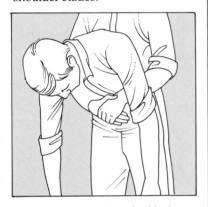

4. If this does not clear the blockage, stand behind the casualty with your arms clasped around his chest at the level of the lowest ribs. Lean the casualty's head forward and push your clasped hands strongly upwards into his chest. Repeat this procedure several times. This procedure can be used with children, but the pressure must be minimal
5. If this does not work, try to move the obstruction with your fingers. Take extreme care if using this method with a baby. Only use it if you can see the obstruction and there is no risk of pushing it further downwards
6. If this fails, send for medical help
7. After recovery, check pulse and breathing and treat for shock (see *Emergency Techniques, p374*) if necessary.

COLD AND CHILLING
Prolonged exposure to low temperatures may lead to a dangerous and a progressive drop in body temperature, particularly in the old or very young – the condition is known as hypothermia. The casualty may gradually slide into stupor, unconsciousness, and finally death.

Babies become quiet and lose their appetite. The chest and stomach will feel cold, but the hands, feet and face may look pink.

Adults become sluggish and confused. Mental and physical processes are impaired while the skin looks pale, and sometimes bluish. The sufferer may lose consciousness: breathing will be shallow and the pulse weak.

ACTION—BABIES
For babies, immediate medical help is required. Meanwhile you can help by warming the baby with your own body heat. Get into bed with the child and snuggle round him. The gradual warmth of skin-to-skin contact will begin to relieve the problem.

ACTION—ADULTS
1. First prevent further heat loss, then gradually restore the normal temperature. Send for medical help
2. If the casualty is outside, provide any shelter you can, wrap the casualty in blankets or use your own body warmth to warm him
3. If the casualty is young, place him in a warm bath and give him a warm, sweet drink. Do not give a bath if the casualty is elderly
4. If the casualty is old, place him in warm surroundings, give him a warm, sweet drink and wrap him in warm clothes and blankets
5. Do not give elderly casualties hot water bottles or electric blankets – blood will surge away from the vital organs and heart failure may result
6. Do not give alcohol.

COMA *See Unconsciousness.*

CONCUSSION *See Head Injuries.*

CONVULSIONS
Convulsions are uncontrollable fits of muscle spasm, in which the limbs twitch, the eyes roll and there may be loss of consciousness. In babies they are sometimes caused by heatstroke or associated with a high fever; in adults, epilepsy is the usual cause, though convulsions may be seen after a drug overdose.

In babies and small children, any convulsion lasting for more than two or three minutes or in which breathing stops should be considered a medical emergency. Send for medical help immediately. The symptoms are twitching limbs; rolling eyes; a red, congested face; frothy spit; and an arched back with the breath held.

The most common cause of a convulsion in an adult is epilepsy. There are two forms of epilepsy, known as 'petit mal' and 'grand mal'. The symptoms of petit mal are lack of awareness of surroundings and pallor, with fixed and staring eyes; on recovery, the sufferer has no recollection of the event. It is rare to see convulsions in petit mal.

In grand mal, the sufferer may be warned of an impending attack by an 'aura' and so be able to take steps to minimize its effects. Nevertheless there may be loss of consciousness, with rigidity and the twitching of limbs; the sufferer may bite his tongue, producing frothy, blood-stained spittle as a result; he may lose control of his bladder and bowel functions.

ACTION – BABIES
1. There is no effective First Aid treatment for a child who is having convulsions
2. Stay with the child, and make sure that he does not injure himself on any sharp object. Cool the child if there is a high fever
3. Loosen any tight clothing and make sure that he has plenty of air
4. Do not attempt to restrain the casualty
5. Do not put anything in the casualty's mouth in an attempt to stop him biting his tongue
6. After the fit has passed, lay the casualty in the recovery position (see *Emergency Techniques p375*)
7. Send for medical help.

ACTION – ADULTS
1. If possible, loosen tight clothing
2. Do not try to restrain the casualty
3. Do not try and insert anything in the casualty's mouth in order to prevent him from biting his tongue
4. Stay with the casualty and protect him from injury
5. When the casualty has relaxed, wipe the froth from his mouth and check the airway for vomit or any other obstruction
6. Place the casualty in the recovery position (see *Emergency Techniques, p375*)
7. Make sure that clean clothing is available when the casualty recovers consciousness
8. Make sure that the casualty consults his doctor.

CORONARY *See Heart Attack*

CRAMP
A prolonged and painful contraction of a muscle caused by a lack of salt and body fluids. Cramp may result from vigorous exercise, sweating, diarrhoea, vomiting or low temperature, and is often experienced at night.

ACTION
1. Stretch the affected muscle as much as possible by straightening it – if there is cramp in the back of the calf, place one hand on the heel and the other on the toes. Push the foot
continued p386

CHILDBIRTH

It is extremely unlikely that you will ever have to deliver a baby and unwise to attempt to do so, unless medical help is totally unavailable. The following techniques are for use only in the event of such an emergency.

Remember, above all, that childbirth is a natural event, so your aim should be to interfere with the natural process of birth as little as possible. Before you attempt to do anything yourself, you should contact the emergency services and ask for an ambulance. Give as many details as you can about the pregnancy as clearly as possible.

The first stage of labour normally begins with the mother-to-be complaining of a low back ache or pain. This is accompanied by a discharge of blood-stained mucus from the vagina. This indicates that the birth canal has cleared ready for birth and that the cervix has dilated.

The first contractions of labour now commence, moving down the abdomen like a wave every 10 to 20 minutes.

The contractions occur naturally and the mother should not attempt to add to their force. Encourage her, however, to empty her bladder and bowels at an early stage, if she has not done so already. The process may continue for some time – up to 24 hours in the case of a first child, but, on average, around 10 hours in subsequent pregnancies. All that can be done at this stage is to get the mother to lie down and reassure her.

Towards the end of the first stage, however, the contractions gradually speed up and become more painful. There will also be a sudden discharge of clear fluid from the vagina – either in a sudden burst, or a constant trickle. This, the 'breaking of the waters', is perfectly normal. It means that the sac surrounding the baby in the womb has broken. Dry off the fluid gently with a clean towel.

The second stage of labour follows the 'breaking of the waters'. The contractions speed up, until they occur every two minutes or so. Their force also increases and the mother feels an irresistible urge to push down and strain with them. As the baby is now on the way, this should not now be discouraged. The second stage lasts, on average, for an hour for a first baby and slightly less for subsequent ones. It is now the mother needs your help.

ACTION – DELIVERY
1. Support the mother with pillows so that she is in a sitting position
2. Bring her legs up and ask her to grasp her knees

PREPARING FOR BIRTH

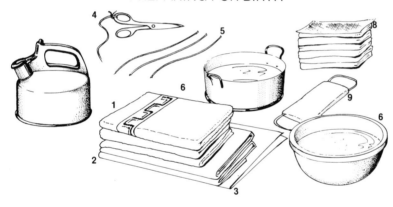

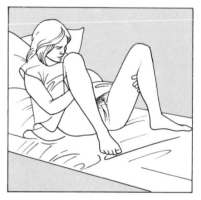

3. Ask her to bend her head forward with each contraction
4. As each contraction passes, encourage her to lie back and relax
5. As each contraction begins, the mother should breathe in, out, and in again and hold her breath. This exercise, which she will have practised at ante-natal classes, adds to the strength of the contraction
6. If the mother has an involuntary bowel movement, clean the area, wiping away from the birth canal
7. Constantly reassure and encourage the mother
8. In a normal delivery, the crown of the baby's head will appear at the entrance to the birth canal, receding between contractions with more of the baby appearing with each subsequent contraction. Birth is now imminent.
9. Ask the mother to stop pushing and pant vigorously instead. If birth is hurried, there may be damage to the mother's tissues
10. The mother may push gently between contractions
11. As the head emerges, support it gently in the palm of your hand, as it must not be allowed to emerge

Your first task is to keep the mother calm, so you must remain calm yourself. Remember that birth takes time; there is no need to panic. You will need the following items:
1. A soft, clean towel or blanket in which to wrap the new-born baby.
2. Another clean sheet, blanket, or some towels to cover the top part of the mother's body. You should ask her to remove any clothes that make her feel uncomfortable; the sheet will thus help her to keep warm
3. A clean sheet – preferably waterproof – to cover the surface on which the mother will lie
4. A pair of scissors to cut the umbilical cord. These should be sterilized in boiling water for 10 minutes. It is useful to tie string to the handles, so the scissors can be easily removed
5. Three pieces of thin string, each 23 cm (9 in) long. Sterilize these, too, for 10 minutes
6. Two basins or bowls of water that

has been boiled for cleaning purposes. Keep these covered until they are needed
7. Some cloths or swabs. These will be needed to clean the mother and the baby's face
8. Sterile gauze
9. Sanitary towels, sterilized dressings.

If you do not have all the right materials, improvise. Remember everything you use must be scrupulously clean. Lack of hygiene means the risk of infection, which will endanger the lives of both mother and baby. Keep anyone with a sore throat or a cold well away. Wear a surgical mask, or improvise one with a clean handkerchief. Scrub your hands, nails and forearms thoroughly under a jet of running hot water for four minutes before delivery starts. Do not dry your hands. Repeat the process as necessary during delivery.

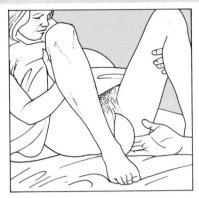

suddenly. Do not try to pull the
head out of the canal

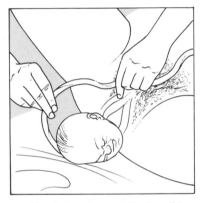

12. Check that the umbilical cord is
not around the baby's neck. If it is,
gently ease it over the neck. Do not
pull on the cord

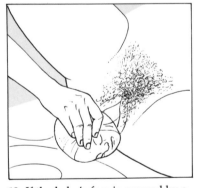

13. If the baby's face is covered by a
membrane, part it and pull it off
gently with your fingers. The
membrane could stop the baby
breathing
14. The baby will now slide out of
the birth canal. Do not try to pull the
baby out. Support it under the
armpits. Do not pull on the
umbilical cord
15. The baby will be slippery, so grip
the ankles with a cloth and lift
gently, holding it upside down for a
few moments. Use your other hand
to wipe any blood and mucus away
from its face. Open the mouth

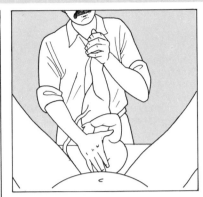

16. At this stage, most babies cry. If
not – and there is no sign of
breathing – blow gently into the
mouth and nose. Watch the chest to
see if breathing starts; if nothing
happens, check that the airway is
not blocked by mucus. If it is, place
a piece of gauze over the mouth and
nose, place your mouth over the
gauze and suck the mucus out. Start
artificial respiration, if necessary.
Never smack the baby

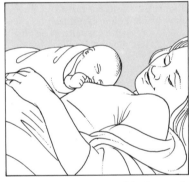

17. Wrap the baby in a blanket and
place it on the mother's abdomen.
Take care not to pull the umbilical
cord – this is still attached to the
mother. Let the baby suck at the
breast, if the mother feels able to
suckle it
The third stage of delivery involves
dealing with the afterbirth. This is
expelled from the womb by mild
contractions some 10 to 30 minutes
after delivery has been completed.

ACTION – AFTERBIRTH
1. Wait for the placenta to separate
from the womb. When the
contractions indicate this is
imminent, get the mother to put her
knees up and apart, hold her breath
and push. Do not pull at the
placenta or umbilical cord
2. Keep the placenta intact and do
not throw it away. A doctor must
check that it is complete, as
otherwise the mother may face
complications later
3. Do not cut the umbilical cord,

unless there is no prospect of
medical help for some time. If this is
the case, tie the pieces of string you
prepared earlier around the cord
10 cm (4 in), 15 cm (6 in) and 20 cm
(8 in) from the baby's navel. Knot

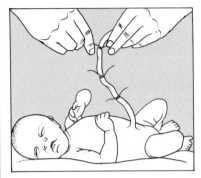

the pieces of string firmly, especially
the one nearest the baby. If this is
not tightly tied, the baby could bleed
to death when the cord is cut

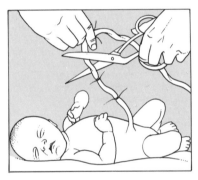

4. Using the sterilized scissors, cut
the cord between the two pieces of
string further from the baby's navel.

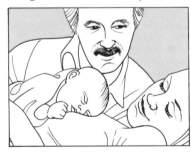

Dress the cut end with a sterilized
dressing and secure it by tying a
folded nappy cloth around the baby.
Check for bleeding after a few
minutes
5. Clean up the mother, make her
comfortable and encourage her to
relax. Place a sanitary towel or clean
cloth over the vagina, as it is normal
for a small amount of bleeding to
occur at this stage. If this looks
severe, massage the abdomen just
below the navel to encourage the
womb to contract. Continue the
massage until medical help arrives.

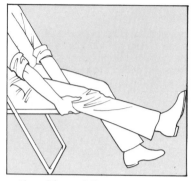

continued from p383
as far towards the front of the leg as you can
2. Once the muscle has started to relax, massage it vigorously
3. A drink of slightly-salted water may help to stop the cramp returning.

CUTS AND SCRATCHES
Minor cuts and scratches rarely need medical attention. Blood clots form quickly in a healthy person, and the small flow of blood before the cut seals helps to carry away most of the dirt. You should, however, make sure that anybody who has been cut or grazed by anything dirty, or who has been in contact with the soil or an animal, consults a doctor – an anti-tetanus injection may be necessary.
See also Wounds and serious bleeding.

ACTION
1. Wash your hands
2. Remove any obvious dirt, grit or foreign body from the cut
3. Cleanse the cut, using gauze or sterilized cotton-wool moistened in a little diluted disinfectant and working away from the cut
4. Dry the wound carefully and apply the appropriate dressing
5. Do not apply antiseptic creams, as these only seal in dirt and germs
6. If the cut oozes pus, or is sore and inflamed, consult your doctor.

DIABETIC EMERGENCY
Sufferers from diabetes are unable to absorb sufficient sugar from their diets because they are deficient in the hormone insulin. To live a normal life, they must take insulin or drugs regularly and control their sugar intake carefully.
  Occasionally, an error is made, or regulation becomes impossible. Lack of sugar, or an excess of insulin may suddenly lead to an insulin coma (hypoglycaemic coma), whose symptoms are confusion, shock, and loss of consciousness. Alternatively, a lack of insulin and an excess of sugar may lead to a diabetic coma (hyperglycaemic coma) whose symptoms are a more gradual onset,

flushed dry skin; breath that smells like nail-varnish remover, and loss of consciousness.

ACTION
1. Send for medical help immediately
2. If the casualty is conscious and confirms that he has diabetes and that he lacks sugar, give him something sugary to eat or drink
3. If the patient is unconscious, treat accordingly – *see Unconsciousness*
4. Do not give sugar to an unconscious diabetic – there is a strong chance that you will make his condition worse.

DISLOCATION *See Bones.*

DISORIENTATION *See Mental Disturbance.*

DROWNING
Anyone who is in difficulties in water may be drowning, or about to drown. If you are a good swimmer, and have been trained in life-saving techniques, attempt a rescue. If you know that the water is shallow and safe, wade out to the casualty. Otherwise, mark his position, throw a line or life-belt and get help.
  As soon as the casualty is on dry land, or has reached shallow water in which it is safe to do so, start artificial respiration (*see Emergency Techniques, pp370-375*).

ACTION
1. If the casualty is breathing, coughing, choking or vomiting, get him out of the water and place him in the recovery position
2. If the casualty is not breathing, but still in the water, start artificial respiration as quickly as possible. Do not worry about water in the lungs. It is generally easier to use the mouth-to-nose method
3. If necessary, empty the lungs of water by turning the casualty face down and compressing the whole chest. Gravity can also be used by forcing the casualty's head down.
4. If the casualty is not breathing *see Emergency Techniques, pp370-375*.
5. Once breathing is restored, place the casualty in the recovery position, treat for shock and hypothermia.
6. Send for medical help. The casualty must go to hospital.

DRUG OVERDOSE *See Poisoning.*

DRUNKENNESS *See Alcohol.*

EAR INJURIES
Foreign bodies in the ear can cause temporary deafness and, if they penetrate deeply, can damage the eardrum. Symptoms include pain

and impaired hearing.
  Never poke anything into the ear in an attempt to dislodge a suspected foreign body – such probing may perforate the eardrum. Try pouring warm oil or water into the ear drop-by-drop, with the head tilted away from you. After a few minutes, tilt the head towards you. As the oil or water runs out, it may bring the foreign body with it. If this fails, consult a doctor.

ELECTRIC SHOCK
Do not touch a casualty who has had an electric shock until you are sure that the electric current has been switched off.
  If this proves impossible, push the casualty away from the source of the current with something that is non-conductive – anything made of rubber, cloth or dry wood. A rolled-up newspaper, or even the casualty's own clothing, if it is dry, will prevent the transmission of the current to your own body. This should be attempted only if ordinary domestic current is the source of the shock. If the casualty is in contact with a high-voltage supply, such as an electricity pylon, do not attempt first aid. Summon medical help immediately and notify the police.

ACTION

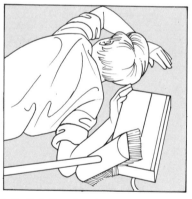

1. Switch the electric current off, or move the casualty from the source of the current
2. Follow the standard procedures for emergency resuscitation (*see Emergency Techniques, p370-375*)
3. Treat for shock
4. Check the casualty for burns and treat accordingly (*see Burns and Scalds*).

EPILEPSY *See Convulsions.*

EXPOSURE *See Cold & Chilling.*

EYE INJURIES *See facing box.*

FAINTING
A temporary reduction in the supply of blood to the brain will cause a

temporary loss of consciousness. The reason for this may be a shock, fright or exhaustion, suddenly standing up (especially after a hot bath) or a long period of standing still.

Often the casualty feels faint before actually becoming unconscious – he becomes dizzy, starts sweating and his face becomes pale. At this stage a faint may be avoided if you sit the casualty down and place his head between his knees.

ACTION

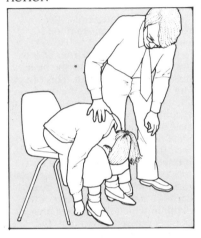

1. Lay the casualty gently on the ground, raise his legs and support them

2. Loosen any tight clothing and make sure that the casualty has plenty of air

3. If the casualty appears to have difficulty in breathing, place him in the recovery position *(see Emergency Techniques, p375)*

4. When the casualty regains consciousness, reassure him, then give small sips of cold water, and then a hot, sweet drink when he has fully recovered. Do not give alcohol

5. If the casualty is unconscious for more than two or three minutes, treat as for unconsciousness – *see Unconsciousness.*

FALLS *See Unconsciousness, Head Injuries, Bones.*

FINGERS AND TOES
An injury to a finger or toe – when, for example, a finger is trapped in a car door, or something heavy is dropped on to a toe – can be extremely painful. There may be bleeding under the nail and swelling; eventually the nail may drop off.

ACTION
1. Put the finger or toe under the cold-water tap. This will help to reduce the swelling

continued p388

EYE INJURIES

The eye is an extremely sensitive instrument, so all eye injuries are potentially serious. As well as the pain and inflammation such injuries cause, there is always the chance that the eyeball will be penetrated, so increasing the risk of possible infection. The commonest cause of injury is a foreign body in the eye. Dust, grit and loose eyelashes can all adhere to the surface of the eyeball or get caught under the eyelid; blows or flying fragments of glass, metal and grit can cut or bruise the surface of the eye.

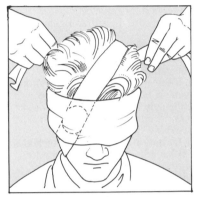

An eye that has been torn, punctured or damaged by a blow should be protected with a sterile eye pad, secured by a bandage. The pad will help absorb the blood and fluid that may leak from the wound, as well as protecting the injury from infection. Keep the sound eye still, since moving it will cause the injured eye to move, so exacerbating the injury. Seek immediate medical help.

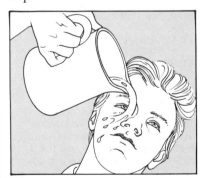

To deal with chemical damage, flush the eye with clean, cold water for at least 15 minutes. It may be necessary to hold the eye open, or for the casualty to place the head in water and blink continuously. Cover the eye with an eyepad and get medical help. Do not apply eye ointment.

If there is a foreign body in the eye, ask the casualty not to rub it. Sit the

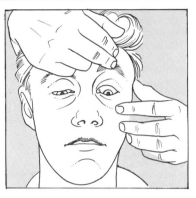

casualty in a chair facing a light and tilt the head back. Standing behind the casualty, steady the head with one hand and separate the lids of the affected eye with the other. Examine the eye carefully. When you locate the body, wash the eye

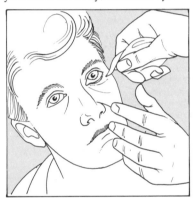

out with clean water, or use a moistened swab or the corner of a handkerchief to remove it. If it is embedded, seek medical help.

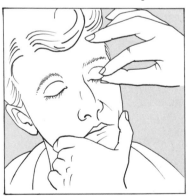

If the foreign body is trapped under the upper lid, ask the casualty to look down, rather than up. Take hold of the eyelashes and pull the eyelid downwards and outwards, so that the lashes can brush the object away. If this fails, try blinking the eye under water to float the object off it.

continued from p387
2. Give domestic painkillers
3. Consult your doctor – he may make a small hole in the nail to release the pressure
4. If the injury looks serious enough for it to be likely that the nail will eventually fall off, put a plaster round it. This will reduce the possibility of the nail being pulled off accidentally, and allow time for the nail to grow back underneath.

FISH-HOOKS
A fish-hook lodged in the skin is best removed by a doctor. However, in an emergency, you may need to remove one yourself. A pair of pliers will be necessary.

ACTION

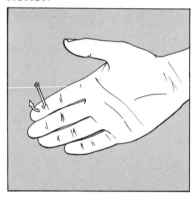

1. Push the hook through the skin so that the barb can be seen

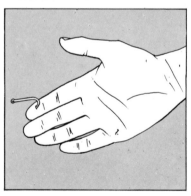

2. Cut the barb off with a pair of pliers
3. Pull the remainder of the hook back through the flesh and out through the point of entry
4. Wash the wound thoroughly with soap and water, and watch for signs of infection over the next few days
5. Apply a dressing, and keep an eye on the casualty in case of shock (*see Emergency Techniques, p375*).

FITS *See Convulsions.*

FOOD POISONING
Acute abdominal pain often accompanies an attack of food poisoning. The sufferer may suddenly feel ill, and almost immediately experience pain, diarrhoea and vomiting.

In mild cases the poisonous food passes through the system and the problem clears up quickly, but, even so, weakness and tiredness may persist. Rest is advisable.

ACTION
1. Do not leave a person who is vomiting alone, and, using the appropriate emergency technique, make sure that the airway is clear so that vomit cannot be inhaled
2. Do not give the casualty any medicines unless they have been prescribed by a doctor
3. Make sure the sufferer gets plenty of rest
4. If possible, save a sample of the food that you suspect is the cause of poisoning for examination
5. If the symptoms persist for more than six hours, or appear to be unusually serious, call for medical help – persistent vomiting and diarrhoea may lead to severe dehydration, a condition which is particularly dangerous for children and the elderly.
See also Poisoning.

FOREIGN BODIES
Foreign bodies – particles of dust, grit, insects or indeed anything that is not naturally a part of the human body – may be swallowed, inhaled or become lodged in the eyes, ears nose or any other orifice.

To deal with swallowed or inhaled objects, *see Choking*, with foreign bodies in the ear, *see Ear injuries* and with foreign bodies in the eye, *see Eye injuries*. Never attempt to remove foreign bodies from the nose. Send for medical help.

FRACTURES *See Bones.*

FROSTBITE *See Cold & Chilling.*

GAS
Some types of gas are deadly poisons, but others are not. All gases likely to be encountered in domestic first aid, however, are highly inflammable. Never use a naked flame in the vicinity of gas.

ACTION
1. If the casualty is lying in a gas-filled room, open all doors and open or break windows
2. If another person is present, tell him to wait outside in case you are overcome by the gas (if possible, tie one end of a rope around your waist and leave the other end with him). Take several deep breaths, hold the last and enter the room
3. Carry the casualty out of the room and place him gently on the ground in the recovery position (*p375*)
4. Follow standard emergency procedures (*see Emergency Techniques pp370-375*)
5. Summon medical help and notify the police.

HAEMORRHAGE *See Cuts & Scratches, Wounds & serious bleeding.*

HEAD INJURIES
After a blow to the head, a casualty may lose consciousness, have concussion, suffer from compression or suffer from a combination of all these problems. Head injuries can be extremely dangerous, so immediate medical attention is essential.

Concussion results from a blow strong enough to shake the brain around inside the skull. This can be the result of a blow to the head, on the point of the jaw, or a fall from a height. The casualty may become pale and clammy and breathe shallowly. Consciousness may be lost, though not necessarily immediately, and there may be a loss of memory.

Sometimes a blow to the head causes a depressed fracture of the skull, in which the affected area of bone is pressed down onto the tissue of the brain. This is compression, an extremely serious condition, which can develop as long as two days after the casualty has apparently fully recovered from the initial accident.

Immediate medical help is essential. The casualty will have a flushed face, noisy breathing and one or both of his pupils will be dilated. He will lose consciousness, but not necessarily immediately.

ACTION
1. Maintain breathing, using the appropriate method of artificial respiration, if necessary (*see Emergency Techniques pp370-375*).
2. If the casualty is breathing normally, place him in the recovery position. The body should be laid on the appropriate side so that any fluid released by the injury can drain from the ear
3. Keep a constant watch on the casualty's breathing and be prepared to start or restart artificial respiration at any time
4. Send for medical help.

HEATSTROKE
Prolonged exposure to the heat of the sun, especially in young children, may affect the body's temperature-controlling mechanisms, causing heatstroke. The symptoms are a temperature of 40°C (104°F); flushed, dry skin:

vomiting, sometimes a loss of consciousness. The problem can usually be avoided by limiting exposure to the sun, wearing a sun hat, and by increasing the intake of fluid and salt.

ACTION

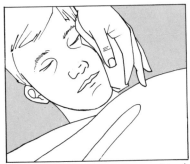

1. Strip the casualty and wrap him in a cold, wet sheet in order to bring down body temperature
2. If the casualty is unconscious, place him in the recovery position (*see p375*)
3. Try to create a current of air around the casualty by fanning
4. Take the temperature regularly. Once it has fallen replace the wet sheet with a dry one. Keep checking the temperature in case it starts to rise
5. Send for medical help.

HERNIA

A hernia, or rupture, occurs when the muscles and tissues of the abdominal wall have become so weakened that a part of the intestine protrudes through the wall. This process may take place gradually, or suddenly without warning.

The swelling may be painless, but sometimes causes severe discomfort and vomiting. Occasionally the piece of intestine is strangled by the pressure of the muscles surrounding it. This is an extremely serious condition and requires immediate treatment.

ACTION
1. Do not attempt to reduce the swelling under any circumstances
2. Lay the casualty gently on the ground
3. If the casualty vomits, place him in the recovery position (*see p375*)
4. Send for medical help.

HEART ATTACK

Heart attacks occur when the heart stops pumping. This can happen as the result of the death of a section of heart muscle, or the blockage of one of the arteries supplying the heart muscle with blood. The severity of heart attacks may vary; in mild cases, sometimes the victim is not aware that he has suffered an attack.

If, however, the heart attack is serious, the casualty will suffer from the following symptoms at various stages. These are a sudden constricting pain in the chest; an ashen-grey or bluish-grey face; bluish lips; closed eyes (if the eyelids are opened, pupils will be unnaturally large); no pulse; loss of consciousness; cessation of breathing.

Immediate action is essential, so emergency first aid should be started at once (*see Emergency Techniques pp370-375*). Remember, however, never to start heart massage if you can detect a pulse, no matter how weak this is. It is also worth noting that a constricting pain in the chest, which may spread into the jaw and left arm, can be the forerunner of a heart attack. The pain is sometimes associated with pallor, blue lips and a clammy skin, and is brought on by exertion or excitement.

This condition is known as angina pectoris. The casualty may have suffered from angina before and carry tablets to control it. Check to see if this is the case, then send for medical help.

HICCUPS

Hiccups, repetitive spasms of the diaphragm that cause a gulp of breath to be taken, are rarely a serious problem, but can cause considerable discomfort. If they persist for more than an hour, or are a frequent occurrence, you should consult your doctor – they may be a sign of a more serious problem.

Everybody seems to have their own cure for hiccups. Among the most common are drinking a glass of water and holding the breath with a finger in each ear. One or either of these methods will work on most occasions, but a new technique is at present undergoing medical trials in America. The early signs are encouraging. Cut a small wedge of fresh lemon, soak it in Angostura Bitters, then swallow the wedge quickly.

HYPOTHERMIA *See Cold & Chilling.*

KISS-OF-LIFE *See Emergency Techniques p370.*

LOSS OF CONSCIOUSNESS *See Unconsciousness*

MENTAL DISTURBANCE

It is almost impossible for a layman to know whether or not a casualty is suffering from mental disturbance. Send for medical help.

In the case of a person who looks likely to attempt suicide, you can help as long as you are sure that you

are in no danger. You should, of course, send for professional assistance as soon as it is practical to do so. However, you can make a valuable contribution if you keep the potential suicide talking. Stay calm and confident, and concentrate on listening sympathetically.

MUSCLE STRAIN

An injury to a muscle in which the muscle fibres are stretched or torn. Otherwise known as a 'pulled muscle', the injury is a common sports hazard.

The symptoms of muscle strain include a sudden, sharp pain associated with a loss of power in the muscle and tenderness.

ACTION
1. Make sure that the casualty has no other injury, such as a bone fracture
2. Gently massage the injured muscle. This will help to relieve pain

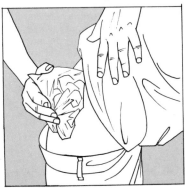

3. As soon as possible after the injury, apply ice to the affected muscle

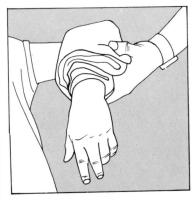

4. Later, apply heat – a hot towel or a hot bath will help
5. If in doubt, or if the injury seems serious, treat it as a fracture and send for medical help.

NOSEBLEEDS

Nosebleeds may be directly caused by a blow or by illness, but also can occur spontaneously as the result of a ruptured small blood vessel in the nasal cavity. Some people are more prone to nosebleeds than others, but the condition is not caused by high blood pressure.

ACTION

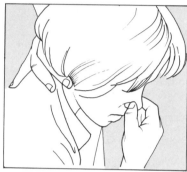

1. Ask the casualty to lean his head forwards not backwards, and pinch his nostrils together
2. Have a bowl handy to catch any blood that may escape
3. The nosebleed should stop after about 10 minutes – if it does not, repeat the procedure above, and apply an ice pack or cold compress to the nose
4. If this does not work, seek the advice of a doctor, who may decide to cauterize the nasal blood vessels.

OVERDOSE *see Poisoning.*

PAIN *See Abdominal Pain.*

POISONING

Poisoning is usually the result of swallowing, inhaling or injecting an injurious agent. Some poisons act directly on the digestive system, others are first absorbed into the body and then act on the nervous system. The latter are more dangerous, because the effects are not immediately visible. In both cases prompt treatment is extremely important.

ACTION

1. Send for medical help
2. If the casualty is conscious, or the evidence is at hand, try to identify the drug or poison and, again if possible, keep a specimen of it for the doctor
3. Wipe any of the drug or poison away from the casualty's mouth and lips
4. If you establish that the substance was corrosive, as in the case of an acid, try to dilute it as much as possible by giving the casualty water or milk. Do not force liquids on to an unconscious casualty
5. Do not try to make the casualty sick in cases of corrosive poisoning
6. If the casualty is conscious and can confirm that the poison was not

corrosive, make him vomit—stick your finger down his throat and wiggle them around until he is sick. Make sure that no vomit is inhaled
7. Never try to induce vomiting with emetics such as a salt solution
8. If the casualty is unconscious, or loses consciousness, place him in the recovery position, check that the airway is clear and be ready to give artificial respiration (*see Emergency Techniques pp370-375*).

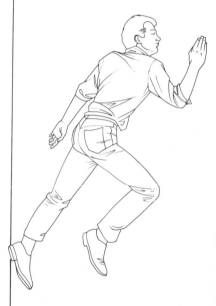

PULLED MUSCLE *See Muscle Strain.*

ROAD TRAFFIC ACCIDENT

At the scene of a road traffic accident, your first priority must be to ensure that your actions do not lead to further accidents. Follow the procedures below carefully.

ACTION

1. Stop your car – or a passing car, if you are on foot – in a safe place. Dim the headlamps and point them at the scene of the accident. Switch on hazard-warning lights. Put out any cigarettes in case there is escaping petrol
2. Place a red warning-triangle 50 paces back down the road from the scene of the accident, in a place where it can be seen by oncoming drivers
3. If possible, clear any debris from the road
4. Approach the scene of the accident and switch off the engine of any car involved
5. Check the victims. Do not move them unless there is imminent danger of fire or explosion
6. Treat the most seriously injured victim first (*see Emergency Techniques, pp370-375*)
7. Unless emergency treatment is required by any other casualty, tell

the next passer-by to find a telephone, call the emergency services and ask for 'ambulance'. The location of the accident, the number of casualties involved and their situation should be relayed clearly and precisely
8. Continue treating the casualties until help arrives
9. Do not give alcohol or any stimulants. Do not smoke or use naked lights.

RUPTURE *See Hernia.*

SCALDS *See Burns & Scalds.*

SLIPPED DISC *See Back injuries.*

SPRAIN

A sprain is the result of a tear or an over-stretching of the ligaments surrounding and supporting a joint. The joint is painful, cannot support weight and starts to swell – after a while bruises may appear.

ACTION

1. Lie the casualty down gently. Raise the affected joint and support it with cushions or a pillow
2. Remove any clothing covering the joint and apply an ice pack or cold compress for a few minutes
3. Bandage the joint. Check the bandage at intervals and loosen it if swelling continues
3. If the sprain seems serious, or there is any possibility of a fracture, treat it as you would a bone fracture and send for medical help.

STINGS *See Bites & Stings.*

STOMACH PAIN *See Abdominal Pain.*

STRAIN *See Muscle Strain.*

SUFFOCATION *See Emergency Techniques, pp370-375.*

SUNBURN *See Burns & Scalds.*

UNCONSCIOUSNESS

Unconsciousness can occur for many reasons. When treating an unconscious casualty, always remember two points. Never try to force drink down the throat of an unconscious casualty in a misguided attempt to bring him round. Never leave a casualty who is unconscious on his own, except to obtain medical help. Return to the casualty as quickly as you can.

ACTION

1. Follow standard emergency routines (*see pp370-375*)
2. Make sure that any casualty consults his doctor, even if he recovers naturally.

WOUNDS AND SERIOUS BLEEDING

Wounds are divided into two categories – open, when blood escapes from the body, and closed, when blood escapes internally from the circulatory system. In the latter case, there may be no visible signs of bleeding, with the exception of bruises under the skin in some instances.

In all cases, the priority is to stop the bleeding as soon as possible. Continuous blood loss can lead to death. The body will be taking its own steps to help you in your task, as the blood-clotting factors work to clot the blood, while the blood pressure drops to restrict the blood flow. Always seek medical help.

There are several types of open wound, incisions, lacerations, grazes and contusions among them. Treat as below, except for special cases.

ACTION

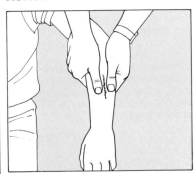

1. Apply direct pressure to a large wound to stop the bleeding by squeezing the sides of the wound together firmly with your fingers. Alternatively, place a dressing or towel on the wound and apply pressure. Keep this pressure up for 15 minutes, or until the flow of blood decreases and a clot begins to form. Do not apply pressure to a scalp wound in case of a skull fracture. Bandage it and wait for medical help.

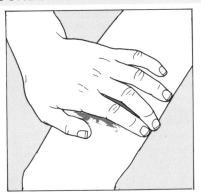

2. If the wound is small enough, you may be able to deal with the bleeding by simply placing your fingers over the wound and applying firm pressure.

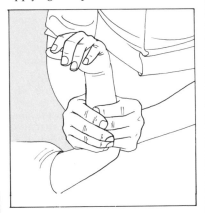

3. If possible, lay the casualty down, raise the injured part of the body as high as possible, support it and continue to maintain the pressure. Elevation helps to slow down the flow of blood by reducing the blood pressure. Never apply a tourniquet or rubber bandage to restrict the blood supply, for the body tissues could be seriously damaged. It is important to interfere as little as possible with the rest of the circulation while stopping bleeding.

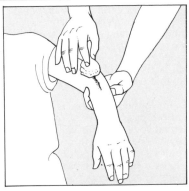

4. Again if possible, clean the edges of the wound after the bleeding has stopped and before bandaging it. The aim is to remove loose dirt, which could cause infection, but it is vital not to disturb the blood clot which will have formed. Use a swab and warm water.

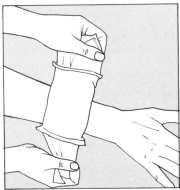

5. Apply a sterile unmedicated dressing to the wound, making sure it extends well beyond the wound's edges. Press it down firmly and secure it with a bandage. Alternatively, use a piece of gauze, cotton wool and a bandage. Never place cotton wool directly on to a wound and do not use adhesive dressings or plasters, which may disturb the clot when it is removed.

Direct local pressure is the best method of controlling bleeding. Indirect pressure can be used only to control arterial bleeding and never for longer than 15 minutes. Locate the appropriate pressure point — the branchial artery in the arm, or the femoral artery in the thigh. To compress the former, slide your hand under the arm and press up and in to push the artery against the bone. To compress the latter, bend the casualty's knee, locate the artery in the groin and press it against the rim of the pelvis.

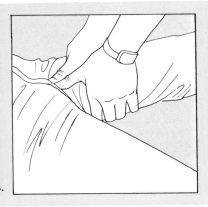

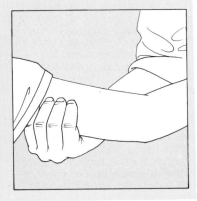

WOUNDS AND SERIOUS BLEEDING

6. If bleeding continues, with blood seeping through the bandage, apply another dressing on top of the first one and bandage again. Do not remove the first dressing and bandage – you may break up the clot that will have started to form.

If the wound has a large foreign body embedded in it, never attempt to remove it. Not only will you damage the tissues surrounding the wound if you try to pull it out; it may be restricting the bleeding by plugging the wound. Small surface foreign bodies, however, can be rinsed or wiped off.

ACTION

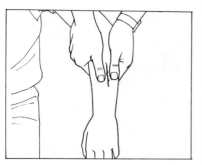

1. The first step is to control the bleeding. Do this by applying direct pressure to the edges of the wound, squeezing them together alongside the foreign body. Once the bleeding has been controlled, gently place a piece of gauze over the wound and around or over the foreign body. Do not use medicated gauze.

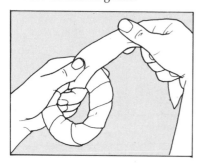

2. Make a ring bandage, as shown in *Bandages and Dressings*, and place it carefully around the wound. Alternatively, pads of cotton wool may be used, but you may need a second layer of gauze. When making the ring or building up the padding, remember the aim is to make it high enough to stop the next bandage from putting pressure on the foreign body.
3. Secure the ring bandage in place with a diagonally applied roller bandage, taking care not to apply any pressure to the foreign body.

Start by passing the bandage under the limb and up over the pad, avoiding the protrusion. Continue until the ring is secure. If possible, raise the affected limb – this will lower the local blood pressure, so restricting the flow of blood – and immobilize it. Ask the casualty to maintain this position and get immediate medical help.

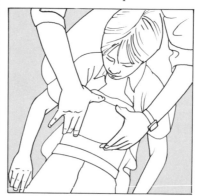

In the case of a puncture wound, remember that the opening may be deceptively small in relation to its depth. While the flow of blood may be reduced as a result, dirt may have been carried to the full depth of the wound, so carrying the risk of a potentially serious infection developing. As long as the blood flow is not too heavy, do not attempt to staunch it – the flow will help to clean out the wound – and let it clot in its own time. When the bleeding has stopped naturally, wash the wound with a swab and warm water and cover it with a clean, dry dressing. Always call in a doctor – if the wound is serious or was made by something dirty, an anti-tetanus injection will be necessary.

In the case of a stab wound to the chest – or a deep chest wound – there may be an additional problem. Such a wound can be extremely serious, since the lungs may be punctured. If this is the case, you will be able to hear air passing in and out of the wound as the casualty breathes, while there may be blood-stained bubbles at the site of the wound. This is an emergency – send for medical help at once.

ACTION – CHEST WOUNDS
1. Seal the wound immediately with the palm of your hand and support the casualty in a half-sitting position, twisting the body so that the weight is on the injured side. This will aid breathing
2. Cover the wound with an airtight, sterile, unmedicated dressing to

make a substitute for the lungs' natural seal. Secure this in place
3. If the cause of the injury is still in place – a knife may be left in a stab wound, for instance – do not remove it. It will be acting as a plug and its continued presence will reduce blood loss and so help to lessen shock. Bandage around it
4. Treat for shock and arrange immediate removal to hospital. If the casualty becomes unconscious, place in the recovery position (*see Emergency Techniques p375*).

Internal bleeding can occur as the result of a blow, a fracture, or a crush injury. It can also be caused by various medical conditions, such as a stomach ulcer. It is often extremely difficult to detect – there may be blood in the sputum, urine or faeces, but this may take some time to appear, if at all. If you know that a casualty has sustained a severe blow to the body, assume there is internal bleeding and act accordingly. The risk is especially high in children, who have less blood to lose than adults. Characteristic signs are pallor, coolness at the extremities, a rapid, weak pulse and shallow breathing, sickness and thirst, and tenderness at the site of the blow.

ACTION – INTERNAL BLEEDING
1. Send for medical help
2. Lie the casualty down gently, the head lowered and to one side to aid the flow of blood to the brain. Wrap the casualty in blankets and, if possible, raise the legs and support them in order to assist the return blood flow to the heart
3. Do not give anything to eat or drink
4. Loosen any restricting clothing, such as a collar or tie
5. Treat for shock. If the condition of the casualty deteriorates before medical help arrives, start resuscitation (*see Emergency Techniques pp370-375*).

Many minor wounds are relatively easy to treat. Normally, the blood flow stops quickly, and your aim is therefore to clean and dress the wound as soon as you can to minimize the risk of infection. You should always wash your hands before starting treatment. Protect the wound with a temporary sterile pad and clean the surrounding skin. Then gently clean the wound itself, using more than one swab if necessary, and dab it dry when you have finished. Dress the wound with an adhesive plaster, or a sterile dressing and bandage.

Safety in the home

Safety in the home is one of the most important elements of preventive medicine. By taking simple precautions and actions, you can minimize the risk of household accidents and injuries, particularly to babies and young children.

ACTION CHECK LIST – BABIES AND CHILDREN

* Keep polythene bags well out of reach. Children can suffocate if they pull such bags over their heads.
* Never leave your baby alone with a bottle in case he or she chokes on the feed. Never give peanuts to a small child for the same reason.
* Keep small objects, such as buttons and coins, out of a baby's reach. Babies put such things in their mouths and can easily swallow them.
* Check that cots and playroom equipment are well-made and safe.
* Keep a baby's dummy on a short string. Long strings can strangle a baby.
* Keep kettles, kettle flexes and tea or coffee pots well out of reach. The hot liquids will scald.
* Never drink anything hot with a child on your lap.
* Never carry hot drinks over a child's head.
* Never let table cloths extend over the edges of tables in case a child pulls at them. Similarly, keep hot drinks away from table edges.
* Always check the temperature of bath water. Children can be easily scalded.
* Never leave a baby or small child alone in the bath.

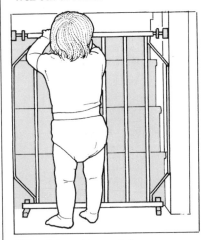

* Keep pan handles turned inwards when you are cooking. Alternatively fit a safety guard around your cooker.
* Make sure windows are fitted with child-proof safety catches.
* Keep balcony doors firmly locked.
* Always use the harness in a baby's high chair and fit a harness if the chair is not equipped with one.
* Keep all medicines well out of reach and always lock your medicine cupboard.
* Never use old soft drink bottles for storage of poisonous or corrosive chemicals and cleaners.
* Protect all fires with fireguards.
* Keep lighters and matches out of reach.
* Make sure children's night clothes are flame-resistant.
* Keep petrol and paraffin away from children.
* Keep hot irons – and their flexes –well out of reach.

* Fit safety gates on stairs.
* If practical, fit safety glass to windows to which children have easy access.
* If your child wears glasses, have the lenses made from plastic, or splinter-proof glass.
* Keep sharp tools, such as knives and scissors, away from small children.
* Make sure toys are without points or sharp edges.
* Do not let small children carry or drink out of glasses – always use plastic cups or mugs.
* Never let a child wander into the street unaccompanied by an adult. Teach the basic rules of road safety as soon as a child is old enough to understand them.
* Encourage your child not to show off by riding a bicycle with 'no hands'.
* Check your child's bicycle regularly for safety. Pay particular attention to lights, tyres, brakes and chains. If your child cycles at night, make sure reflective clothing is worn.

* Always make sure your child wears a seat belt in a car. A baby should always travel in a special baby seat in the back, while young children should use special child harness.

ACTION CHECK LIST – ELECTRICITY

* Make sure that your wiring is in good condition and that your plugs are properly connected. Never connect more than one appliance to the same plug.
* Always unplug a television set or a radio, and disconnect aerials at night and at times when the appliances will be left unattended.
* The only plug in the bathroom should be for a shower or for an electric razor. It should be professionally installed and specially insulated.

ACTION CHECK LIST – FIRE

* All open fires should have a strong guard, preferably fixed to the wall, in order to keep coal and logs in and children out.
* Never try to put out a household fire with water, unless you are sure that the electricity has been switched off at the mains.
* Make sure that all ashtrays are empty and all electrical appliances switched off and unplugged before you go to bed.
* Never pour anything inflammable on to a fire.

ACTION CHECK LIST – GARDEN AND GARDEN-TOOLS

* Never leave tools lying around.
* Keep all chemicals, such as fertilizers and weed-killers, locked up. Label all bottles clearly.
* Make sure that children cannot fall into barrels or a pond – a child can drown in just a few inches of water.
* Keep wiring away from the blades of a mower or shears.
* Never leave a bonfire unattended unless it is in an incinerator.
* Wear gloves and goggles or a mask when working with chemicals, a sander or a saw.

ACTION CHECK LIST – KITCHEN AND HOUSE

* Have a foam fire-extinguisher available and check it regularly.
* Remember the risk of fire when cooking with oil.
* Your kitchen and bathroom, should be fitted with a non-slip floor.

First aid box and medicine cupboard

When you administer First Aid – even for the most minor of accidents – you undertake certain responsibilities.

You must first of all assess the condition of the casualty and identify the main problem. You must then give the most immediate and appropriate form of treatment and then, depending on circumstances, arrange for the casualty to receive medical aid. Your responsibilities end only when you have handed over the casualty to trained medical personnel. You can help them still further by keeping a clear record of what you found and what you have done, so they can take this into account in their treatment of the injury or injuries.

In order to cope with the day-to-day responsibilities of First Aid, every home should have a properly-equipped First Aid box and a medicine cupboard. While bandages and dressings can be improvised in an emergency, it is far more preferable to have everything to hand that you might need. This section tells you what types of medicine, bandages and other items of useful First Aid equipment you should possess, so that you are prepared for most eventualities. You will also find information on ways of avoiding domestic accidents – one of the major causes of fatalities each year. By studying the Home Safety check list and acting on it, you will reduce the risk of accidents affecting your family.

A good First Aid box *(right)* should contain at least 10 individually wrapped adhesive dressings, a sterile eye pad and attachment and several triangular and roller bandages. Remember that roller bandages come in specific widths – to suit fingers, hands and feet, arms, legs and the trunk of the body – so it is a good idea to have at least one of each. You should also include a box of assorted plasters, for minor cuts and grazes, and surgical tape for sticking down the edges of dressings. You will also need some sterilized cotton wool, for cleaning wounds, eye ointment, safety pins, scissors and tweezers. Other optional extras include finger bandages – special bandages shaped like a finger tip – and some gauze.

A medicine cupboard *(left)* should contain some soluble aspirin – the soluble variety is preferable to pills because some people find it difficult to swallow the latter – and some junior aspirin, or paracetamol mixture, for children. Use both as pain-killers. You will also need anti-histamine cream for insect bites and stings, antacid powder or tablets for indigestion, calamine lotion to soothe sunburn and bites, and kaolin mixture. This is suitable for adults and children, whereas kaolin-and-morphine is only suitable for adults. The mixture should be thrown away and replaced every six months. Finally, you will need an antiseptic solution – follow the instructions for its use carefully, as it may need diluting – and a thermometer.

The contents of your First Aid box and medicine cupboard should always be kept out of the reach of children. Dressings, for instance, are useless if not sterile, while medicines can be positively harmful, if swallowed at random. Always buy medicine bottles with 'childproof' tops. If you have finished a course of pills and there are some left over, return the unused pills to your doctor. Finally, never take medicines prescribed for other people.

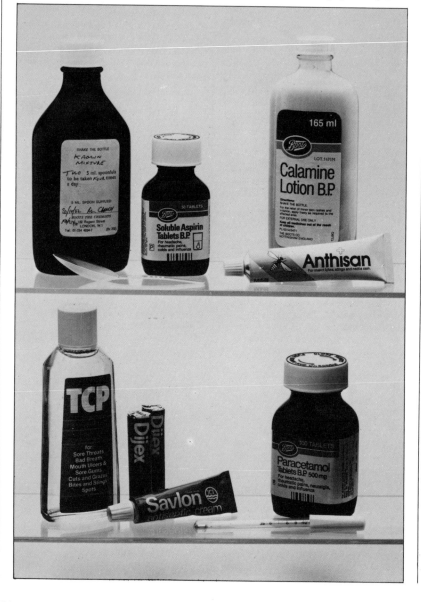

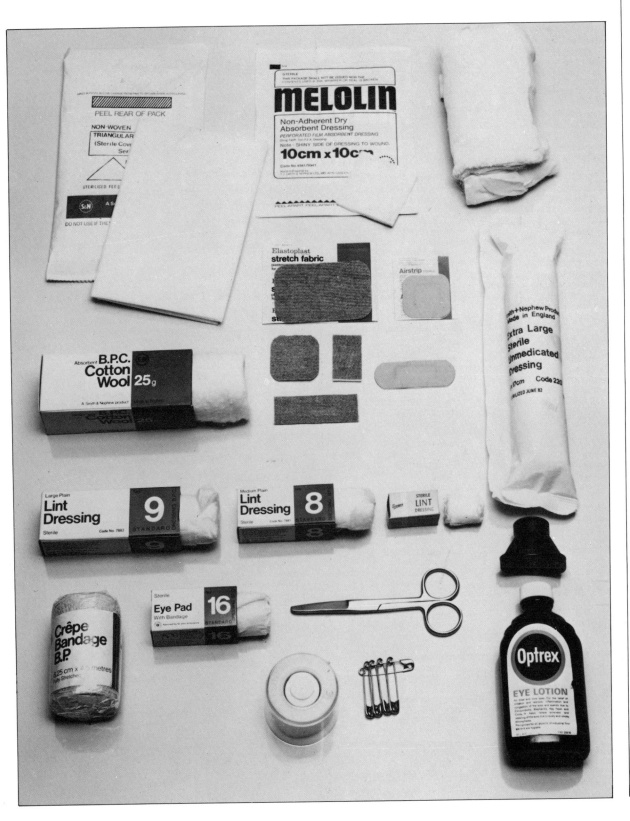

Index

Bold page numbers refer to main articles or entries. Page numbers in italic refer to illustrations.

404

Useful addresses

The organizations listed here can help you find out more about many medical and health problems. In addition, the Family Centre of *Good Housekeeping*, National Magazine House, 22 Broadwick Street, London W1 is always pleased to help with readers' queries, but please enclose a stamped, addressed envelope.

ADDICTION

ACCEPT
Alcoholism Community Centres for Education, Prevention and Treatment,
Western Hospital, Seagrave Road, London SW6 1RZ
ACTION ON SMOKING AND HEALTH (ASH)
27-35 Mortimer Street, London W1N 7RJ
AL-ANON FAMILY GROUPS
61 Great Dover Street, London SE1 4YF
AL-ATEEN
61 Great Dover Street, London SE1 4YF
ALCOHOLICS ANONYMOUS
PO Box 514, 11 Redcliffe Gardens, London SW10 9BQ
DRUGS INFORMATION AND ADVISORY SERVICE LTD
111 Cowbridge Road East, Canton, Cardiff
GAMBLERS ANONYMOUS
17/23 Blantyre Street, Cheyne Walk, London SW10
HELPING HAND ORGANISATION
8 Strutton Ground, London SW1P 2HP
NATIONAL COUNCIL ON ALCOHOLISM
3 Grosvenor Crescent, London SW1X 7EE
RELEASE
1 Elgin Avenue, London W9 3PR
STANDING CONFERENCE ON DRUG ABUSE (SCODA)
3 Blackburn Road, London NW6 1XA
TURNING POINT
8 Strutton Ground, London SW1P 2HP

ADOPTION

BRITISH AGENCIES FOR ADOPTION AND FOSTERING
11 Southwark Street, London SE1 1RQ
PARENTS FOR CHILDREN
222 Camden High Street, London NW1 8QR

ALLERGY

ACTION AGAINST ALLERGY
43 The Downs, London SW20 8HG

ALTERNATIVE MEDICINE

BRITISH ACUPUNCTURE ASSOCIATION
37 Peter Street, Manchester M2 5QD
BRITISH CHIROPRACTORS ASSOCIATION
120 Wigmore Street, London W1
BRITISH COLLEGE OF NATUROPATHY AND OSTEOPATHY
6 Netherhall Gardens, London N3

THE BRITISH HOMOEOPATHIC ASSOCIATION (BHA)
27a Devonshire Street, London W1N 1RJ
BRITISH HYPNOTHERAPY ASSOCIATION
67 Upper Berkeley Street, London W1H 7DH
BRITISH SOCIETY FOR MUSIC THERAPY
48 Lanchester Road, London N6 4TA
SCHOOL OF HERBAL MEDICINE
148 Forest Road, Tunbridge Wells, Kent TN2 5EY
THE SOCIETY OF TEACHERS OF THE ALEXANDER TECHNIQUE
3b Albert Court, Kensington Gore, London SW7

ANOREXIA NERVOSA

ANOREXIC AID
The Priory Centre, 11 Priory Road, High Wycombe, Bucks
ANOREXICS ANONYMOUS
24 Westmoreland Road, Barnes, London SW13

AUTISM

NATIONAL SOCIETY FOR AUTISTIC CHILDREN
276 Willesden Lane, London NW2 5RB

ARTHRITIS

ARTHRITIS CARE
6 Grosvenor Crescent, London SW1

ASTHMA

ASTHMA RESEARCH COUNCIL
12 Pembridge Square, London W2

BACK TROUBLE

BACK PAIN ASSOCIATION
31-33 Park Road, Teddington, Middlesex
SPINAL INJURIES ASSOCIATION
126 Albert Street, London NW1

BLINDNESS

ASSOCIATION OF BLIND AND PARTIALLY SIGHTED TEACHERS AND STUDENTS
36 Town Row, West Derby, Liverpool
ASSOCIATION OF TALKING NEWSPAPERS
Peter Craddock, Honorary Secretary, 36 Circular Road, Castlerock, Co. Londonderry
BRAILLE CORRESPONDENCE CLUB
Social Services Department, Civic Centre, Newcastle upon Tyne NE1 8PA
LONDON ASSOCIATION FOR THE BLIND
14-16 Verney Road, London SE16 3DZ
NATIONAL FEDERATION OF THE BLIND OF THE UNITED KINGDOM
20 Canon Close, Rayners Park, London SW20 9HA
NATIONAL LEAGUE OF THE BLIND AND DISABLED
Tottenham Trades Hall, 7 Bruce Grove, London N17 6RA
NATIONAL LIBRARY FOR THE BLIND
Cornwell Road, Bredbury, Stockport SK6 2SG

NATIONAL MUSIC FOR THE BLIND
(also known as Radio Churchtown)
2 High Park Road, Southport, Merseyside PR9 7QL
OPTICAL INFORMATION
Walter House, 418-422 Strand, London WC2R 0PB
PARTIALLY SIGHTED SOCIETY
Breaston, Derbys DE7 3UE
ROYAL COMMONWEALTH SOCIETY FOR THE BLIND
Commonwealth House, Heath Road, Haywards Heath, West Sussex RH16 3AZ
ROYAL NATIONAL INSTITUTE FOR THE BLIND
224 Great Portland Street, London W1N 6AA
ST DUNSTAN'S
PO Box 58, 191 Old Marylebone Road, London NW1 5QN
TELEPHONES FOR THE BLIND
Secretary, A Chudley, Mynthurst, Leigh, Surrey
UNITED KINGDOM GUIDE DOGS FOR THE BLIND ASSOCIATION
Alexandra House, 113 Uxbridge Road, London W5 5TQ

BLOOD DISORDERS

ANTHONY NOLAN BONE MARROW APPEAL
St Mary Abbots Hospital, Marloes Road, Kensington, London W8 5LQ
THE HAEMOPHILIA SOCIETY
PO Box 9, 16 Trinity Street, London SE1 1DE
LEUKAEMIA RESEARCH FUND
43 Great Ormond Street, London WC1N 3JJ
THE LEUKAEMIA SOCIETY
Mrs J Pankhurst, Hamlyns View, St Andrews Road, Exeter EX4 2AF
ORGANISATION OF SICKLE CELL ANAEMIA
200a High Road, Wood Green, London N22

CANCER

CANCER AFTERCARE AND REHABILITATION SOCIETY
Lodge Cottage, Church Lane, Timsbury, Bath
CANCER INFORMATION ASSOCIATION
Marygold House, Carfax, Oxford OX1 1EA
CANCER PREVENTION SOCIETY
102 Inveroran Drive, Bearsden, Glasgow G61 2AT
CONTOUR
2 Hans Road, Knightsbridge, London SW3 1RX
MARIE CURIE MEMORIAL FOUNDATION
124 Sloane Street, London SW1X 9BP
MASTECTOMY ASSOCIATION
25 Brighton Road, South Croydon CR2 6EA
NATIONAL SOCIETY FOR CANCER RELIEF
Michael Sobell House, 30 Dorset Square, London NW1 6QL
TENOVUS CANCER INFORMATION CENTRE
90 Cathedral Road, Cardiff CF1 9PG
WOMEN'S NATIONAL CANCER CONTROL CAMPAIGN
1 South Audley Street, London W1Y 5DQ

CHILDREN

ACTION RESEARCH FOR THE CRIPPLED CHILD
Vincent House, North Parade, Horsham, West Sussex RH12 2DA
AID FOR DOWN'S BABIES, EDINBURGH
13 Lovedale Road, Balerno, Midlothian EH14 7DW
THE ASSOCIATION FOR CHILDREN WITH HEART DISORDERS
11 Millthorne Avenue, Clitheroe, Lancs
ASSOCIATION OF PARENTS OF VACCINE DAMAGED CHILDREN
2 Church Street, Shipston on Stour, Warwickshire CV36 4AP
BRITISH GUILD FOR SUDDEN INFANT DEATH STUDY
Pathology Department, Royal Infirmary, Cardiff CF2 1SZ
CHILD POVERTY ACTION GROUP
1 Macklin Street, Drury Lane, London WC2
CONTACT A FAMILY
16 Strutton Ground, Victoria, London SW1P 2HP
CHURCH OF ENGLAND CHILDREN'S SOCIETY
Old Town Hall, Kennington Road, London SE11 4QD
DOWN'S CHILDREN'S ASSOCIATION
Quinborne Centre, Ridgacre Road, Birmingham B32 2TW
THE FOUNDATION FOR THE STUDY OF INFANT DEATHS
5th Floor, 4 Grosvenor Place, London SW1X 7HD
INVALID CHILDREN'S AID ASSOCIATION
126 Buckingham Palace Road, London SW1W 9SB
LADY HOARE TRUST FOR PHYSICALLY DISABLED CHILDREN
7 North Street, Midhurst, West Sussex GU29 9DJ
NATIONAL ASSOCIATION FOR DEAF/BLIND AND RUBELLA HANDICAPPED
311 Grays Inn Road, London WC1X 8PT
NATIONAL ASSOCIATION FOR GIFTED CHILDREN
1 South Audley Street, London W1Y 5DQ
NATIONAL ASSOCIATION FOR THE WELFARE OF CHILDREN IN HOSPITAL
Exton House, 7 Exton Street, London SE1 8UE
THE NATIONAL CHILDMINDING ASSOCIATION
13 London Road, Bromley BR1 1DE
NATIONAL CHILDREN'S BUREAU
8 Wakley Street, Islington, London EC1V 7QE
THE NATIONAL DEAF CHILDREN'S SOCIETY
45 Hereford Road, London W2 5AH
NATIONAL SOCIETY FOR MENTALLY HANDICAPPED CHILDREN AND ADULTS (MENCAP)
123 Golden Lane, London EC1Y 0RT
NATIONAL SOCIETY FOR THE PREVENTION OF CRUELTY TO CHILDREN
1 Riding House Street, London W1P 8AA
PRE-SCHOOL PLAYGROUPS ASSOCIATION (PPA)
Alford House, Aveline Street, London SE11 5DH

THE STILLBIRTH AND PERINATAL DEATH ASSOCIATION
37 Christchurch Hill, London NW3 1JY
VOLUNTARY COUNCIL FOR HANDICAPPED CHILDREN
8 Wakley Street, Islington, London EC1Y 7QE

CHIROPODY

INSTITUTE OF CHIROPODISTS
59 Gloucester Place, London W1
SOCIETY OF CHIROPODISTS
8 Wimpole Street, London W1

COELIAC DISEASE

COELIAC SOCIETY
PO Box 181, London NW2 2YA

COLITIS AND CROHN'S DISEASE

NATIONAL ASSOCIATION FOR COLITIS AND CROHN'S DISEASE (NACC)
3 Thorpefield Close, Marshalwick, St Albans, Herts AL4 9TJ

COLOSTOMY

COLOSTOMY WELFARE GROUP
2nd Floor, 38/39 Eccleston Square, London SW1V 1PB

CYSTIC FIBROSIS

CYSTIC FIBROSIS RESEARCH TRUST
Alexandra House, 5 Blyth Road, Bromley, Kent BR1 3RS

DEAFNESS

THE BRITISH ASSOCIATION OF THE HARD OF HEARING
6 Great James Street, London WC1N 3DA
BRITISH DEAF ASSOCIATION
38 Victoria Place, Carlisle CA1 1HU
THE BRITISH TINNITUS ASSOCIATION
c/o 105 Gower Street, London WC1E 6AH
NATIONAL CENTRE FOR CUED SPEECH
London House, 68 Upper Richmond Road, Putney, London SW15 2RP
NATIONAL DEAF-BLIND HELPER'S LEAGUE
18 Rainbow Court, Paston Ridings, Peterborough PE4 6UP
NATIONAL UNION OF THE DEAF
32 Little Ealing Lane, London W5 4EA
THE ROYAL ASSOCIATION IN AID OF THE DEAF AND DUMB
27 Old Oak Road, Acton, London W3 7HN
ROYAL NATIONAL INSTITUTE FOR THE DEAF
105 Gower Street, London WC1E 6AH

DENTAL HEALTH

BRITISH DENTAL HEALTH FOUNDATION
26 Ravensdale Avenue, London N12 9HS

DIABETES

THE BRITISH DIABETIC ASSOCIATION
10 Queen Anne Street, London W1M 0BD

DISABILITY

THE CULTURAL SOCIETY OF THE DISABLED
10 Warwick Row, London SW1E 5EP
DISABILITY ALLIANCE
96 Portland Place, London W1N 4EX
DISABLED DRIVERS ASSOCIATION
Ashwellthorpe Hall, Ashwellthorpe, Norwich NR16 1EX
THE DISABLED HOUSING TRUST
6 Oakenfield, Burgess Hill, West Sussex
DISABLED LIVING FOUNDATION INFORMATION SERVICE
364 Kensington High Street, London W14 8NS
DISABLEMENT INCOME GROUP
Attlee House, 28 Commercial Street, London E1 6LR
NATIONAL BUREAU FOR HANDICAPPED STUDENTS
40 Brunswick Square, London WC1N 1AZ
NATIONAL FUND FOR RESEARCH INTO CRIPPLING DISEASES (ACTION RESEARCH FOR THE CRIPPLED CHILD)
Vincent House, Springfield Road, Horsham, West Sussex RH12 2PN
PHAB (PHYSICALLY HANDICAPPED AND ABLE BODIED)
42 Devonshire Street, London W1N 1LN
THE ROYAL ASSOCIATION FOR DISABILITY AND REHABILITATION
25 Mortimer Street, London W1N 8AB
THE SENIOR CONSELLOR FOR DISABLED STUDENTS
The Open University, Walton Hall, Milton Keynes MK7 6AA
SEXUAL AND PERSONAL RELATIONSHIPS OF THE DISABLED
The Diorama, 14 Peto Place, London NW1 4DT
SPECIALIST GROUP FOR THE DISABLED
The British Computer Society, 29 Portland Place, London W1N 4HU

DWARFISM

ASSOCIATION INTO RESEARCH INTO RESTRICTED GROWTH
Charles Pocock, 4 Laburnum Avenue, Wickford, Essex

DYSLEXIA

BRITISH DYSLEXIA ASSOCIATION
Church Lane, Peppard, Oxfordshire RG9 5JN
DYSLEXIA INSTITUTE
133 Gresham Road, Staines, TW18 2AJ
HELEN ARKELL DYSLEXIA CENTRE
14 Crondace Road, London SW6 4BB

EDUCATION AND EMPLOYMENT

ASSOCIATION OF BRITISH CORRESPONDENCE COLLEGES
4 Chiswell Street, London EC1Y 4UR

THE EMPLOYMENT FELLOWSHIP
Drayton House, Gordon Street, London WC1H 0BE
THE NATIONAL INSTITUTE OF ADULT EDUCATION
198b De Montfort Street, Leicester LE1 7GE

ELDERLY

AGE CONCERN ENGLAND
Bernard Sunley House, 60 Pitcairn Road, Mitcham, Surrey CR4 3LL
AGE CONCERN SCOTLAND
33 Castle Street, Edinburgh
AGE CONCERN WALES
1 Park Grove, Cardiff, S Glamorgan
AGE CONCERN N IRELAND
128 Great Victoria Street, Belfast 2
HELP THE AGED
32 Dover Street, London W1A 2AP
THE PRE-RETIREMENT ASSOCIATION
19 Undine Street, Tooting, London SW17 8PP

EPILEPSY

BRITISH EPILEPSY ASSOCIATION
Cowthorne House, Bigshotte, New Wokingham Road, Wokingham, Berkshire RG11 3AY
SCOTTISH EPILEPSY ASSOCIATION
48 Govan Road, Glasgow G51 1JL

FRIEDRICH'S ATAXIA

FRIEDRICH'S ATAXIA GROUP
12c Worplesdon Road, Guildford, Surrey GU2 6RW

GLAUCOMA

INTERNATIONAL GLAUCOMA ASSOCIATION
King's College Hospital, Denmark Hill, London SE5 9RS

HEART DISEASE

BRITISH HEART FOUNDATION (BHF)
102 Gloucester Place, London W1H 4DH
THE CHEST HEART AND STROKE ASSOCIATION (CHSA)
Tavistock House North, Tavistock Square, London WC1H 9JE

HOMOSEXUALS

CAMPAIGN FOR HOMOSEXUAL EQUALITY
PO Box 427, Manchester M60 2EL
LESBIAN LINE
BM Box 1515, London WC1N 3XX
PARENTS ENQUIRY — COUNSELLING FOR PARENTS OF YOUNG GAYS
Rose Robertson, 16 Hornley Road, Catford, London SE6 2HZ

HUNTINGTON'S CHOREA

ASSOCIATION TO COMBAT HUNTINGTON'S CHOREA
Borough House, 34a Station Road, Hinckley, Leics LE10 1AP

ILEOSTOMY

ILEOSTOMY ASSOCIATION OF GREAT BRITAIN AND IRELAND (IA)
Amblehurst House, Chobham, Woking, Surrey GU24 8PZ

URINARY CONDUIT ASSOCIATION (UCA)
8 Coniston Close, Dane Bank, Denton, Manchester M34 2EW

INFERTILITY

CHILD
Farthings, Gaunts Road, Pawlett, Nr Bridgewater, Somerset
NATIONAL ASSOCIATION FOR THE CHILDLESS (NAC)
Birmingham Settlement, 318 Summer Lane, Birmingham B19 3RL

KIDNEY DISEASE

THE BRITISH KIDNEY PATIENT ASSOCIATION (BKPA)
Bordon, Hants
NATIONAL FEDERATION OF KIDNEY PATIENTS' ASSOCIATIONS
c/o Mrs Margaret Jackson, Acorn Lodge, Woodsetts, Worksop, Notts
THE RENAL SOCIETY
64 South Hill Park, London NW3 2SJ

LARYNGECTOMY

THE NATIONAL ASSOCIATION OF LARYNGECTOMY CLUBS
Fourth Floor, 39 Eccleston Square, London SW1V 1PB

LEPROSY

BRITISH LEPROSY RELIEF ASSOCIATION (LEPRA)
Fairfax House, Causton Road, Colchester, Essex CO1

LIMBLESS (AMPUTEES)

BRITISH LIMBLESS EX-SERVICEMEN'S ASSOCIATION
Frankland Moor House, 185/7 High Road, Chadwell Heath, Essex
BRITISH AMPUTEE SPORTS ASSOCIATION
Dr J R Mirrey, Leachim Heights, Redhill Common, Redhill, Surrey

MENTAL HEALTH

BRITISH ASSOCIATION FOR THE RETARDED
Pembridge Hall, 17 Pembridge Square, London W2 4EP
INSTITUTE OF MENTAL SUBNORMALITY
Wolverhampton Road, Kidderminster, Worcestershire DY10 3PP
MENCAP — THE SOCIETY FOR MENTALLY HANDICAPPED CHILDREN AND ADULTS
123 Golden Lane, London EC1Y 0RT
THE MENTAL AFTER CARE ASSOCIATION
Eagle House, 110 Jermyn Street, London SW1Y 6HB
THE MENTAL HEALTH FOUNDATION
8 Hallam Street, London W1N 6HD
MONGOLISM/DOWN'S CHILDREN'S ASSOCIATION
Quinborne Community Centre, Ridgacre Road, Quinton, Birmingham B32 2TW
NATIONAL ASSOCIATION FOR MENTAL HEALTH (MIND)
22 Harley Street, London W1N 2ED
NATIONAL SCHIZOPHRENIA FELLOWSHIP
78/79 Victoria Road, Surbiton, Surrey KT6 4NS

PHOBICS SOCIETY
4 Cheltenham Road, Chorlton-cum-Hardy, Manchester
M21 1QN
SCHIZOPHRENIA
ASSOCIATION OF GREAT
BRITAIN
Tyr Twr, Llanfair Hall,
Caernarfon, Gwynedd LL55 1TT
SCOTTISH SOCIETY FOR THE
MENTALLY HANDICAPPED
13 Elmbank Street, Glasgow
G2 4QA

MIGRAINE

BRITISH MIGRAINE SOCIETY
178a High Road, Byfleet,
Weybridge, Surrey KT14 7ED
THE MIGRAINE TRUST
45 Great Ormond Street, London
WC1N 3HD

MOTOR NEURONE DISEASE

MOTOR NEURONE DISEASE
ASSOCIATION (MND)
c/o Mrs Kate White,
25 Rickfords Hill, Aylesbury,
Bucks

MULTIPLE SCLEROSIS

ACTION FOR RESEARCH INTO
MULTIPLE SCLEROSIS (ARMS)
71 Gray's Inn Road, London
WC1X 8TR
THE MULTIPLE SCLEROSIS
SOCIETY
288 Munster Road, Fulham,
London SW6 6AP

MUSCULAR DYSTROPHY

MUSCULAR DYSTROPHY
GROUP OF GB
Nattrass House, 35 Macaulay
Road, London SW4 0QP

MYASTHENIA GRAVIS

BRITISH ASSOCIATION OF
MYASTHENICS
Hon. Sec: Mrs M Rivett,
38 Selwood Road, Brentwood,
Essex

PAGET'S DISEASE

NATIONAL ASSOCIATION FOR
RELIEF OF PAGET'S DISEASE
413 Middleton Road,
Rhodes, Middleton,
Manchester

PARKINSON'S DISEASE

PARKINSON'S DISEASE
SOCIETY
36 Portland Place, London
W1N 3DG

PHENYLKETONURIA

NATIONAL SOCIETY FOR
PHENYLKETONURIA AND
ALLIED DISORDERS (NSPKU)
14 Newfound Drive, Cringleford,
Norwich NR4 7RY

POLIO

BRITISH POLIO FELLOWSHIP
Bell Close, West End Road,
Ruislip, Middlesex

PREGNANCY, CONTRACEPTION, ABORTION

BRITISH PREGNANCY
ADVISORY SERVICE
Aysty Manor, Wootton Wawen,
Solihull, West Midlands B95 6BX
BROOK ADVISORY CENTRE
233 Tottenham Court Road,
London W1
FAMILY PLANNING
ASSOCIATION
27/35 Mortimer Street,
London W1
MARIE STOPES HOUSE
103 Whitfield Street, London W1
NATIONAL ABORTION
CAMPAIGN
374 Grays Inn Road, London WC1
THE NATIONAL CHILDBIRTH
TRUST
9 Queensborough Terrace,
London W2 3TB
PREGNANCY ADVISORY
SERVICE
13 Charlotte Street, London W1
THE ASSOCIATION FOR POST
NATAL ILLNESS
7 Gowan Avenue, Fulham,
London NW6

RHEUMATISM AND ARTHRITIS

THE ARTHRITIS AND
RHEUMATISM COUNCIL FOR
RESEARCH
41 Eagle Street, London WC1
BRITISH RHEUMATISM AND
ARTHRITIS ASSOCIATION
6 Grosvenor Crescent, London
SW1X 7ER

NATIONAL ANKYLOSING
SPONDYLITIS SOCIETY
6 Grosvenor Crescent, London
SW1X 7ER

SPASTICS

ASSOCIATION OF THE
PARENTS AND FRIENDS OF
SPASTICS
Rotary Centre for Spastics, 7
Queen's Crescent, St George's
Cross, Glasgow G49 9BW
CENTRE FOR SPASTIC
CHILDREN
61 Cheyne Walk, London SW3
SPASTICS SOCIETY
12 Park Crescent, London
W1N 4LQ

SPINA BIFIDA

ASSOCIATION FOR SPINA
BIFIDA AND
HYDROCEPHALUS
Tavistock House North, Tavistock
Square, London WC1H

SPORTS AND RECREATION

ADVISORY PANEL ON
WATERSPORTS FOR THE
DISABLED
c/o The Sports Council, 70
Brompton Road, London
SW2 1EX
ASSOCIATION FOR BLIND
AND DISABLED RADIO
AMATEURS
Radio Society of Great Britain, 45
Doughty Street, London WC1
THE BRITISH ASSOCIATIONS
OF SPORTING AND
RECREATIONAL ACTIVITIES
OF THE BLIND
5 Curzon Road, Thornton Heath,
Surrey
BRITISH CORRESPONDENCE
CHESS SOCIETY
90 Headstone Road, Harrow,
Middlesex HA1 1PE
BRITISH DEAF SPORTS
COUNCIL
140 Green Lane, Cookridge,
Leeds LS16 7JQ
THE BRITISH SKI CLUB FOR
THE DISABLED
Corton House, Corton, Nr
Warminster, Wilts
THE BRITISH SPORTS
ASSOCIATION FOR THE
DISABLED
Haywards House, Ludwig
Guttman Sports Centre, Stoke

Mandeville, Harvey Road,
Aylesbury, Bucks HP21 8PP
CAMPING FOR THE DISABLED
c/o David Griffiths, Mobility
Information Service, Copthorne
Community Hall, Shelton Road,
Shrewsbury or 1 Mallory Road,
Oswestry, Shropshire SY11 2OJ
GREAT BRITAIN WHEELCHAIR
BASKETBALL LEAGUE
18 Wroxall Drive, Grantham,
Lincolnshire NG31 7WQ
HANDICAPPED ADVENTURE
PLAYGROUND ASSOCIATION
Fulham Palace, Bishops Avenue,
London SW6 6EA
RIDING FOR THE DISABLED
National Headquarters, National
Agriculture Centre, Stoneleigh,
Kenilworth, Warwickshire
CV8 2LY

TUBERCULOSIS

BRITISH THORACIC
ASSOCIATION
30 Britten Street, London SW3

WEIGHT WATCHERS

WEIGHT WATCHERS (UK) LTD
Group Therapy Classes, 635 Ajax
Avenue, Slough

OTHER USEFUL ADDRESSES

THE BRITISH RED CROSS
SOCIETY
9 Grosvenor Crescent, London
SW1X 7EJ
INVALIDS AT HOME
Mrs J Pierce, 23 Farm Avenue,
London NW2 2BJ
JEWISH WELFARE BOARD
315-317 Ballards Lane, London
N12 8LP
LEONARD CHESHIRE
FOUNDATION
26-29 Maunsel Street, London
SW1P 2QN
NATIONAL ASSOCIATION OF
CITIZENS ADVICE BUREAUX
110 Drury Lane, London
WC2B 5SW
PATIENT'S ASSOCIATION
11 Dartmouth Street, London
SW1H 9BN
RAPE
Rape Crisis Centre, PO Box 42,
London N6 5BU
Tel: 01-340 6913/6145 (24 hours)
THE SAMARITANS
17 Uxbridge Road, Slough
SL1 1SN

BIBLIOGRAPHY

The publishers acknowledge their indebtness to the following publications that were consulted for reference:
Bailey & Love's Short Practice of Surgery — AJ Harding Rains, HD Ritchie (HK Lewis); *A Companion to Medical Studies* — R Passmore, JS Robson (Blackwell Scientific); *Diseases of Children* — Hugh Jolly (Blackwell Scientific); *Davidson's Principles and Practice of Medicine* — J Macleod (Churchill Livingstone); *A Short Textbook of Medicine* — JC Houston, CL Joiner, JR Trounce (Hodder & Stoughton); *Clinical Pharmacology* — DR Lawrence (Churchill Livingstone); *An Introduction to Human Physiology* — JH Green (Oxford University Press); *Concise Medical Dictionary* (Oxford University Press); *Hutchinson's Clinical Methods* — R Bomford, S Mason, M Swash (Baillière Tindall); *Everywoman* — D Llewellyn-Jones (Faber); *Fundamentals of Obstetrics and Gynaecology* — D Llewllyn-Jones (Faber); *A Concise Textbook of Biochemistry* — SP Datta, JH Ottoway (Baillière Tindall); *Human Embryology* — MJT Fitzgerald (Harper & Row); *The Human Heart* — B Phibbs (CV Mosby); *British National Formulary* — British Medical Association & Pharmaceutical Society of Great Britain; *Pregnancy* — G Bourne (Cassell); *F/40 Fitness on 40 Minutes a Week* — M Carruthers, A Murray (Futura); *A Family Guide to Common Ailments* — J Gomez (Hamlyn); *Price's Textbook of the Practice of Medicine* — (Oxford University Press); *Textbook of Human Anatomy* — WJ Hamilton (Macmillan); *Hamilton Bailey's Physical Signs in Clinical Surgery* — A Clain (John Wright); *Jamieson's Illustrations of Regional Anatomy* — R Walmsley, TR Murphy (Churchill Livingstone); *Gray's Anatomy* — TB Johnston, J Whillis (Longman); *Essential Exercises for the Childbearing Year* — E Noble (John Murray); *A Textbook of Surgery* — DA Macfarlane, LP Thomas (Churchill Livingstone); *A Guide to Housesurgeons in the Surgical Unit* — GJ Frankel, C Ludbrook, HAF Dudley (Heinemann Medical); *Tabor's Medical Dictionary* — (FA Davis).